Measurement in health promotion and protection

[redacted]

Cover design by Maria Josephy Schoolman

World Health Organization
Regional Office for Europe
Copenhagen

Measurement in health promotion and protection

Edited by

T. Abelin
Z.J. Brzeziński
Vera D.L. Carstairs

WHO Regional Publications, European Series No. 22

ICP/HST 101/s04

Measurement in health promotion and protection /
edited by T. Abelin, Z.J. Brzeziński, Vera D.L. Carstairs
Copenhagen : WHO. Regional Office for Europe, 1987
WHO Regional Publications. European Series ; No.22
ISBN 92-890-1113-0
Health Promotion — Health Status —
Health Surveys — Health Status Indicators —
Health Planning

ISBN 92 890 1113 0
ISSN 0378-2255

CONTENTS

PART II. METHODS OF MEASUREMENT

PART III. EXAMPLES AND APPLICATIONS OF MEASUREMENTS

Editorial Board

Contributors

T. Abelin
Professor and Director, Institute for Social and Preventive Medicine, University of Berne, Switzerland

Christa Altenstetter
Professor, Political Science, Graduate School and University Center, City University of New York, NY, USA

A. Alzate
Professor of Epidemiology, Faculty of Health, Universidad del Valle, Cali, Colombia

K. Lange Andersen
Professor, Head of Postal Medical Services, Laboratory of Environmental Physiology, Oslo, Norway

P.A. Baghurst
Senior Research Scientist, Division of Human Nutrition, Institute of Animal and Food Sciences, CSIRO, Adelaide, Australia

H. van Balen
Chef de service, Unité de recherche et d'enseignement en santé publique, Institut de médecine tropicale Prince Léopold, Antwerp, Belgium

R.N. Basu
Director, National Institute of Communicable Diseases, Delhi, India

E. Berkanovic
Professor of Behavioural Sciences and Health Education, School of Public Health, University of California, Los Angeles, CA, USA

R.P. Bernard
Director of Epidemiology in Human Reproduction, International Federation for Family Health and International Association for Maternal and Neonatal Health, Geneva, Switzerland

B. Bissegger
Statistical Analyst, Federal Statistical Office, Division for Sociocultural Statistics, Berne, Switzerland

Madeleine Blanchet
President, Government of Quebec, Ministry of Social Affairs, Council of Social and Family Affairs, Sillery, Canada

D.H.J. Blom
Netherlands Institute for Preventive Health Care, Leiden, Netherlands

L. Breslow
Professor of Public Health and Director of Cancer Control Research, Division of Cancer Control, Jonsson Comprehensive Cancer Center, Los Angeles, CA, USA

Z.J. Brzeziński
Professor and Head, Department of Epidemiology and Health Programming, National Institute of Mother and Child, Warsaw, Poland

Vera D.L. Carstairs
Assistant Director (Statistics and Research), Information Services Division, Common Services Agency for the Scottish Health Service, Edinburgh, United Kingdom

C. Castillo-Salgado
Professor of Social Medicine, Autonomous University of Mexico, Mexico

J. Catford
Professor of Health Education and Health Promotion and Director, Welsh Heart Programme, Cardiff, United Kingdom

J.R.H. Charlton
Lecturer in Medical Statistics, Department of Community Medicine, St Thomas's Hospital Medical School, London, United Kingdom

A. Colvez
Epidémiologiste, Chargé de recherche, Institut national de la santé et de la recherche médicale, Le Vésinet, France

W.E. Coonan
Director, South Australian Health Development Unit, Adelaide, Australia

W. Dab
Observatoire régional de santé d'Ile-de-France, Paris, France

J.K. Davies
Senior Research Officer, Scottish Health Education Group, Health Education Centre, Edinburgh, United Kingdom

J. Dennis
Research Fellow, Health Services Research Unit, University of Kent, Canterbury, United Kingdom

P. Draper
86 Ashburnham Grove, Greenwich, London, United Kingdom

T. Dwyer
Senior Lecturer in Epidemiology, School of Public Health and Tropical Medicine, University of Sydney, Australia

F. Falkner
Professor, Maternal and Child Health, School of Public Health, University of California, Berkeley, and Professor, Pediatrics, School of Medicine, University of California, San Francisco, CA, USA

Gerda G. Fillenbaum
Research Associate, Sandoz Purposive Archiving Project, Center for the Study of Aging and Human Development, Duke University Medical Center, Durham, NC, USA

Virginie H. des Fontaines
Département de médecine préventive et sociale, Faculté de médecine Saint-Antoine, Paris, France

G. Davis Gammon
Clinical Assistant Professor, Depression Research Unit, Department of Psychiatry, Yale University School of Medicine, New Haven, CT, USA

M. Goldberg
Professeur, Université Paris V, GERSS, U88, Institut national de la santé et de la recherche médicale, Paris, France

B.M. Greenwood
Medical Research Council Laboratories, Fajara/Banjul, Gambia

R. Guerrero
Professor of Epidemiology, Department of Social Medicine, Faculty of Health, Universidad del Valle, Cali, Colombia

Martha E. Harnly
Research Associate, Medical Research Institute of San Francisco at Pacific Medical Center, Institute of Cancer Research, San Francisco, CA, USA

A.S. Härö
Kallionlaita 2, 02610 Espoo 61, Finland

M.A. Heasman
Director, Information Services Division, Common Services Agency for the Scottish Health Service, Edinburgh, United Kingdom

F.J. Henry
International Centre for Diarrhoeal Disease Research, Dhaka, Bangladesh

B.S. Hetzel
Chief, Division of Human Nutrition, Institute of Animal and Food Sciences, CSIRO, Adelaide, Australia

H. Howald
Head of the Research Institute, Swiss School for Physical Education and Sports, Magglingen, Switzerland

Sonja M. Hunt
Research Unit in Health and Behavioural Change, University of Edinburgh, United Kingdom

W.A. Jedrychowski
Professor, Department of Epidemiology, Institute of Social Medicine, Medical School, Cracow, Poland

Karen John
Associate in Research, Depression Research Unit, Department of Psychiatry, Yale University School of Medicine, New Haven, CT, USA

S.B. Kar
Associate Dean and Chairman, Professor of Behavioural Sciences and Health Education, and Professor, Population and Family Health, School of Public Health, University of California, Los Angeles, CA, USA

J. Krupinski
Director, Mental Health Research Institute, Melbourne, Australia

P.A. Lamarche
Programme Planning Officer, WHO Regional Office for Europe, Copenhagen, Denmark

W. van Lerberghe
Unité de recherche et d'enseignement en santé publique, Institut de médecine tropicale Prince Léopold, Antwerp, Belgium

D.R. Leitch
Division of Human Nutrition, Institute of Animal and Food Sciences, CSIRO, Adelaide, Australia

Hermione Lovel
Lecturer, Health Care Planning and Evaluation, Institute of Child Health, University of London, United Kingdom

B. Marti
Department of Social and Preventive Medicine, University of Berne, Switzerland

I.W. McDowell
Director, Health Care Research Unit, Epidemiology and Community Medicine, University of Ottawa, Canada

J. McEwen
Reader, Department of Community Medicine, King's College School of Medicine and Dentistry, London, United Kingdom

S.P. McKenna
ACR Epidemiology Research Unit, University of Manchester, United Kingdom

P. Mercenier
Chef de service, Unité de recherche et d'enseignement en santé publique, Institut de médecine tropicale Prince Léopold, Antwerp, Belgium

C. Montoya-Aguilar
Chief, Monitoring Implementation and Effectiveness, World Health Organization, Geneva, Switzerland

D. Morley
Professor, Tropical Child Health, Institute of Child Health, University of London, United Kingdom

D. Nabarro
Senior Lecturer, Department of International Community Health, Liverpool School of Tropical Medicine, United Kingdom

V. Navarro
Professor of Health Policy, School of Hygiene and Public Health, Johns Hopkins University, Baltimore, MD, USA

A. Nissinen
Department of Epidemiology, National Public Health Institute, Helsinki, Finland

H. Noack
Institute for Social and Preventive Medicine, University of Berne, Switzerland

D. Nutbeam
Assistant Director, Welsh Heart Programme, Cardiff, United Kingdom

P. Puska
Professor, Department of Epidemiology, National Public Health Institute, Helsinki, Finland

M. Mujibur Rahaman
Associate Director, Nutrition Programme, International Centre for Diarrhoeal Disease Research, Dhaka, Bangladesh

L.M. Ramström
Director-General, National Smoking and Health Association, Stockholm, Sweden

O.I. Rojas
Director-General, Hospital Universitario del Valle "Evaristo Garcia", Cali, Colombia

J. Rutenfranz
Professor, Institut für Arbeitsphysiologie, Universität Dortmund, Federal Republic of Germany

D.D. Rutstein
Ridley Watts Professor Emeritus, Department of Preventive Medicine, Harvard Medical School, Boston, MA, USA

S. Sastrawinata
Chairman, Coordinating Board of Indonesian Fertility Research, and Executive Secretary, International Federation for Family Health, Bandung, Indonesia

E. Schach
Research Associate and Head, Division of Applications, University Computing Centre, Dortmund, Federal Republic of Germany

Jotna Sokhey
Directorate-General of Health Services, Nirman Bhawan, New Delhi, India

R.N. Srivastava
Professor, Department of Social and Preventive Medicine, MLB Medical College, Jhansi, India

Ann R. Taket
Lecturer in Health and Health Care, Department of Clinical Epidemiology, London Hospital Medical College, and Department of Geography and Earth Science, Queen Mary College, University of London, United Kingdom

M.C. Thuriaux
Epidemiologist, Epidemiology and Statistics, WHO Regional Office for Europe, Copenhagen, Denmark

Gill Tremlett
Institute of Child Health, University of London, United Kingdom

J. Tuomilehto
Department of Epidemiology, National Public Health Institute, Helsinki, Finland

K. Uemura
Director, Division of Epidemiological Surveillance and Health Situation and Trend Assessment, World Health Organization, Geneva, Switzerland

B.L. Verma
Department of Social and Preventive Medicine, MLB Medical College, Jhansi, India

S.S. Wali
Department of Medicine, Ahmadu Bello University, Zaria, Nigeria

Myrna M. Weissman
Professor, Psychiatry and Epidemiology, Depression Research Unit, Department of Psychiatry, Yale University School of Medicine, New Haven, CT, USA

G.Z. Williams
Director, Institute of Cancer Research, Medical Research Institute of San Francisco at Pacific Medical Center, San Francisco, CA, USA

Foreword

*In health, as in any other area, measurement is essential in knowing where we are and where we are going. The first joint publication of the International Epidemiological Association (IEA) and the WHO Regional Office for Europe in 1979 (*Measurement of levels of health, *European Series No. 7) provided information on concepts and processes in the measurement of health and thus addressed mainly the first of these issues. At the IXth Scientific Meeting of the IEA in 1981, a sequel was proposed, to deal with the measurement of improvements in health through programmes of disease control and through health promotion. This book should provide the people responsible for such programmes, and those who attempt to measure the impact of health programmes, with the beginnings of a resolution of the second issue, an indication of where we are going.*

Concepts and tools of measurement in health progress have developed rapidly during the time (1982–1985) required for the preparation of the manuscript. In many instances, descriptions of the concepts or methods were less easy to obtain than illustrations of their everyday use in health promotion and the improvement of health. Since the problems of improving and promoting health apply throughout the world, these illustrations have been sought from developing and developed countries alike.

Concurrently with the development of the manuscript, the Member States of the World Health Organization began to assess their progress towards the goal of health for all. In the European Region, this implied the development of regional targets and indicators, so that the detailed evaluation would cover the specific problems of the Region and the proposed solutions, an important part of which is health promotion. The evaluation of progress towards health for all in the European Region of WHO has already brought to light the dearth of appropriate indicators that transcend the traditional indicators of mortality and morbidity in such areas as disabilities, lifestyles, the impact of environmental health, and the role of the community in the definition and development of health services. The experience gained in the last five years is closely reflected in some of the contributions to the third part of this book; the two final chapters, on the role of indicators and on the new health promotion programme in the Regional Office, are a particular indication of the close relationship of the philosophy behind this book to the concepts and applications of health for all.

J.E. Asvall
WHO Regional Director
for Europe

Preface

Measurement in health has long played an important role among the activities of the International Epidemiological Association, as clearly shown in the book published jointly by the World Health Organization and the International Epidemiological Association in 1979. The measurement of health promotion has in recent years been a central issue in scientific meetings of the International Epidemiological Association. The present book continues and updates work on these concerns.

The book reviews the overall concepts of health and health promotion, as well as the important process of promoting health and its social and political implications. Methods of measuring health, essential for health care planning and evaluation, are presented. The final part of the book includes a number of examples of the use of such measurements for assessing progress in health and monitoring the results of specific health promotion programmes.

The goal of the World Health Organization and its Member States is the achievement of health for all; it is hoped that this book will help everyone involved in implementing health promotion activities, in monitoring their results and thus working towards this goal. For epidemiologists, this publication should exemplify one of the most important uses of epidemiology.

J. Mosbech
President
International Epidemiological Association

Acknowledgements

The planning of this publication began at a workshop on positive health indicators held during the IXth International Scientific Meeting of the International Epidemiological Association in 1981. The contributions of the participants in this workshop to the preparation of this volume are greatly appreciated.

The Editorial Board wishes to acknowledge the assistance of Professor W.W. Holland, Department of Community Medicine, St Thomas's Hospital Medical School, London, and Dr T. Purola, Department of Social Policy, University of Helsinki, who provided many useful suggestions during the early stages of the work.

In addition, the Editorial Board thanks Mr R. Anderson, Institute for Social Studies in Medical Care, London; Dr L. Breslow, School of Public Health, University of California; Dr Ilona Kickbusch, Regional Officer for Health Education, WHO Regional Office for Europe; Professor M. Manciaux, Université de Nancy 1, Faculté "B" de médecine de Nancy; and Dr K.L. White for their assistance in reviewing the manuscripts and for their many suggestions, which were an invaluable help in the production of this book.

Introduction

The Member States of the World Health Organization have agreed on the goal of health for all by the year 2000. To attain this, their governments must work both to reduce inequalities in health status and to improve the overall health status of their populations; individuals and communities should increasingly be involved in the development of their own health, adopting healthier lifestyles and behaviour patterns and playing an increasing part in the provision and development of their health services.

To find out whether the efforts to achieve health for all are producing the desired improvements, it will obviously be necessary to measure the changes in the health status of individuals and hence of communities brought about by the implementation of health policies, programmes and activities. Epidemiological measurements are an important set of tools in this kind of assessment; they will also help health planners and health practitioners at all levels to appreciate the nature and size of health problems and the programmes required to overcome them. This approach has, however, rarely been used until now to measure *changes* in health status in a positive sense and to relate these changes to specific policies and interventions. The instruments needed for this type of dynamic application have not been adequately identified in the past and are often unfamiliar to those responsible for decisions about health at national, regional or local levels.

Traditionally, measurements of health have tended to concentrate on mortality, morbidity and other manifestations of ill health, measuring progress by the reduction in negative factors and outcomes. A joint publication by the International Epidemiological Association (IEA) and WHO was explicitly directed towards providing measurements of health rather than covering the "measurements of ill health that have dominated the field of health indicators used for evaluation of health status".[a] It was aimed towards measuring health status rather than towards measuring change and improvement, however, and did not specifically consider the measurement aspects of the programmes for the promotion and protection of health.

---

[a] *Measurement of levels of health.* Copenhagen, WHO Regional Office for Europe, 1979 (WHO Regional Publications, European Series, No. 7).

The quantitative determination of national plans and programmes has become increasingly accepted as part of the routine management of health resources. In developing countries particularly, the management of limited and scarce resources has always required the careful selection and application of reliable measurements, to permit the rational choice of activities and the optimal use of resources. Planning that does not take into account such evaluative measurements often leads to grandiose programmes that cannot be maintained owing to lack of funds, and whose impact on the overall health of the population is at best negligible and sometimes negative. The methods of measuring health exemplified in this earlier publication therefore met with considerable interest in developing countries, although the book was originally written with the problems of Europe in mind.

At the IXth International Scientific Meeting of the IEA held in 1981 in Edinburgh, WHO and IEA convened a workshop at which they agreed to publish a further volume that would address the measurement of improvements in health and try to link these improvements with developments in health policy, social policy and other relevant areas. This book would also review the actions taken at the individual or population level to promote and protect health, and examine how both processes and outcomes can be assessed quantitatively.

The purpose of the present book is thus threefold: to develop the conceptual framework of health promotion and protection; to discuss the measurement of activities directly or indirectly related to the promotion or protection of health; and to present examples of measurements in use or in the course of development. It deals with a wide range of activities that affect health, including personal lifestyles and behaviour, environmental conditions, and activities aimed at the protection of individuals and communities and at those living conditions that affect our health, and with social and political aspects of change. This book should assist countries and regions to develop and evaluate strategies to reach their goals of improving and protecting the health of their people.

From a theoretical point of view, the approaches to health promotion, health protection and measurement are applicable equally to developing and to developed countries. Some of the measures will, however, in practice need to be adapted from country to country, depending on the local health priorities and the information base available, as well as the particular patterns of health problems and sociocultural factors, while others will be universally applicable. The local availability of resources will also limit the use of more complex and costly measurements. Although the authors of Parts I and II of this book are mainly from the northern hemisphere (though often with experience of health work in developing countries), the illustrations and applications in Part III include contributions from developing countries to a larger extent than was the case in the earlier publication.

The book is primarily aimed at people in health departments who are responsible for health management and policy development, and in particular those most concerned with health promotion policies and their evaluation. It is hoped that it will create a greater understanding of the possible uses of quantitative methods for identifying problems, setting targets and assessing progress towards these targets. This publication should also be of interest to scientists concerned with the development of measurements in epidemiology, health services or social policy, who need to identify areas where further work is needed or where new methods should be investigated, and also to those responsible for training health workers, so that future generations are aware of the developments and applications of the measurement of health changes.

The book is in three parts. Part I clarifies the concepts of health and health promotion, discusses the main processes that lead to improved health and suggests the areas of health promotion and protection in which measurement is possible and relevant. Part II has more of a textbook function and includes chapters on how to measure the principal dimensions of health and processes of health promotion and protection. After reading each chapter, administrators and others who do not have particular expertise in the field of measurement should be able to define the concepts and assess the possibilities of measurement in this field. Researchers should view this Part as a summary of measurement options in various fields of health promotion and protection, although inevitably it has not been possible to cover extensively some of the more complex measures currently being developed. In Part III, specific examples of the application of measurements to achieved or potential improvements in health are presented, including discussions of successes and failures, and some recent developments, both theoretical and practical, are described.

Concepts such as health, health promotion and health protection have as yet no clear and widely accepted definition. The prevailing usage of the terms at any time will reflect the sociocultural and institutional framework within which they are found. In Chapter 1 concepts of health and health promotion are discussed, and a working definition of health promotion is given. The working authors have emphasized different aspects of health promotion according to their experience. In the overall framework of the book, however, health promotion is meant to comprise all efforts to protect, maintain and improve health.

Part I

Concepts

1. Concepts of health and health promotion

H. Noack

The Problem

Concepts of disease and medical care, health and health promotion do not exist in a sociocultural, institutional and political vacuum. They reflect the values, beliefs, knowledge and practices shared by lay people, professionals and other influential groups.

Worldwide, health is defined in negative terms as the absence of disease. Progress in medical science and technology over the last 100 years has produced an immense body of knowledge that allows us to specify distinct diseases in ever greater detail, explain their underlying mechanisms and use many forms of intervention to prevent and treat them and to minimize distress, suffering and disability. The vast organizational complexes called health care systems that exist in many countries have become a source of growing and serious concern, despite their unquestionable contribution to the cure of disease and the care of the sick.

As most of these concerns are well known, only the main symptoms of what has been referred to as "health crisis 2000" *(1)* will be mentioned here. In the developed world, these are the growing numbers of "new deaths" due to diseases of the cardiovascular system and the respiratory system, cancer and accidents; the increasing prevalence of diseases of lifestyle; the problem of the elderly and the mentally ill; the health cost of poverty and unemployment; the health consequences of pollution; specialization and subspecialization in medical care; the growing cost of medical technology; poor planning and unbalanced allocation of health resources; and the uncontrolled rise of health care expenditure in many countries. In the developing world, large proportions of the population suffer from a high prevalence of ill health and die prematurely, a situation that is largely due to a serious shortage of food and poor living conditions (*(2)*, see also Chapter 8.6).

A new health consciousness among large segments of the population and new health movements can be observed in a growing number of countries. At least in part they seem to reflect concern about the apparent or real health crisis. WHO has launched a global strategy for health for all by the year 2000 *(3)*, which calls for a reorientation of health policy and health services and for new priorities in the distribution of health resources. A common element in these efforts is that they are aimed at the promotion of positive health.

Positive health, however, is an elusive concept *(4)*. There are no sufficiently homogeneous lay definitions of it nor any consistent professional or scientific definitions. Major textbooks of clinical medicine *(5)* and public health *(6)* place heavy reliance on negative terms. Authors on the philosophy of modern medical science *(7,8)* have traced several conceptual and semantic problems in defining health. While disease is considered an evaluative and explanatory concept for the purpose of diagnosis, prognosis and therapy, health is seen as a normative and holistic term. "Health and disease are not symmetrical concepts ... And, while there are many diseases, there is in a sense only one health ..." *(8)*.

Quite obviously, any attempt to define positive health raises a number of problems. One is that there are certain limitations to the study and identification of the "causes" of good health. This means that contrary to the prevention and treatment of disease, it is not easy to specify and justify health promotion strategies or methods, at least from a scientific point of view. Furthermore, because under these circumstances it tends to be difficult to agree on useful operational definitions of health, it is also difficult to evaluate health promotion activities or programmes. Such difficulties, as well as related scientific and practical problems, can only be touched on in this chapter but most of them cannot easily be resolved. The purpose of this chapter is to review, analyse and clarify the concepts of health and health promotion, and to discuss their practical relevance.

The Socioecological Paradigm of Health

According to Kuhn's theory of progress in science *(9)*, scientific disciplines pass through stages of "normal science", in which the scientific community shares a particular paradigm (the paradigmatic stage), and stages where paradigms are changing ("pre-normal stage", "crisis" and "revolution"). A paradigm is a conceptual framework that determines which situations are viewed as legitimate scientific problems or puzzles. Associated with a paradigm is a basic assumption about the nature of the problem (e.g. in astronomy: "The sun is the centre of the universe") as well as a general agreement about a common terminology and about methodological issues such as measurement techniques, procedures for testing hypotheses and formal rules of theory construction.

As several authors have indicated *(10–13)* in the medical and health sciences it seems that we are currently witnessing the beginning of a shift from a stage of normal biomedical science towards a stage where a more global perspective, such as a socioecological paradigm, may eventually replace the biological paradigm, ideally by integrating it. A considerable body of scientific research and relevant theory has already been accumulated by more recent disciplines and by multidisciplinary fields that strongly support the psychosocial and ecological perspective and provide elements for the new paradigm: biomedical epidemiology and community medicine *(6,14,15)*, medical sociology and social epidemiology *(16–18)* and psychosomatic medicine *(19)*. Quite obviously, a shift in medical paradigm, as indicated here, has certain implications for the concepts of health and disease as well as for health promotion and prevention. This can be seen by a brief look at the history of medical science and practice.

The roots of western medical science lie in the Hippocratic tradition, a system of medical thought and practice flourishing around 400 BC on the Greek island of Cos. According to this system, wellbeing or ill health were conceived as resulting from an equilibrium between environmental factors such as winds, temperature, water, soil and food, and an individual's way of life, i.e. his or her eating, drinking and sexual habits as well as work and recreational behaviour. This "external" balance between man and his environment was assumed to determine his internal balance, an equilibrium between the four humours of the human body: blood, phlegm, black bile and yellow bile. Within this paradigm clinical practice was meant to assist nature's healing forces, and public health care the prediction and control of the community's health problems by understanding the human ecosystem *(11,20)*.

Interestingly, the main elements of Hippocratic thought — health as a state of balance and the importance of both human and environmental factors — were developed earlier by traditional Chinese medicine. According to Chinese thought, the human body was conceived as a system of interrelated components that have a natural tendency to maintain a state of dynamic balance. Imbalance or illness were thought to result from a number of factors such as poor diet, lack of sleep, lack of exercise, or disharmony within the family or society *(21,22)*. Thus both the Hippocratic and the traditional Chinese paradigms had essentially ecological frameworks. The world and the human beings within it were viewed as wholes that tended to remain in a state of balance, because of their dynamic nature.

The world view that has decisively shaped modern science and technology — commonly referred to as the mechanistic or Cartesian paradigm emerging in the sixteenth century — is a radical departure from the thinking of antiquity. The entire universe, including the body of all living creatures, was viewed as a huge mechanical machine functioning like a clock with great precision according to mathematical laws. To discover these laws, man had to apply the analytical method and study their component parts. Understanding these laws allowed man to master and control nature. Unlike plants and animals, human beings were thought to be inhabited by a rational mind that was separate from the body but connected to it through the pineal gland in the brain *(22)*.

As pointed out by several authors *(12,23)* modern medicine with its undeniable achievements and its limitations — as well as the underlying biomedical paradigm — rests largely on the Cartesian view of the world. Neglect of the human environment and the division between mind and body have allowed medical scientists and physicians to focus almost exclusively on the human organism and its parts, especially during the last 100 years. According to the biomedical paradigm, disease is a "temporal or permanent impairment in the functioning of any single component, or of the relationship between components making up the individual" *(24)* or — more succinctly — "the breakdown of the machine, and the doctor's task is the repair of the machine" *(12)*.

From both a practical and a health policy point of view, the conceptualization of disease itself is of no particular concern. More important are the causal factors and the mechanisms that explain disease and that must be influenced in order to prevent or control it. It is interesting to note that throughout the seventeenth and eighteenth centuries, long before the advance of biomedicine, social medicine was considered to provide a theoretically and practically relevant framework that will be referred to here as the sociomedical paradigm. As shown in Rosen's fundamental work on the evolution of social medicine *(25)*, this paradigm has deep historical roots in antiquity and in mediaeval times.

According to the sociomedical paradigm, there is a clear link between the prevalence of health or ill health in any given population, and socioeconomic and sociocultural factors. During the period of early capitalism in Europe with its rapid industrialization and urbanization, poverty and the adverse living and working conditions of the lower classes were seen to account for their poor health and high rates of premature death. Insufficient nutrition, poor housing, inadequate hygiene, the extremely long working day, lack of recreation and the noxious effects of work itself were identified as the most deleterious influences on health and wellbeing. A relatively clear notion of the physiological consequences seemed to exist already, as these factors were assumed to distort physical development and lower bodily resistance to epidemic diseases. Beginning in the eighteenth century in France and later also in Germany and the United Kingdom, a growing number of empirical studies, which were made possible through the introduction of surveys and statistical methods, lent support to the sociomedical paradigm *(25)*.

In the middle of the nineteenth century social reformers, politicians, administrators and liberal physicians strongly demanded that health should become the concern of society, and medicine was considered to be a social science. Towards the turn of that century medical sociology was perceived as an important new field of study, both in Germany and in the United States. The task of medicine was seen as to intervene in social and political life, to remove the unjust socioeconomic and environmental conditions that hampered both the life and the health of the lower classes. Within general frameworks such as social hygiene and social therapy, the concept of social medicine was very broad indeed. It was regarded as a comprehensive strategy including not only sanitary but also social reform, and also as a discipline that was concerned not only about access to and provision of medical care, but also about prevention of disease and accidents and about health education *(25)*.

Owing to the growing success of biomedicine, but perhaps also to the partial improvement of living and working conditions in the major industrialized countries towards the end of the nineteenth century, the movement of social medicine lost most of its momentum. Bacteriology was seen as providing the ultimate medical truth *(25)*. Microbiologists began their highly successful programme that identified microorganisms as the specific agents of most known infectious diseases. Germ theory and with it the "doctrine of specific aetiology of disease" *(26)* were developed, a theoretical framework that since then has been used to explain the cause of a large number of other diseases by specific agents such as radiation, noise, physical stress, chemical compounds, alcohol, cigarette smoke and air pollution, often with moderate success *(6)*. Within this framework health essentially means the absence or low level of such disease agents in the physical environment.

Yet very soon the weaknesses of germ theory and of the doctrine of specific agents were pointed out. Communicable diseases seemed to involve not only infectious agents but also factors such as nutrition, working and living conditions, education and income *(25)*. It was concluded that microorganisms are a necessary but not a sufficient condition for the development of an infectious disease, and that a crucial role is played by the susceptibility of individuals (and therefore by host factors). Subsequently, immunological resistance was discovered, which provided the scientific basis for a new area of disease prevention through immunization or vaccination, and also of clinical immunology *(11)*.

In a far more general sense the notion of resistance has since become a most powerful concept, in particular resistance to physical and psychosocial stressors and other potential risks to health. According to this framework, the maintenance of health requires a sufficient level of specific or generalized resistance resources to cope with disease agents and other risks to health *(16)*. Furthermore, the introduction of the concept of host resistance has helped to replace the deterministic single-factor doctrine of disease causation by a probabilistic framework that is in accordance with current scientific thinking.

Along with the development of psychosomatic medicine, medical sociology and social epidemiology over the last few decades, resistance and susceptibility have themselves become phenomena of growing clinical and scientific interest. On the basis of a fairly large amount of empirical evidence it can be concluded that stress and coping are major links between the influence of environmental conditions on the individual and his or her level of ill health or health. Under normal circumstances people tend to adapt to their physical and social environments and cope with demands in such a way that they can maintain their physiological, emotional and cognitive balance. However, particular situations or events (e.g. poverty, malnutrition, physical exhaustion, loss of social support, personal loss) that may be experienced as stressful, tend to increase general susceptibility and hence the risk of loss of balance and hence of disease. Which disease a person succumbs to may well depend on genetic and acquired constitutional factors as well as on the specific interaction between the person and the environment *(16,26)*.

Within this framework two considerations appear to be important. First, health or ill health does not depend merely on social and environmental factors and an individual's resistance gives him or her a more or less stable predisposition to a particular disease. Health or ill health also depends on his or her physical and psychological potential to cope effectively with internal (e.g. bodily) and external demands. Second, most diseases are likely to be the result of many interacting conditions: external as well as internal factors, contributing (e.g. precipitating) and predisposing factors. Thus, quite contrary to the doctrine that diseases have specific causes most conditions of ill health — and, as a logical consequence, of good health as well — have heterogeneous origins *(16,19)*.

Strong support for a multifactorial, socioecological paradigm of health comes from epidemiological research on chronic disease, in particular studies of cardiovascular morbidity and mortality. Although the issue is far from resolved, large cross-sectional and longitudinal studies of populations that differ in their exposure to risks, as well as large-scale intervention trials, clearly indicate the importance of several risk factors in the development of coronary heart disease, in particular high blood pressure, overweight, a high level of serum cholesterol, cigarette smoking and lack of physical activity *(27)*. In a nine-year follow-up study it was shown that mortality from all causes of death was significantly related to a number of high-risk practices such as smoking cigarettes, consuming too much alcohol, being physically inactive, being obese or underweight and sleeping fewer than seven or more than eight hours per night. There was an inverse relationship between all these practices and longevity. A significant relationship was also found between mortality and the size of the social network and the nature of social relationships *(28)*.

There is overwhelming evidence today that the conditions and the prevalence of health and disease vary enormously between and within the regions of the world. The strikingly higher rates of morbidity and mortality in the less developed countries of the south, compared with the highly developed countries of the north, are generally explained by a serious shortage of food and by extensive poverty due to socioeconomic and political developments. The higher prevalence of poor health and chronic disease among lower social classes and minority groups in developed countries *(29,30)* has to some extent been accounted for by their living and working conditions, which may produce excessive physical and psychosocial stress and foster lifestyles that are not conducive to health (*(31)*, see also Chapter 8.6).

Thus a socioecological paradigm is a suitable framework for explaining the conditions and causes of health and ill health and for guiding health-related activities as well as health and social policy. Obviously, such a paradigm will have to integrate the biomedical, the psychosocial and the sociomedical perspectives.

Concepts and Definitions of Health

Given a socioecological paradigm, which parts of the concept of health are relevant to the concept of health promotion? To answer this question several definitions or notions of health, originating from expert, professional and lay people or groups will be reviewed, and then what the author considers to be the key parts of a working definition of health will be discussed.

Probably the best known definition of health is that given in the WHO Constitution:

> Health is a state of complete physical, mental and social well-being and not merely the absence of disease or infirmity *(32)*.

Describing health as a general value, this definition was perhaps intended neither to serve as a framework for formulating goals of health policy nor for deriving operational definitions of health. Nevertheless, it has been criticized for several reasons, one being that it conceptualizes health as a normative state, as an ideal goal that can be approached but never attained *(8,24)*. Other criticisms are that in this definition the ambiguous concept of health is replaced by the equally ambiguous notion of wellbeing *(8)*, and that "complete" wellbeing is difficult to measure *(33)*. Another serious objection is the wide scope of the concept of health which, according to Antonovsky *(16)*, reflects "the quintessential expression of medical imperialism, of the assumption that everything in life falls in the jurisdiction of the health care system and of those who control that system". Still other critics have remarked that health is not a state but a task *(34)*, a means to an end such as the fulfilment of role obligations *(10)*.

Concepts of health as a process, an activity or a potential are emphasized in the following statements. Thus, health has been conceived as:

> ... a *modus vivendi* enabling imperfect men to achieve a rewarding and not too painful existence while they cope with an imperfect world *(35)*;
>
> ... the imputed capacity to perform tasks and roles adequately *(36)*;
>
> ... the power to live a full, adult breathing life in close contact with what I love — I want to be all that I am capable of becoming *(37)*.

Health as an activity or potential is also emphasized in the following:

> It is in our choice of lifestyles that we can most affect the way we enjoy health as a way of life *(1)*;
>
> ... an experience of well-being resulting from a dynamic balance that involves the physical and the psychological aspects of the organism, as well as its interaction with its natural and social environment *(22)*.

At least two of the criticisms of the WHO definition seem to apply to these definitions as well. They are made up of concepts that are difficult to define and even more difficult to measure. It will therefore be instructive to consider an operational definition of health that avoids these shortcomings.

As one of the key elements of his theory of salutogenesis — so far perhaps one of the very few theoretical frameworks attempting to explain why people stay healthy in spite of the ubiquity of pathogens — Antonovsky *(16)* proposes a health continuum from ease to dis-ease. People may move along that continuum either in the direction of ease (salutogenesis) or in the direction of dis-ease (breakdown), depending on their capacity or lack of capacity to manage states of tension caused by exogenic or endogenic stressors. The ease/dis-ease continuum is operationally defined as a space with four dimensions or facets that have four or six discrete values each.

1. Pain (with four values from "no pain at all" to "severe pain" as felt by the individual).

2. Functional limitation (with four values from "no limitation at all" to "severe limitation" for the performance of life activities as defined by the individual).

3. Prognostic implication (with six values from "no acute or chronic condition" to "serious acute and life-threatening condition" as defined by the professional health authorities).

4. Action implication (with four values from "no particular health-related action" to "active therapeutic intervention" required, as seen by the health authorities).

Although this definition allows the measurement of levels of health, especially in the grey zone of mild forms of ill health, it is not free of problems. Thus, wellbeing (ease) is reduced to the absence of pain or limitation. Other symptoms or psychological feelings, however, such as weight loss, temperature, chronic fatigue, emotional distress or their absence may be equally important. Furthermore, this definition of health/ill health mixes personal or lay and professional judgements. For practical reasons, this may limit the use of the measurement. Finally, the concept of an ease/dis-ease continuum seems to suggest a single health/ill health dimension, whereas health and ill health are more appropriately viewed as representing several dimensions or various discrete characteristics of a complex system with two extreme hypothetical states, namely complete balance and total breakdown.

Having reviewed expert or professional definitions of health, lay concepts will also be considered. It seems that so far, at least in western culture, not many efforts have been made to study what lay people mean by health and how they explain it. However, in several studies undertaken in Europe and North America *(4)* quite similar concepts were found. Although they may be biased in terms of both social class and culture, some of the findings of a study by Herzlich *(38)* that can be considered the classical study in this field will be summarized here. The health concepts reported are based on extensive interviews with 80 adults in France, half of them middle class and half of them professional people.

According to this study, health and illness reflect opposing views of both conditions and ways of life. Health is seen as entirely endogenous and it is associated with unrestrained nature, life in the country and personal activity. Illness, on the other hand, is entirely exogenous, a product of the forced and constrained life in the city, expressing itself in personal inactivity. The various lay concepts of health have been combined into three broad categories: health-in-a-vacuum or "being"; reserve of health or "having"; and health as an equilibrium or "doing".

> Health-in-a-vacuum is simply the absence of illness. Health is strictly speaking not something positive, it's simply not being ill. The fact of not having a body, so to speak, if it doesn't bother you in any way, health is basically an absence, it isn't anything positive, it's rather a negative thing.
>
> ... the reserve of health expresses an organic–biological characteristic as such ... It may be good, less good or poor, and may also vary according to the kind of life the individual leads; one may build up one's reserve of health or break into it. This capital asset of vitality and defence may increase or dissipate ... [It] does not consist only of resistance to illness, it also appears as the "substructure" of the other types of health.
>
> Equilibrium ..., both in its presence and in its absence, represents an autonomous experience; one feels that one has equilibrium or that one has lost it ... [It comprises] physical well-being, plenty of physical resources, absence of fatigue, psychological well-being and evenness of temper, freedom of movement and effectiveness in action, good relation with other people ... [However] ... there is no such thing as perfect health, it's much more a matter of being able to keep a balanced life ... To be slightly ill, for example, to have a tendency to bronchitis isn't to be in bad health ... I am in good health when I am in equilibrium, when I feel myself capable of doing what I want *(38)*.

Towards a Working Definition of Health

The definitions and concepts of health reviewed here reflect quite different cultural and institutional backgrounds as well as social and political orientations. Despite such differences, however, they have several common elements. They show that health is a holistic concept, in accordance with the Old English *hal* from which it derives, meaning whole *(33)*. Furthermore, these definitions indicate that health is a complex, multidimensional concept. The common themes referring to several such dimensions are: health as the absence of symptoms, illness or disability; health as a positively valued psychological experience; health as balance or equilibrium within oneself and with the environment; health as a capacity or potential to pursue personal goals and to cope with environmental and social demands; or health as the process of goal-directed action or as the process of effective coping.

The question is, which of these meanings should be incorporated into a working definition of health that is relevant to the concept of health promotion? Before advancing a proposal for such a working definition it will be useful to clarify two problems. One is related to the well known issue of the health/disease dichotomy, which is not a useful concept in this context as already indicated. Health and disease are considered as states or processes that are socially defined: generally health refers to non-deviance and disease to deviance from certain institutional or sociocultural norms that tend to vary. Furthermore, health and disease will be defined either medically by doctors or other health professionals, or through social interaction and lay consultation by the people involved *(39)*.

The other problem is whether one should require a concept of health to be measurable. The author feels that to require this confuses the notion of a general concept that is culturally and socially defined, with the notion of an operational definition. An operational definition such as Antonovsky's *(16)* ease/dis-ease continuum may well be useful or even necessary in the context of a theory or of an evaluation study. As a general requirement it would, however, reduce the meaning of the global concept of health to one of many possible specific meanings and thereby exclude most of it. Of course, single dimensions of the global concept can and often will have to be measured, in the medical as well as in the psychological, sociological or epidemiological sense of measurement.

Turning now to a proposal for a working definition of health, it is necessary to introduce briefly the general theoretical framework in which the author has chosen to formulate this proposal, namely the systems perspective. This perspective seems to be most suitable because it fits the socioecological paradigm of health and accounts for one of its central meanings, dynamic balance or equilibrium. The discussion will draw mainly on Miller's fundamental work on living systems *(40)* and in part on Capra's thinking *(22)*.

According to the systems perspective, living systems such as societies, social organizations, human beings and animals form a hierarchy of interdependent units where the higher-level system is made of lower-level subsystems. With regard to human health and disease, it is useful to see individuals as parts of social units such as families or other primary social groups which in turn form subsystems of larger sociocultural, economic and political systems embedded into an even more global societal and ecological system. Individuals, on the other hand, are made of smaller interacting components such as cognitive system, affective system, circulatory system, digestive system or reproductive system, each defined by its particular function in relation to the individual as a whole person.

Within such a hierarchy, health can be defined as a state of dynamic balance — or more appropriately as a process maintaining such a state — within any given subsystem, such as an organ, an individual, a social group or a community. This balance can partly be explained as the result of the individual's or the community's autonomous capacity for self-organization, self-renewal or self-repair due to automatic mechanisms of positive and negative feedback *(22)*. In addition, dynamic balance also depends on the ability of a person or group to interact with their social, cultural, economic, natural and technical environments, in a meaningful and successful way, e.g. through exchange, communication, work, and social and political action. Health is thus viewed as a dynamic characteristic of the individual, the social group or the socioecological system: it is clearly associated with the activities of such systems as a whole or of their component parts. For instance, many parameters of man's subsystems, such as heart rate, blood pressure, endocrine activity, blood sugar level, brain waves, psychological mood or the information processed in the cognitive system, tend to oscillate permanently between an upper and lower limit, and they also change over time, often in terms of particular rhythms.

Under normal conditions, when individuals are adapted to their environment and the environment doesn't impose any unusual risks or demands on them, they will be able to maintain an internal dynamic balance and thus health. Even an imbalance not exceeding a certain level and duration will be tolerated or controlled. However, changes in the environment or "self-initiated" internal change beyond such a level and duration will upset the balance, leading to a state that is associated with shifts in certain system parameters. If these parameters are pushed to their extreme values, according to systems thinking, a state of stress is reached that manifests itself in a well known pattern of physiological responses and often in psychological distress. Structural changes may also result, leading either to better adaptation of the individual to the environment (e.g. through immunity or learning), or to the breakdown of the system as in the case of ill health *(41)*.

Whether an individual will be able to control stress or fall into a state of imbalance depends not only on the nature of the situation and the "fit" between individual and environment, but also upon his or her potential to control it or cope with it. From a system's point of view, coping potential is thus an important health resource and therefore an aspect of health itself.

It can be assumed that coping potential and the process of coping itself are very much determined by the capacity of the subsystems of the individual to react adequately and effectively. This will be possible if they are flexible and can mobilize sufficient resources, and if system parameters can take on extreme values, at least temporarily. Under such conditions, for example, a temporary high heart rate, high blood pressure or high level of cognitive activity may indicate that the individual has great flexibility and thus sufficient coping potential.

Quite often, however, coping with adverse environmental conditions is not limited to individual activity, but involves social action and interaction. Furthermore, in developed countries it seems that large parts of the population have adopted individual or collective patterns of coping with the stresses of daily life and work that are known as major risk factors of chronic mass disease (in particular overeating, smoking and excessive drinking) *(27,28)*. In developing countries, on the other hand, substantial population groups manage to survive with an extreme shortage of food and without the elementary facilities of life *(2)*.

On the basis of these considerations, two *key dimensions* of health can be defined: health balance and health potential. Both dimensions seem to integrate much previous thinking as well as important conclusions drawn from research and practical experience, and they are relevant to the level of both the individual and the community.

At the level of the individual, health balance is a process or an internal state that is customarily taken as a dynamic equilibrium, as already discussed. Normally, lay people will experience such a state either as the absence of physical and psychosocial needs, symptoms, illness or disability, or in a positive sense as physical, psychological or social wellbeing, depending on their sociocultural background and personal health-related experiences. Health professionals, on the other hand, will define health balance in terms of physiological and/or psychological and behavioural parameters, that usually vary between certain accepted norms and form particular patterns over time. Thus, subjective or professional judgements of negative or positive health and of its established biological parameters can serve as indicators of health balance of individuals. More complex indices can be developed, for example by combining subjective and medical parameters as suggested by Antonovsky for the ease/dis-ease indicator *(16)*.

At the community level, health balance also reflects dynamic balance, but as related to the characteristics of a particular population, such as the experiences and activities of people and the interactions among them. The health balance of a community may be assessed, for example, through household surveys by subjective ratings of the level of wellbeing, health-related activities, absence of sickness or disability *(42)*; by epidemiological indicators such as the stability of morbidity over time, relationships between birth rate and mortality or between the demand for and use of health services *(43)*. More complex indices can be developed on the basis of such measurements and by using stochastic models, e.g. measurements of the level of health and quality of life *(44)*.

The second key dimension of health, health potential, is not just a particular condition specific to a given time or situation, but an important and relatively stable prerequisite of health balance. Health potential refers to either the capacity or the particular type of interaction between person and environment that is required to maintain such an equilibrium and to reestablish it when it is lost.

At the individual level health potential can, for example, mean good nutritional status, immunological resistance to infectious agents, physical fitness, emotional stability, adequate health knowledge and attitudes, or a healthy personal lifestyle and an effective pattern of coping with psychosocial stress. For several of these variables physiological indicators or psychological and sociological measurements are available. However, more global indicators of health potential, e.g. of physical status, general coping potential, lifestyle patterns and self-help resources, would seem to be quite useful.

In the community, health potential refers to the capacity required or to the activities undertaken to prevent health imbalance and to maintain or re-establish health balance. Important elements of a community's health potential are the scope and efficacy of health policy and administration; the proportion of the budget allocated to health promotion, prevention and social welfare; the levels of employment, income and social security; the quality of housing and the safety of the physical and technical environment; the adequacy of living conditions and of nutrition. Other important factors are access to health, education and other public services; health beliefs, health practices and recreational activities; and social and cultural activities and services. A number of measurements and indicators have been used or suggested to assess the very many different aspects of health potential, for example, of health policy and public health resources, employment and social welfare, collective health attitudes and lifestyles, level of social integration and social support (*(28,42)*, see also Chapter 8.6).

Health balance and health potential can be considered as key dimensions of a working definition of health, because they integrate the important aspects of the socioecological paradigm and lend themselves to operational definitions of more specific concepts or parameters. It is also important to note that health potential is a critical condition of health balance, an essential general health resource.

Health Resources and Health Risks

Having discussed health balance and health potential as important characteristics of the socioecological system, what conditions are known to affect health in a significant way?

As emphasized by several authors *(4,16)* so far very little research has been undertaken to determine what is conducive to positive health, and the process of salutogenesis has rarely been studied. Nearly all scientific work has focused on the causes of disease and on pathogenesis, perhaps for very good reasons. To specify health-promoting conditions and processes the author will draw mainly on disease-related epidemiological, sociomedical and clinical knowledge and, in addition, on a good deal of common sense. Although this may somewhat limit the strength of the argument, it does not seem to be a serious problem. As health and disease are not distinguished as dichotomous categories and accept both a negative and a positive definition of health, much of epidemiological and social science research about the relationship between environmental, personal and behavioural variables on the one hand and about risk factors and the incidence of disease on the other *(6,18,28)* is highly relevant here. This also holds true for a great deal of clinical experience and research *(5,19)*. Space does not allow these issues to be considered in any detail.

Another perhaps more serious problem lies in the fact that both health balance and health potential are complex concepts that refer to characteristics of social, cultural, biological and ecological systems. Thus, variables that are isolated and defined in order to study or alter a specific segment of such a system cannot be analysed easily and manipulated on the basis of a simple cause–effect relationship. There is always the difficulty of deciding how these variables might interact with factors that are not included, and there are seldom clear-cut criteria telling how "to close or lock up the system" *(15)*.

These considerations are of considerable practical relevance as most attempts at health promotion or the prevention of disease are interventions into goal-directed and self-controlling socioecological systems, that often show a high degree of dynamic balance and possess a considerable potential for "neutralizing" any kind of intervention. In industrialized countries, the attempt to influence certain aspects of lifestyle such as cigarette smoking, overeating or the regular use of analgesics through health information campaigns is perhaps a good example. Unless such efforts are supported by politics, economic forces, sociocultural values and relevant social networks, their effect is likely to be small. Of course, a systems approach is not always necessary, as for example in the case of poverty or of man-made environmental hazards to health such as toxic chemical substances, physical pollutants or specific work-related risks. Here a straightforward socioeconomic or ecological analysis will generally be sufficient to pinpoint the problem.

To provide at least a general answer to the question raised at the beginning of this section, the author has summarized what according to some of the literature *(1,4,6,16,28,31,45)* appear to be the most important factors influencing health (Table 1). A distinction is made between health-supporting factors, called health resources, and health risks, a category comprising all conditions and processes that affect health in a negative way.

Table 1 is self-explanatory and does not require any additional comments. Instead, an example will illustrate how it might be used. Physical health, more specifically the problem of maintaining or restoring "normal" body weight, will be considered. From the perspective of the biological system, this can be taken as a problem of the relationship between the input of matter and the output of energy, controlled by adequate nutrition and perhaps physical activity. In the context of the interaction between environment and person, however, as for example in lifestyle counselling, several additional factors would have to be taken into account. Relevant in such a situation might be the health-related knowledge and attitudes of the people concerned, their actual eating and drinking habits and perhaps their stress at home or at work. Further important factors might be socio-economic conditions such as income and access to adequate food. As a health policy issue, aspects of the social, cultural, economic, natural and technical environments will be of interest (besides the health values, the lifestyle and the income of the social groups concerned) and primarily the production, distribution, price, sale and quality of food and perhaps also of alcoholic drinks.

Concepts of Health Promotion

Using the concepts dealt with in the previous sections, health promotion can now be considered in a more systematic way. It is important to note that health promotion is a relatively new and not yet clearly defined term that seems to have largely replaced the very old concept of hygiene.

The meaning of health promotion overlaps considerably with the meaning of prevention. Customarily, three levels of prevention are distinguished *(33)*:

> Primary prevention can be defined as the promotion of health by personal and community-wide efforts, e.g., improving nutritional status, physical fitness, and emotional well-being, immunizing against infectious diseases, and making the environment safe.
>
> Secondary prevention can be defined as the measures available to individuals and populations for the early detection and prompt and effective intervention to correct departures from good health.
>
> Tertiary prevention consists of the measures available to reduce impairments and disabilities, minimize suffering caused by existing departures from good health, and to promote the patient's adjustment to irremediable conditions. This extends the concept of prevention into the field of rehabilitation.
>
> An epidemiologic interpretation of the distinction between primary and secondary prevention is that primary prevention is aimed at reducing incidence of

disease and other departures from good health, secondary prevention aims to reduce prevalence by shortening the duration, and tertiary prevention is aimed at reducing complications.

The main difference between the concepts of disease prevention and health promotion seems to be one of focus rather than one of overall perspective. Whereas prevention is a disease-related concept health promotion is a health-related one. It is for this reason that the author sees no sense in trying to define a boundary between them.

In the rest of this chapter, health promotion is taken as the more general concept. Health promotion is meant to comprise all efforts directed at the protection, maintenance and improvement of health potential, and hence of health balance. As health potential and health balance are closely interrelated aspects of the socioecological system we are concerned with in human health and of the people who belong to it, any health-related effort will generally affect both of them. It seems useful, however, to exclude from the concept of health promotion all clinical activities such as medical diagnosis, treatment and patient care. This leads to an important clarification: whereas self-care, medical treatment and patient care aim essentially at a better health balance, the main goal of health promotion is to maintain or improve health potential. (For a more comprehensive discussion of health promotion see Chapter 15.)

In agreement with other authors *(21,31)* two major types of health promotion are distinguished here: the individual health approach and the community health approach. The individual health approach aims directly at improving an individual person's health potential. As a consequence, he or she is expected to change his or her health behaviour and lifestyle and to help improve health-related aspects of the social, cultural, economic, natural and technical environments. Thus, the personal health approach lies in the tradition of clinical intervention, counselling and face-to-face education *(21)*.

The community health approach, on the other hand, is primarily directed towards improving the socioecological health potential: the health resources of the economic, social, cultural, natural and technical environments. It is assumed that this will have a positive impact on people's physical conditions, health risks and lifestyles and consequently on their individual health potential. The community health approach thus follows very much the tradition of social medicine and public health *(6,25)*.

On the basis of some of the literature in the field *(4,6,21,46)* the major goals and strategies of both the individual and the community approach, as they relate to the different subsystems of the socioecological system (Table 2), have been reviewed. They will be outlined in the following paragraphs, without going into too much detail.

As already indicated, the primary aim of the individual health approach is to strengthen the individual person's health potential so that he or she will be able to cope more effectively with environmental demands, psychosocial stress and health problems or health risks. Three somewhat different strategies may be chosen: strengthening the body through adequate nutrition

Table 1. Summary of health resources and health risks

System	Health resources	Health risks
Person		
Biological system	Good nutritional status, immunity	Malnutrition, susceptibility to infections
Cognitive system	Ego identity, positive health attitudes, adequate health knowledge	Inappropriate health attitudes and misinformation
Whole person	Emotional stability, physical fitness	General vulnerability
Health-related behaviour		
Habits	Healthy personal habits	Smoking, excessive drinking, overeating, lack of exercise
Work	Fulfilling and unstressful work	Overwork, stressful and dangerous work
Recreation	Sufficient sleep and recreation	Insufficient recreation and sleep
Sociocultural system		
Health culture and practices	Positive health-related values, norms, lifestyle, religion	Unstable, health-related values and beliefs, unhealthy lifestyles
Social network	Social integration, social ties	Social isolation, lack of social support

System	Health resources	Health risks
Sociocultural system (contd)		
Work organization and job system	Availability of work, positive work climate, job satisfaction	Unemployment, work stress, job dissatisfaction
Health services, schools, social institutions	Adequate and accessible health care and social services, health education	Lack or inaccessibility of health and social services or health education
Socioeconomic structure	Adequate material resources, income, social security	Lack and uneven distribution of resources
Physical–biological environment		
Physical resources	Adequate food supply, safe consumer goods	Insufficient and unhealthy food, easy access to cigarettes, alcohol, drugs
Micro-environment	Adequate housing and communication, safe water and transportation, waste disposal	Inadequate housing, crowding dangerous traffic conditions
Macro-environment	Healthy climate, preservation of nature	Environmental pollution, exploitation of nature

Table 2. Overview of concepts of health promotion

System	Health promotion: personal approach
Person	
Biological system	Adequate nutrition, immunization
Cognitive system	Health information, education counselling
Whole person	Exercise, training, social activity
Health-related behaviour	
Habits	Healthy life habits
Work	Fulfilling and unstressful work
Recreation	Sufficient rest and recreation
Sociocultural system	
Health culture and practices	Positive health beliefs, knowledge and lifestyle
Social network	Social integration and social support
Work organization and job system	Awareness of stressful conditions, participation in improvement
Health services, schools and social institutions	Appropriate use of services, participation in health activities
Socioeconomic structure	Participation in health policy
Physical-biological environment	
Physical resources	Avoidance of unhealthy food and products
Micro-environment	Awareness of need for adequate housing, safe roads, participation in improvement
Macro-environment	Awareness of damage to environment, participation in improvement

Health promotion: community approach	System
	Person
Good nutritional status, immunity	Biological system
Ego identity, adequate health attitudes and knowledge	Cognitive system
Emotional stability, physical fitness	Whole person
▲	**Health-related behaviour**
Healthy life habits	Habits
Fulfilling and unstressful work	Work
Sufficient rest and recreation	Recreation
▲	**Sociocultural system**
Health propaganda, mass information, health education programmes	Health culture and practices
Information networks, support of self-help	Social network
Employment policy, improvement of work safety, environment	Work organization and job system
Health and education policy and planning	Health services, schools and social institutions
Economic and social policy	Socioeconomic structure
	Physical-biological environment
Policy and legislation related to food, tobacco, alcohol, drugs, consumer products	Physical resources
Urban planning, provision of housing, safe water, waste disposal	Micro-environment
Policy and legislation related to pollution control and preservation of nature	Macro-environment

and immunization against infectious diseases; improving health motivation and health knowledge through information, education or counselling; and supporting the whole person's health potential through physical exercises, training, social and cultural activities.

Besides immunization, the crucial health promotion strategy is often considered to be health education both as an interpersonal and as a community-related effort. It is argued that effective health education will make it possible to change health-related behaviour and lifestyle and thus reduce the burden of "modern disease". Quite often, such a view rests on the assumption, sometimes a strong philosophical stance, that autonomous man is the master of his destiny and therefore responsible for his health or ill-health. A substantial amount of analytical work and empirical research suggests, however, that such a view greatly underestimates the cultural, social and economic pressures on individuals. It must be concluded that modifications of health behaviour and lifestyle can be expected if suitable changes also take place in personal development and socialization as well as in the social conditions of daily living and work *(6,18)*. There is growing evidence that at least cardiovascular health can be improved through community-based health promotion programmes, of which health education is an integral part *(27)*.

A somewhat more realistic aim of health education may thus be to help people interact with their environment so that they can reflect and attempt to modify health-related values and practices, develop more adequate social skills and strengthen emotional and social ties with other people. Health education may further aim at making people aware of and informing them about the need for more appropriate housing, safer roads and a less polluted environment, about proper nutrition and the quality of food, about the relationship between lifestyle, work stress and health, and about the appropriate use of health and social services. Thus, to improve health potential, health education may address people's skills at analysing their lifestyle and the system they live in, and at acting in a more healthy and health-conscious way.

The community health approach differs considerably from the personal health approach, in terms of both goals and strategies. As indicated in Table 2, it is directed towards many different segments of the social, cultural, economic, natural and technical environments. It therefore involves a relatively broad range of political, legislative and administrative strategies and means. Starting from the most general level of the socio-ecological system, the natural and technical environments, it can be seen that this approach may include the formulation and implementation of policies in a variety of fields: preservation of nature and pollution control; urban development and housing, waste disposal and traffic safety; production, taxation and sale of food and of products affecting the health of the people.

At the level of the social, cultural and economic environments, a community health approach may, for example, aim at integrating economic and social policy, health and education policy, and employment policy and legislation related to occupational health. Some of the primary goals of such efforts should be to maintain or help establish adequate health services and health education programmes, healthier working conditions, information networks and facilities for self-help groups, health information campaigns and community-based health programmes.

The overall aim of any community-oriented health promotion programme will, of course, be to improve the health potential of the community as a whole, besides reducing health risks and hazards. It is clear that the goals, strategies and means will differ markedly from one region or country to another. Whereas in many less developed countries health promotion programmes must be directed urgently towards the improvement of the very elementary conditions of living, in developed countries health promotion should address the negative consequences for health of industrialization, high technology, the bureaucratic organization of many aspects of social life and the distribution of wealth.

It must be emphasized that the community approach and the individual approach are not alternative health promotion strategies. Ideally, any systematic effort towards the better health of individuals would be an integrated element of a comprehensive community-oriented, socioecological strategy.

Conclusion

Today, concepts of health and health promotion can most fruitfully be analysed and discussed in the context of a socioecological paradigm. On the basis of such a paradigm health has been defined in terms of two interrelated aspects of the socioecological system and the people belonging to it, health stability and health potential.

Health balance refers to the maintenance of the physical, psychological and social balance of any social group or individual, health potential to the group's or individual's capacity to cope with environmental and psychosocial demands or stresses. Whereas the treatment of an individual's imbalance and the re-establishment of balance are the main concerns of self-care and medical care, health promotion aims primarily at improving health potential and thereby at maintaining health balance.

Health balance and health potential can be measured by a number of established clinical, epidemiological, psychological and sociological indicators both at the level of the community or of any other social group and at the level of the individual person. However, more complex and more sensitive indicators are desirable. They should allow the assessment of health potential as well as health balance in social groups and communities and the measurement and evaluation of the effect of health promotion programmes.

In aiming to improve health potential, health promotion may be undertaken either to strengthen health resources or to reduce the health risks of individuals, groups or the whole community. The individual health approach attempts to strengthen the physical and psychosocial health potential of individuals and, as a desired consequence, individual lifestyle and certain environmental health resources, particularly through immunization, health education and counselling. The community health approach is directed towards the improvement of economic, cultural, social, natural and technical health resources, and thereby towards the improvement of the personal lifestyle and health potential of individuals and social groups. It uses a large variety of political, legislative and administrative strategies and means.

Because the health problems in the developing countries differ vastly from those in developed countries, entirely different aims, strategies and means of health promotion are called for. In large parts of the Third World the greatest possible effort must be made to fight hunger and to improve living conditions. In many developed countries, on the other hand, health promotion should help to reduce the negative consequences for health of large-scale technological development, including unhealthy lifestyles. All such efforts will be the more effective, the better individual or small-group approaches to foster autonomous health activities are integrated into a comprehensive community framework. The most promising strategy — if there is such a strategy at all — is likely to be one combining comprehensive health promotion efforts and health care policy into a truly socioecological health strategy.

References

1. **O'Neill, P.** *Health crisis 2000.* London, William Heinemann Medical Books, 1983.
2. **Banerji, D.** *Poverty, class and health culture in India.* New Delhi, Prachi Prakashan, 1982.
3. *Global strategy for health for all by the year 2000.* Geneva, World Health Organization, 1981 ("Health for All" Series, No. 3).
4. **Anderson, R.** Health promotion: an overview. *European monographs in health education research,* **6**: 1–126 (1984).
5. **Weatherall, D.J. et al.** *Oxford textbook of medicine.* Oxford, Oxford University Press, 1983.
6. **Last, J.M.** *Public health and preventive medicine.* New York, Appleton Century-Crofts, 1980.
7. **Burns, C.R.** Diseases versus health: some legacies in the philosophies of modern medical science. *In:* Engelhardt, H.T., Jr. & Spicker, S.F., ed. *Evaluation and explanation in the biomedical sciences.* Dordrecht, D. Reidel, 1975.
8. **Engelhardt, H.T., Jr.** The concepts of health and disease. *In:* Engelhardt, H.T., Jr. & Spicker, S.F., ed. *Evaluation and explanation in the biomedical sciences.* Dordrecht, D. Reidel, 1975.
9. **Kuhn, T.** *The structure of scientific revolutions.* Chicago, University of Chicago Press, 1968.
10. **Ahmed, P.I. et al.** Toward a new definition of health: an overview. *In:* Ahmed, P.I. & Coelho, G.V., ed. *Toward a new definition of health.* New York, Plenum Press, 1979.
11. **Catalano, R.** *Health, behavior and the community.* Oxford, Pergamon Press, 1979.

12. **Engel, G.L.** The need for a new medical model: a challenge for biomedicine. *Science,* **196**: 129–136 (1977).
13. **Noack, H. & Müller, H.R.M.** Morbidity, illness behaviour and the medical model. *In:* Noack, H., ed. *Medical education and primary health care.* London, Croom Helm, 1980.
14. **McKeown, T.** *The role of medicine.* London, Nuffield Provincial Hospital Trust, 1976.
15. **Morris, J.N.** *Uses of epidemiology.* Edinburgh, Churchill Livingstone, 1975.
16. **Antonovsky, A.** *Health, stress, and coping.* San Francisco, Jossey-Bass, 1981.
17. **Brown, G.W. & Harris, T.** *Social origins of depression.* London, Tavistock, 1978.
18. **Mechanic, D.** *Medical sociology.* New York, The Free Press, 1978.
19. **Weiner, H.** *Psychobiology and human disease.* New York, Elsevier North-Holland, 1977.
20. **Dubos, R.** Hippocrates in modern dress. *In:* Sobel, D.S., ed. *Ways of health.* New York, Harcourt Brace Jovanovich, 1979.
21. **Burkitt, A.** Health education. *In:* Clark, J. & Henderson, J., ed. *Community health.* New York, Churchill Livingston, 1983.
22. **Capra, F.** *The turning point.* London, Fontana Paperbacks, 1983.
23. **Susser, M.** *Causal thinking in the health sciences.* New York, Oxford University Press, 1973.
24. **Polger, S.** *Health, International encyclopedia of the social sciences.* New York, MacMillan & Free Press, 1968, Vol. 5.
25. **Rosen, G.** The evolution of social medicine. *In:* Freeman, H.E. et al., *Handbook of medical sociology.* Englewood Cliffs, Prentice-Hall, 1979.
26. **Dubos, R.** *Mirage of health.* New York, Harper & Row, 1959.
27. **Winkelstein, W., Jr. & Marmot, M.** Primary prevention of ischem c heart disease: evaluation of community interventions. *Annual review of public health,* **2**: 253–276 (1981).
28. **Berkman, L.F. & Breslow, L.** *Health and ways of living.* Oxford, Oxford University Press, 1983.
29. **Klein, S.D.** Class, culture, and health. *In:* Last, J.M., ed. *Public health and preventive medicine.* New York, Appleton Century-Crofts, 1980.
30. **Townsend, P. & Davidson, N., ed.** *Inequalities in health. The Black report.* Harmondsworth, Penguin Books, 1982.
31. **Castillo-Salgado, C.** Assessing recent developments and opportunities in the promotion of health in the American work place. *Social science and medicine,* **19**: 349–358 (1984).
32. *Basic documents,* 35th ed. Geneva, World Health Organization, 1985.
33. **Last, J.M.** *A dictionary of epidemiology.* Oxford, Oxford University Press, 1983.
34. **Illich, I.** *Limits to medicine.* Penguin Books, 1976.
35. **Dubos, R.** *Man, medicine and environment.* New York, Praeger, 1968.
36. **Parsons, T.** Definitions of health and illness in the light of American values and social structure. *In:* Parsons, T., ed. *Social structure and personalities.* New York, The Free Press of Glencoe, 1964.

37. **Robinson, K.** What is health? *In:* Clark, J. & Henderson, J., ed. *Community health.* New York, Churchill Livingstone, 1983.
38. **Herzlich, C.** *Health and illness.* London, Academic Press, 1973.
39. **Freidson, E.** *Profession of medicine.* New York, Harper & Row, 1970.
40. **Miller, J.G.** *Living systems.* McGraw-Hill, 1978.
41. **Henry, J.P. & Stephens, P.M.** *Stress, health and the social environment.* New York, Springer-Verlag, 1977.
42. **Cartwright, A.** *Health surveys in practice and in potential: a critical review of their scope and methods.* King's Fund Publ. Office, London, 1983.
43. **Murnaghan, J.H.** Health indicators and information systems for the year 2000. *Annual review of public health,* **2**: 299–361 (1981).
44. **Leu, R.E. et al.** Die quantitative Erfassung von Gesundheitszustand und Lebensqualität, illustriert am Beispiel von Psoriasiskranken, Institut für Sozialwissenschaften, Basel (in press).
45. **Kahn, L.R.** *Work and health.* New York, John Wiley & Sons, 1981.
46. **Clark, J. & Henderson, J.** *Community health.* New York, Churchill Livingstone, 1983.

2. Approaches to health promotion and disease prevention

T. Abelin

Insights into the factors affecting health and into the causes and natural history of many diseases have led to an increasing understanding of how health can be promoted and diseases prevented. Although some of the most valuable rules of hygiene date back thousands of years, the scientific basis of health promotion and disease prevention was established mainly during the nineteenth and twentieth centuries. Some well known examples are:

— active immunization against many infectious diseases;

— the importance of keeping drinking-water free of pathogens;

— the identification of vectors of infectious diseases;

— the role of iodine and fluoride in the prevention of goitre and dental caries;

— the role of vitamins, protein, fibre and other food constituents in a balanced diet;

— the carcinogenic effect of ionizing radiation;

— the harmful effect on cardiovascular health of hypercholesterolaemia, high blood pressure, smoking and other risk factors;

— the role of smoking in the causation of lung cancer, myocardial infarction, chronic bronchitis, emphysema and several other diseases;

— the improvement in the prognosis for several forms of cancer and other diseases by early detection and treatment.

Looking at this list superficially, one would expect health promotion and disease prevention to be easy enough to accomplish just by telling people what immunizations to get, what to eat and what to drink, which habits to adopt and which to avoid. According to one school of thought, it would then be the people's own responsibility to follow or ignore the advice.

Unfortunately, a health promotion approach based on this attitude does not improve the health of the majority of people. What is needed is a more differentiated analysis of the determinants of human health. This analysis has to take the biomedical factors into account, but also consider how these factors interact with a complex system of social, biological and physical influences. Based on this type of analysis, more specific approaches to health promotion and disease prevention have been developed.

A simple model that can visualize many of these influences has been known for a long time: the epidemiological model of interaction of host, agent and environment. In this model, developed in the context of the fight against infectious diseases, the host element is thought of in terms of biological susceptibility (or resistance) to disease; the agent is a microbial organism capable of causing specific pathological changes in the susceptible host; and the environment is understood as contributing to causation by determining whether the agent is able to multiply and maintain its pathogenicity outside the host, to reach the host and to cause infection. Based on this model, there are three major approaches to infectious disease control: improving host resistance by immunization and proper nutrition; eliminating or reducing the agent by measures of personal and environmental hygiene; and creating an environment that discourages the agent from multiplying and spreading by measures of sanitary engineering and vector control. Depending on the nature of the ecological balance that determines the spread of disease, one or other of these approaches may be the crucial one for a given disease in a given situation. Thus, the major approach in the control of gastrointestinal infections is the strict separation of sewage and drinking-water by sanitary engineering methods and through the chemical treatment of drinking-water supplies. In malaria control after the Second World War, major advances were made in the elimination of vectors by the use of residual insecticides, whereas it is now known that insecticide use has major disadvantages. Emphasis now is, or should be, placed on the health implications of creating new environments as a result, for example, of the construction of dams or the creation of artificial lakes. At the same time, malaria prevention by medication — that is, by increasing host resistance — has become the method of choice in specific situations.

The host–agent–environment model of disease causation has also been used successfully in the control of nutritional deficiency and of many occupational diseases in industrialized countries. Here, as in the case of infectious disease control in the same areas, it has usually been possible to restrict health protection and disease prevention to the application of technical measures, without having to interfere significantly with deeply rooted personal habits or social dynamics.

Today, health promotion and disease prevention have become a more complex task in most parts of the world, because the reasons for not applying the well known methods appropriately are intricately interwoven with the entire social and political situation. In those countries where infections and nutritional deficiency are still the foremost public health problems, poverty, lack of education, dependence on food grown elsewhere, all against a background of adverse political conditions, make it almost impossible to apply measures that would work under more favourable circumstances. Health promotion measures and those leading to the long-term improvement of social and economic conditions, have to go hand in hand in these situations. It is not sufficient to act unilaterally on health-related problems, nor to limit one's efforts to people at high risk; rather, the whole community has to be involved in a joint effort that gives a continuing sense of collaboration and participation to everybody and leads to the long-term improvement of general living conditions. In some situations, specifically health-related measures may even have to be given second priority to start with, while top priority is given to such efforts as the improvement of housing, literacy and public education.

In industrial countries as well, the factors that favour health and those that cause the prevailing diseases (such as cancer and heart disease) are intimately interwoven with deeply rooted social, economic and political conditions. Depending on the nature of these relationships, different approaches to health promotion and disease prevention are appropriate and effective. In well designed programmes, aspects of several of these approaches will have to be combined. The purpose of this chapter is to present these approaches briefly, and to look at their rationale and particular features. The model on which this presentation is based, and which is also at the origin of some of the concepts presented in Chapter 1, evolved as a useful frame of reference, when a new concept of health promotion and disease prevention was being developed for a highly industrialized country *(1)*. But the examples will show that it is also applicable to the less developed parts of the world.

Factors influencing Health

It was shown in Chapter 1 that health can be understood as depending on a state of balance between the individual and his or her physical and social environment. This balance is affected on the one hand by the individual's health potential or ability to cope with environmental challenges, and on the other by the type and degree of environmental stress. Fig. 1 shows the different types of host and environmental influences, in elaboration of the classical host–agent–environment model of disease causation. The lower box represents the factors of the physical–biological environment distinguishing between the general and the personal environment. The upper box shows factors of health-related behaviour in terms of lifestyle and personal habits. These have changed radically during this century, and are known today to play a significant role in strengthening one's health or causing disease. Here again, a distinction between the collective level and the individual level is made, which will facilitate the classification of health promotion approaches.

The box marked "sociocultural system" reminds us that an individual's behaviour has to be seen in the context of the dynamics of the social groups to which he or she belongs. To some extent, people's lifestyle and behaviour are influenced by their family, their friends and their neighbours. But there are more anonymous influences that may be related to economic interests (advertising, mass media) or to cultural factors and customs. It will be almost impossible for many individuals to adopt healthy lifestyles against

Fig. 1. Factors that influence levels of health

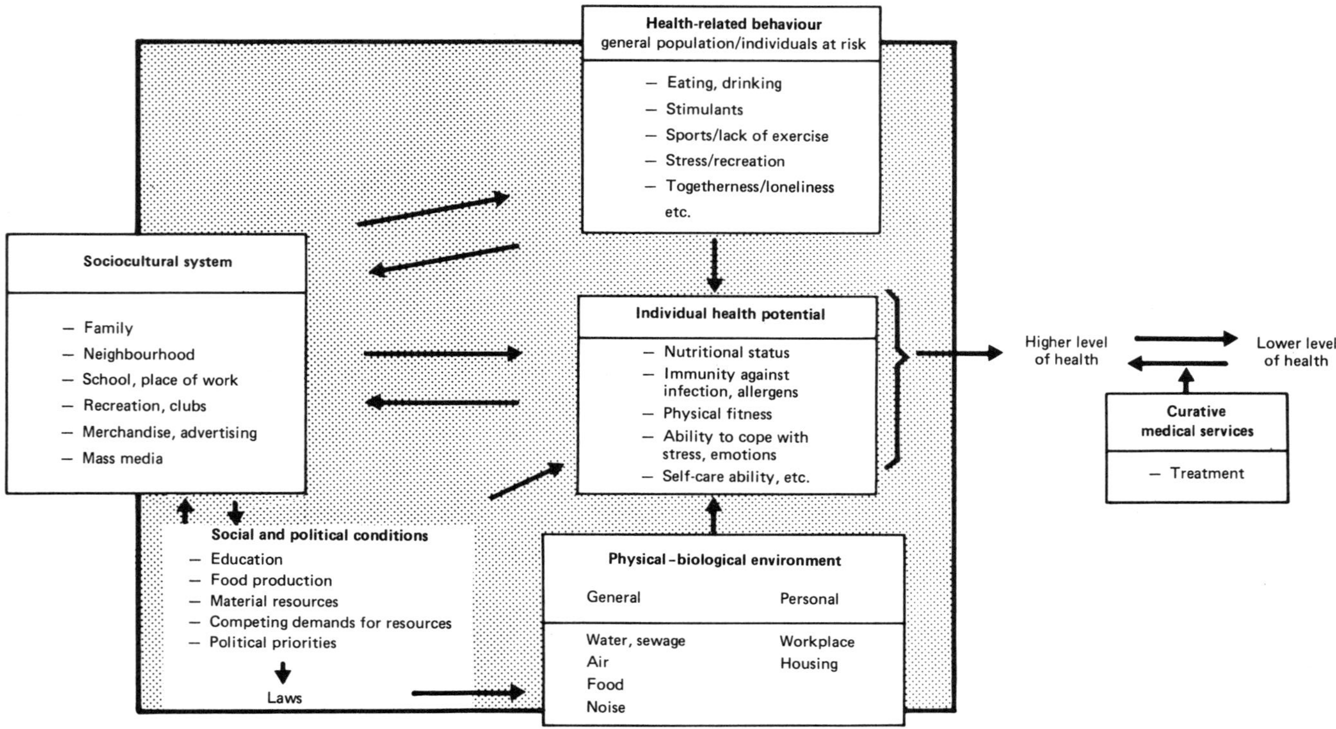

the stream of these forces. On the other hand, very positive movements influencing individual behaviour have reached individuals from their social environment.

In the shaded background social and political conditions determine to what degree health promotion measures will be taken and to what degree they will be able to reach their goals.

Finally, the right hand box shows the role that curative medical care has as a resource to influence the level of health. Its interventions are welcome when the health balance has been severely disturbed and when the health potential of the individual and his or her immediate environment is insufficient to restore health. Health services do not, however, compare with the many interactions of man with his environment in determining his level of health.

Approaches to Health Promotion and Disease Prevention

Based on this model, the different approaches to health promotion and disease prevention become readily apparent. But it also becomes apparent that no single approach will be sufficient to do justice to the complex network of factors, and that in designing programmes the issue will not be to choose between approaches, but to determine the most promising combination of approaches.

In Fig. 2 these approaches are shown in relation to the personal and environmental factors just identified.

Medical and related services

Whereas health promotion is a matter for the whole community and takes place mostly outside medical practice, disease prevention is a typically medical activity. This is particularly true where high-risk individuals are identified and brought under special preventive care. Nevertheless, the strategies of involving physicians and other medical professionals in preventive work differ markedly depending on local circumstances. In particular, physician density, but also such factors as insurance coverage of preventive attention and the availability of non-medical preventive services play an important role.

Where the density of medical professionals is low, such as in most of the less developed countries, the best use of their services is made through a referral system in which nonprofessional health workers identify high-risk individuals (and families) using clearly defined criteria and refer them to physicians or other specialized agencies for professional attention. This approach, known as the "risk approach" in health care, has been particularly successful in preventing maternal and neonatal deaths through the identification of high-risk pregnancies, but its potential includes many other areas of preventive medicine as well *(2)*.

The situation is rather different in most industrialized countries, where physician and hospital bed density is high, and where the issue is not so much that of the delegation of activities to nonprofessionals, but rather that of the distinction between tasks to be performed by the family physician

Fig. 2. Approaches to health promotion based on factors that influence levels of health

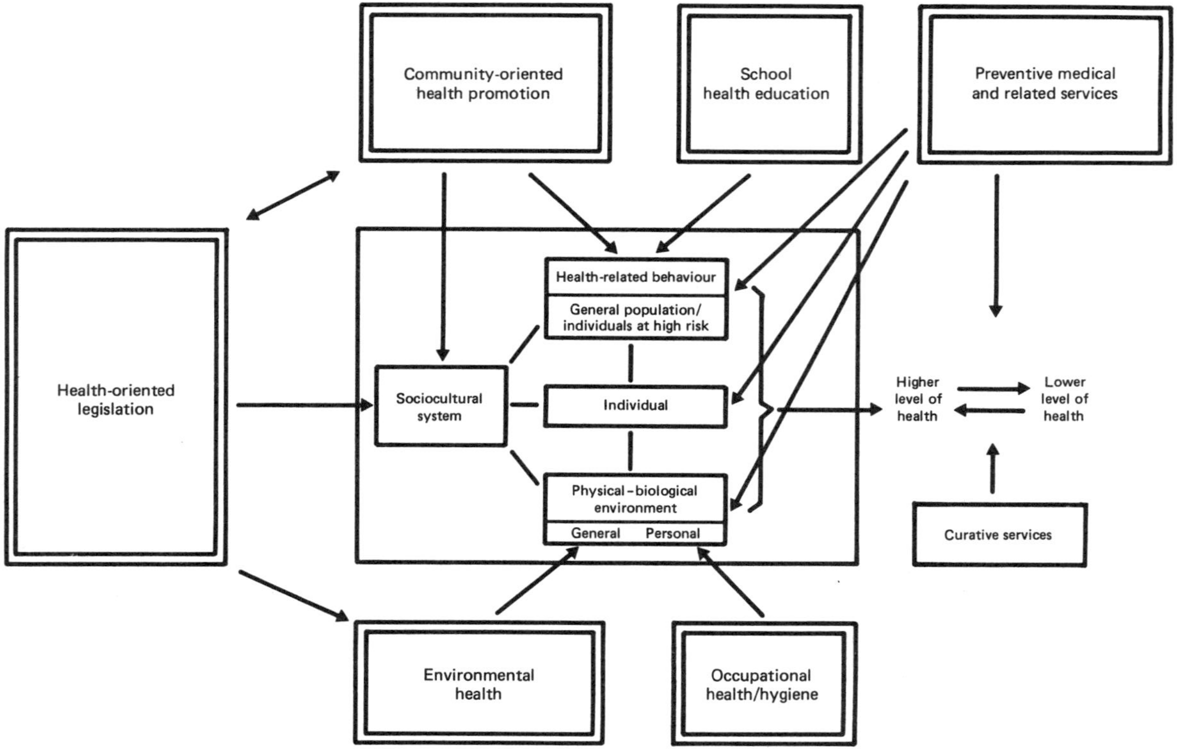

versus specialized agencies and by medical versus nonmedical professionals. But what are typically medical activities?

Some of the features of medical practice have traditionally been the one-to-one relationship between physician and patient, the problem-orientation of the doctor's actions, and the application of particular diagnostic and therapeutic techniques. This is why in industrial countries medical practice deals with those tasks of health promotion and disease prevention where the particular circumstances of individuals have to be taken into account (such as in health risk appraisal and risk factor correction) or where medical techniques have to be applied (such as in immunization, desensitization and early detection of disease). Table 1 gives an overview of health promotion and disease prevention activities in medical practice.

Table 1. Health promotion and disease prevention activities in medical practice

Purpose	Activity
To increase health potential	Immunization
	Desensitization
	Preventive medication
	Advice on personal hygiene
To reduce personal risk	Appraisal of individual risk situation
	Analysis of possibilities for risk reduction
	Advice and support in changing behaviour, working conditions, living conditions, etc. of people at high risk
To prevent progress of pathological processes	Early detection and correction

Whereas all these activities can be incorporated into medical practice, some of them such as immunization, health risk appraisal, early detection of pathological processes and guidance towards behavioural change may be more effectively organized in other settings, taking advantage of specialized know-how or mass procedures. Activities in these areas are discussed in more detail in Chapter 3.

Health education

Of course, health education begins in the home, where parents teach their children the basics of personal hygiene and how to avoid hazards. The education of parents may have a supportive effect, but those parents who need support most usually do not participate. Therefore, in so far as parents are not sufficiently prepared for this task, be it by lack of education, by neglect, because they fail in their role as exemplars, or because new information does not become available to them, school health education is the most important approach for reaching children. The objectives of school health education programmes must be explicitly stated, so that the most appropriate contents and methods can be chosen and success can be measured. A recent publication on smoking and children *(3)* demonstrates how health education not only consists of the transmission of knowledge, but is just as much concerned with values, attitudes and skills. The following list of contents, however incomplete, shows how wide-ranging health education is:

— transmission of knowledge and understanding of the body;

— transmission of knowledge about health hazards;

— practice of healthy habits (personal hygiene, exercise, food habits, drinking habits, etc.);

— consumer education (e.g. shopping for food, analysis of cigarette and alcohol advertising);

— practice of psychological and social competence such as resisting peer pressure (to smoke, drink, take drugs), coping with interpersonal conflict and relaxation techniques.

Many of these subjects are not included in the regular curricula of training programmes for school teachers and adult education mediators. Specialized services are therefore required to prepare supporting materials and introduce the subjects into the educational system. At the same time, the rules and regulations of the educational system should ensure that health education principles and subjects are integrated both into the school curriculum and into everyday school life.

Community-oriented health promotion

In both less developed and industrialized countries, experience has shown that a purely individual approach to health promotion, such as by trying to change the behaviour of those at increased risk, will rarely suffice to improve significantly the health status of the population. The main reason is that people tend to develop their lifestyles as members of groups and followers of group leaders, rather than as isolated individuals. Therefore, in community-oriented programmes it is the leaders who have to be convinced of the usefulness of the health messages and prepared to carry the less active members of the community with them in improving their health situation. As the leaders of a community and their families rarely belong to the groups at highest risk, they would tend to be left out in programmes that are aimed at individuals at risk rather than at the community as a whole. It is not possible here to look at the features of community-oriented health promotion in any detail. The concepts and principles relevant here have been discussed by a WHO working group and are presented in Chapter 15. As will be shown in Chapter 4.1 an important point is participation of the members of the community, not just passively in programmes organized for them, but in setting priorities, making decisions and planning and executing their own health-related activities. The art of health promotion in the community is to get existing groups to direct their efforts towards health-related goals, rather than to create new organizations that would have to compete with existing ones. This is achieved by person-to-person contact between health promotion animators and members of the community, using the techniques of community development and community social work, supported by local community leaders, health professionals and the mass media.

In many parts of the world, community health promotion programmes are still in the stage of experimental projects, where large samples of the population are examined in detail and trends of risk factors and disease are compared with those in control communities. But as their success becomes increasingly evident *(4)*, more programmes will be introduced on a routine basis and scientific evaluation will have to be replaced by surveillance programmes that use simpler measurements of the process of health promotion and indicators of intermediary success, besides observation of long-term disease rates. Examples of such measurements will be presented in Chapter 5.

Environmental health

Unlike community-oriented health promotion, measures of environmental hygiene such as the provision of safe food and sufficient and safe water supplies have been among the classical elements of public health programmes for many years. When new environmental hazards such as ionizing radiation were discovered several decades ago, the time-tested concepts of regulation and control could be applied to them as well. Today, food and water control, radiation protection, wastewater treatment and garbage disposal have become routine activities in most industrialized countries, although new developments such as the introduction of new types of food processing, the importation of food from distant parts of the world and new uses for ionizing radiation require the constant adaptation of measurement techniques, the introduction of new surveillance schemes and a constant international exchange of experience.

While developments may be fairly well under control in many parts of the world, this is certainly not the case in some of the poorer countries, where the hot climate favours contamination, but where a tight network of public health laboratories would be too expensive. In this situation priority has to be given to measures such as the provision of sufficient quantities of drinking-water, the use of simple devices for water chlorination at individual wells and a system of rapid distribution of perishable food, while a programme of surveillance based mainly on the health status of the population has to ensure that weak points are rapidly detected.

Another aspect of health protection, where the problems of regulation and control have not yet been solved, concerns air and water pollution caused by industrial waste, automobile exhausts and other products of modern life. In a number of countries environmental protection laws have been passed, but in general there remains a conflict between economic and health considerations. This is a problem not only for highly industrialized countries, but very much also for many countries of the Third World who are trying to introduce industries while saving on investments in pollution control. Here, as in the case of bacterial contamination of food, milk and water, careful surveillance is needed both of pollutants and of the health status of the population.

A third aspect is to ensure an environment suitable for healthy living. This includes measures to avoid the development of breeding grounds for disease vectors, to create recreational areas and to ban advertising of harmful products.

Occupational health

Unlike the control of contamination and pollution in the general environment, occupational health hazard control requires an individualized approach that takes into account the particular characteristics of each workplace. Depending on the type of work, emphasis is on adapting the workplace to the needs of the human organism (ergonomics) or psyche (occupational psychology), or on applying the principles of occupational safety. Recently the workplace has also been used to carry out programmes of health promotion and disease prevention unrelated to the particular hazards of the workplace, and it has been demonstrated that morbidity and mortality can be reduced significantly if sufficient effort is put into such programmes *(5)*.

The coverage of enterprises by occupational health services varies considerably within and between countries, depending on such factors as the type of legislation and the size and type of enterprise. In addition the type of service differs and often emphasis is on health examinations and medical interventions in case of accidents rather than on the provision of healthy working conditions. Quantitative assessment of the services provided and comparison with other enterprises and other regions is used in stimulating progress towards more active health promotion programmes for the workplace.

Health-oriented legislation

Health promotion activities may be rather futile, if they exist in isolation and are not supported by a legislative framework based on the recognition of health as a highly valued priority. An indirect effect of legal support may be greater credibility for those involved in health promotion work, but more importantly, laws are the main formal tool of society to regulate life in the interests of its members' wellbeing. In Table 2, where several types of legislation are distinguished, it becomes clear that not only do the laws inside the health system have health consequences, but so do the laws regulating our environment, natural resources and living conditions.

Of course, no generally valid classification scheme is possible because wide differences exist in the type of service provided by governments and the private sector, and because certain tasks, such as environmental control, may be assigned to agencies inside or outside health departments. Nevertheless, Table 2 may serve as a checklist to identify areas where health

Table 2. Various kinds of law that have an effect on health

Type of legislation	Examples inside the health system	Examples outside the health system
Regulatory	Health professions Health insurance Health services Epidemic control Environmental control	Labour Housing, zoning Transport Energy School curriculum Production, advertising and sale of harmful products (tobacco, alcohol)
Setting up and financing of government activities	Public health laboratories Health education agencies Health statistics agencies	Food supplement programmes
Fiscal		Taxation on cigarettes, alcohol
Subsidiary	Support of nongovernmental programmes	Agricultural subsidies

promotion should be a guiding principle of legislation. As an example of how stimulating it can be to assess the state of legislation in a given area of health promotion and to make international comparisons, reference is made to a recent WHO publication on smoking control *(6)*. One of its major conclusions is that it is advantageous for countries to introduce comprehensive legislative packages on smoking control including a ban on advertising, the regulation of sales, the declaration of harmful substances, restrictions on smoking in public places and at the workplace, smoking education, as well as fiscal and economic measures, rather than to include these measures separately in sectorial legislation. Another conclusion is that smoking control legislation is urgently needed in the less developed countries, if they want to be spared a destructive epidemic of smoking-related chronic diseases a few years from now.

Planning of Health Promotion Programmes

Each of the approaches discussed in this chapter requires its own institutional infrastructure, specialized personnel and technical support. In addition, when specific goals in the framework of health promotion and disease prevention are to be reached, an overall goal-oriented programme is needed that specifies the weight given to each particular approach, the coordinating procedures, the goal-specific scientific support and the funding.

In Table 3 this principle is illustrated by examples from two distinct areas of health promotion work. In the first example the subject is smoking control, which is the concern of several WHO recommendations *(8)*. The targets are to reduce tobacco consumption by 50% and to increase the rate of nonsmokers to 80% (or maintain it at 80%).

The second example is the control of protein-energy malnutrition (PEM) and diarrhoea in Third World urban slum children. The targets are to reduce PEM in infants of 1–4 years by 75%, to reduce the rate of diarrhoeal episodes, and to increase breastfeeding of 6 months and more to 50%. Parallel experience in a community-oriented health promotion programme in South America and in health promotion work in Europe has made it clear that many of the relevant approaches and practical problems are very similar regardless of the cultural, economic and health context in which the programmes take place. It can be expected that in the Third World as in Europe, the dynamics of a programme can be stimulated by establishing quantitative goals and measuring progress periodically. The goals in the last column of Table 3 and some of the details of health promotion activities were derived from case studies in different parts of the world made available in a recent publication on nutritional intervention strategies *(9)*, whereas other activities are based on personal experience.

As Table 3 shows, almost all activities in one programme find their logical counterpart in the other. The methodologically trained professionals needed to carry out certain approaches are the same in both cases: teachers (for school health education), psychologists (to supervise guidance in behaviour change), community social workers (to activate the community) and public relations professionals (for radio and television support). A problem common to both industrialized and less developed countries is that health professionals and those professionals mentioned above often find it difficult to collaborate because their frames of reference, priorities and approaches to problem solving are very different. Whereas health professionals would regard community development work as an instrument to reach specific health goals, their collaborators may tend to consider the health aspects of their programmes as good starting points for arriving at general development. To avoid misunderstanding and conflict they must all state clearly what their goals are at the outset of a programme.

Assessing the Situation and Evaluating Progress

The measurement of health and health promotion will be discussed more thoroughly in Chapter 5. Nevertheless, as measurement is an integral part of health promotion, certain considerations will be mentioned in the present context as well.

When health promotion is taken seriously, it is not done blindly. Rather, goals have to be set that relate to the current health situation; programmes have to be designed that take the local circumstances into account; and progress has to be monitored, both in terms of the health goals and of intermediary goals related to the execution of the programmes. This requires measurement at several levels.

Measurement of levels of health

Before programme goals can be set for improving the level of health, the health situation has to be known. If the community is to participate in health promotion, not only do those aspects of health that are considered important by the health experts have to be assessed, but so also do any additional needs considered important by the members of the community. As the classification of levels of health is related to human physiology and psychology rather than to local circumstances, standard methods of measurement have evolved, some of which will be discussed in the second part of this book.

Health is so intricately interwoven with lifestyles and living conditions that the process of improving a population's health is very slow, requiring years if not decades for significant changes to appear. This has to be taken into account when progress in health promotion programmes is being assessed. Only those parameters that can realistically be expected to change within a given time period should be reviewed. Government and other funding agencies have to be aware of this and not expect rapid improvements in levels of health, despite the rapid feedback often required.

Assessment of lifestyles and environmental influences

As shown in Table 3, health promotion programme goals are stated in terms not only of health itself, but also of health-related habits and environmental parameters. Here again standardized methods of measurement can be used. In some areas such methods have been established and widely recognized *(10)*, whereas in others they have only recently been recommended *(11)* or need further elaboration.

Assessment of determinants of lifestyles

Health promotion programmes aimed at changing lifestyles require a thorough knowledge of the cultural background, social structure and dynamics of the target communities. When these are known, intermediary goals can be set, such as the number of contacts with community leaders, the type and number of people supporting certain activities and the number of people participating in the programmes. Again it will be necessary both to assess the initial situation and to monitor progress; but owing to the diversity of situations, it would be hard to find standardized measurements that would be meaningful everywhere, and in many situations the most meaningful approach will be to create and apply *ad hoc* measurement criteria. The same holds true even more distinctly when political and legal contexts are to be assessed and when progress is to be monitored in this area.

Table 3. Approaches to reaching health promotion goals as illustrated by two examples

Approaches to goals through:	Goals in smoking control	Goals in control of protein-energy malnutrition (PEM)
Medical and related services		
Medical practice	Advice on smoking cessation by the family doctor *(7)*	Identification of PEM-children by health promotors
Related services	Smoking cessation clinics	Nutrition recovery centres
Health education		
Schools	Smoking education programmes *(3)*	Nutrition education programmes
Parent education	Smoking cessation support for pregnant women	Parents working in nutrition recovery centre kitchens Mothers participating in breastfeeding promotion groups
Community-oriented health promotion		
Community groups	Nonsmokers' rights groups	Mediator-led home gardening groups; breastfeeding promotion groups Groups for community management of nutrition recovery centres
Community events	Nonsmoking days Autograph hours with nonsmoking sports champions	Booths at community fairs serving soya beans dishes
Mass media	Publicity in support of the goal	Publicity in support of the goal

Approaches to goals through:	Goals in smoking control	Goals in control of protein-energy malnutrition (PEM)
Environmental health		
Environmental hygiene		Construction of sanitary units
Pollution control	Indoor smoking restrictions	
Health-oriented living space	Ban on cigarette advertising	Ban on public advertising for infant formulas
Occupational health	Smokefree workplace; time off for cessation groups	Time off for breastfeeding
Legislation	Laws on taxation, advertising, indoor smoking, funding of educational programmes	Laws on food supplement programmes; programmes promoting economic independence

Conclusion

The enormous changes in living conditions brought about by developments such as mass production, mass communication and urbanization, and the widespread inability to subordinate these conditions to human needs, are an increasing challenge to human health. It took several decades of epidemiological research and repeated drawbacks in superficially conceived health promotion campaigns to understand how strongly interrelated human health and the prevailing social conditions are. As a logical consequence, health promotion and the (re-)adaptation of lifestyles and living conditions to biologically and culturally determined human needs cannot be separated. As Chapters 4.1, 4.2 and 4.3 show, this process requires the participation of the community as a whole and a political process in which health and health promotion are valued as a pace-setting priority both inside and outside the traditional boundaries of the health system.

This is not to say that health promotion activities are only meaningful when they involve man and society in radical change. On the contrary, health promotion activities can be an important element in breaking the vicious circle in which poverty, lack of education, political impotence and despair keep man from attaining self-fulfilment and wellbeing; or in which material abundance leads to boredom, purposelessness, apathy and an overflow of stimuli, dependence, addiction and self-destruction. These processes are known today, and it is particularly in the area of health and health promotion that changes in the right direction have a realistic chance of success.

In this chapter a system to classify the influences on health has been used that shows the current approaches to health promotion in a systematic order. Depending on particular needs and situations, certain approaches will get more emphasis than others. But whatever the approach, it can be expected that the measurement of needs as a basis for formulating quantitative goals will be an indispensable motivation and that the quantitative demonstration of progress towards health will be a forceful incentive to carry on with the effort.

References

1. **Société suisse de médecine sociale et préventive.** Organisation de la prévention primaire en Suisse "Modèle Prévention 83". *Sozial- und Präventivmedizin,* **28**(3–4): 181–184 (1983).
2. **Backett, E.M. et al.** *The risk approach in health care with special reference to maternal and child health, including family planning.* Geneva, World Health Organization, 1984 (Public Health Papers, No. 76).
3. **Wake, R. et al.** *A manual on smoking and children.* Geneva, International Union Against Cancer, 1982.
4. **Puska, P. et al.** Change in risk factors for coronary heart disease during 10 years of a community intervention programme (North Karelia project). *British medical journal,* **287**: 1840–1844 (1983).
5. **Kornitzer, M. et al.** Belgian heart disease prevention project: incidence and mortality results. *Lancet,* **1**: 1066–1070 (1983).

6. **Roemer, R.** *Legislative action to combat the world smoking epidemic.* Geneva, World Health Organization, 1982.
7. **Russell, M.A.H. et al.** Effect of nicotine chewing gum as an adjunct to general practitioners' advice against smoking. *British medical journal,* **287**: 1782–1785 (1983).
8. WHO Technical Report Series, No. 636, 1979 (*Controlling the smoking epidemic*: report of the WHO Expert Committee on Smoking Control).
9. **Underwood, B., ed.** *Nutrition intervention strategies in national development.* New York, Academic Press, 1983.
10. *Guidelines on studies in environmental epidemiology.* Geneva, World Health Organization, 1983 (Environmental Health Criteria, No. 27).
11. *Guidelines for the conduct of tobacco smoking surveys of the general population.* Geneva, World Health Organization, 1983 (unpublished document WHO/SMO/83.4).

3. Some fields of application for health promotion and disease prevention

L. Breslow

Use of the Terms "Health Promotion" and "Disease Prevention"

This chapter is concerned with activities in the health system that are specifically directed towards health promotion and disease prevention. Excluded from consideration here, therefore, are the many factors outside the health system that bear on health and are sometimes regarded as elements of disease prevention. These factors, considered more closely in Chapters 4.2, 8.4 and 8.6, include adequate income level, good housing and proper education; certainly, when they are grossly deficient, health often suffers. Parts of the population in industrially developed countries, as well as in developing nations, still lack these essentials for good health. Even within the health system, most activities fall beyond the limits of this chapter because they are directed to the diagnosis and treatment of illness rather than to health promotion and disease prevention. Again, such activities may contribute a great deal to health but not in the way dealt with here.

The definition of health promotion and disease prevention as used in this chapter will be in accordance with the concepts presented in Chapter 1. Although they do have different meanings, there is some overlap, and hence the terms are often used in the combined form: health promotion and disease prevention.

Disease prevention consists of measures designed to prevent disease, e.g. vaccination against poliomyelitis and not smoking cigarettes to reduce the risk of lung cancer. Active immunization to prevent the occurrence of specific infectious diseases is typified by smallpox eradication and the great progress that has been made against diphtheria, measles and many other such diseases. In the case of non-infectious agents of disease, such as toxic chemicals, however, we are not dealing with such highly specific relationships as that between a particular virus and the corresponding disease. For example, cigarette smoking is causally related not only to lung cancer, but also to other chronic lung conditions, coronary heart disease and bladder cancer. Lung cancer, for its part, may result from exposure to asbestos, ionizing radiation and chromate as well as to cigarette smoke. Causal relationships in the case of toxic chemicals thus tend to be far more complex than the relatively simple forms characteristic of infectious agents. For that reason, it has become usual to express the non-infectious disease agent relationships in terms of risk. Thus, both avoiding the occurrence of poliomyelitis and reducing the risk of lung cancer are examples of disease prevention.

Health promotion, on the other hand, consists of measures that strengthen a person's health potential or reserves. Such reserves include, for example, cardiovascular fitness and sound teeth. Some individuals appear biologically capable of surviving to about 80–90 years in good health. Both obvious and subtle congenital deficiencies may impair that ability. More important here, certain measures may enhance the likelihood of reaching the ninth decade of life in good health. These measures constitute health promotion. For example, good nutrition during infancy promotes health by strengthening resistance to infection. Maintaining cardiovascular fitness helps individuals ward off damage to the heart and blood vessels from many unknown causes. Proper care of the teeth and gums tends to preserve good teeth, which aid digestion and thereby promote health.

Conceptually, health promotion and disease prevention do overlap. Thus, immunization may be regarded as strengthening the reserves against a disease such as influenza, as well as specifically preventing the infection. Including sufficient iron in the diet may be regarded as strengthening the body against, or specifically preventing, iron-deficient anaemia. Where the measures are directed towards the avoidance of particular diseases, the term "prevention" seems more appropriate; where the measures contribute to health in a more general sense, "health promotion" may be the preferred term. In any event, the two are closely related, especially in so far as activities in the health system are concerned.

Achieving Optimum Nutrition

About 4000 years ago, a Chinese physician prescribed "cereals for energy, fruits for accessory. Animals for benefit, vegetables for supplement".[a] With a broad interpretation of the word "animal", that prescription for diet could hardly be improved today. Sigerist observed that Galen's idea of hygiene was "a correct amount of food, drink, sleep, wakefulness, sexual activity, exercise, massage, etc." *(1)*. Hippocrates some 2500 years ago, in his treatise on *Airs, waters and places,* recommended that physicians ascertain "the mode in which the inhabitants live and what are their pursuits, whether they are fond of drinking and eating to excess, and given to indolence, or are fond of exercise and labor, and not given to excess in eating and drinking" *(2)*.

Since ancient times, physicians and others concerned with public health have thus emphasized the importance of diet, as well as other aspects of living, in the preservation and promotion of health. Despite progress in medical science as well as in agriculture, industry and trade, a gross lack of

---

[a] **Xa Da-dao**, personal communication, 1981.

sufficient food continues to be a major problem in many developing countries. Together with certain infectious diseases, chronic starvation is still a principal cause of death in much of the world. Solving that problem must therefore remain high on the international health agenda.

In the developed nations, on the other hand, we appear to be entering a new era of health problems in which nutrition is involved in different ways. For many decades, biochemists and other medical scientists have been building up extensive knowledge about the macronutrients: protein, fat and carbohydrates. Elucidating their roles in the growth and functioning of the human body has been a signal achievement of medical science. Delineating the importance of the micronutrients, particularly the vitamins and trace elements, has proceeded in a parallel fashion. At first, this took the form of epidemiological investigation, as in the case of James Lind's discovery that citrus prevented scurvy and of Joseph Goldberger's finding that meat and milk would prevent pellagra. Chemical studies subsequently confirmed that vitamin C (ascorbic acid) and niacin were the essential nutrients involved. Approximately the same pattern led to the discovery that iodine was the nutrient that prevented goitre and to knowledge of other micronutrients.

During the second half of the twentieth century, epidemiologists, clinicians and laboratory scientists turned their attention to more chronic and subtle conditions than the gross infections and nutritional deficiencies that had previously occupied the spotlight. Another surge of effort in our time is revealing more about the relationship of food to health. Protein deficiency leading to kwashiorkor has been stressed in the developing nations, but recent advances go far beyond starvation in the ordinary sense and the specific nutritional deficiencies that were identified in earlier periods.

Ushering in the new era of nutritional knowledge was the discovery of an association between coronary heart disease and a high-fat diet. That finding stimulated vigorous inquiry into its possible import. While the significance of the association is not completely clear, there is now a substantial consensus that consumption of a diet with 30–40% fat, and especially a diet high in animal fat, is a major factor in the recent epidemic of coronary heart disease. That epidemic has affected people in the industrialized nations severely, particularly middle-aged men among whom it has progressed to cause more than a third of all deaths. Besides nutrition, of course, other factors such as high blood pressure and cigarette smoking have been identified as being involved in the rise in deaths from coronary heart disease. In fact, its multifactorial origin is a prototype for understanding the causes of the chronic diseases generally.

There is substantial evidence that excessive consumption of animal fat leads to high blood cholesterol levels which are an important factor in coronary heart disease. On this basis, several dietary intervention trials have been carried out by health systems to reduce high blood cholesterol. While some of these trials have succeeded in lowering cholesterol levels, the evidence that this has had an impact on coronary heart disease is less convincing. Meanwhile, however, in certain countries such as the United States, where the consumption of animal fat and corresponding cholesterol levels (and other risk factors for coronary heart disease) have declined, mortality from the condition has fallen dramatically. On the other hand, in some countries of eastern Europe, for instance, where animal fat consumption appears to be rising, mortality from coronary heart disease has increased.

These data on high animal fat consumption as a factor in coronary heart disease have been accumulating over several decades. During the past few years, evidence has emerged that essentially the same dietary pattern may be involved in breast cancer and possibly other cancers. A US National Academy of Sciences report *(3)* has concluded that:

> . . . of all the dietary components it studied, the combined epidemiological and experimental evidence is most suggestive for a causal relationship between fat intake and the occurrence of cancer. Both epidemiological studies and experiments in animals provide convincing evidence that increasing the intake of total fat increases the incidence of cancer at certain sites, particularly the breast and colon and, conversely, that the risk is lower with lower intakes of fat . . .
>
> . . . It is not now possible, and may never be possible, to specify a diet that would protect everyone against all forms of cancer. Nevertheless, the committee believes that it is possible on the basis of current evidence to formulate interim dietary guidelines that are both consistent with good nutritional practices and likely to reduce the risk of cancer. These guidelines are meant to be applied in their entirety to obtain maximal benefit.
>
> 1. There is sufficient evidence that high fat consumption is linked to increased incidence of certain common cancers (notably breast and colon cancer) and that low fat intake is associated with a lower incidence of these cancers. The committee recommends that the consumption of both saturated and unsaturated fats be reduced in the average US diet. An appropriate and practical target is to reduce the intake of fat from its present level (approximately 40%) to 30% of total calories in the diet. The scientific data do not provide a strong basis for establishing fat intake at precisely 30% of total calories. Indeed, the data could be used to justify an even greater reduction. However, in the judgement of the committee, the suggested reduction (i.e. one quarter of the fat intake) is a moderate and practical target and is likely to be beneficial.
>
> 2. The committee emphasizes the importance of including fruits, vegetables and whole grain cereal products in the daily diet. In epidemiological studies, frequent consumption of these foods has been inversely correlated with the incidence of various cancers. Results of laboratory experiments have supported these findings in tests of individual nutritive and nonnutritive constituents of fruits (especially citrus fruits) and vegetables (especially carotene-rich and cruciferous vegetables) . . .

The excessive consumption of refined sugar as a factor in dental caries and the possibility that lack of fibre may be involved in bowel cancer exemplify the continuing need for close attention to carbohydrate intake, as well as to protein and fat.

Standards for vitamin intake were first formulated to prevent the classic deficiency diseases such as scurvy and rickets. The recommended daily allowances are now being reviewed. For example, the estimated requirement for vitamin C has recently been raised from 45 mg to 60 mg, with much larger amounts advocated by some. Vitamin A and/or its precursors in vegetables appear to be, and are being studied as, a possible factor against certain forms of cancer.

Besides the vitamins and minerals (calcium, phosphorus, magnesium, iron, zinc and iodine) for which standards have long been established, other micronutrients are being found that are important for maintaining human health. These include vitamin K, biotin and pantothenic acid, trace elements such as copper, fluoride, manganese, chromium, selenium and molybdenum, and the electrolytes sodium, potassium and chloride.

Characteristic of this "second round" of nutrition advance is the search for optimum quantities, not only for the minimum essential. Thus, too little or too much caloric intake in relation to energy expenditure may lead to people being underweight or obese, both of which can adversely affect health. Excessive fluoride causes mottling of tooth enamel; too little leaves the teeth highly vulnerable to caries. Amounts of about 1–2 g sodium per day seem necessary, and much larger amounts (over 5 g) appear to be related to high blood pressure, but the ideal for most individuals is not yet clear.

Thus, an effort is being made to define the optimum quantities of various nutrients, as well as the types of food in which they occur, to maintain and enhance health. The health system will be increasingly occupied with this matter.

Avoiding Self-inflicted Hazardous Substances

While industrialization in the developed world has obviously brought many benefits, early contact with relative affluence has also given rise to certain health hazards.

It has been shown that what constitutes adequate nutrition is receiving renewed interest, with emphasis on optimum rather than minimum requirements for health. Eating too much and getting fat or eating too much of certain nutrients can significantly damage health, just as starvation and other nutritional deficiencies can cause severe or even fatal illness. Among the earliest to quantify the adverse impact of obesity, insurance company actuaries in the 1930s set higher life insurance premiums for individuals whose weight was substantially above "normal".

The newly acquired ability to buy enough food leads some people to eat too much. The newly affluent were the first to get fat and suffer the health consequences and the increased life insurance premiums. As "money in the pocket" spread to larger and larger segments of the population, obesity followed. Only after some decades of experience do people learn to restrict their intake in a more properly balanced diet.

Modern health systems have recently begun to give this aspect of health maintenance appropriate attention. As Hippocrates did 2500 years ago, we are recognizing that excessive indulgence in food, and particularly fat, is a hazard to health.

How to achieve a truly balanced diet, one that maximally promotes and protects health, is a great challenge to the health systems of industrialized nations. It is necessary to consider both excesses and deficiencies equally, because more and more people have the opportunity to eat too much.

Recent affluence also leads to the consumption of various hazardous substances. Most notable in the twentieth century has been cigarette smoking. The respiratory and enteric pathogenic organisms that were responsible for the great epidemics of the nineteenth century were discovered only during the second half of the century. Comparably, the cigarette was discovered to be the main cause of the major diseases of the twentieth century only during the second half of the century. In the case of microorganisms, of course, exposure came mainly from the environment over which the individual had little influence, whereas cigarette smoking reflects a more individual choice in a milieu that favours the habit.

With the spread of information about the health effects of cigarette smoking, tens of millions of people throughout the world have stopped smoking and untold millions have never started. While public health leaders have played some role in these developments and physicians have been among the first to quit, the health system as a whole has yet to become substantially engaged in helping to curtail one of the most important, current preventable causes of illness and death. Greater understanding is needed of the processes involved in acquiring and giving up the habit of cigarette smoking, and of the skills required to help people deal with the problem.

Alcohol, though often associated with food, has no known nutritive value except its calories, whose intake may unfortunately deter those who imbibe too much from eating valuable foods. Alcohol sedates the higher cortical centres and, by loosening social inhibitions mediated there, appears to stimulate people when they drink. Larger amounts adversely affect the nervous system generally. Gross impairment of function, e.g. the ability to drive an automobile, occurs with blood levels of 100 mg per 100 ml; measurable impairment is evident at much lower levels. Loss of competence due to alcohol consumption causes many deaths from traffic and other accidents and other forms of violence. Alcohol also has a direct toxic effect on the nervous system, liver and other organs.

While these effects are reasonably well known, the health system has responded only sluggishly to the challenging, preventable health damage caused by the excessive use of alcohol. Whereas cigarette smoking is a modern phenomenon, any amount of which damages health, drinking alcohol in various forms extends back to antiquity. Also, in facilitating social intercourse and possibly in other ways, the moderate consumption of alcohol may have some beneficial effect, although its nature and extent are by no means clear.

On the one hand, alcohol is associated with food and, on the other, with drugs. The use of drugs has accelerated recently in the industrialized nations. Although it is common to differentiate sharply between drugs used legitimately in the health system and those obtained illicitly outside that system, the distinction may be somewhat artificial. Opiates prescribed by physicians are valuable in relieving pain, and perhaps not used generously enough for that purpose; sometimes though, even among physicians themselves, they cause harmful addiction. Beyond the health system, opiates such as heroin may lead to addiction and damage health through recreational use. Other drugs are used by the health system as tranquillizers and sedatives. Again, excessive prescription may be harmful, and their use with only tangential or no connection to the health system has become widespread and dangerous. During the past couple of decades, the extensive use in some countries of cannabis and other drugs for their psychoactive effects has caused some clear-cut damage and some potential adverse but ill-defined effects.

The rapid increase in both the creation and the use of hazardous substances during the twentieth century poses some serious problems for the health system. The optimum amounts of nutrients, alcohol and drugs, and the circumstances of their consumption, remain to be further elucidated. In the case of cigarettes, most people would say that zero is the ideal amount. The health system is being called upon increasingly to help individuals and communities achieve the optimum use of drugs.

Enhancing Bodily Resistance to Pathogenic Agents

Bacteria, viruses and other microorganisms have always plagued mankind. Jenner's discovery of smallpox vaccination opened the way to success in combating the communicable diseases they caused. Thereafter, and especially after Pasteur's demonstration of their infective nature, medical science has marched steadily towards their conquest. The health system that emerged during the late nineteenth and early twentieth centuries celebrated its greatest triumphs in overcoming one communicable disease after another.

Establishing individual immunity was a key strategy. Taking advantage of the body's ability to develop a resistance to specific organisms, medical scientists found ways to eliminate the pathogenic organisms' capacity to cause disease and, at the same time, to preserve their capacity to stimulate resistance, i.e. immunity. Applying these techniques led to control of disease after disease. Smallpox eradication has undoubtedly been the greatest achievement in the history of health systems. Success in this venture required much more than basic scientific knowledge and the technology derived from it. Other important factors included a well designed strategy, international commitment to, and cooperation in, the mission, and the exercise of organizational and diplomatic skill.

While great progress has been made, certain segments of the population are still not well protected by the available immunizing agents. For example influenza vaccine, despite its inadequacies, could be of tremendous benefit to the elderly if health systems could make it systematically available. The experience gained in smallpox eradication and in other communicable disease control campaigns provides the basis for further advances in the enhancement of resistance to pathogenic organisms. The technology and expertise of developed nations should be made more fully available to developing nations to secure the entire world against communicable diseases.

It is also possible to stimulate resistance against pathogenic agents other than microorganisms. Certain allergens, for example, provoke asthma and possibly other conditions in hypersensitive individuals. Although the cause and mechanisms of such disorders are far less well understood than in the case of communicable disease, it is known that some of the people affected can be helped by desensitization. Determination of the particular allergens — dog dander, house dust, pollen, moulds, etc. — that are responsible for some asthma attacks has permitted the creation of agents that can enhance the resistance of hypersensitive individuals to attacks. While by no means fully effective and still cumbersome to use, this anti-allergen approach is one means of dealing with a common set of disorders.

Building up resistance to certain carcinogenic agents likewise appears to be a possibility. As noted earlier, vitamin A and its precursors seem to inhibit the development of malignancy in the lung and some other sites. Presumably they do this by enhancing tissue resistance to the malignant process in a similar manner to the way they generally enhance the body's structure and function. Studies now under way may disclose the extent and mode of this action.

Some investigators have long suspected that certain forms of cancer have a viral cause or at least a cause related to that kind of biological activity. Support for this line of thought is now coming from the epidemic of acquired immune deficiency syndrome (AIDS). The bodily defences are apparently weakened in some manner that allows the development of disease, sometimes in the form of Kaposi's sarcoma. Although not yet well formulated, an obvious approach is to try to enhance the body's resistance, i.e. to counter the pathological process.

These examples of hypersensitive and malignant disorders indicate the way in which it may be useful to apply the idea of immunity to conditions other than those caused by the classical microorganisms for which the concept was originally developed. The mechanisms are different but similar. Enhancing resistance to pathogenic agents may have a great future, and health systems should devote attention to this possibility while using immunizing agents already available to complete the control of diseases caused by microorganisms.

Minimizing Exposure to Deleterious Environmental Circumstances

Eating properly, avoiding hazardous substances and enhancing bodily resistance to pathogenic agents, as noted above, are important ways of promoting health and preventing disease. However, they all depend ultimately on individual action.

Another approach to the promotion of health and the prevention of disease, i.e. through environmental measures, circumvents these inherent difficulties. This approach takes into account man's biological capacities and vulnerabilities and aims to establish conditions of life that protect health.

Several categories of agent — microorganisms, chemicals and physical agents — encountered in the natural or the increasingly man-made environment can injure health. Protecting people against microorganisms that are a continuing threat to their health may be achieved by the various means considered earlier. Erecting environmental barriers to exposure, however, is another highly effective way of preventing communicable diseases. These barriers include treating sewage carrying human discharges that may be infectious, avoiding groundwater contamination, eliminating pathogenic microorganisms in drinking-water by chlorination or other means, pasteurizing milk, safeguarding food against contamination with microorganisms, and controlling the vectors of viral and parasitic diseases such as mosquitos and snails. All these measures reduce the individual's risk of exposure without depending on the individual's participation.

Experience gained through the sanitary control of the environment has facilitated the prevention of disease, the development of barriers against the growing array of hazardous chemicals produced by industry and the controlled use of chemicals (such as fluoride) in the environment to promote health. To safeguard people against toxic chemicals, e.g. in groundwater used for domestic purposes, health systems have established monitoring systems similar to those already in use to keep watch on microorganisms. In the case of toxic chemicals, the surveillance extends from the water itself to the surrounding ground and to the source of discharge. As yet, of course, these monitoring schemes are by no means as systematic as those in general operation for the observation of water's bacteriological quality, but they are expanding. If such surveillance detects that the water supply is contaminated it triggers engineering and other responses to minimize the potential damage to people's health. Increasingly, too, regulations are being adopted that prevent the spillage of dangerous chemicals into water supplies. In sanitation, we are thus moving from a bacteriological to a toxicological era.

It is also necessary to consider how the environmental use of chemicals can promote health. Increasing the fluoride content of drinking-water to the optimum level for resistance to dental caries is an example. Again, there is a parallel with the addition of chlorine to kill pathogenic organisms.

Physical agents are likewise coming into prominence as agents of disease, with ionizing radiation a prime example. During the early part of the twentieth century, soon after the discovery of medical and industrial uses for X-rays, radium and other sources of ionizing radiation, it became clear that they were damaging people's health. Further experience, including long-term follow-up of people exposed to the effects of nuclear explosions, has established the extensive damage that can be done to people's health by ionizing radiation.

Studies of dose–response indicate a linear relationship between radiation and cancer (and some other effects). Hence, it must be presumed that even the small amount of radiation received in each of the tens of millions of chest X-ray examinations performed annually in the world carries some risk. For that reason, the amounts of radiation used for such purposes and the number of such examinations deserve continuing scrutiny. Health considerations also enter into the expanding use of ionizing radiation in, for example, nuclear plants for producing energy.

Efforts to minimize people's exposure to chemical and physical, as well as microbiological, agents of disease focus on the various places that exposure can occur, such as the home and the workplace. Attention must increasingly be given to the potentially deleterious effects on health of man-made or man-converted natural products. It may be instructive to consider one type of product, asbestiform fibres, to illustrate a major, current environmental health problem. Workers who have been exposed to asbestos during mining and processing for construction and industrial purposes suffer lung cancer, mesothelioma, pulmonary fibrosis and other adverse health effects. Similar effects have been noted among those exposed to the clothing of these workers in their homes and among those living down-wind from asbestos processing plants, presumably because of exposure to the same asbestos material. Now consideration is being given to the possible damage to health caused by exposure to asbestos fibres in drinking-water, homes and public buildings where the material has been used in construction, and even in the ambient air. As yet, evidence of adverse effects from these relatively small exposures is weak, but the age and other characteristics of those exposed in these ways, and the fact that effects may occur as long as 50 years or more after exposure, indicate the need for continuing study. Furthermore, man-made fibres have been introduced to accomplish the same industrial purposes as asbestos and to avoid exposing workers and others to natural asbestos fibres. Yet these man-made fibres apparently have many of the same properties. Which of asbestos's properties are responsible for its effects on health? How long must those exposed to the man-made fibres be observed in order to ascertain whether these fibres will have the same effects? These and related questions confront those responsible for protecting people against such environmental hazards.

Incorporating Health Concerns into Education

Civilization advances mainly through education, which serves the purpose not only of enriching the lives of those fortunate enough to acquire it but also of aiding their productive participation in society. This practical aim is becoming ever more important. Closely related to that aim is education for health. Obviously, both the individual and society will benefit.

Nations establish various levels of education (typically, primary, secondary and higher education) to enhance people's lives both culturally and productively. The extent of education is generally accepted as a measure of social progress.

Specific attention to health in education has slowly been increasing over the years, with appreciation of the fact that good health can raise the effectiveness of education itself as well as the opportunity for cultural advance and social productivity.

Education for health in the school system has taken the form of physical fitness regimens, as well as aiding young people to understand what can be accomplished by individual action to prevent disease and promote health. Exercise periods during the day and sports after school exemplify the efforts of the educational system to promote health and physical fitness. In some countries, these efforts have included mass participation in sports. There is a danger however that, as has happened in some countries, resources are focused on developing an elite corps of athletes even at a relatively early age, and their prowess is merely observed by the mass of students whose own physical fitness is neglected.

Schools can also play a prominent role in developing knowledge and attitudes about behaviour that affects health, e.g. cigarette smoking, alcohol use and nutrition. Not only in the classroom, but also in the lunchroom and through teachers and extracurricular activity, young people may be assisted to develop healthy lifestyles. New programmes screen schoolchildren for height, weight, blood pressure, blood cholesterol levels, vision, hearing, etc., as a basis for teaching young people how to maintain their health.

Cultivation of a social milieu that supports health-promoting behaviour at an early age, not just book learning, is an ever more significant aspect of school health education. Studies in some countries show that cigarette smoking, physical inactivity, alcohol use and overeating often start in childhood and may persist into adult life with an adverse impact on health. Hence, those concerned about public health are turning their attention to the potential for health promotion by building resistance against these habits and strengthening more favourable ones during the school years.

Adults, too, of course, can learn to adopt habits that are conducive to health and to give up those that lead in the opposite direction. For example, tens of millions of people throughout the world who were addicted to cigarettes have given them up, physical exercise is becoming more popular, and dietary patterns are improving in some countries. These and many other signs show that adults can be influenced to adopt habits that support health. Although habits are not altered easily, many individuals do change them. What influences adults to adopt more healthy lifestyles, however, is not clear. As in childhood, their social milieu seems to be a strong factor. Adults who do change their habits apparently require knowledge, motivation and, especially in difficult cases, skill. For example, overcoming obesity may be facilitated not only by knowledge of the hazard and a desire to lose weight, but also by learning how to deal with the craving for food.

Cultivating the knowledge, motivation and skills to lead healthy lifestyles among adults is an extremely subtle task. Apart from a few enthusiasts, physicians have largely avoided it on several grounds: a sense that their efforts are not very successful, too little time left over from what they see as their primary commitment (caring for the sick), and little or no compensation for the counselling involved. It does appear, however, that physicians are themselves adopting habits conducive to health and may begin to take a more active role with regard to their patients.

Public health workers are turning their attention to the matter, trying to reach the public mainly through the mass media, other channels of information, clinics and community campaigns. Policy options to combat cigarette smoking include, for example: prohibition, nowhere seriously advocated; restriction of smoking areas in various places of work and recreation; reduction of tar, nicotine and other hazardous substances in cigarette smoke; restrictions on advertising cigarettes; public information; education, particularly in schools; aid to people who want to quit; taxation and other economic measures; export and import policies; and research *(4)*.

While the tendency in health work is generally to intervene, both with individuals and in communities, it is important to make careful observations before trying to develop healthy behaviour in people. People do follow habits that are, more or less, good for their health. Rather than merely testing what may favour more healthy lifestyles, it may be useful to study why and how some people, for example, lose weight, stop cigarette smoking, etc. With such understanding, it may be easier to educate others to do the same.

Orienting Medical Services towards Greater Emphasis on Health Promotion and Early Detection and Correction of Disease States

Since antiquity, the physician's primary mission has been to heal the sick. A secondary theme has always pervaded his work however, namely studying and teaching health. The word "doctor", often used to signify physician, is ultimately derived from a classical root meaning "to teach". That aspect of the history and practice of the physician betokens the side of his work concerned with health promotion rather than disease care.

In recent decades, more and more medical services are concentrating on maintaining health, not just responding to patients' complaints. One may see that thrust in, for example, some areas of psychiatry and paediatrics where practice emphasizes a partnership with the patient in maintaining and enhancing health. Any particular disease problems may be handled within this framework of care. Some physicians are extending the framework into the care of adults generally, young and old and of both sexes.

The notion of health promotion and disease prevention as a basis for medical service has long been expressed in some countries as an annual check-up. Unfortunately vague as to content, the annual check-up has only recently come under extensive and serious examination. During the 1970s in North America, several professional bodies as well as individuals identified specific elements for lifetime health monitoring. They noted the possibility of dividing a lifetime into age periods, such as pregnancy, infancy, early childhood, later childhood, adolescence, young adult life, young middle age, older middle age, old age and advanced old age. For each of these times in life, one may identify specific health goals, professional services and health protection "packages" designed to prevent disease and promote health *(5,6)*.

The professional services in such an approach are of two types: first, physical procedures to ascertain features of health status, such as blood pressure; and second, counselling, about nutrition for example. These professional services deal with health risk indicators, which can be anatomical, physiological, chemical, bacterial, immunological and behavioural. Achieving the optimum in these parameters may accomplish both the secondary prevention of disease, i.e. the early detection and prompt handling of disease processes to avoid progression, and the promotion of health.

Anatomically, one can discern obesity, breast lumps that may mean cancer, pulmonary lesions (by X-rays) and cervical dysplasia or carcinoma *in situ* (by microscopy), among other signs of danger to health. Every sign should, of course, be followed both with appropriate diagnostic tests and with appropriate care for the secondary prevention of disease and the promotion of health.

Physiological examinations of cardiovascular and pulmonary function, such as with electrocardiography and measurement of forced expiratory volume, reveal highly important health reserves that may need to be enhanced, or the early stages of disease whose progression may be prevented. Other bodily systems, such as the eye and the ear, may be approached in a similar fashion.

Chemical tests may reveal conditions such as hyperlipidaemia or glucose intolerance that deserve the same kind of attention as that suggested by anatomical and physiological surveillance.

Bacteriuria and a positive tuberculin test are examples of bacteriological conditions that require attention. Although bacterial infections are becoming relatively less important health problems in developed countries, they are still important to health in many parts of the world.

Immunological bases for health now extend far beyond the well established practices for preventing childhood communicable diseases. Antigens against the various influenza viruses are being used with partial success in the elderly. Also as noted earlier, strengthening resistance through desensitization to certain agents of asthma has become feasible though far from perfect. Perhaps the most exciting current front for immunological approaches to preventing disease and promoting health is in cancer research. Advances in molecular biology with techniques for investigating virus–cell relationships and in other aspects of cancer research open up the opportunity to explore immunity principles for cancer prevention.

Behavioural factors in health, as noted already, deserve the educational system's attention. Medical services can also influence behaviour in a healthy direction. Enhancing health and preventing certain diseases is possible in so far as the medical services can identify behaviour that puts health at risk and counsel people to modify such behaviour. So far, the medical services have focused on behaviour that is grossly antagonistic to health, e.g. severe alcoholism and extreme overeating, just as medicine still tends to concentrate on full-blown disease rather than its early physical manifestations.

From brief consideration of these health parameters — anatomical, physiological, chemical, bacterial, immunological and behavioural — it is evident that medical services can be substantially reoriented towards the part of the spectrum that has been neglected historically but is now receiving more attention. It precedes the diagnosis and treatment of disease that has largely occupied the medical services. It includes the promotion of health (i.e. strengthening bodily reserves for living), the primary prevention of disease (i.e. the avoidance of disease), and the secondary prevention of disease (i.e. the early detection of disease and action to prevent its progress into typical clinical form).

This concept of health promotion and disease prevention (primary and secondary) pertains to individuals. It thus differs from the concept that presents health promotion as the development of social circumstances, e.g. educational and environmental, that favour health.

In the concept advanced here, the promotion of health and the primary and secondary prevention of disease are on the same spectrum with the diagnosis and treatment of disease, all pertaining to individuals. The current health situation calls for the reorientation of medical services towards the health part of the health-disease spectrum, for the incorporation of health concerns into education and for the minimization of exposure to deleterious environmental circumstances. Vigorous pursuit of all three modalities — medical, educational and environmental — is necessary for the most effective approach to health.

References

1. **Sigerist, H.C.** *Landmarks in the history of hygiene.* London, Oxford University Press, 1956.
2. **Bernarde, M.A.** *Our precarious habitat.* New York, W.W. Norton Company, 1973.
3. **Committee on Diet, Nutrition and Cancer, National Research Council.** *Diet, nutrition and cancer.* Washington, DC, National Academy Press, 1982.
4. **Breslow, L.** Control of cigarette smoking from a public policy perspective. *Annual review of public health,* **3**: 129–151 (1982).
5. **Breslow, L. & Somers, A.R.** The lifetime health monitoring program. *New England journal of medicine,* **296**: 601–608 (1977).
6. **Canadian Task Force on the Periodic Health Examination.** The periodic health examination. *Canadian Medical Association journal,* **121**: 1–46 (1979).

4. The process of health promotion

4.1 The role of participation in health promotion — *A.S. Härö*

Participation *versus* the Medical Model of Disease

An important consideration in planning and evaluating health promotion activities is that the conceptual framework of health promotion lies outside the traditional medical model of disease and disease-oriented services. In the medical model the physician plays the active part as an expert in disease, whereas the person concerned remains in a passive role. This applies to curative medicine, where it is most obvious, but even in such aspects of disease prevention as immunization and early detection the people concerned depend on their doctor's advice and interventions, and assume the role of passive clients. Furthermore, diseases rather than people are the focus of activities in the medical model. Only in recent years has an extended concept of illness developed, where the consequences for the patient in terms of impairment, disability and handicap are also considered *(1)*. In the nursing model *(2)* the orientation is more towards the patient as an individual than towards specified diseases. Nevertheless these are merely extensions of the basic medical model, because their underlying assumption is one of expert care providers and lay care receivers.

In recent years this model has been modified to take into account the role played by patients in complying with treatment and actively contributing to their own rehabilitation. However, although this model recognizes that the patient can learn, the basic assumptions or paradigms underlying the medical model have still been retained: namely, that according to an unwritten contract, the patient trusts the physician with decisions, and with the technical acts considered necessary by expert opinion. By another extension the medical model has been applied to groups of individuals with collective health problems such as epidemics. But again, the assumption has been retained that medical experts determine the actions to be taken, whereas the main role of the population is a passive one.

The Participatory Model

As shown in Chapter 1, the paradigm underlying health promotion distinguishes itself clearly from that on which disease-oriented medical care is built. Health is defined not merely as the absence of disease, but as a state of balance between man (with his potential and weaknesses) and his physical and sociocultural environment. As the balance is a dynamic one, man has to play an active role in it. He can strengthen the balance by increasing his health potential or reserves, or by assuring optimal concordance between actions to meet his own needs and those to meet the needs imposed by his environment. In other words, man has to participate actively in all aspects and stages of health promotion, as he is at the same time subject and object in the process.

An important step towards recognizing the role of participation in health promotion was the development of the concept of primary health care. The principles of primary health care were very carefully formulated in the Alma-Ata Declaration in 1978:

> Primary health care is essential health care ... made universally accessible to individuals and families in the community through their full participation and at a cost that the community and country can afford ... It forms an integral part both of the country's health system, of which it is the central function and main focus, and of the overall social and economic development of the community. *(3)*

Much attention has been given to "participation" in this statement. This reflects the view that the greatest chance of improving health is to involve the whole community in health promotion and the prevention of illness. There is much evidence to show that this is the only successful way. WHO has for some time stressed that health should be *by* the people, not *for* the people.

Forms of Participation

At the level of principles both professional and lay people agree that community involvement is important. But when considering how this should be done in practice their opinions differ. As a rule, professionals, especially physicians, accustomed to having a dominant expert role, believe that laymen can be involved only by following the advice they are given. Politicians are not sure how the public can be involved in such a way that there is a proper balance between informal and formal arrangements. Opinions also differ markedly about the incentives that could motivate and mobilize large numbers of people. There are many alternative ways of organizing participation which, at least in theory, satisfy the minimum requirements. In this area the concepts are not clear and the objectives often contain more verbosity than essential facts.

The critical issue is the role of participants. There is no sense in being active if there is no possibility of influencing the volume, orientation and location of services. The prerequisite for the full participation of the community is that formal authorities and professional experts should delegate enough decision-making powers to the other participants. What is enough and what is the correct balance depend on circumstances and tradition.

It is almost impossible to discuss the general principles of participation without relying on some models or theoretical images of how participation can be made effective. This depends largely on the concept of health and disease. Historically, public health boards or ministries became important once the principles of how to fight contagious diseases were properly understood. Their general idea of participation consisted of the experts (medical, social and technical) knowing what should be done. The laymen's role was to follow advice and orders for the common good. This approach is closely related to the medical model, but applied to collective actions. The area of interest was limited to a few diseases and sanitation control. The problems were treated as the physician treats a patient, and the health board took care that the community complied.

Another way of organizing participation is to set up planning boards responsible for cooperation and dialogue between service users and providers. The providers are usually represented by experts, and the users by the leaders of the community. When building hospitals or considering other major investments the dialogue can be very useful. But even in this case the experts dominate, the area of interest is narrow and real participation is minimal. Also planning boards are a temporary arrangement and do not guarantee any continuous dialogue between users and providers.

The model that most completely corresponds to the full participation advocated by WHO involves delegating responsibility as well as power to the community. When doing this it is important to find a mechanism that can really function in a way that keeps the whole population continuously involved. The task is to develop communities into active units that can take care of their own problems. In principle, developmental goals are not limited to health matters only, but include such general issues as learning how to stand on one's own feet and be responsible for basic services. The continuity of the relationship facilitates innovative solutions for the future too, when circumstances may have changed.

Political Aspects of Participation

It is inherent in the concept of participation that political issues will develop when it is put into action. More generally, the paradigms underlying health policy determine to a marked extent how the authorities and especially the professional groups will react. If the narrow concept of health (absence of illness) dominates, the political discussion will have a tendency to be limited to traditional medical services, to their volume and location. Equity may be labelled as a ridiculous issue here because no society can afford to provide the whole spectrum of advanced medical interventions to everybody in need. On the other hand, the limited extent to which these types of intervention benefit health is easy to show. By contrast, in an inclusive health concept the positive aspects such as the road towards equity are underlined. A healthy environment, the way of life and, of course, prevention in a more narrow sense are expected to diminish the burden of sicknesses and thus to minimize the need for highly specialized curative services.

This may be resented by those who are devoting their lives to the provision of these services and who may try to find political support for traditional health policies. But the more important political question is how participation, as practised in the context of health promotion, fits into the prevailing political system.

The traditional public health boards and even planning committees represent relatively politically conservative solutions. On the other hand, to make health, broadly defined, into the responsibility of laymen is a major political move. In this model the professional experts are "resources", ready to respond to people's needs as seen by laymen, rather than advisers to professional decision-makers. The planning activities work from the bottom up, rather than from the top down guided by central authorities *(4)*. The key words are delegation and development. But whereas the delegation of power and responsibilities presupposes a formal organizational structure that satisfies requirements about representativeness, authority and stability (as will be discussed more amply in Chapter 4.2), the prevailing political and organizational structures often do not easily allow a concept of participation to be put into effect.

Measurement Aspects of the Participatory Model

It is exceptional for measurements to be made solely out of curiosity. Pure interest in knowledge can motivate individual researchers and scientific institutions, but when societal organizations introduce measurements, the reasons are usually practical: examination of the current situation, trends, costs, coverage and many other facts is needed to evaluate achievements and to plan future action.

Measurements in the form of studies, surveys and more or less routinely collected statistics are only apparently neutral and "scientific". In reality they depend on a framework, or model, which is constructed on the basis of subjective elements, such as values, ideas and ways of approaching problems. There are health situations where the model to use and the type of measurements to be applied are self-evident. This may be the case in the control of specific diseases, where the medical model is a suitable basis for assessing needs and providing services, and where a standard classification of diseases *(5)* can provide the basis for assessing the incidence and prevalence of disease.

Just as any other model, the participatory model remains theoretical without measured facts, but measurement in the context of the participatory model is more difficult to conceptualize than in the context of the medical model. Whereas in the medical model, biological parameters are of interest, what needs to be measured in the participatory model are parameters such as knowledge, attitudes, motivation and behaviour, and even the more complex parameters of community dynamics. As a consequence — and because the participatory model is of recent origin — there is a shortage of facts and knowledge. In this situation active policies can only be developed with measurements when possible and feasible, while the gaps are filled with careful reasoning and common sense. The paradox is that in this context the use of an exaggeratedly careful "scientific" approach may take too long to provide the necessary timely insights, and that as a consequence questionable ideas may be introduced uncritically as a basis for action. Thus, occasional mistakes cannot be avoided when the participatory model is used, but they can be corrected in due course if sufficient emphasis is given to continuous evaluation.

Conclusion

As pointed out in Chapter 1, Kühn's theory of science *(6)* postulates that scientific progress is associated with the acceptance of new paradigms. Similarly in health promotion, progress can be expected to be related to the introduction of new approaches and new ways of looking at things. An important element is the replacement of the traditional medical model by a participatory health model based on the realization that health is determined more strongly by people's way of life and their interaction with the environment than by biomedical expertise and services.

However, the delegation and development approach requires an active, well trained society and especially competent leaders. It needs a training that can take a long time when the starting level is low and the traditions unfavourable. But it may be the only way towards the physical, mental and social wellbeing of the community as a whole, and thus needs to be given a chance.

References

1. *International classification of impairments, disabilities and handicaps.* Geneva, World Health Organization, 1980.
2. **Riehl, J.P. & Roy, S.C.** *Conceptual models for nursing practice,* 2nd ed. New York, Appleton CC, 1980.
3. *Primary health care: report of the International Conference on Primary Health Care, Alma-Ata, USSR, 6–12 September 1978.* Geneva, World Health Organization, 1978 ("Health for All" Series, No. 1).
4. **Rifkin, S.B.** The role of the public in the planning, management and evaluation of health activities and programmes, including self-care. *Social science and medicine,* **15A**: 377–386 (1981).
5. *International classification of diseases,* 1975 Revision. Geneva, World Health Organization, 1977, Vol. 1.
6. **Kühn, T.S.** *The structure of scientific revolutions.* Chicago, Chicago University Press, 1970.

4.2 Valuing health: social and political implications — *P. Draper & J. Dennis*[a]

The extent to which a government values the health of its population can be gauged from analyses of policy objectives and their relationship to actual policies. The translation of health-oriented objectives into health-promoting policies depends, in part, on the style and machinery of the political system.

Different Objectives

Attempting to produce health-promoting rather than illness-creating policies challenges the general supremacy of economic objectives in policy-making. Governments pursue a number of different economic objectives — stable prices, a favourable balance of payments, constant growth and full employment for example — which normally override health and other social objectives. Of these different economic goals, perhaps the most central to our concerns because of its pervasiveness and its link with the idea of progress is constant growth.

The assumption of a direct relationship between economic growth and human welfare is faulty for three reasons. First, indiscriminate or unplanned economic growth typically has some adverse consequences for health *(1)*. Second, where growth is a major objective the precedence given to economic considerations often pre-empts efforts to improve health. Third, the gross national product (GNP) has various inadequacies as an indicator. Many writers, including Abel-Smith & Leiserson *(2)*, have commented on the misleading character of GNP from a health or wider social perspective. Some of their criticisms are considered here.

First, GNP accounting is based only on activity that is marketed and recorded. Thus, goods exchanged or services given without payment are excluded. For example, neither the care given to the elderly by their families nor the benefits of breastfeeding are counted. (In passing, it may also be noted that much of the economic activity that is not disclosed to the authorities for tax or other reasons, the "hidden economy", is also excluded.) In developing countries the routine collection of information may be very patchy, thereby necessitating considerable guesswork and increasing the possibility of errors.

Second, GNP (or GNP per capita) discloses nothing about the distribution of income within any country. Thus, a decline in the income of already poorly-fed and poorly-housed groups could be masked by a rise in income elsewhere in society. Conversely, there could be an improvement in the poorest levels of nutrition, housing or sanitation without a corresponding rise in the average level of income.

---

[a] John Dennis was supported by a grant from the Health Education Council.

Third, GNP is measured only in terms of money and therefore tells us little about social utility. An increase in the number or severity of road accidents will *increase* GNP through the resultant replacement or repair of vehicles. Clearly, this is not indicative of an increase in welfare. Similarly, no distinction is conventionally made between the results of investment in a cigarette factory, for example, or of investment in a new bakery for wholemeal bread.

The rejection of GNP as a measure of welfare, even if widespread, would not mean that more health-sensitive objectives would inevitably emerge. Economic objectives maintain their supremacy in a variety of ways despite such criticism.

In developing countries greater provision of health care may be rejected on the grounds that resources should instead be concentrated where they will result in the greatest increase in production. Such action rests on the view that welfare can best be served by achieving economic growth and *then* allowing the benefits (including health services) to trickle down to the rural and other impoverished sectors of the population. This economistic approach contrasts strongly with a basic needs strategy, that is with a development strategy that makes human health and welfare its prime objectives. This strategy recognizes that health is not a commodity that can be bought with health services at a fairly late stage in development. Rather, the objective of health for all is best pursued by making health objectives part of the overall development strategy. As Abel-Smith & Leiserson *(2)* point out "Health-improving activities range much wider than the provision of health services". Thus, poverty, nutrition, land tenure, irrigation and urbanization, for example, are seen, in part, as health problems and planning proceeds with this in mind.

One might think that the relatively affluent industrialized countries would have sufficient economic security (despite the recession) to take greater account of health objectives. Yet the protection of the sick or needy and the promotion of health have been sacrificed to economic objectives.

In the United Kingdom, for example, this has been characterized by the government as "fighting inflation" or "getting the economy right" before improving social services. Criticizing the lack of progress in coordinating social policies, the Black report *(3)* on inequalities in health commented:

> No doubt this is attributable to the precedence currently given not only by the government but by other bodies to economic over social objectives in policy, to a failure to appreciate the interrelatedness of policies, but above all to the stultifying effects of public expenditure control which has dominated all attempts of planning during the mid and late 1970s.

If health is valued it clearly should be much more central in policymaking; economic policy cannot be allowed to override health objectives.

Different Policies

In considering how the content of policy reflects — implicitly or explicitly — the priority given to health, it is instructive to look at sectors outside the health services. The importance of the wider environment for public health is increasingly recognized. In this section we will examine the nature of various policies, thus illustrating their importance for health. Brief examples will be given from five different sectors: transport, energy, agriculture, employment and defence.

Transport policy

What are the features of a transport policy that demonstrate that health is being valued? In a nutshell the key issues are equity, that safety measures effectively attempt to prevent accidents, that damaging stress and pollution (including noise) are minimized and, more positively, that pleasant and valuable physical activity, such as walking or cycling, is encouraged. In practice then, a society that values health will have a transport policy that distributes the ability to travel equitably, includes such measures as speed restrictions on roads and requires the use of safety equipment such as seat belts and motorcycle helmets. Lead in petrol will also have been phased out. More fundamentally, the policy will also favour the development of safer, more energy-efficient and nonpolluting forms of transport such as waterways and rail. The provisions for cyclists, especially the separation from motorized traffic by cycleways and cycle routes, are also a good test of a health-promoting transport policy.

Energy policy

When energy policy is considered, some of the same principles are at work. An energy policy that values health will demonstrate equitable distribution, low accident rates, low pollution and high levels of conservation. There will be a strong interest in researching and developing renewable forms of energy, such as solar power, because of their potentially low accident rates and low pollution. Energy conservation is also an important indicator because it helps reduce energy production and hence accidents and pollution.

Agricultural policy

The agricultural sector presents some ready examples of policies that demonstrate scant regard for health, for example policies that subsidize sugar production or even more extreme, tobacco growing. Since 1975, the Norwegian government has provided some illustrations of the difficulty of trying to develop agricultural and food policies that reflect a concern for health. They attempted to increase people's consumption of fruit, vegetables and cereals and reduce their consumption of fat *(4)* and while there have been some gains there have also been problems. The difficulties encountered have often been economic: resistance was met, for example, because of the effects on the cost of living.

Employment policy

A health-promoting employment policy is one that rejects widespread unemployment because of the damaging psychological and other effects of involuntary unemployment, and because of the positive case for most people to have socially useful work that is safe and for which they are paid. The kind of thinking behind such a policy is illustrated by this comment from an editorial in the *British medical journal (5)*:

> Before the end of the century with increasing automation agriculture, mining, power generation, and manufacturing will occupy no more than one-fifth of the population available for work. Government planners should be taking account of these realities and looking for ways of expanding the service industries and government enterprises if we are to see any end to massive unemployment.

Employment policy will need to take account of such structural changes in patterns of employment. At their most fundamental these changes may require a revision of the work ethic. A health-promoting employment policy would currently incorporate measures such as job-sharing and opportunities for education at all ages, perhaps through a mechanism similar to sabbaticals.

Defence policy

What would constitute a defence policy that reflected a strong concern for health? The extravagant use of resources and the dangers in current defence policies have been recognized by many people, including health workers, and by the World Health Organization, for example in the Declaration of Alma-Ata. Health-sensitive defence policies would demonstrate effective interest in at least three areas: in disarmament, in research into conflict resolution and in non-violent resistance to aggression *(6,7)*.

From this sketch of the different kinds of policy that emerge if health is valued, it will be seen that a comparative analysis of policies in various countries and the assessment of trends reflecting the effects of these policies would permit some measurement of the extent to which a policy is health-promoting.

It will also be seen from this sketch that profound and pervasive social implications would follow from the implementation of such policies. At a simple level for example, a successful attack on smoking would have repercussions not only in the agricultural sector but also in shipping, in manufacturing and particularly in retail distribution. Similarly, a nutritional policy that resulted in a significant reduction in sugar consumption would have a major impact on sugar-based economies such as those of Mauritius and the West Indies. The impact on the social life of communities, from changes of the kinds discussed in other sectors such as energy or employment, would be large and far-reaching. Similarly, it can be expected that some changes would be vigorously resisted by various powerful vested interests. A comprehensive approach to health policy is required to take account of the repercussions and the difficulties of implementation.

There is another reason why a comprehensive approach to health policy is called for and this lies in the interrelatedness of policies. Nutrition, for example, is much affected by the decisions of many different government departments as well as by the activities of the private sector. That a shift towards health-promoting policies calls for better coordination has been widely recognized in recent years. For example, in a review by the Organisation for Economic Co-operation and Development of integrated social policy in Austria *(8)*, the investigating team said:

> One of the essential preconditions for the realisation of a comprehensive health policy as it has been conceived in Austria is improved coordination and integration at all levels and among all the functions concerned. This objective, important for the effectiveness and economic efficiency of health policy and health-related policies, is being pursued in Austria in a pragmatic manner from various angles. Further substantial progress will depend, however, to a large extent on the elaboration of a comprehensive national health development plan embracing all relevant areas and including policies, institutions, action programmes and measures coming under the competence of many different authorities or organisations.

Similarly, the British working party that was set up to investigate continuing inequalities in the health of different social groups, commented in the Black report *(3)*:

> Our recommendations reflect the fact that the reduction in health inequalities depends upon contributions from within many policy areas, and necessarily involving a number of government departments. Our objectives will be achieved *only* if each department makes its appropriate contribution. This in turn requires a greater degree of co-ordination than exists at present.

Different Politics

The realization that to value health it is necessary both to reorder economic and social objectives and change policies will not, of itself, ensure that this happens. The task is not simply a question of defining and embracing new objectives and then generating appropriate policies. For at least two reasons these changes will often require a different type of politics, a new way of conducting public affairs.

In the first place, the complexity and interrelatedness of policy areas will probably necessitate some new machinery of government. Experience in many countries shows that government departments tend to be insular, giving little time or effort to collaborate with other departments relevant to their work. There are many ways in which the government machinery could be transformed, though not without resistance.

In an imaginative article, Lipton *(9)* describes what he thinks might be a speech of some future minister of health. The minister, Lipton speculates, holds the view that "the prior need was not 'more' skills or capital for 'growth', but a more efficient transformation of human power (including skills and capital) into human welfare". To achieve this, the minister would create a special Cabinet committee on positive preventive health, including the ministers of many government departments, hoping thus to reduce the boundaries of demarcation between conventional ministries. This imaginary Cabinet committee, very similar to that proposed in the Black report, would be just as difficult to achieve as other reforms in government machinery. Changes are not easy but they can and do happen.

In the United Kingdom, a recent consultation paper on health and social services *(10)* makes some other suggestions. The study group sees some advantage in giving the task of providing health and social services to a single administrative authority, on a trial basis at least. For some countries this would be an uncontroversial proposal, while for others it would not be. The study group further suggests that:

> in framing their own actions and policies, therefore, Government Departments would be required to assess and detail their impact on health. The Chief Scientist in the Cabinet Office would be required to present an annual, published report to Parliament detailing the health impact of government policies.

A second reason why a different type of politics will be required is that current patterns pay too little attention to participation, a subject treated more thoroughly in Chapter 4.1. Far from simply being the creation of the liberal 1960s, suitable for rejection as a passing fad, the idea of participation has a long history. It is important for those with an interest in health for two reasons: its direct effect on health and, through its role in creating successful changes, its indirect effect.

The argument for participation based on its indirect effects is clear though rarely stated. With evidence from the literature of industrial sociology, the contention is that for changes to be successfully implemented the people affected have to be committed to the change. Such commitment can be generated through the participation of those involved in relevant decision-making. Thus, successful changes in policies for health reasons will be helped by participation. While national changes would currently be impractical objects for direct involvement, there are considerable opportunities at local level. Indeed it could be argued that local approaches to change from the bottom up are preferable, since there is a greater chance of appropriate policies being devised. A high level of participation in local affairs may also create an irresistible pressure for national decisions to take account of local feeling.

Valuing health implies that the psychological and social states of individuals are thought important. Writers on industrial organization have long been concerned with the psychological consequences (such as apathy and submissiveness) of work situations in which staff have little control over the tasks they perform. There have thus been many studies of job satisfaction and participation, and of these Blumberg *(11)* writes:

> there is hardly a study in the entire literature which fails to demonstrate that satisfaction in work is enhanced or that other generally acknowledged beneficial consequences accrue from a genuine increase in workers' decision making power. Such consistency of findings, I submit, is rare in social research.

The authors feel that just as participation at work encourages job satisfaction, so valuing health (life satisfaction or fulfilment) requires that a more participatory style of politics be created.

Given the evidence of dissatisfaction with existing institutions and processes the problem is the development of political systems in which it will be easier to participate. The report of the Committee on Public Participation in Planning *(12)* is an important example of what can be attempted when sufficient effort is put into this problem. Assessments of the range and depth of political activity among its citizens could provide a society with a measure of the vitality of its political system.

The establishment of a participatory system should not be expected to lead to immediate and widespread participation. In the first place, the skills of acting together rather than being acted upon will take some time to learn. As Pateman *(13)* puts it in a seminal book:

> in the contemporary theory of democracy it is the participation of the minority elite that is crucial and the non-participation of the apathetic, ordinary man lacking in the feeling of political efficacy, that is regarded as the main bulwark against instability.

The experience of this theory in operation has to be unlearned. The contrary experience, that individual political activities can have some effect, could be learned at the workplace or in the community. Skills learned and experience gained at this level could be very relevant at the national level.

The success of the transition towards more participatory styles rests though on the early involvement of those who will carry out their civic duties within the new system. In this seemingly hopeless situation, where participation can only come about through participation, the writings of Freire *(14)* are most helpful. Although he worked with illiterate people, his methods are relevant for all politically less developed cultures. He describes his pedagogy of the oppressed as something that:

> must be forged *with*, not *for* the oppressed (be they individuals or whole peoples) in the incessant struggle to retain their humanity. This pedagogy makes oppression and its causes objects of reflection by the oppressed, and from that reflection will come their necessary engagement in the struggle for their liberation.

While his language may be more suited to conditions in some parts of the world than others, the message for educationalists is supported by those who have a "community development" approach to social problems, the essential elements of which are very similar to Freire's.

Conclusion

Some would argue that a different type of politics is a prerequisite for attempts to put into operation the valuing of health. It seems likely that without it, objectives will not fully reflect health considerations and policies will only be partially successful. Nevertheless, there are ways of improving health that depend less on changes in politics, pollution control for example. A measure of the importance attached to valuing health is the extent to which such generally recognized problems are being effectively tackled now.

References

1. Draper, P. et al. Health and wealth. *Royal Society of Health journal,* **97**(3): 121–126 (1977).
2. **Abel-Smith, B. & Leiserson, A.** *Poverty, development and health policy.* Geneva, World Health Organization, 1978 (Public Health Papers, No. 69).
3. **Townsend, P. & Davidson, N., ed.** *Inequalities in health. The Black report.* Harmondsworth, Penguin, 1982.
4. **Milio, N.** Promoting health through structural change: analysis of the origins and implementation of Norway's farm-food-nutrition policy. *Social science and medicine,* **15A**: 721–734 (1981).
5. Monetarism and health. *British medical journal,* **285**: 914–915 (1982).
6. **Boserup, A. & Mack, A.** *War without weapons.* London, Pinter, 1974.
7. **Roberts, A., ed.** *The strategy of civilian defence.* London, Faber, 1967.
8. *Integrated social policy: a review of the Austrian experience.* Paris, OECD, 1981.
9. **Lipton, M.** From protective health to national recovery? *Institute of Development Studies bulletin,* **9**(2): 54–62 (1977).
10. **Social Democratic Party.** *Fair treatment: social democracy in the health and social services.* London, SDP Policy Department, 1982.
11. **Blumberg, P.** *Industrial democracy: the sociology of participation.* London, Routledge & Kegan Paul, 1968.
12. *People and planning:* report of the Committee on Public Participation in Planning. London, HM Stationery Office, 1969.
13. **Pateman, C.** *Participation and democratic theory.* Cambridge, Cambridge University Press, 1970.
14. **Freire, P.** *Pedagogy of the oppressed.* Harmondsworth, Penguin, 1972.

4.3 The political, economic and institutional prerequisites of legislation and planning in support of health promotion — *C. Altenstetter*

By many standards of comparison and statistical measures of health, severe disparities are found between north and south in health status, coverage and benefits, medical, health and social services, physical and manpower infrastructures, and investments in technological hardware. Differences in morbidity and mortality rates among social groups and geographical areas persist across WHO regions and within individual countries *(1,2)*. Those regions most favoured according to standard health indicators, such as the European Region of WHO, include the most industrialized, urbanized and polluted countries. In consequence, the high levels of economic development and living standards attained in these countries have become the focus of growing concern about new and severe health-related problems, which are nonetheless also relevant to other, in particular less industrialized, countries.

Despite specific differences, several experiences are shared by most countries. First, the macro policy-making system that anticipates and responds to old or new health problems is typically highly institutional and bureaucratic. But many areas of decision-making, which had been considered outside the centre stage of politics, have become politicized. In many instances, the methods and practices of conflict resolution and management are deeply entrenched and often run counter to the need for innovation and problem-solving *(3)*.

Second, the problem-solving abilities of statutory agencies and other government institutions vary widely. Contrary to some views, such abilities are more a function of excellent diagnoses of the nature and scope of health problems and the quality of proposed remedies, reinforced by the political willingness to act, than they are a function of forms of government and administrative organization or even control through the ownership of institutions and centres. Some ways of dividing government authority and the territorial allocation of responsibilities for programmes can enhance operational abilities, but at other times they are a considerable hindrance. Moreover, problem-solving abilities do not depend in a strict sense on formal planning apparatuses or on national health plans, even though plans can help identify priorities, specify steps for action, and suggest timetables for reaching targets. The realization of targets depends on a myriad other factors, many of which are entirely beyond the scope of health planning. Above all, achievements require expertise in a variety of skills, diverse manpower and organizational abilities that should be, but often are not, available nationally, regionally or locally.

Third, decision-making about the promotion and implementation of health programmes is not well synchronized structurally and politically in most countries. A considerably longer time than national decision-makers usually allow for implementation is needed before programmes show any effects, positive or negative. After decisions on national policy are made, it takes 2–5 years or more before the necessary procedural, regulatory and/or organizational changes are made. Ironically, precisely when implementation machinery is finally in place to carry out a health policy, national decision-makers begin to change the policy or alter some of its elements, and the problems of administrators and implementers start all over again.

Fourth, problem-solving requires actions and strategies that are not limited to legal, organizational and territorial boundaries. However, problem-solving operates in a world where many of the conditions conducive to cooperation and coordination do not exist and where such relationships and processes have not developed. There are several reasons why cooperation and coordination across policy sectors do not occur in many countries. The constitutional and legal allocation of authority and responsibility to different government levels and ministries often dates back many decades. Tunnel vision and highly streamlined official lines of communication, in countries that have traditions of central authority in policy-making and administration, are hardly conducive to cooperation and coordination. Old routines and practices are fairly resilient and resurface, directly and indirectly, in health policy-making processes even though the political and institutional frameworks may have changed over time. Often new mechanisms coexist with several layers of behavioural and institutional routines and practices. This is true especially in countries that have experienced changes of regime. Every country irrespective of regime type and administrative organization invariably has legacies of one kind or another, and today's governmental and ministerial divisions of labour, competence, and authority are seldom oriented to the multidimensional nature of health issues.

A Health Policy Perspective

To discuss concepts of health and list the main processes promoting action in support of health, some framework for assessment must be established. Not everything in health and health promotion involves elements of policy. Many significant issues are strictly personal or group-related, and many others are beyond the scope of health policy. Nevertheless, issues and dimensions of policy will come into play in realizing progress through mechanisms proposed by global and national strategies for the achievement of health for all by the year 2000. The health for all strategy relies on such mechanisms as multiprogramme efforts, contributions by many policy sectors to health, and the coordinated development of national policy for the promotion of health *(4)*.

Concepts involved in health policy and policy processes

Unlike fairly uniform and unambiguous concepts in medicine, public health, epidemiology, computer technology and other disciplines, those associated with health policy and policy processes involving health promotion are not standard and clear-cut concepts. They are heterogeneous and highly complex because they refer to multiple, diverse and mostly qualitative dimensions of public and private activities in health. Typically these concepts refer to macro phenomena, in contrast to most concepts used in the disciplines mentioned above, which usually relate to micro phenomena. Herein lies one primary source of confusion. Correspondingly, policy measures designed to promote health are broader in scope and more controversial. They are less precise and predominantly of a qualitative and descriptive nature. Hence they are wide open to different interpretations and judgements.

But leaving aside political and theoretical explanations, there are additional sources of confusion. Language is a major culprit. The concept of "policy" is difficult to translate into one equivalent term even when functional equivalents of what is meant by policy exist in different political cultures and systems. When the concept of "politics" is used interchangeably with "policy", because separate terms do not exist in other languages to communicate the essence of both activities or dimensions, confusion is compounded.

Politics and policy

Although politics and policy defy simple definitions, a few clarifications will be offered but there will be no attempt to solve problems of interpretation and judgement. Political science studies micro and macro politics as major fields of enquiry and provides, for example, two standard formulations of macro politics: (*a*) politics is the "authoritative allocation of values" *(5)* through the use of legitimate power, authority and rules *(6)*; (*b*) politics relates to the question of who gets what, when and how *(7)*, which raises issues of conflict among participants. The scope and focus of the study of politics differ from the scope and focus of policy.

Policy content

Policy has been defined as "the projected programme of goal values and practices" *(8)*. This formulation suggests that policy provides rules for action and includes initial goal statements, reformulations through amplification or restriction, or both, and supplementary practices. From this definition it can be inferred that two dynamic elements are inherent in policy: these are substantive content and normative values, and empirical processes. Policy content can be influenced by systematic and informed knowledge in such areas as epidemiology, public health and medicine, all of which can make a contribution to health legislation. But realistically, content is shaped by day-to-day politics, values and belief systems, and institutional arrangements. All three elements are highly value-laden and in interacting with one another they can severely bias policy-making in the promotion of health. Therefore legislation should not be considered neutral; instead, it should be viewed as the end product of a highly political process. As a response to existing problems, legislation essentially reflects how policy-makers have defined those problems and how they will define health promotion in the future. But a definition of this kind may be highly inadequate: it may be too broad or too specific. In short, although legislation has considerable potential for solving problems related to health, it also has the potential for creating errors, inadequate responses and palliatives rather than solutions.

Health promotion

Given the wide range of countries, it is conceivable that the promotion of health will be defined differently throughout the world. One country may define it by drawing on the considerable input received from experts and knowledgeable individuals in health as well as the typical participants in legislative processes. Another country may equate the definition with obtaining additional funds and other resources. A third country may launch two national strategies: a strategy of persuasion designed to influence and alter personal lifestyles and behavioural patterns, and a strategy of regulation designed to control, for example, the tobacco- and alcohol-producing industries. Finally, a country may be guided by considerations of what is considered best for the political system: a decision not to disturb the present relationship of political and institutional forces and not to alter the relative position of ministries or government departments concerned with individual aspects of health promotion.

Policy processes

Policy processes, like policy content, are deeply rooted in political and economic forces and existing institutional frameworks. In addition to considering these structural–developmental elements, there are other ways of viewing policy processes. They can refer to prelegislative processes but are not limited to them. They can include legislative and post-legislative activities. Whatever the major activity of a particular phase, politicians, government leaders, top health bureaucrats, health planners, party and interest group elites, self-help groups and others play different roles as policy actors.

There is general agreement *(9, 10)* that the significant phases of the policy processes are (*a*) problem definition, (*b*) agenda setting, (*c*) policy formulation, (*d*) policy adoption or legislation, (*e*) implementation, and (*f*) evaluation. It is generally understood that each phase gives prominent exposure to an exclusive set of policy actors and is typically confined to selected institutions. In addition, because of differences in the kinds of politics played and the problems to be resolved, each phase makes contributions to aspects of health policy or to implementation that are different from those made by the other phases.

This understanding of the policy process is a dynamic way of viewing how the division of legitimate authority into branches of government (legislative, executive and judicial) impinges on policy-making and implementation. Invariably most political systems have institutionalized the principle of the division of power. Therefore legislators, health bureaucrats, planners and courts, in isolation from or in coalition with other interests, have been found to define and formulate aspects of health policy and to shape policy processes in one way or another. Although details of policy may be decided in separate processes and contexts, they all contribute to what is considered a health policy in a given case. Furthermore, federally structured political systems experience additional and complex phases of the policy process because the authority to decide health policy and the responsibility to carry it out may be divided between levels of government. Irrespective of federal or nonfederal systems, the authority to make decisions on health promotion and the responsibility to carry out related programmes are typically separated. This fragmentary system has important consequences for policy development and implementation, as will be discussed in more detail in other sections of this chapter.

What can be learned from this?

To recapitulate: an understanding of the properties of a policy universe for health promotion, in contrast to other imaginable universes relating to health, is essential and should therefore be amplified. First, the notion of dichotomy between politics and administration and, by implication, the existence of separate and independent spheres of influence are inadequate for capturing the realities of policy-making and implementation. Politicians and bureaucrats — civil servants and other policy actors — are involved in policy-making, and they make distinct contributions *(11,12)*. But despite a shift in policy formulation and development from the legislative to the executive branch, technocratic channels or coordinating mechanisms or both, politics continues to play a role in shaping policy content and policy processes in post-industrial societies in the east and the west, the north and the south. Although contemporary politics is an important determinant of policy content and policy processes, it is only one of many such influential forces.

Second, according to the theory of the division of power into different branches of the government, the actors involved in policy processes should respect organizational, jurisdictional and territorial boundaries. Moreover, such processes should be limited to political or administrative or judicial domains and should be sequential. In practice, policy processes do not respect boundaries. Instead, they are cross-cutting, overlapping, and frequently reversible.

Third, political and institutional contexts exert a significant and independent influence on policy content that can be adequate to solve a problem and can produce the best solution. But policy content often mirrors the political preferences of the actors and consequently may provide only the second-best response to health promotion.

A final point needs to be made. The findings of health policy research may be supportive or critical of policy content. They may also confirm or be critical of established processes. Whatever the main interest is, health policy research, in contrast to much health services research, is concerned with macro phenomena that consist of political and institutional elements and arrangements. That policy may have manifestations at the micro level does not nullify this claim. In fact, most solutions and actions in support of health promotion lie somewhere on a macro–micro continuum, but with each step from macro to micro analysis the causal texture of observations differs. These points may be obvious, but when health research is contrasted with biomedical research, they are often overlooked.

The Nature and Substance of What is Needed for Progress in Health

Any progress in health beyond present levels and scopes, whatever these may be in individual countries, requires political and organizational problem-solving strategies in practically all countries and often redefinitions of procedural rules. Mechanisms of intersectoral policy-making and implementation outlined in the strategy for health for all by the year 2000 are examples of new strategies.

The key argument of this chapter then is that the political authority to make and define health policy and the division of operational responsibilities between many policy actors (governmental and private) to carry them out are at the heart of any progress in health through new legislation and planning. Moreover, differences in the command of political and institutional resources and privileged access to national policy-making processes, including the proposed coordinating mechanisms, give members of certain policy sectors and subsectors considerable authority and influence, which are denied to representatives of other sectors and lay people. The central issues are raised in the following questions. Are advocates of health promotion members of ministries and institutions that identify and define problems for legislation and planning? Do they command sufficient political resources to influence governments to respond to emerging health problems and to sponsor measures to solve them? Do they occupy strategic positions in old or new political and institutional mechanisms? If they do, can they really ensure the faithful implementation of their decisions? Because of the considerably different political contexts in countries, answers will vary widely but the same questions apply to every country.

General Prerequisites for Health outside the Health Sector

Future directions that should be taken to improve the preconditions of health outside the health system have been identified. According to WHO *(13)*:

> To reach [the targets for health for all in Europe by the year 2000], much will have to be done to improve specific health-related aspects of lifestyles, environmental conditions and health care, but such improvements will have little effect if certain fundamental conditions are not met. Without peace and social justice, without enough food and water, without education and decent housing, and without providing each and all with a useful role in society and an adequate income, there can be no health for the people, no real growth and no social development.

The same considerations will also apply outside Europe. Available knowledge in different areas of human experience, sharpened perceptions of problems and acute awareness of political issues should provide further guidance in pinpointing the future directions and specifying the preconditions of health. However, proposing appropriate processes to achieve these objectives and discussing the thousands of individual decisions on policy and programme operations that are needed in many policy sectors in each country are beyond the scope of this chapter. The author will therefore focus first on why it is still important in the 1980s to be concerned about preserving past achievements in health, and then discuss a few macro structural conditions that are the fundamental prerequisites for the promotion of health.

There are growing indications that all countries — with controlled or free market economies, affluent or less affluent, northern or southern — are at a crossroads where individually and collectively they are reconsidering previous national health strategies and priorities. Several reasons account for this reassessment. In the past two decades, the national level of decision-making has been regarded as the best and most suitable one for allocating national resources in most countries. The existing ministerial organization and the territorial assignment of authority and responsibilities supported the centre's predominance. Health planning and health programming further concentrated decision-making at the centre. But since the Alma-Ata resolution of 1978, which focused on primary health care and decentralization, the validity of the centre's predominance, the desirability of centralization, and the centre's capacity to respond to the entire range of health problems at their source have been fundamentally questioned. Despite the apparent movement in this new direction, the realization of many requests for intersectoral policy-making and new legislation and planning efforts pull in the opposite, i.e. the old, direction of centralization.

Undoubtedly, countries will have to do more with less because of the present economic circumstances and the continued growth of health expenditure despite efforts to control costs *(14)*. Under these conditions, the crucial issue for health advocates is not necessarily how to obtain more funds, physical, technological and manpower resources, and other capacities, but to avoid becoming the victims of the competition for restricted funds and losing further ground in relation to other policy sectors such as defence. A process of curtailing resources and transferring them from health and social services is already under way in many countries with conservative, socialist, or social–liberal political leadership. Nor has eastern Europe been spared budgetary problems. However disquieting the restriction of resources may be, it may also set free dormant creative and innovative forces.

Undoubtedly, priorities in health and other policy areas need to be set now more than ever. But this is likely to intensify fierce competition for a proportion of a shrinking economic pie and provoke a struggle to protect past achievements, acquired rights, services and resources. Political resistance must be expected to new legislation and planning geared specifically to redistributing resources from established priorities and patterns of political authority, and the responsibilities associated with the management of those priorities, when government resources are more circumscribed than they were 10 or 20 years ago. Resistance — manifest or latent or both — to the redistribution of resources is bound to come from all those groups, organizations (public and private) and governments (provincial and municipal) to whom proposed legislation and planning may pose a threat and a loss of influence and funds.

The relationship between economics and politics is highly complex. In past decades economics has been the overwhelming determinant of the allocation and distribution of money in many countries. As long as funds were available, hard choices were not necessary. Generally, one may wish that political consideration should have or should regain primacy over economic considerations in determining priorities in health, but the ascendancy of politics is by no means likely. The structural conditions of government and policy-making concerning health remain the same even if economic and social conditions are critical and whether the leadership is oriented to reform or the *status quo*. Not surprisingly, to balance the books and to appeal to the public for applause, regime support or re-election, many governments behave in similarly pragmatic ways. Generally guided by short-term considerations, they often support decisions that may be sensible in the short term but not in the middle and long terms.

As already stated, legislation is the product of political processes that do not always produce the most adequate or rational responses. Such processes enable established political forces and institutions, that control strategic positions for the formulation of priorities and strategies, to play crucial roles in most countries irrespective of particular political–ideological circumstances. New mechanisms for intersectoral policy coordination and implementation will hardly remain immune to the influence of dominant forces and interests.

The Macro Structural Conditions of Mechanisms for Health Promotion

The coordinated development and implementation of national health policy are essential parts of the strategy for achieving health for all. Coordination through the managerial process for national health development and national health development networks is an attempt to rationalize allocative and distributive decision-making and implementation that typically cut across policy sectors, government levels and public and private sector lines *(4, 10)*. The purpose of this section is to offer a few promising approaches to an understanding of these structural conditions.

From a cross-national perspective several classes of structural issue that bear upon the functioning and effectiveness of these mechanisms can be distinguished. Such issues can serve as guides to decision-makers and problem-solvers in identifying the emergence of problems.

Functions and structures of coordinating bodies

Many governments (central and regional) have expanded the scope of what are considered to be health issues and have honed the tools for implementation in political debates, legislation and planning. Correspondingly, many governments have set up national councils, commissions, interagency committees and coordinating networks in health and other areas. Their purpose is to ensure the rational use of resources by setting priorities and targets for health and other policy sectors. Indeed, concerted action and joint implementation strategies have been common approaches adopted by many countries over the past few decades or so. They are still considered major avenues for the promotion of health in the future as well as sources for the innovation and rationalization of policy.

The meaning of these developments is not unequivocal. Governments and individuals may actually make similar assessments. Governments and perhaps their agencies need justifications for their activities, and individuals may require plausible explanations of their observations of changes or improvements (perceived or actual). However, the issue of whether the cause of changes can be attributed to policy actions and interventions is considerably more complex than can be discussed here. But other developments are clear. They have led to the growing structural interdependence of the health sector and other policy sectors *(15,16)*. Like health issues, other domestic policy fields such as environmental management *(17)* have been defined more broadly and comprehensively. Increasing interdependence has led in varying degrees to the dependence of some sectors and the success of the strategies adopted *(18)*. The reasons for growing interdependence range from the realization that expertise and technical assistance needed to be obtained from other sectors, to the realization of the need to share limited resources with other jurisdictional and territorial divisions of policy-making and implementation. Past developments have produced another by-product, namely, considerable resistance to any overtures for cooperation and coordination, because both activities may reduce funding and lead to the loss of political clout and authority and hence of some autonomy *(15,18)*. Why? The control of political, economic and administrative resources within the macro policy-making system is not exercised equally by all policy sectors.

When, because of structural conditions, much energy is spent on political manoeuvres and efforts to build coalitions and seek consensus in the government realm and in commissions and bodies, the area for action, in contrast to that of political and substantive debate, may shift elsewhere. Whether, in consequence, the quality of policy content or that of joint action is always improved is by no means clear. Assessments of this kind depend on specific countries and on which considerations — political or substantive ones — have been given primary attention and priority.

Coordination of policies for health subsectors

Within the health sector, some countries have been successful in coordinating national policies for individual health subsectors — private medicine, hospital medicine, self-help approaches, alternative ambulatory services, home health care, manpower, training, and health insurance. But progress in other sectors has slowed down considerably. In other countries, efforts to integrate these policy areas have hardly begun.

On an operational level, health planning has attempted to integrate hitherto piecemeal and disjointed approaches to health and medical services. But progress differs widely internationally. Debates about health planning have gone through several international cycles. A first cycle started in the early 1970s *(19)*. A second cycle began from the mid- to the late-1970s *(20,21)*. This cycle is still in progress. Individual countries have passed through domestic cycles similar to the international ones. Initial enthusiasm about particular approaches has given way to some disillusionment and the moderation of expectations about what planning could or could not accomplish given certain structural conditions of government and administration.

Problems of "overcrowded" policy sectors

Many policy sectors in industrialized countries are said to be overcrowded. An overcrowded policy sector is a result of increased and diverse political demands on policy-makers. Alternative groups want to participate in setting national priorities and be included in relevant processes of policy development, coordination and implementation. The extent of overcrowdedness is considered a complicating factor for national action and administration *(12)*. In the light of the many groups interested in some or all aspects of health promotion, the issue of overcrowdedness and its effects are highly relevant to the promotion of health in many countries.

National differences and consequences for organizational change

From a cross-national perspective, it is essential not to view intersectoral policy-making and implementation from the political and organizational perspectives of a few countries in the world. Proposing organizational changes as solutions, on the basis of inferences drawn from atypical or unique country cases and unique scenarios, can be misleading and may prove to be disappointing. Such changes may work fairly well in the context of one country but may not work at all in others because of differences in cultural and social patterns and political and administrative practices. Power, authority and rules governing the political game are neither absolutes nor constants. Nor are they predictable within countries. In this context, the qualitative differences in the observations of scenarios concerned with policy issues or with the delivery of services and care cannot be overemphasized.

Public and private sector interests

The findings of much applied policy research have emphasized the operational difficulties involved in distinguishing between public and private activities and public and private interests even in countries where the private sector is relatively unimportant. But at least in countries where strong elements of both sectors exist, participants from different sectors and institutions usually participate in mechanisms reflecting the goals of the strategy for health for all. This mix of participants contributes to the development of priorities and targets. Participants usually include, in addition to the relevant ministries, academics and the legal profession, management and trade union elites, church and other groups. They sit on councils or coordinating committees and are members of networks. How and where to draw lines between sectors, bureaucratic segments or interests or both are questions that are extremely difficult to resolve in the abstract. In many instances these lines have become completely blurred *(22)*. When aspects of implementation are examined, these lines are even less distinct *(23)*. Consequently, rather than make a case for the necessity of separate policy sectors, distinct segments, or interests inferred from some questionably formal criteria, it would be better for programme designers and health planners to become more sensitive to this kind of overlap of diverse interests when projecting the effectiveness of joint actions and measures to promote health. The political and institutional realities, in contrast to the legal notion of reality, will determine whether the promotion of health is encouraged or discouraged.

Conclusion

All the elements described are the structural features and conditions of the policy-making and implementation of health in many countries. Undoubtedly, all the aspects and circumstances discussed are not present in each country; but in those where a few are present, such factors, independently and jointly, are likely to generate considerable dynamics and political and administrative cross-pressures that can serve as the bases for health promotion. But their final effects cannot be predicted. Consequently, how supportive or disruptive these interacting elements prove to be is not a question of theory or of design but one of empirical enquiry.

Intersectoral Mechanisms

Many aspects of intersectoral mechanisms are highly ambivalent, administratively and politically complex, and deeply rooted in institutional legacies of protecting turf or building empires. Above all, their functioning is little understood. From a policy perspective, demands for intersectoral cooperation and coordination lead to a paradox: for political reasons you are damned if you ask for cooperative and coordinative strategies from other ministries; for reasons of problem-solving you are damned if you don't ask for them. A similar paradox applies to national health councils and intersectoral core groups as proposed by the managerial process for national health development.

The institutionalization of consultative, cooperative and coordinative relations among different policy sectors and intersectoral core groups is already high in some countries, and they are functioning quite well. Such relations are only just emerging in other countries. Several conditions conducive to cooperation have been identified *(18,24,25)*:

— the fewer the participants the higher the chances that they will cooperate;

— the less cooperation required among ministries and agencies the better the relationships;

— the less change that is involved the greater the likelihood of consensus and decision-making;

— the greater political support and shared goals among policy sectors the more likely it is that they will cooperate and make joint decisions;

— the fewer programme elements or programmes that have to be shared with other ministries the greater the probability that policy sectors will cooperate;

— the fewer resources needed from other ministries the greater the likelihood of cooperation;

— the greater the gains (political and administrative) for all participating units, ministries and sectors the better the chances of cooperation.

Conditions that stimulate or discourage cooperation also apply to coordination. But political and administrative coordination is a more complex activity. Some conditions seem to favour intersectoral coordination: first, when there is an overall consensus on goals and on cultural, ethical and medical values that are considered for adoption; second, when political and administrative benefits from intersectoral coordination accrue to all participating ministries, so that no policy sector and no ministry loses and all gain from such a government approach; third, when overall and final responsibility for national health policy lies with the top government authority or office, or alternatively with one of the multisectoral committees mentioned in the strategy for achieving health for all by the year 2000. All three conditions are highly desirable but are unlikely to be present simultaneously in the real world.

Additional structural conditions that may hinder or reduce the effectiveness of intersectoral decision-making bodies vary in the extent to which they are linked to the highest political authority or to a powerful ministry, or both. The extent of this closeness to or, conversely, distance from a powerful centre enhances or diminishes opportunities for joint decisions in support of health promotion. But the responsibilities of national health councils or networks vary considerably. Because they often compete with regular government and administrative channels, multisectoral councils or committees have deliberately been given advisory or consultative responsibilities. Some have consultative and others have advisory responsibilities only. Some have final decision-making authority over policy and programme operations, including responsibility for monitoring and evaluation. If such responsibilities have been authorized, recommendations by a council can be expected to be accepted automatically by the highest legitimizing political authority. If intersectoral bodies have advisory responsibilities only, however, recommendations can easily be changed or ignored by the government. In essence, the inability of advisory bodies to give binding political and legal force to their recommendations should be considered a derivative weakness. When consultation is the main *modus operandi* and a body lacks proximity to important policy-makers, the potential of intersectoral decision-making to achieve meaningful results is weak and hence questionable.

Some of these situations are often found in western polities but not exclusively so. Many countries have not given their national health council ultimate authority. Nor has any final policy-making authority been given to a nucleus within an intersectoral network. Consequently, opportunities for political manoeuvres are to be seized, no doubt by the more influential political forces in both the membership network and the larger political community. In the light of the composition of these councils or committees, it should be expected that some participants will have more power, authority and influence than others because participation as such does not secure authority or influence. Nor does it secure access to the inner circles. In fact, participants can be either core members or marginal ones.

Additional opportunities to influence measures taken to promote health exist in the implementation phase. Policy decisions and decisions on operational programme details are not identical. National coordinating bodies are primarily interested in policy issues, not administrative and regulatory details. They are not concerned with overview and enforcement functions. Often they are not allowed to address these issues because an enterprise of that kind would pose a threat to the regular administrative offices concerned with one or more aspects of administration. Moreover, contrary to widespread views, for policy performance in support of health promotion, aspects of implementation, monitoring and evaluation are as important as the initial decisions on policy. More importantly, decisions of either kind are not self-executing. Someone somewhere needs to act on them. That action will be taken in the normal course of events should not be taken for granted.

Conclusion

It follows from this discussion that the effectiveness of actions and strategies in support of health promotion is influenced by a myriad diverse and mostly unpredictable factors. Action research based on a policy perspective can be critical of policies and processes. As is the case for action research in other fields, action research designed to promote health has been inspired by a set of theories, and it uses concepts and methods from multiple disciplines. This research orientation, both in terms of units and levels of analysis, is not, however, synonymous with standard research on health services.

Promising prognoses of the effects of actions to promote health require not only correct diagnoses of health problems but also the correct identification of the political and institutional macro frameworks in which the actions will be carried out. Unfortunately, the acquisition of the knowledge on which to base a solid understanding of this complex matter has rarely received the specific attention of health policy-makers and researchers. Consequently, the conclusion of much health research lacks institutional and multi-institutional analyses *(26)* that could have highlighted which conditions and mechanisms of health promotion are likely to produce favourable or unfavourable results. Such knowledge is indispensable, for it forms the foundation for determining how to design programmes and interventionary tools to improve health promotion. Proposals not based on this knowledge may well yield less than satisfactory outcomes.

References

1. *Evaluation of the strategy for health for all by the year 2000: seventh report on the world health situation. Vol. 5, European Region.* Copenhagen, WHO Regional Office for Europe, 1986.
2. *The work of WHO 1984-1985. Biennial report of the Director-General to the World Health Assembly and to the United Nations.* Geneva, World Health Organization, 1986.
3. **Altenstetter, C., ed.** *Innovation in health policy and service delivery: a crossnational perspective.* Cambridge, MA, Ölgeschlager, Gun & Hain, 1981.
4. *Formulating strategies for health for all by the year 2000.* Geneva, World Health Organization, 1979 ("Health for All" Series, No. 2).
5. **Easton, D.** *A framework for political analysis.* Englewood Cliffs, NJ, Prentice-Hall, 1965.
6. **Dahl R.** *Modern political analysis,* 2nd ed. Englewood Cliffs, NJ, Prentice-Hall, 1970.
7. **Lasswell, H.** *Politics: who gets what, when, and how?* New York, World Publishing, 1958.
8. **Lasswell, H. & Kaplan, A.** *Power and society: a framework for political inquiry.* New Haven, CT, Yale University Press, 1950.
9. **Dror, Y.** *Public policy-making re-examined.* Scranton, PA, Chandler, 1968.
10. *Managerial process for national health development: guiding principles.* Geneva, World Health Organization, 1981 ("Health for All" Series, No. 5).
11. **Aberbach, J.W. et al.** *Bureaucrats and politicians in western democracies.* Cambridge, MA, Harvard University Press, 1981.
12. **Grant Jordan, A.** Iron triangles, wooly corporatism and elastic nets: images of the policy process. *Journal of public policy,* **1**(1): 95–123 (1981).
13. *Targets for health for all: targets in support of the European regional strategy for health for all.* Copenhagen, WHO Regional Office for Europe, 1985.
14. **Mach, E.P. & Abel-Smith, B.** *Planning the finances of the health sector. A manual for developing countries.* Geneva, World Health Organization, 1983.
15. **Kohn, R.** *Coordination of health and welfare services in four countries.* Copenhagen, WHO Regional Office for Europe, 1979 (Public Health in Europe, No. 6).
16. **Hokenstad, M.C. & Ritvo, R.A., ed.** *Linking health care and social services: international perspectives.* Beverly Hills, Sage Publications, 1982.
17. **Schæfer, M.** *Intersectoral coordination and health in environmental management.* Geneva, World Health Organization, 1981 (Public Health Papers, No. 74).
18. **Scharpf, F.W.** Interorganizational policy studies: issues, concepts and perspectives. *In:* Hanf, K. & Scharpf, F.W. *Inter-organizational policy-making.* London, Sage Publications, 1978.

19. *European Conference on National Health Planning.* Copenhagen, WHO Regional Office for Europe, 1974 (unpublished document EURO 4107).
20. **Pan American Health Organization and US Department of Health, Education and Welfare.** *Health planning, an international view.* Report of an international workshop, Copenhagen, 1977.
21. *Planning and management for health:* report on a European Conference. Copenhagen, WHO Regional Office for Europe, 1986 (EURO Reports and Studies, No. 102).
22. *Review of status of national health development networks/centres: with special reference to WHO support.* Geneva, World Health Organization, 1981 (SHS/81.2).
23. **Hull, C. & Hjern, B.** Policy analysis in mixed economy: an implementation approach. *Policy and politics,* **11**(3): 295–312 (1983).
24. **Rogers, D.L. et al.** *Interorganizational coordination: theory, research and implementation.* Ames, IA, Iowa State University Press, 1982.
25. **Hanf, K. & Scharpf, F.W., ed.** *Inter-organizational policy-making.* London, Sage Publications, 1978.
26. **Holland, W. et al.** *Measurement of levels of health.* Copenhagen, WHO Regional Office for Europe, 1979 (WHO Regional Publications, European Series, No. 7).

5. Conceptual and methodological aspects of measurement in health and health promotion

H. Noack & T. Abelin

Given that health promotion and protection are deliberately planned and guided processes directed towards specified health goals, they can hardly be thought of without some amount of quantitative assessment, and therefore should include measurement as an indispensable tool. The purpose of this chapter is to present a conceptual and methodological basis as well as some practical guidelines for planning and using measurements in this context. It intends to help those involved in health promotion and protection to take better advantage of the opportunities that relevant and sound measurements can provide, but also to make them aware of some of the potential difficulties and limitations of measurement in this field. In this chapter the term "health promotion" will be used in its more general sense and include health protection as well.

Some Basic Concepts

In general terms, measurement can be defined as any procedure that assigns values to objects, persons, responses or events according to some rule.

Measurement in health promotion draws on the behavioural and social sciences, epidemiology and other disciplines dealing with human biology and ecology. Thus, the range of phenomena and attributes that may be measured in this field is very wide indeed, comprising both subjective and objective factors and processes, as well as continuous and discrete variables. Hence, different types of measurement scales are relevant, and several basic properties of measurements need to be considered.

It is customary to distinguish four major types of measurement scale, which will be described briefly *(1)*.

Nominal scale. This scale arranges items (objects, persons, attributes, responses, etc.) to be measured into a set of unordered and mutually exclusive qualitative categories such as nationality, region, place of birth, skin colour or method of intervention. A particular value is arbitrarily assigned to each of these categories. In the case of a category with two alternatives (e.g. male/female, healthy/ill) one speaks of a dichotomous scale.

Ordinal scale. Items are classified into ordered qualitative categories. Examples are sociological variables such as social class or level of social support, psychological variables such as degree of subjectively perceived health balance or of depression, and clinical variables such as the medically defined severity or stage of a disease. Values (e.g. 1, 2, 3, etc.) are generally assigned to express the increasing quality of an attribute of interest. But differences between values are merely differences in qualitative order and not natural or other meaningful distances.

Interval scale. Values are assigned to items with a natural or otherwise meaningful distance between them. Thus, a particular distance between two values in one part of the scale expresses the same distance between two values in some other part of the scale. Examples are Fahrenheit or Celsius temperature, year of birth, or time according to classical physics.

Ratio scale. This is an interval scale with a meaningful or "true" zero point. Ratios between values are meaningfully defined so that a particular value can be said to be so many times more or less than another value. Examples are absolute temperature, height, weight, blood count, income, number of health/disease events in a given population over some period of time (morbidity or mortality rate).

As this brief outline indicates, the numerical values of the four types of measurement scale have quite different properties. This is important when data are statistically analysed and interpreted, as the following example may illustrate. Let us assume that in evaluating a health education programme two kinds of outcome measure were considered: first, psychosocial variables such as level of subjective wellbeing, life satisfaction, perceived success in coping with job or life stresses, and judged duration of healthy activities during the last week (e.g. hours of jogging, gardening, talking to friends); second, biomedical variables such as body mass index, serum cholesterol, blood sugar level, heart rate and blood pressure after particular cognitive and physical tests. Now, on the basis of the biomedical variables that have interval or ratio-scale properties it would be possible to calculate exact change scores for each individuum, but not so on the basis of the psychosocial measures which represent nominal or ordinal scales. This is not to say, however, that the biomedical would be more relevant than the psychosocial data, but only that they provide a different kind of information.

This example can also be used to introduce briefly some other important properties of measurement, to which reference will be made again in Chapter 6. The first one, validity, refers to the extent to which a given instrument or test measures what it purports to measure. Thus, both a subjectively perceived level of wellbeing and a body mass index may be considered valid outcome measurements of health education despite their different scale properties.

Three further criteria, accuracy, precision and reliability, refer to different aspects of the degree of exactness of measurement. Accuracy is defined as the degree to which a measurement reflects a true value. For example, when a measurement of a person's weight of 70 kg is considered to be accurate, another measurement of the same person recorded as 71.333 kg would be more precise although — if faulty — it would not be accurate. Precision is not always required in measurement: for instance it may be sufficient to record events by age in completed years rather than in years and months, although for infant deaths, days, weeks and months may be relevant. The level of precision required will depend on the use to be made of the data. Finally, reliability refers to the degree to which a measurement is stable, i.e. gives the same result when repeated *(1)*.

Measurements used in the assessment and evaluation of health promotion programmes commonly need to be sufficiently valid, accurate, precise and reliable. But two additional criteria will usually be important: measurements should also be economic, that is provide a satisfactory amount of information relative to their costs; and they should be acceptable to those who will provide and use the information collected. Although all these properties of measurements can themselves be measured and quantified, the final decision about the needed quality of measurements always involves value judgements. Of course, the values of such measurement properties will often vary, depending on the perceived needs in health promotion as well as on the political and sociocultural context. For this reason it will not always be easy to reach a consensus on the required validity, accuracy, reliability, precision, economy and acceptability of a set of measurements selected to assess, for example, health potential or certain aspects of health promotion processes.

Because many concepts in health promotion, particularly the concept of health itself, are complex, multidimensional phenomena, still another property of measurements needs to be considered, namely their complexity. In epidemiology as well as in the quantitative social sciences a distinction is often made between measurements that differ in level of complexity, for example between health statistics, health indicators and health indices as measurements of health (Fig. 1).

In a recent review of the literature *(2)*, health indicators were defined as measurements selected from the larger pool of health statistics because they have the power to summarize or represent several statistics, or to serve as useful proxy measures for relevant information. In general they represent one class of data only (e.g. mortality or morbidity but not the two together). Examples given are indicators of survival (e.g. infant mortality rate, maternal mortality rate) and indicators of healthfulness of life (e.g. a list, in order of frequency, of the 10–15 most commonly reported health problems in the population; the number of persons with sick days per 1000 persons per year; the volume of sick days per 1000 persons in the last 14 days; the proportion of persons with less than the minimum food intake; literacy rates for male and female adults).

Fig. 1. A suggested hierarchy of health measures

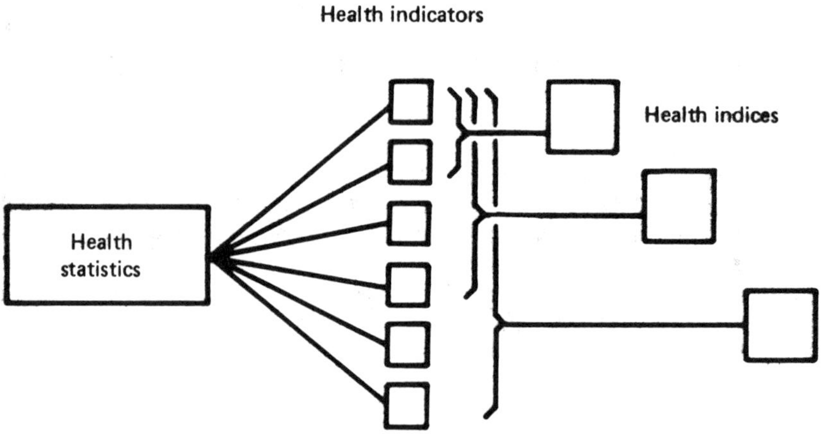

Source: **Murnaghan, J.H.**. *(2)*.

Health indices, on the other hand, refer to the more complex, multidimensional measurements or scales and are often composed of several individual indicators *(2)*. An example is the index "disparity reduction rates" which is composed of the infant mortality rate, life expectancy at year one, and the literacy rate of a given country or population group. These are indicators that can generally be calculated for most countries and that express important dimensions of social wellbeing. Another example is gross national product.

Although some progress has been made in this field in recent years *(2,3)* the development of widely applicable measures and indicators of health still seems to be in its infancy, and there is an unquestionable need for extensive research and developmental work.

The Process and Context of Measurement of Health and Health Promotion

The general purpose of measurement in health promotion is to serve as a tool in programmes or activities that aim at a higher level of health potential and hence of health balance. In Chapter 1 health balance is defined as a state of dynamic equilibrium that an individual or a social group tends to experience under "normal" conditions. An individual person interacting with his or her environment may express such a state as the absence of symptoms, illness or disability and/or as physical, psychological and social wellbeing; in a community it may reflect a low degree of social disruption due to ill health. Health potential, on the other hand, is defined as the capacity for or the particular types of health-related behaviour that are required to maintain this dynamic equilibrium or to re-establish it when it is lost.

It is important to note that both concepts reflect static properties or resources of the system concerned, as well as dynamic properties or processes. Thus, health potential refers to resources such as adequate income, housing and nutrition, physical fitness, emotional stability and social integration, and indicates a certain degree of stability of these qualities; but it also refers to health-related processes such as maintaining a healthy lifestyle and participating in community health programmes and in social and political activities directed towards the improvement of health resources.

To consider the more specific purposes as well as the content and certain methodological aspects of measurement in this field, health promotion will be conceptualized by using a general framework of rational social planning and decision-making *(4)*. Accordingly health promotion can be viewed as an activity consisting of four steps.

1. Assessment of the situation and identification of needs and goals.

2. Specification of a policy, a programme or a plan of actions that are thought to achieve these goals.

3. Implementation, management and monitoring of the programme or plan.

4. Evaluation of the programme's outcome and impact on the larger environment.

These steps are generally thought of as elements of a cyclical or cybernetic process in which measurement and evaluation imply reassessment of the situation, redefinition of objectives, redesign of the programme, re-evaluation of its outcome and so forth. Within such a framework, the measurement of health and of the resources and processes associated with health may serve three general purposes: (*a*) the identification of health promotion needs, (*b*) monitoring of health promotion programmes or activities, and (*c*) evaluation of their efficiency, effectiveness and impact. Any measurement may be made once or regularly, and it may be part of a specific health promotion programme in the community or of national health surveillance and monitoring of change.

Obviously, the settings where such programmes generally take place vary in many ways, within and particularly between countries. Thus, they vary with regard to the distribution of power and resources, to political and sociocultural traditions, values and practices as well as to the level of health potential and health balance within different strata of the population such as different social classes. In spite of such differences in the settings of health promotion, however, it seems useful to consider four of its common elements: a given health promotion programme or intervention; health potential as the primary goal of health promotion; health balance as a condition of the system concerned that is specific to a particular time and situation; measurement and evaluation (Fig. 2).

The first element, the health promotion programme or intervention, could be centred on the individual, such as immunization, health counselling or a training course in coping with specific demands, or it could concentrate on the community, such as employment policy, pollution control or health propaganda in the mass media. These efforts are intended to have an impact on the second element, health potential. The intended change of health potential may either consist of improved health resources (or correspondingly lowered health risks), of strengthened health-promoting processes, or both. As further indicated in the conceptual model, a change of health potential is expected to have an effect on the third element, health balance. Finally, measurement and evaluation would represent essential elements of feedback and monitoring. Thus, if a particular health education programme improves psychological health resources (e.g. coping skills) and health-promoting processes (e.g. actual coping behaviour), the resulting overall change in health potential (e.g. increased resistance to life strain) is likely to improve health balance (e.g. indicated by lowered physiological risk factors or subjectively perceived wellbeing). Based on measurements of health balance it could be decided whether the health education programme needs to be changed or not.

It follows from the social and cybernetic nature of this process that planned and monitored change in health potential and health balance cannot be viewed as a linear chain of cause and effect in any mechanistic or deterministic sense. Any health promotion programme or activity is an intervention into a complex social, economic or ecological system that tends to maintain a particular level of internal dynamic balance, mainly through

Fig. 2. A conceptual model of the health promotion process

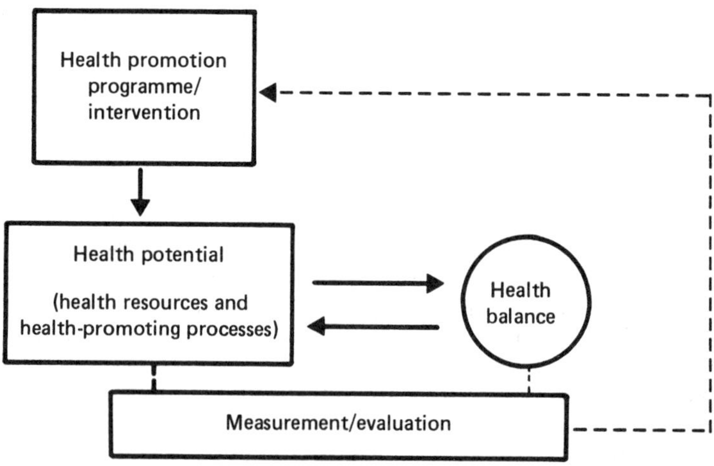

feedback and adaptive mechanisms. Such an intervention is likely to result in some permanent improvement of health potential and health balance if the intended changes correspond with the system's growth and development. For example, a health education programme is most likely to be effective if it produces changes in health behaviour that meet personal needs and accord with sociocultural values, and if such changes do not conflict with political, economic and social pressures — in other words if it is part of a widely supported and comprehensive health promotion policy or plan.

Within such a frame of reference, the purpose of measurement will be either to assess and evaluate those attributes of health potential and health balance that reflect the intended or expected changes within the complex dynamic system in which health promotion takes place, or to monitor the programme elements and activities that were defined as operational goals when the programme was conceived. To accomplish this requires both knowledge and understanding of the system, a suitable health promotion programme and sufficient resources, and also a certain degree of planning of the measuring itself.

More specifically, in the process of planning measurements in this field, three questions need to be answered.

1. How does the measurement contribute to the goals of health promotion and what use will be made of the information to be collected?

2. What are the most relevant dimensions or variables of the measurements?

3. What measuring instruments or procedures are best suited to collect such information and from what sources can it be obtained?

There are, of course, many possible health promotion programmes and a large variety of political, sociocultural and institutional settings for such programmes. It would therefore be neither possible nor meaningful to give detailed answers to these questions. What seems to be useful, however, is to illustrate and discuss the important steps in planning measurements of health balance, health resources and the health promotion process.

Planning Measurements of Health Balance

As emphasized before, health is a complex, multidimensional concept. Any plan to measure health, therefore, requires a clear conceptualization of the specific focus of either health potential or health balance or both. Using several examples, three important steps in the planning of measurements of health balance will first be discussed and illustrated: (*a*) determine the purpose of measuring health balance, (*b*) specify the content of the envisaged measurements, and (*c*) select measurement procedures and sources of data. In doing this, some of the inherent difficulties will also be outlined.

The purpose of measuring health balance

When planning measurements of health balance the most central question is usually "What is the information being collected for?". As already indicated such information may be needed for the identification of health promotion goals or targets, for surveillance of health and monitoring of change, and for the evaluation of specific health promotion programmes, and perhaps also for health services research or other kinds of social science research. A further question might be "Who is going to use the information provided and how will it be used?". For example, the kind of information and hence the nature of the data needed and perhaps even the measurements to be made may be rather different if used by policy-makers, administrators, health professionals, health educators, industrialists or the mass media.

The content of measurements of health balance

What dimensions or attributes of health balance will be most relevant to the purpose of measurements, and which variables, statistics or indicators will reflect them as closely as possible? In any health promotion programme hundreds of variables could be relevant and they may fall into one or more of the following categories: (*a*) biomedical parameters (e.g. weight, blood count, blood pressure); (*b*) psychological measures (level of psychological development of children, subjective wellbeing, level of anxiety or depression); (*c*) sociological indicators (degree of social integration or of social role performance); (*d*) healthiness of life (morbidity rate, disability rate); (*e*) survival or length of life (life expectancy, maternal mortality rate). If the progress of specific health promotion activities is to be monitored together with the promotion programme itself, indicators should be used that are likely to reflect those specific aspects of health balance that are most likely to be affected by the programme. On the other hand, for the long-term surveillance of health balance in the population, more complex indices may be better. The crucial and most difficult question always tends to be one of validity "How many and which measurements should be selected and on what basis?". Obviously, in most situations time and money will be the critical factors in such a decision, in addition to previous research results, experience and, of course, common sense.

The selection of measurement procedures and of sources of data

The next important question generally tends to be "What measuring procedures should be used and what are appropriate sources of data?". Clearly, one should always check whether data are already available or existing records can be used. If this is not the case a wide range of clinical, epidemiological and social science methods are at our disposal, including observation methods, standardized tests, questionnaires and interview. Depending on the availability of data and the particular method to be used, a variety of sources of data may be considered: vital events registers, population and household censuses, routine health services records, epidemiological surveillance data, sample surveys, disease registers and sources in sectors other than health (see also Chapter 9). One may also have to decide whether professional or trained lay people should collect the data or whether self-report instruments might be adequate. Besides validity, accuracy, precision and reliability the most critical issues will often be the accessibility of data and the cost of data collection.

In planning measurements of health, these decisions will, of course, not be made in the sequence in which they have been presented here, as they tend to be interrelated. Although it is not their intention to enable the reader to plan measurements of health balance, the authors hope they have shown that measurements of health should always be planned with sufficient care and, if possible, with the help of experienced personnel.

Planning Measurements of Health Resources

Quite often it is not health balance itself that will be of interest, but what has been defined as one of its most important conditions, namely health resources. To measure health resources it is useful to conceptualize the process of health promotion, for example by using a model like the one shown in Fig. 2. This means making an assumption or stating a hypothesis about the links between a particular health promotion programme or intervention, health potential and health balance. On the basis of such a hypothesis a sufficiently clear concept of relevant health resources can be formulated, given a particular goal of the health promotion effort.

Similar to the approach outlined in the previous section, several important aspects of planning measurements of health resources will now be discussed and illustrated, and attention drawn to some of the inherent difficulties.

The purpose of measuring health resources

Again, the most central question is likely to be "What is the information being collected for and who is going to use it?". In the context of health promotion, the purpose of measuring health resources may be to identify health promotion needs and goals and to set priorities, it may be strategic planning in terms of the specification of a plan of action, the allocation of resources and its implementation, or it may be the monitoring and evaluation of such a plan. As before, different groups of people with different interests may be using such information, e.g. politicians and health administrators, health professionals and educators and perhaps lay people participating in the process, and they may be interested in different kinds of data.

The content of measurements of health resources

Which dimensions, variables and categories are likely to be most relevant to the intended purpose of the measurements? Here the number of potential variables tends to be even greater than in the case of measuring health balance. The following list gives an overview but it is not meant to be exhaustive: (*a*) aims, scope and coordination of health policy (e.g. formulation of specific health promotion targets and of a multisectorial approach to environmental health); (*b*) improvement of conditions in the biological–physical environment (level of pollution control, supply of safe water); (*c*) socioeconomic health resources (material wealth, income, employment, social security); (*d*) health promotion and preventive measures (proportion of GNP spent on health promotion and prevention, existing programmes in health education and occupational health); (*e*) nature and amount of social support of individuals (quality and size of social network); (*f*) lifestyle and health culture (pattern of eating habits and of physical activity, of sleep and recreation, of health-related values and beliefs); (*g*) health-related skills (health knowledge, competence, attitudes); (*h*) physical health resources (nutritional status, physical fitness, immunization status, lack of organic pathology). Given a particular set of goals and a certain amount of time and other resources, it will generally require some effort to select a sufficiently valid set of variables.

The selection of measurement procedures and sources of data

Having identified a set of variables of the health resources to be measured, it can be decided how they are to be measured and what sources of data are to be used. Again, limitation of money and time will be crucial factors, besides certain properties of the measurements.

Planning Measurements of Health Promotion Processes

In the preceding chapters a large variety of health promotion programmes and activities has been presented ranging from the rather general, such as setting political priorities and community involvement in health promotion and protection, to the more specific such as immunization and health education. Many of these processes are slow and will not have immediate effects, especially when changes in the socioeconomic and sociocultural conditions of health and of human behaviour are concerned.

It may not be satisfactory to restrict assessment in this field to measurement of more or less stable properties such as health resources and health balance. Rather, it may be more fruitful to monitor the process of health promotion and protection directly, by measuring relevant dynamic aspects or processes such as events and participation in health education and the distribution of health information, or laws and regulations enforced, tests performed and sanitary conditions improved in the field of health protection.

Frequently, a relatively low level of measurement, such as nominal or ordinal scales, and moderate precision will be sufficient. Nevertheless, quite often this type of measurement will be indispensable for obtaining continuing feedback about health promotion programmes and thus enable decision-makers to reassess them whenever needed.

The purpose of measuring health promotion processes

Planning health promotion programmes implies that certain goals or operational targets are being set, e.g. in terms of reaching a particular proportion of the population with some message or in terms of changing health-related behaviours of a defined population group in a specified way. If such targets are not stated explicitly, it will be difficult to measure and judge the intended progress, and the opportunity to learn from previous experience may be forfeit. If, however, programme targets are stated explicitly, this will provide an essential condition for feedback and self-regulation mechanisms; measurements and experiences can be judged accordingly and corrections be made to the programme if indicated.

The primary purpose of measuring health promotion processes is thus to provide a sufficiently accurate account of what is being done and what is going on, to make it known to others and to ensure that the quality of the programme is being maintained or improved, throughout the target area and during the whole programme period.

The content of measurements of health promotion processes

Ideally, quantitative assessment and evaluation should be an integral part of any health promotion programme and should be planned together with the programme. Logically, the content of measurements of processes will always depend on their specific nature and may be related to one or several of the following dimensions: (*a*) political decision-making and resource allocation in fields such as environmental health, public health information and health counselling; (*b*) level of coordination of health promotion and protection programmes; (*c*) nature and number of health promotion events taking place in a given region or community; (*d*) kind and level of participation of groups and persons in important health promotion activities; (*e*) content and numbers of health information materials distributed among particular populations; (*f*) degree of mass media coverage of health promotion activities; (*g*) number of installations, factories and public places inspected by the health authority within a given period of time; (*h*) amount of waste, pollutants or hazardous substances removed from the physical environment and from industrial products. Obviously, these categories merely provide examples and other aspects of health promotion processes can easily be identified depending on the goals and nature of the programmes.

The selection of measurement procedures and sources of data

In well designed and well managed health promotion programmes all essential events and activities would be documented, e.g. by records on planning activities, courses or programmes, on the nature and degree of participation of people, on the acceptance of programmes and on the experiences gained. Such records will allow for periodic semi-quantitative accounts of the processes of interest. When, in addition, the level of awareness of health promotion in the population or their active participation is to be measured, sample surveys may be necessary.

Whether professional people or institutions will have to be contracted or trained volunteers can be considered sufficiently competent to collect the data, e.g. by carrying out household or telephone interviews, will always depend on factors such as the purpose of measurements as well as the financial resources and the time available. Involving volunteers may, of course, have the advantage of strengthening the community's awareness and/or responsibility for health promotion and protection.

To be able to evaluate the impact of health promotion programmes on specific political, social or psychological processes the design of the assessment tends to be crucial. Thus, it will quite often be necessary to perform measurements before and after the implementation of a health promotion programme. In such situations, it may be advisable to consult or to co-operate with professional personnel. It must, however, be emphasized that measurements in health promotion need not be, and often cannot be, research instruments, but should — as already pointed out — be considered as integrated elements of health promotion programmes.

Some Fundamental Issues in Measuring Health and in Health Promotion

Many of the approaches to health promotion and protection, as well as to measurement, outlined in this book, rely on a general philosophy of social change that has been referred to as social engineering and must be interpreted as mechanistic and technocratic. According to such a philosophy whole social–biological systems, or parts of these systems, such as social groups and individual people can be changed or modified in a more or less rational and practicable way. The mechanisms by which this can be accomplished are assumed to consist of two essential steps: first, the specification of goals or targets that describe intended future states of such systems; and second, the selection and employment of interventions or methods that are known or at least expected to be suitable to reach these targets.

Whether, in a given field of health promotion, the social engineering approach can be considered effective and efficient and hence successful is not a matter of belief or speculation, but is primarily an empirical question which, in principle, can be answered on the basis of information collected through measurement. But the use of such information will ultimately always be part of a more general process of reasoning and judgement. Thus, on the basis of the available empirical evidence it may be decided to what degree an observed change (e.g. in lifestyle) can be attributed to a particular health promotion activity (e.g. a community health education programme) or to other underlying mechanisms (e.g. a secular trend towards more healthy behaviour). But as causal inferences cannot generally be drawn in a strict sense in this field, such a decision will often also depend on philosophical positions and ideological views.

As has been pointed out in Chapters 1, 4.1 and 4.3, as well as in this chapter, health promotion activities are always interventions into complex societal and ecological systems. The way they function and change may be explained by historical, economic, sociocultural and biological processes. Any mechanistic view of such processes and any technocratic approach to alter them must be considered reductionist and hence insufficient or even misleading. This has consequences for the conceptualization of both the health promotion process and the function of measurements within such a process.

In the health promotion process, it is important to conceptualize the two key elements adequately, namely the health goals or targets and the interventions that are assumed to achieve them. Thus, health targets should not be viewed as more or less constant goal values that have been set once and forever as in cybernetic machines, and the interventions should not be confused with treatments that are imposed on social groups or individuals by some external force. On the contrary, targets and interventions will be viewed more adequately as social perspectives and activities, which may or may not be shared by those responsible for a particular health promotion programme and by those participating in it. Measurement may, of course, serve several functions, depending on what the targets and interventions are, how much consensus on specific targets and intervention procedures exists among those involved, and what kind of information they request.

For example if, according to a biological model, environmental hygienists propose to treat drinking-water from nearby supplies by a well known technical procedure to keep the concentration of pathogenic microorganisms at a minimal level and if they receive sufficient economic and practical support, it will suffice to measure the concentration of indicator bacteria in water samples at regular intervals. If, however, political representatives define the lowering of cardiovascular morbidity and mortality by new community-based health promotion programmes as a priority target (political model) and if this involves a process of activation and mobilization in the population (participatory model, see Chapter 4.1), measurements may at first have to concentrate on very different issues. For example, measurement of a programme's acceptance within the community, or measurement of changes in health attitudes or behaviour and of other parameters should perhaps first be used to evaluate and monitor health promotion efforts. Only when this has been accomplished to a satisfactory degree may it be meaningful to measure change in morbidity and mortality.

As illustrated by these examples, the function of measurements will largely depend on what information is needed, for what purpose and by whom. As has been pointed out several times in this chapter, these are fundamental questions that require specific and careful answers. Only if such answers can be given by those involved in the health promotion process will it be possible to decide what level of validity, accuracy, precision and reliability the intended measurements should have, and only then will it be possible to judge whether a particular measurement would be acceptable and economic.

Conclusion

Although measurement in health promotion and protection can draw on a fairly large body of well established epidemiological and social science knowledge and methodology, it is still a rather novel, multidisciplinary field. Undoubtedly, there is a substantial lack of useful conceptual tools, comprehensive theory and relevant experience.

This situation seems to explain, at least in part, why measurement activities in health promotion are often relatively isolated, improvised efforts rather than clearly conceptualized and integrated elements of planned health promotion programmes. It may also explain why it is still a difficult task to choose between the vast and growing number of potentially useful measurements and indicators of health potential and health balance.

In this chapter, several basic concepts related to the measurement of health and health promotion have been introduced, and the reader has been provided with some practical guidelines that may assist him or her in evaluating and perhaps choosing among the many measurement instruments presented in Part II of this book. The reader will hardly go wrong in approaching such problems if he or she is guided by three questions: What information is needed? Who is going to use it? And how?

References

1. **Last, J.M.** *A dictionary of epidemiology.* Oxford, Oxford University Press, 1983.
2. **Murnaghan, J.H.** Health indicators and information systems for the year 2000. *Annual review of public health,* **2**: 299 (1981).
3. *Development of indicators for monitoring progress towards health for all by the year 2000.* Geneva, World Health Organization, 1981 ("Health for All" Series, No. 4).
4. **Rein, M.** *Welfare planning, International encyclopedia of the social sciences.* New York, Macmillan, 1968, Vol. 11 & 12.

Part II

Methods of measurement

6. Measurement: what and how?

Z.J. Brzeziński

Measurements directly or indirectly related to health range from simple counts of certain events or objects to complex scales and comprehensive indices *(1)*. Certainly, recognition of simple events or objects may also vary in complexity. Frequently such events as the occurrence of a disease should match strict definitions and criteria and these in turn involve a more or less complicated measuring procedure. The scope of such measurements is too wide for detailed presentation. Since one is concerned here with the promotion of health and the prevention of illness rather than with cure, promotion and prevention will be the main criteria for inclusion.

Health results from the interplay between an individual or a population and a combination of environmental influences. Therefore planning for health promotion and illness prevention should take into account both the biology and behaviour of individuals and populations and a variety of biological, physical, chemical, cultural and socioeconomic factors of the environment. This complexity is recognized in the ambitious global health programme known as health for all by the year 2000, initiated by the Thirtieth World Health Assembly in 1977 and further developed at the Alma-Ata Conference in 1978 *(2)*. This was the base for the formulation of the global strategy *(3)* and the setting of targets.

The main target of the programme is the attainment by all citizens of the world by the year 2000 of a level of health that will permit them to lead a socially and economically productive life. This requires improvements in many areas, starting with basic living and working conditions, including housing, sanitation, nutrition, employment, healthy lifestyles and a safe environment, and ending with adequate health care. The programme calls for the multisectoral, multiprofessional involvement and active participation of the community as a whole and each person in the community as an individual.

Scope of Measurements in Health Promotion and Protection

The development of programmes aimed at health promotion and protection, as well as the monitoring of their implementation, progress and outcome or benefit, require a broad spectrum of various categories of measurement. Some of them are needed to identify and quantify each problem, others to describe its determinants. One also needs appropriate measurements of the content and process of intervention, and finally, the measurements of changes resulting from it to learn if a given programme has attained its expected targets. However, the same measurement can often serve several purposes in the same programme, for example, to identify and quantify a problem and to indicate the degree of its reduction. Accordingly, measurements can be classified and grouped in various ways.

For the purpose of Part II of this book measurements are considered from two points of view, as they relate to health and as they are involved in health promotion and protection.

The first approach starts with measures of child growth and development and continues through physiological indices of physical function and measurements of psychosocial state and function. The next chapter deals with aspects specific to measuring the health of the elderly. Considerations of complex indices of health status follow.

The last two chapters are concerned with measures showing the lack of health, such as sickness, disability and death, and showing how these events can be used as measurements of programmes that promote and protect health.

The section devoted to measurement in health promotion and protection begins with an assessment of promotion and protection at the personal level. The next two chapters present measurements of behaviour that is conducive to good health and people's involvement and participation in activities that promote and protect health. The following chapters present measurements related to the protection of a healthy environment, the provision and management of services, and finally, areas of social policy outside the health sector that affect health and the assessment of priorities accorded to health promotion.

The last section of Part II is devoted to the development of information systems to support health programmes.

Existing Gaps

In spite of a wide range of presently available measurements many areas are not fully covered, and further development is needed. One would like to have more and better indicators of levels of performance, both social and physical, showing the level of health reserve we all have at any age and in any state of health. Measures of physical functional level and disability need further development for both individuals and populations. Existing measures of activity of daily living or task performance require improvements in standardization and comparability.

A wider use of physiological indices of physical function should also be made. Not enough is available for measuring the psychosocial state in terms of ability to cope with major life events. The components of wellbeing need to be better identified and measured. This kind of measurement is needed not only to assess the quality of life but also as an integral part of any evaluative procedure in promotive, preventive and curative interventions.

Measurements providing information on the availability and use of facilities in a given society, that according to current knowledge increase the health of populations, are also inadequate. The same may be said about measurements dealing with protection from environmental hazards. Although there is fragmentary information on the presence and levels of a number of pollutants, it is difficult to relate them to well defined populations to assess the proportion of people enjoying an environment free from a given hazard.

Another area that calls for further development is health behaviour. The current measures of behaviour conducive to health are in most cases crude and scanty. A similar situation exists with attitudes to the management of an individual's health. Most of the information available does not go beyond crude indicators such as the use of certain screening services, annual check-ups or antenatal care clinics.

The scope and content of information on various aspects of primary care are also far from satisfactory. The availability, accessibility and acceptability of services are most frequently measured by resource-to-population allocation and use ratios. However, measures of time, cost and distance, which are considered to present barriers to the use of services, are rarely available. Also, utilization measures are not always available in a format that can be related to the availability of services. Measurements of self-care and family care, or the use of alternative sources of care outside the health system are almost nonexistent.

In addition to the development of new measurements, better use could be made of some available at present. For example, one can use mortality data, instead of calculating the traditional mortality rates, to assess the number of years to be gained if death from a given cause or causes could be prevented. This has the advantage of giving greater weight to deaths at younger ages, thus permitting better assessment of the importance of mortality from a particular disease. Similarly, cumulative measures of morbidity or disability may indicate time free from disease or disability gained by eliminating a particular kind of illness. This approach has the additional value of providing more informative data to people who are less familiar with health statistics.

Basic Characteristics of Measurements

Previous remarks show the wide scope of problems related to health promotion and the prevention of ill health. The arsenal of possible measurements applicable to this field is similarly wide. They have been developed by different technical disciplines, each with its own peculiarities and requirements. The selection of an appropriate measurement or battery of measurements depends on the information the measurements are supposed to provide and the nature of the problem being investigated. In selecting a measurement it is also important to examine its characteristics to make sure that its limitations do not disqualify it from use for a particular purpose.

The validity of a measurement is expressed by the degree to which it measures what it is intended to measure. It is a fundamental requirement, since, unless this criterion is met, the relevance of the results to the problem studied can be questioned *(4)*.

Reliability is expressed by the degree of stability shown when a measurement is repeated under similar conditions. Therefore, the more reliable a measurement procedure is, the more likely it is that the results can be replicated. Certainly the ideal reproducibility of measurements is hardly possible, and the degree of reliability depends on the divergences between observers and measuring instruments, as well as the stability of the attribute being measured *(4)*.

Accuracy is expressed by the difference between the measured value and the true value of the attribute in question. In many instances this condition is difficult to satisfy, especially if one cannot take a direct measurement. For example, blood pressure is measured indirectly by using a sphygmomanometer and cuff. The resulting measurements are highly correlated with the actual arterial blood pressure but there is no absolute one-to-one relationship *(5)*.

The sensitivity and specificity of a simple or complex test should be considered when measuring a disease or condition. A test to diagnose a disease for instance will achieve some correct results (true positives (a)) and true negatives (d)) and some incorrect results (false positives (b) and false negatives (c)). The sensitivity of such a test is appraised by the number of persons who are affected and detected by the test (a) over the number of affected persons in the population (a + c):

$$\frac{a}{a+c} \times 100.$$

Specificity is measured by the number of persons who are not affected and in whom the test was negative (d) over the number of unaffected persons in the population (b + d):

$$\frac{d}{b+d} \times 100.$$

To assess specificity and sensitivity one needs to have a reference measurement and a diagnostic procedure of known validity. Usually an improvement in sensitivity leads to lower specificity and decisions about specificity and sensitivity required depend on the character and purpose of the study.

The feasibility of measurements is the main barrier to a wider use of many available measurements. It may be due to costs and organizational problems or to the attitude of people on whom the measure is to be performed. Therefore one should consider both the simplicity and the acceptability of measurements to be used.

The fundamental problem of measurements is to what extent they are properly representative of the phenomenon measured. If one is interested in the prevalence of a certain disease or condition in a population, it is usually impossible to examine all the people in it. Similarly, to assess the level of air pollution in an area, it is equally impossible to measure the pollution at all possible points in that area. Measurements are, therefore, performed only on a part of the population or only at certain points of that area. Then one must ask whether the results obtained are truly representative. If a disease or condition depends on age and the part of the population examined includes a greater proportion of elderly than the target population as a whole, then the prevalence of the disease will be overestimated. If the level of air pollution varies from place to place and the measurements are taken in a place that is more polluted than the rest of the area, they will not properly reflect the actual conditions. Therefore appropriate techniques to select a population or other samples should be used to ensure the representativeness of the measurements *(6)*.

Variations occur in the subsequent readings of instruments, at the same place, from place to place and over time, that originate from sources other than variation in the measured variable. Similar variations occur in observers and laboratory work. If these variations occur at random, then, although they affect the precision of the estimate, they will not produce results that depart systematically from the true values. If an instrument or observer makes a systematic error, however, the results will be biased. Bias may also originate from other sources, such as the lack of representativeness of a sample. In surveys, bias may arise from non-participation, because non-participants may differ significantly in many respects from the rest of the sample (see Table 1).

Table 1. Comparison between participants and non-participants regarding variables obtained from public registers

	Participants (N = 365)	*P*	Non-participants (N = 172)	Total sample (N = 537)
Civil status				
Married (%)	71		36	60
Unmarried (%)	21	<0.001	44	28
Divorced (%)	7		19	11
Widowers (%)	1		1	1
Annual salary (median SKr)[a]	52 100	<0.01	42 300	49 300
Number of sickness benefit days (2 years median)	8	<0.001	45	13
Sickness benefit spells (number, median)	2	<0.001	4	
Born abroad (%)	17	<0.001	34	22
Registered for intemperance (%)	13	<0.001	35	20

[a] SKr 4.50 = US $1.00 (November 1975).

Source: **Bergstrand, R. et al.** *(7)*.

Quality Control

Measurement errors are unavoidable, no matter where and by whom measurements are taken. The purpose of quality control in measurement is, therefore, not to eliminate errors, but to reduce them as much as possible or at least to an acceptable level *(8)*. The actual design of quality control procedures for data depends on the kind of study and measurement used, but it should always provide information on the magnitude of variation and its sources. Also, all possible sources of bias should be examined and evaluated.

References

1. **Rosser, R.** Issues of measurement in the design of health indicators: a review. *In:* Culyer, A.J., ed. *Health indicators.* Oxford, Martin Robertson, 1983.
2. *Primary health care*: report of the International Conference on Primary Health Care, Alma-Ata, USSR, 6–12 September 1978. Geneva, World Health Organization, 1978 ("Health for All" Series, No. 1).
3. *Global strategy for health for all by the year 2000.* Geneva, World Health Organization, 1981 ("Health for All" Series, No. 3).
4. **Last, J., ed.** *A dictionary of epidemiology.* Oxford, Oxford University Press, 1983.
5. **Reid, D. & Holland, W.W.** Measurement in health care studies. *In:* Holland, W.W. & Karhauser, L., ed. *Health care and epidemiology.* Henry Kimpton Publishers, 1978.
6. **Cochran, W.G.** *Sampling techniques.* New York, John Wiley & Sons, 1964.
7. **Bergstrand, R. et al.** Bias due to non-participation and heterogenous sub-groups in population surveys. *Journal of chronic diseases,* **36**(10): 725–728 (1983).
8. **Friberg, L. & Vahter, M.** Assessment of exposure to lead and cadmium through biological monitoring: results of UNEP/WHO global study. *Environmental research,* **30**: 95–128 (1983).

7. Measurement of health

7.1 Measures of human growth[a] — *F. Falkner*

Human growth is commonly considered to have started at the beginning of the seven ages of man. The ancient Chinese, in their traditional wisdom, added another age and celebrated a child's first birthday at the time of birth. Today this tradition continues in some parts of the world and may be used for official purposes. Thus a newborn baby is aged one year from birth, and will be two years of age as of 1 January the following year. Age zero years, therefore, does not exist. This recognizes that the most important year of life, albeit short by 12 weeks, has already occurred. Growth continues from conception, not birth, to maturity.

Prenatal Growth

Comparatively little is known about the important 40-week period of prenatal growth. For somatic assessments of fetal growth, we have had to rely on measurements made on fetuses expelled early in pregnancy as a result of induced or spontaneous abortion. Later fetuses are either born too soon, or are too small for their gestational age. Fig. 1 and 2 are examples of available fetal growth curves that have proved generally valuable for clinical use, but they have one serious fault: the assumption that such fetuses may be considered to have grown normally. This doubtful assumption may be justified if the truly prematurely born infant, without any congenital abnormalities, continues to grow normally after birth in exactly the same way as infants born at 40 weeks of gestation.

[a] Parts of this chapter are based on a paper read at a workshop on the introduction of food to infants, sponsored by the International Organization for the Study of Human Development, Berkeley, California, February 1983.

Fig. 1. Birth weight of infants born between 25 and 44 weeks of gestation (mean ±2 standard deviations)

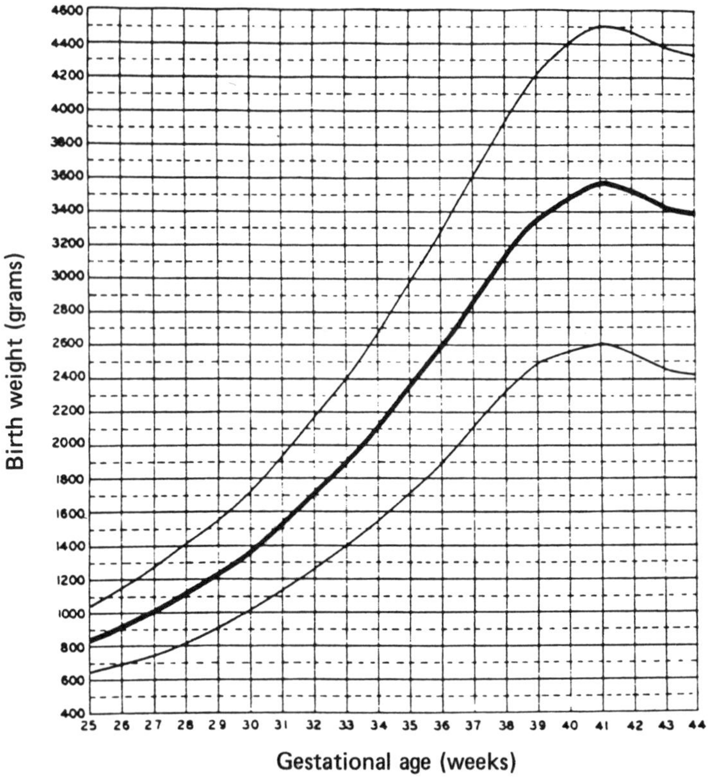

Source: **Usher, R. & McLean, F.** *(1).*

Reliable fetal growth curves related to outcome would be welcomed by many disciplines involved in fetal and infant health. With the advent of non-invasive ultrasound, it should now be possible to measure longitudinally, from 12 weeks of gestation, linear body growth and head circumference, and to continue such measurements after birth for those fetuses born alive. Curves could thus be created by measuring fetuses destined to be full term, destined to be premature and destined to be small for their gestational age. The outcome for each could then be measured after birth, and since it is likely to be different for each group, important indications for intervention and prevention could be revealed.

All infants of low birth weight, particularly those of very low birth weight, are at risk. On escaping from the early risk period in postnatal life, however, prematurely born infants without congenital malformations who

Fig. 2. Length, head circumference and chest circumference of infants born between 25 to 44 weeks of gestation (mean ±2 standard deviations)

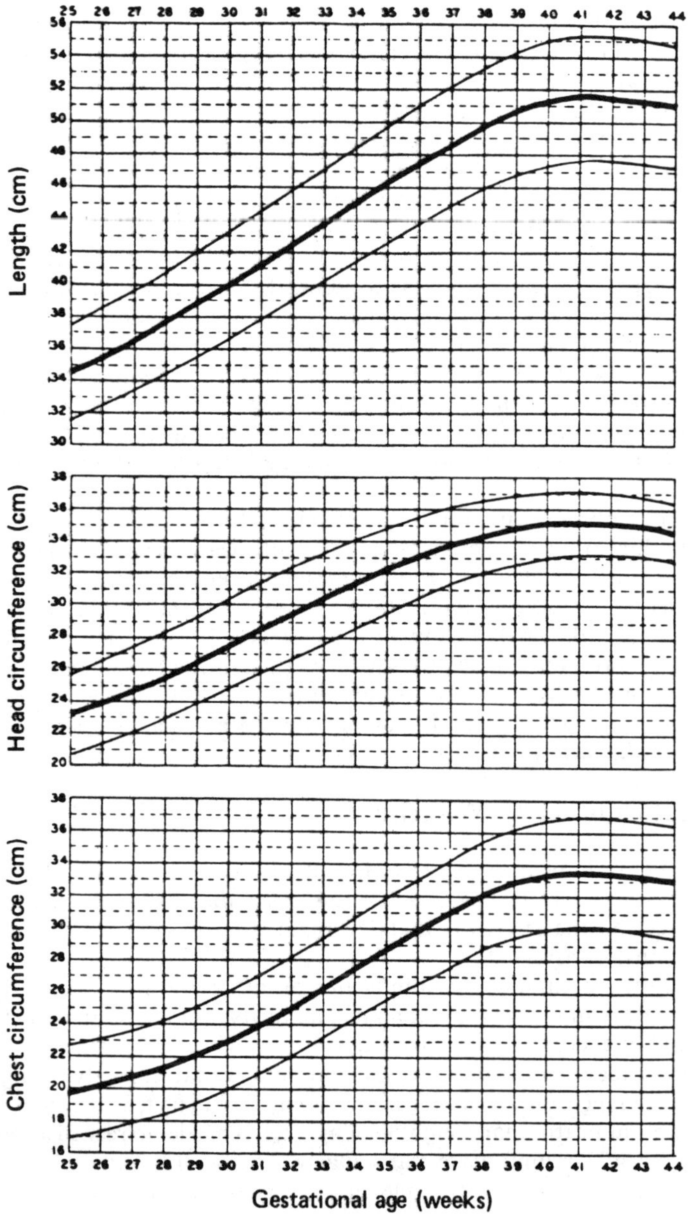

Source: **Usher, R. & McLean, F.** *(1).*

receive reasonable care seem to exhibit catch-up growth and by three years of age have reached the same size as a comparable full-term infant *(2)*. This is not so for small-for-gestational age infants. There appears to be a distribution curve of their size outcome, from those who achieve the same result as the prematurely born infant to those who will remain permanently and irreversibly smaller.

The author has described a pair of monozygous, and thus phenotypically similar, twins born at 39 weeks of gestation *(3)*. One was an infant of low birth weight, half the weight of his twin. Leaving aside a discussion of cause, a summary of outcome for each twin after birth showed that the smaller twin, albeit healthy, had a growth pattern exactly consistent with that of an infant small for his gestational age whose immediate postnatal catch-up was insufficient and by 16 years of age he remained irreversibly and very markedly smaller by many anthropometric measures. Holding the genetic growth factor the same for both boys, the relationship between prenatal growth and postnatal somatic outcome is revealed to be important for non-genetic factors influencing growth.

Much attention to these aspects of prenatal growth and outcome is needed, together with the ability to predict. Smallness may be of little moment, but if associated with, for example stunting of other biological factors such as brain development, smallness becomes an important indicator *(4)*.

In the embryonic period the speed of the fetus's growth is not very great, but the high rate of growth that starts afterwards is due largely to cell multiplication. The number of multiplying cells becomes progressively fewer as the fetus gets older. There is a period of peak velocity of linear growth, just like that in human adolescence, but its time is somewhat uncertain: probably about 20–24 weeks. Then linear growth begins to slow down at birth. Growth in the weight of the fetus follows the same general pattern as growth in length, except that peak weight velocity occurs markedly later, at about 32–34 weeks.

Indicators of Early Maturity

A number of indicators of early maturity are accepted as useful, although these have no agreed overall definition. Since the level of maturity clearly influences postnatal growth and development, the value of some key indicators must be assessed.

The most commonly used indicator of infant maturity is birth weight. This measure indicates more than just maturity, but it is simple to measure reasonably accurately and plays a key role. Data on gestational age, a time-dependent indicator, are less commonly available, partly owing to the difficulty of recording them accurately. Length is, in fact, a more meaningful and stable indicator than weight; but, again, it is harder to record accurately. Finally, head circumference, particularly because of its indication of brain development, is an important indicator and easy to measure.

Clearly, many indicators other than somatic ones are useful and acceptable, but these four seem among the most sensitive. Further, studying the relationships and distributions of such variables, where appropriate, will often lead to more fruitful information than studying just one.

Genetic and Adaptive Factors in Growth

It appears that fetal growth begins to slow down at 34–36 weeks, owing to uterine size, its space for comfortable occupancy now being full. Twins slow down demonstrably earlier, when their combined weight is approaching that of a 36-week singleton fetus.

An entirely hypothetical velocity curve of weight from, for example, the fetus's point of peak growth in weight at 32 weeks to the eighth week of the infant's postnatal life, clearly takes no account of the slowing in growth just described. There must then be catch-up growth in the first eight postnatal weeks, even allowing for normal weight loss after birth, especially for those infants most delayed *in utero*. Therefore, a significant negative correlation exists between birth weight and weight gain in the early postnatal months, as indeed it does for length. The smaller the infant, the more, on average, he or she grows in this period.

This deceleration enables a genetically large infant growing inside a small mother to be delivered successfully. Cattle crosses demonstrate this when a very large female, pregnant by a very small male, has a large calf. Reversing this cross, a small female will have a small calf. Notably, both calves will be the same size after some months and mature to a size about half way between that of their parents. Parenthetically, this endorses the plea of some scientists to create and use growth curves to screen children that are based on what is termed mid-parent stature.

Maternal genetic factors are thought to contribute some 25% of the variation in fetal growth, with the contribution of the paternal genetic factor thought to be much lower. Non-nutritional factors are thought to contribute 50–60% to this variation. The importance of fetal nutrition is not agreed, since under severe conditions of maternal malnutrition, any factor in the mother regulating fetal growth might be expected to act to protect her from serious depletion of nutrient and mineral supplies by slowing down fetal growth. But despite severe maternal malnutrition, nearly normal fetal growth continues, indicating that placental and fetal growth-controlling factors operate normally under these circumstances, possibly by entering maternal circulation and then inhibiting maternal metabolic mechanisms. How is it, then, that the nutrition component of poor and adverse environmental conditions is strongly associated with low birth weight? This is largely due to such factors causing an abnormal and marked reduction in growth rate after 36 weeks, for the mean birth weights of infants born at 36 weeks in many parts of the world under different circumstances are quite similar.

A mother who does not achieve her own growth potential, owing to malnutrition or other adverse environmental factors, is likely to have smaller fetuses and newborn infants. Clearly, two generations or more may be needed to reverse the effects of poor environment on birth size. Mothers of short stature in Guatemala, for instance, had smaller babies than mothers of medium stature. A food supplement given to both samples of mothers during pregnancy increased the birth size of the smaller mothers' infants more than it did those infants of larger mothers, although it did not wholly eliminate the difference *(5)*.

Ecological extremes afford examples of adaptive characteristics in fetal and infant body size, shape and composition. A body shape facilitating the dissipation of body heat would be a beneficial adaptive feature in very hot climates. A linear physique is common in well nourished infants and children in the tropics, and this is thought to be adaptive. The same adaptation may be achieved in different ways, such as the reduced ratio of body mass to surface area found in some American Indians and in the Chinese. At the other end of the climatic spectrum, and contrary to common teaching, Eskimo children have a relatively low skinfold thickness *(6)*. These values, together with estimations of total body fat, are similar to many groups of European children living in temperate climates. Eskimos protect themselves from the environment by their dwellings and clothing, so their physique does not, therefore, reflect the effects of the cold.

People living at high altitudes are subject to both cold and a reduced partial pressure of oxygen in the inspired air. In Peruvian altitudes of over 4000 m, the velocity of fetal and infant growth is comparatively slow, one effect being lower mean birth weights at high altitudes. The ecosystem is probably not conducive to rapid growth, but does each individual adapt to this environment by slow growth, or is a characteristic growth pattern established in the genotype?

The factors influencing the growth of the fetus are complex, numerous, and may be interrelated. In simple terms, they can be listed under genetic, fetal nutritional supply, and other maternal/fetal factors, as well as environmental, utero-placental and fetal factors themselves.

A word on the evaluation of perinatal growth. Three basic periods of perinatal growth should be recognized: intrauterine, or prenatal; transitional; and extrauterine, or postnatal. Prenatal growth standards are needed and have been discussed earlier. In the transitional period, the first 6–12 days of postnatal life are characterized by very large variations and fluctuations, and growth follows no standards. After this period, postnatal growth velocity is distinctly faster than in the prenatal period, so neither can be applied to the other. Separate standards are thus needed to evaluate perinatal growth.

Other Measures of the Growth and Maturity of Children

Body weight is an unstable measurement. Body weight decrements frequently occur; catch-up growth occurs; and when studying the growth of one baby or all babies, particularly in the early months of life, measurements have to be frequent so that the actual pattern of growth can be shown.

During the early days of life there is a 5–10% loss in body weight in healthy infants, due largely to the loss of body water. This normal phenomenon proceeds until the third or fourth day, when weight gain begins, and by the tenth day the birth weight has been regained. As a very rough guide, the birth weight usually doubles in 4–5 months and triples within the first year. The general course of growth is then followed. Interpretation of body weight patterns must always be based on the realization that a gain in weight may indicate growth in fat, bone or muscle, a seasonal effect, catch-up growth, gain in total body water, increased caloric intake and so forth. Body weight patterns, then, may hide important factors.

Important body components or systems may grow very differently and have their own particular growth curves. When a particular tissue or system is being considered, its particular growth pattern should be known in principle and taken into account.

Head circumference is a reasonable indicator of head and brain size. Its velocity curve is very different from that of general growth. A period of rapid incremental growth occurs until birth, and then a marked deceleration begins, although the size of the skull reaches nearly 90% of its adult size by 10 years of age. This measurement may also be used to show the necessity of considering growth patterns within certain age groups or categories of babies and children. Patterns may occur that deviate from normal patterns, yet do not, in themselves, indicate pathological processes.

Height measurement obviously assesses bone growth, which follows the general growth curve. Individual bones in a child, however, may grow at widely different rates, an important factor influencing the final proportions of the body.

Muscle growth is closely similar to the overall pattern of bone growth, but of all the tissues, muscle is the one that develops greatly during the adolescent growth spurt, especially in the male.

Body fat has a complex growth pattern of its own. Fat increases steadily and quite rapidly for about the first nine months of life. A plateau is then reached and soon there is a true loss of fat until about seven years of age. Thus, any curve depicting fat growth must be able to record decreases. At seven years of age, fat is gained once more. In many boys a spurt of fat growth occurs before the general adolescent growth spurt. When the general adolescent spurt of growth begins, including muscle and bone mass, this external fat is stretched over the rapidly growing frame; and there is also an actual loss of fat during adolescence.

Girls follow a different pattern, and in early childhood their fat loss is less than that of boys. Hence, the average female reaches adulthood with more total fat than the average male. Added to these normal patterns are such interrelated factors as overeating and true obesity. The complexity and importance of the growth of fat is clear.

Skeletal maturity is an important indicator of maturity, or developmental age, although the necessity of using X-rays makes it impractical in field conditions. Particularly at times of rapid growth, chronological age is apt to be unhelpful as a marker in an individual child, and maturation of the skeleton or bone age is often more useful.

The length of the skeleton increases by proliferation of cartilage cells in cartilaginous areas, a continuous process from early fetal life that is known as chondroplasia. After vascular penetration of primary and secondary centres, the process of ossification of the cartilaginous areas starts by deposition of osteoid tissue. This is known as osteogenesis. When ossification is complete, by epiphysical closure or fusion, bone growth has ceased. The finality of this cessation has vital importance in considering problems of growth.

In health the two processes are linked very closely even though the relative rates may differ. If dissociation occurs, the final size of the child will be affected. For example, if osteogenesis proceeds apace, while chondroplasia continues at a normal or less rapid rate than osteogenesis, the growth of the skeleton will be diminished and stunting will occur. Put another way, adult stature is determined by the speed of linear growth and by its duration, which is a function of skeletal maturity. The measurement of height is a good practical measure of linear growth, or chondroplasia. The measurement of skeletal maturity or osteogenesis is also clearly important.

X-ray examination reveals the stage of maturity by the use of standards, comparing, for example, the stage of maturation of several ossification centres *(7)*. Since all healthy children eventually reach 100% maturity of any maturational indicator, skeletal maturity provides a good common growth scale. Predictions of growth outcome may also, to some extent, be made by estimating skeletal maturity and relating it to a person's general growth curve.

Velocity of Growth, Growth Standards and Norms

The commonest method of collecting data on human development is the cross-sectional method. Here people are measured once, and mean values of a measure are calculated for various ages. Age differences are usually calculated by comparing mean value of different age groups or by using all individual measures and computing the regression on age. The great majority of the standards used in human biology have been produced from cross-sectional study. These standards in turn form the basis of countless tables of norms, charts and grids. If measures of dispersion, such as percentiles, are added and the samples are reasonably large and representative, then such cross-sectional studies tell us much about human development, mainly as distance data, or average measurements attained at various ages. Cross-sectional studies are inexpensive and comparatively easy to perform, and produce results quickly. They are a vital part of growth studies.

When information is needed on change or velocity over time, however, the cross-sectional study is inappropriate and the longitudinal study must be used instead. In such studies the same people are measured at specific ages over a period of time.

In human development, longitudinal studies can be undertaken from birth to maturity or to the grave. Clearly, the time factor of the study itself virtually prohibits study of one person's whole lifespan. Now that more and more parameters of development may be studied before birth, the longitudinal study of early childhood development can, and should, start in fetal life.

The key to the collection of velocity data is continuity. Even if only two points are available on a curve, the slope of that curve may still indicate a great deal. The desired information will determine the number of points needed and then their separation in time. But good velocity data by no means require an extended period of time.

We usually think in terms of size achieved at various ages, in terms of a baby growing steadily. The word "steadily" reflects a deeply embedded misconception. The changes that occur in the growing person can only be studied and understood if growth is regarded as a continuum, hence the study of velocity growth. These velocities are by no means steady, and the pace of growth varies widely at various ages.

If it is known that a baby weighed 3.0 kg at birth and 6.0 kg at six months, this is useful information but tells only of the weight achieved for age. We can go a step further and say that the baby's weight gain in the first six months of life was 3.0 kg; this is his weight velocity over this time period. If in the next two months he lost weight for some reason and at eight months weighed 5.6 kg, then his weight loss from six to eight months of age was 400 g; note also that the weight gain in his first eight months was 2.6 kg. This immediately shows that when measuring such an unstable factor as weight, frequent measurements may be necessary. In this example, a measurement at birth and one at eight months would not have shown this child's true velocity pattern.

Standards and norms

The debate continues over whether to use one set of growth standards for international purposes, or national standards derived from a privileged sample of the population under study. National standards are often impractical to obtain, although they may be regarded as an ideal. The use of a sample of privileged children has a potential hazard: such a sample may be different genetically from a sample of a less privileged segment of the population.

The world's children, in fact, appear to follow similar growth patterns, although populations of different ethnic and geographical origins have greatly different adult stature and rates of maturation. Thus, children of all ages vary widely in actual stature, and also in the relationship of weight to height. No data exist at present to determine how much variation in size would exist between races, particularly among children under five years of age, if all children lived in optimum conditions.

This leads to the basic question about the use of standards. What is their purpose? Are they to screen an individual child for a growth indicator or to compare one sample of children with another? For the former, ideally, some kind of national standard of the population from which the child comes is required. For the latter, a good representative national sample from another country may probably be used if there is some agreement as to tolerable degrees of deviation from whatever norm is chosen *(8)*.

There is a place for international reference values such as those used in the WHO charts shown in Fig. 3 and 4. These offer a simple and practical approach to health screening by the use of a series of reference values derived from one set of measures, and a value range is selected that most closely resembles that of healthy children in the population concerned. They cover the first five postnatal years.

Fig. 3. Front of the WHO growth chart

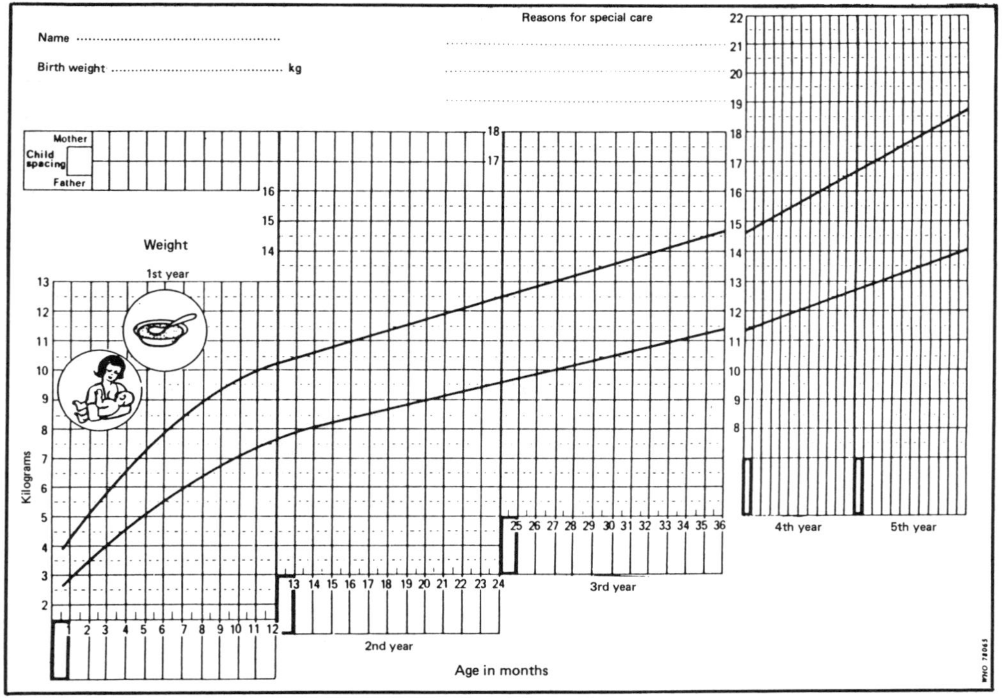

Source: *A growth chart for international use in maternal and child health.* Geneva, World Health Organization, 1978. *Training in recording the child's growth.* Geneva, World Health Organization, 1983 (document EPI/PHW/83/TM.1/Rev.2).

Fig. 4. Reverse of the WHO growth chart

APPOINTMENTS

GROWTH CHART

Health centre		Child's No.
Child's name		
Date first seen	Birthday	
Mother's name		Registration No.
Father's name		Registration No.
Where the family lives (address)		

BROTHERS AND SISTERS

Year/birth	Boy/Girl	Remarks	Year/birth	Boy/Girl	Remarks

IMMUNIZATIONS

TUBERCULOSIS vaccine (BCG) — date: ....
DIPHTHERIA, WHOOPING COUGH, TETANUS vaccine (DPT) Date: 1 dose .... 2 dose .... 3 dose ....
POLIOMYELITIS vaccine (OPV) Date: 1 dose .... 2 dose .... 3 dose ....
MEASLES vaccine — date: ....
OTHER vaccines (specify with date):* *Including tetanus toxoid for the mother

Source: *A growth chart for international use in maternal and child health.* Geneva, World Health Organization, 1978.
Training in recording the child's growth. Geneva, World Health Organization, 1983 (document EPI/PHW/83/TM.1/Rev.2).

To simplify, the indicators of weight, height, and especially weight-for-height up to adolescence and head circumference up to five years of age are the most useful.

Recently some studies have used velocity data for specific purposes. Their great advantage over distance data norms is that the problem of adjusting for age is largely removed. Velocity standards are becoming more available too *(9)*. Fig. 5 gives weight growth velocity curves for boys from birth to three years. Separate curves are used for girls. Fig. 6 and 7 give velocity growth curves of weight for boys and girls, of 2–18 years of age. Curves are also published for length, stature and head circumference.

One example will show the usefulness of this approach, with a warning about its interpretation. It might be decided, with profit, to determine the velocity of weight or height gain, having set certain criteria. Intervention such as nutritional supplements would be indicated if the growth did not achieve the chosen rate. The usefulness of intervention could then be evaluated by continuing to record the pace of growth.

The warning is that although standard velocity curves are appropriately smoothed, even a healthy child's curve over short periods may be anything but smooth, encompassing even the cessation of growth, followed by a catch-up period. Thus, in the above example, criteria for intervention need to obviate the potential for false positives or negatives.

Fig. 5. Percentile velocity curves of six-monthly weight increases in boys, from birth to three years

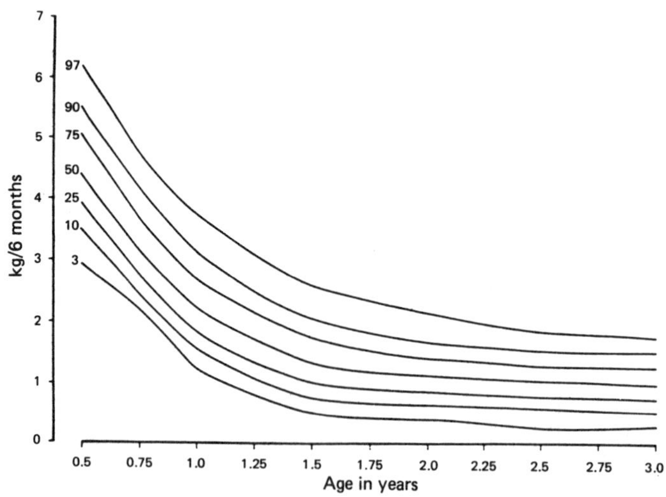

Fig. 6. Percentile velocity curves of six-monthly weight increases in boys, 2–18 years

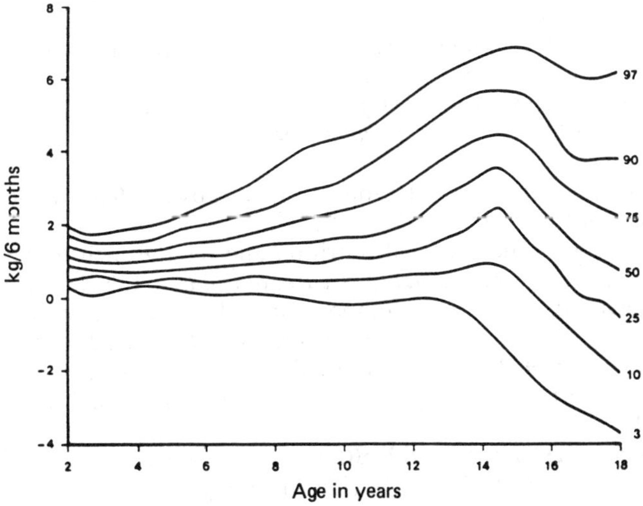

Fig. 7. Percentile velocity curves of six-monthly weight increases in girls, 2–18 years

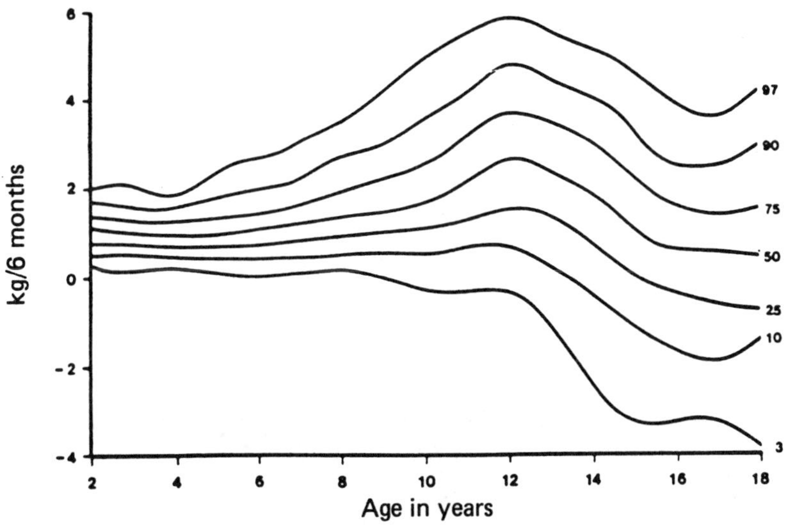

References

1. **Usher, R. & McLean, F.** Intrauterine growth of liveborn Caucasian infants at sea level: standards obtained from measurements in 7 dimensions of infants born between 25 and 44 weeks of gestation. *Journal of pediatrics,* **74**: 901–910 (1969).
2. **Cruise, M.O.** A longitudinal study of the growth of low birth weight infants. *Pediatrics,* **51**: 620–628 (1973).
3. **Falkner, F.** Implications for growth in human twins. *In:* Falkner, F. & Tanner, J.M., ed. *Human growth.* New York, Plenum, 1978, Vol. 1, pp. 397–412.
4. **Falkner, F.** Maternal nutrition and fetal growth. *American journal of clinical nutrition,* **34**: 769–774 (1981).
5. **Lechtig, A. et al.** Maternal nutrition and fetal growth in developing societies. *American journal of diseases of children,* **129**: 434–437 (1975).
6. **Shephard, R.J. et al.** Body composition of the Eskimo. *European journal of applied physiology and occupational physiology,* **32**: 3–15 (1973).
7. **Tanner, J.M. et al.** *A revised system for estimating skeletal maturity from hand and wrist radiographs.* Paris, Centre international de l'enfance, 1972.
8. **National Center for Health Statistics.** Growth charts. *Monthly vital statistics report,* **25**(3): Suppl. (HRA) 76–1120 (1976).
9. **Roche, A.F. & Himes, J.H.** Incremental growth charts. *American journal of clinical nutrition,* **33**: 2041–2052 (1980).

7.2 Physiological indices of physical performance capacity — *K. Lange Andersen & J. Rutenfranz*

Physical performance encompasses all body functions, but some of them are of particular interest in the context of health potential and health promotion, as they enable the individual specifically to master the challenges of his environment and thus to maintain and strengthen his health balance (see Chapter 1). The most widely applied function is the transformation of nutrient into kinetic energy in muscle cells, including the supply functions involved. In view of their central significance, this chapter will be devoted mainly to these functions and their measurement. The discussion will focus on measurements in individuals, but ample reference will be made to methods that are of particular interest to epidemiological application. Examples of such applications and a discussion of their interpretation are to be found in Chapter 11.

Other important functions include those of the visual and auditory senses, and some references to their measurements in the context of health promotion and protection will be given at the end of this chapter.

Physiological Fundamentals

The fire of life. In order to stay alive and function properly, every single cell of the human body must always be supplied with enough energy. Biological oxidation is the most important energy-yielding process. Without a continuous and sufficient flow of oxygen — always governed by the need — the body cannot function properly and health deteriorates. This concept is dramatically demonstrated when the blood supply and consequently the delivery of oxygen is cut off.

Under ordinary life conditions it is the oxygen and not the fuel supply that limits the energy-yielding process. This holds true also for the maintenance of homeostasis during the performance of muscular exercise, when the demand for energy may be many times that at rest. The acceptance of this principle makes it understandable that in the search for an all-over physiological indicator of human functioning, oxygen consumption and use become meaningful measures.

Maximal aerobic power. In terms of maximal oxygen uptake attained during strenuous, but not necessarily exhaustive, muscular efforts, this is widely used as a determinant of physical fitness and has passed the test of time as a meaningful positive indicator of health status. Not only does maximal aerobic power characterize a person's ability to withstand the strain and stress of work, but it also indicates man's ability to cope with environmental stress such as heat, cold and hypoxia at high altitudes.

The oxygen transport system. The chain of transport of oxygen from the air to the cells includes the lungs, the cardiovascular system (central and peripheral) and blood as well as certain biochemical elements of the cells themselves. Exercise testing is widely used in the clinical assessment of functional status for these various elements; measurements and testing procedures depend on the purpose of the test programme.

Adaptation. Maximal aerobic power and related functions of the oxygen transport system are apt to change through adaptation, e.g. through training or increased habitual physical activity. Such an adaptive physiological trend is beneficial for man in general, since it renders him more fit for work, sport and other attractive activities which help in the full enjoyment of life.

Health and physical performance capacity. Physical fitness in terms of maximal aerobic power acquired in youth and maintained throughout life by means of an appropriate pattern of a healthy lifestyle, including habitual physical activity, is thought to have beneficial effects on the cardiovascular, respiratory and locomotor systems as well as on cell metabolism and body functions in general.

Although definite proof that a high standard of physical performance capacity has a beneficial effect on length of life is still missing, epidemiological studies relating physical activity to lowered mortality rates suggest such an effect *(1)*.

There is circumstantial evidence supporting the concept that a high level of fitness goes along with optimal body functions. Fit subjects are physiologically characterized by having a lower heart rate and arterial blood pressure at rest as well as during performance of muscular exercise, which put less stress on the heart of the fit compared to the unfit person *(2,3)*.

Some of the established coronary risk factors are beneficially influenced by fitness, which may contribute to postponing to later years in life the fatal or disabling consequences of ischaemic cardiovascular diseases such as stroke and myocardial infarction. It may therefore be concluded that fitness adds efficiency, pleasure and wellbeing, and probably also years to life *(4–6)*.

Fundamentals of Exercise Stress Testing

The fundamentals of exercise testing have been evaluated by a group of human physiologists and their findings were published by WHO in 1971 *(7)*. No objective measurements made on resting individuals will reveal their capacity to do physical work or predict their maximal aerobic power. Even a simple questionnaire may yield more useful information as to their health status in terms of physical fitness than can be obtained from measurements taken at rest. For example, a low heart rate at rest may indicate a high level of maximal aerobic power, but it may also be a constitutional trait or a sign of disease.

The description of techniques that follows is elementary and limited in scope. They should be carried out only by people who have undergone training in a specialized laboratory. The reader is referred to textbooks of work and exercise physiology for more detailed information *(8–11)*.

Types of ergometer

Ergometers are instruments for measuring work output. Several types are suitable for routine exercise testing:

— bicycle ergometer;

— treadmill;

— steps.

Each of these has its merits and disadvantages, and the type of work task selected for a specific study depends on its purpose and the nature of the population sample.

Bicycle ergometers, which are of use in epidemiological surveys, should be designed for work in the upright position. They have mechanical or electrical brakes.

Electrically braked bicycles provide viscous resistance. Some of the electrically braked bicycles that are commercially available have incorporated a feedback mechanism so that the amount of external work performed is independent of minor variations in the pedalling rate. The main disadvantages of the electrical machines for field studies are the need for electricity and their complexity and cost.

The simpler types of bicycle ergometer with a mechanical braking mechanism are inexpensive, easy to maintain, to calibrate and to operate, and they can be built in any well equipped mechanical workshop to meet the specifications of the investigators. Several types are also commercially available at low cost.

The main drawbacks of bicycle ergometers in exercise testing are the occurrence of fatigue and of pain in thighs and knees which may be intolerable to elderly subjects and to people unaccustomed to bicycle riding. Difficulties in maintaining the prescribed pedalling rate may also be a problem.

The motor driven treadmill allows studies of people's response to walking and running. Treadmills are normally constructed so that both speed and inclination can be varied. Small, portable treadmills that can be used in field laboratories are commercially available. Treadmills have the advantage that the rate of work is constant, is independent of the motivation of the subjects and can be set to any desired work level by adjusting the speed and inclination of the belt. The disadvantages are that the work output cannot be easily calculated and the machines are often noisy and require electrical supply.

Steps have been used that differ greatly in height and modes of performance (single, double, triple and multiple steps). Sturdy construction is essential, and testing is facilitated by bolting the steps to the floor. The facilities of a handrail should be provided, particularly for elderly people. The main disadvantage in using steps is the continuous movement of the arms and head, which creates difficulties when taking physiological measurements. Steps are consequently most useful when physical performance is assessed from measurements of physiological functions during the recovery phase after the exercise period.

Work output can only be calculated with ease and sufficient accuracy from bicycle ergometry and is expressed in watts. When a step test is used work output is assessed by counting the total number of ascents and multiplying this by the subject's body weight. It should be realized that the amount of work performed depends on the weight of the subject, this being in contrast to the use of bicycle ergometry in which the work output is independent of body weight.

Energy expenditure is a fundamental measure in exercise testing and is based on the principle of indirect calorimetry and determination of oxygen uptake.

The classical method of measuring oxygen uptake during muscular exercise includes the collection of expired air into a Douglas bag or tank spirometer, with subsequent metering of the gas volume, followed by an analysis of aliquot samples for the percentage of oxygen and carbon dioxide.

Recently, several instruments have been made available commercially for the collection, metering and analysis of gas from which the relevant variables are computed automatically. These instruments are, however, expensive, difficult to operate and to maintain, and their use should be restricted to controlled environments.

Respiratory variables are always recorded when energy expenditure is measured during exercise. These variables include the volume of air inhaled per breath (Tidal volume), the number of breaths per minute and the total volume of air expired per minute (pulmonary ventilation). These variables relative to oxygen uptake may assess the respiratory mechanisms involved when fitness is impaired.

Cardiovascular parameters such as cardiac output, heart rate and pressure in systemic and pulmonary circulation need to be measured for the analysis of the more fundamental haemodynamic variables. These measurements require invasive methods and their use is therefore limited to specialized hospital laboratories. However, some other circulatory measurements are easily taken and may yield significant insight into cardiovascular functioning during physical activity.

Heart rate may simply be counted during exercise by palpation of the carotid artery or by auscultation of the heart sounds. It is preferable, however, to record exercise heart rate by means of an electrocardiograph. The monitoring of the electrocardiogram (ECG) during an exercise test makes an important contribution to the safety of the test. Telemetry systems for ECG transmission or cardiocorders (miniature ECG tape recorders carried by the subject) have the advantage that they free the subject from the encumbrance of wires and cables.

Blood pressure measured in the brachial artery by the cuff method should be taken whenever possible and recorded because during and after exercise it is an indicator of health status. The use of the cuff method to measure brachial artery pressure during exercise has certain disadvantages. Only systolic pressure can be assessed with reasonable accuracy during the performance of exercise tests.

An *ECG* taken during and after exercise stress testing is widely used in the diagnosis of ischaemic heart disease. It is also used as a health risk indicator because a normal exercise ECG is associated with a low, and an abnormal ECG (particularly ST depressions) with an increased risk of heart attacks.

Exercise Stress Tests in Population Surveys

To measure positive aspects of health on a population basis for the purpose of evaluating fitness and assessing the effect of health promotion programmes, exercise testing has to be simple. Many subjects should be able to be tested within a reasonable period of time. The methods must be acceptable to young and old, whether fit or unfit. Safety precautions, environmental specifications and the preparation of subjects for testing are further described in a manual published by WHO *(7)*.

Many different exercise stress tests have been worked out for measuring physical performance capacity. From a physiological point of view, the test should be selected according to how validly and reliably it measures maximal aerobic power.

Some of the many exercise tests are listed below in order of simplicity ending with the more complex and sophisticated, but also the most valid and reliable, methods.

Single-stage step tests are available in many modifications. An example of this type of physical fitness test is the "Harvard step test" which was used extensively during the Second World War to measure the fitness of military personnel for hard muscular work *(12)*. The method was devised for speed and simplicity of use with large numbers of subjects. A sturdy stepping platform, 50 cm high, a stop watch and a device (metronome or pendulum) for pacing the subjects to the correct rhythm are the necessary apparatus.

The subjects are asked to step on and off the platform 20 times a minute for 5 minutes. The pulse is counted from 1 to $1\frac{1}{2}$, 2 to $2\frac{1}{2}$ and 3 to $3\frac{1}{2}$ minutes after stopping work.

The score is obtained by dividing the duration of the exercise in seconds, multiplied by 100, by twice the sum of the pulse counts during recovery. This test score has been shown to correlate well with the maximal aerobic power *(13)*.

Multistage submaximal to maximal exercises using either a bicycle ergometer or a motordriven treadmill are valid and reliable for assessing maximal aerobic power and related respiratory and circulatory functions.

When *bicycle ergometry* is used, the measurement of oxygen uptake can be omitted with only slight reduction in the accuracy of estimating energy expenditure. This simplification is justified because the range of normal responses in energy expenditure at similar loads is fairly small in individuals who are accustomed to this type of muscular activity. The procedure of choice involves making the subjects exercise at several submaximal exercise stages. Each stage should last for 4–6 minutes to allow for a steady state to develop. The stepwise increased loading can be stopped at target heart rates such as 170 beats per minute for the age group 20–29 years, 160 at age 30–39, 150 at age 40–49, 140 at age 50–59 and 130 at over 60 years. Although these heart rate targets are arbitrary, they rest on the physiological decline in maximal heart rates, and represent a percentage of estimated maximal heart rates (e.g. 85% *(14)*). From a practical point of view these levels are easy to remember. Using this procedure, the test score is expressed as work output corresponding to age-defined target heart rates (W_{170}–W_{160} etc.).

Another way of analysing the data is by plotting the values for work output against the corresponding heart rates. A straight line is fitted, either by eye or by the method of least squares. The line is then extrapolated to the person's predicted maximal heart rate; the corresponding work output is an estimate of the physical work capacity *(15)*.

When a *treadmill* is used in multistage exercise testing, the oxygen uptake has to be measured because the work output cannot be assessed from speed and inclination.

A test to measure *maximal aerobic power* directly starts with a submaximal exercise loading which also serves as a warm-up period. The load is increased stepwise with two or three submaximal stages. Preferably, several strenuous efforts should be made to establish the level at which a further increase in loads does not bring about any further increase in oxygen uptake. This levelling-off in oxygen uptake is taken as the sign that the maximal level has been attained. Any of the three types of ergometer may be used. Running uphill and stepping yield similar results, but bicycling and running horizontally are known to give 5–8% lower values of maximal aerobic power. Although maximal oxygen uptake can be measured with a reasonable degree of accuracy, the procedure is rather time-consuming. The maximal test requires a high degree of cooperation from the subject who must also be motivated to expose himself to maximal or near maximal muscular efforts. This direct determination of maximal oxygen uptake is the method of choice in scientific investigation, but it can be applied only to relatively few people within a reasonable period of time. The complexity and disadvantages of the procedure therefore limit its use in epidemiological research.

ECG at rest and during exercise and arterial blood pressure should be evaluated together with the exercise heart rate for an overall evaluation of circulatory function. Valuable additional information may also be obtained by relating respiratory variables to oxygen uptake.

These simple ways of assessing physical fitness have proved to give valuable information in the following contexts.

1. In the comparison of physical fitness and health status between population groups that differ with regard to lifestyle, occupation, environmental conditions, etc. *(16,17)*.

2. In the evaluation of intervention programmes for the purpose of testing the effect of prevention, health promotion and rehabilitation. This principle is widely applied in athletics to test whether or not a training programme has been effective in improving the physiological status underlying the physical performance capacity *(18)*.

Task Performance Tests

Athletics events are the traditional test of physical performance capacity. Under such conditions fitness can be measured precisely, or estimated subjectively as in gymnastics. The person's performance is the combined result of muscular activity executed by the interaction and coordination of a variety of bodily functions. Motivation plays a decisive role in general.

Most of the widely used physical fitness tests are related to some sort of gymnastic or athletic performance *(19,20)*. To the extent that performance in these tests depends on particular skills, they are not suitable for an analysis of basic physiological functions.

A *12-minute running test* was proposed by Cooper in 1968 *(21)* as an indirect way of estimating aerobic capacity. This test has been widely used owing to its simplicity and practicability. It requires no instruments except a stop watch and can be executed on any ordinary track and field sports ground.

The test score is measured in terms of the distance (in metres) covered by running as fast as possible for 12 minutes. The health hazards of testing people unaccustomed to this type of activity or who may have some medical disorders, should be realized.

The test score has been found to correlate well with the maximal aerobic power in young men and women *(22)*.

Task performance tests aiming at the determination of sensomotor functions such as reaction time, movement coordination, muscle strength, etc. are widely used for occupational purposes. The objectives of these tests are not normally oriented towards health, but they are used to select people for specific work tasks or to evaluate the effect of different training and teaching programmes.

Vision and Hearing Tests

Tests of visual acuity, colour sense and hearing ability (by audiometry) have significant health implications and should be included in programmes devoted to protection against accidents, in noise control programmes and more generally in health studies related to aging.

Hearing test by audiometry

Commonly used clinical tests on the ability to hear the spoken and whispered voice, a coin drop and a watch tick are notoriously poor and subject to many errors in both application and interpretation.

Pure tone audiography is the method of choice for most purposes aiming at screening for hearing disabilities. Many inexpensive apparatuses are commercially available. The results are reliable with a high degree of sensitivity and specificity. A large number of subjects can be tested within a reasonable period of time. Some of the audiometer models can be battery operated, and lend themselves to field studies.

The recording of an audiogram is based on the generation of pure tone sounds. Sound has two fundamental characteristics: frequency, which is measured in hertz (1 Hz = one cycle/second), and intensity level or sound pressure, which is measured in decibels (dB). The definition of sound pressure and the construction of the decibel scale are complicated, and standard textbooks should be consulted for details.

By means of audiography, hearing ability is measured by the application of sound to each ear at different frequencies and sound pressures, usually starting at 250 Hz and testing at octave intervals (octave = doubling of the frequency) up to 8000 Hz. The lowest sound pressure that can be heard at each frequency defines the hearing threshold at that particular frequency. By assessing the threshold at different frequencies an audiogram is constructed.

Audiometry is described in detail in standard textbooks of otorhinology. Guidelines may also be found in textbooks on occupational health practice *(23)*.

Screening tests of vision

Visual acuity or the general ability to see is usually measured by means of a chart on which the optotypes (letters, numbers, etc.) in each line are smaller than those in the line above. This procedure is in principle a two-points discrimination test.

Visual acuity is expressed as a ratio in which the numerator is the test distance, and the denominator is the distance from which the smallest line can be read, e.g. 3/6 – 5/6 – 6/6. The traditional Snellen chart is so constructed that 6/6 (or in decimals 1.0) defines the visual acuity of the normal eye.

The test chart, the distance, the illumination and the contrast between the black optotypes and the white background of the chart must be standardized if the results are to be meaningful. Despite its many drawbacks the Snellen chart continues to be the most widely used measure of visual acuity, requiring no expensive instruments, and can be applied to any population group where normal visual acuity is considered important for safety and the promotion of health.

Accommodation power. The accommodation power of the eye is the ability to focus clearly on objects at different distances, and depends on the function of the eye lens. The accommodation power is in the range of 12–15 diopters in young people, but becomes considerably reduced with age, and may practically be absent in old age. Accommodation is especially important for near visual acuity, and is consequently important for productive work and for health in general.

Accommodation power is usually measured either by moving a test object away from the eye and bringing it gradually closer until images begin to blur, or by holding a test chart with several sizes of optotype at a given distance. Commonly used test charts require the examinee to read aloud the smallest types seen clearly when holding the chart at a distance of 50 cm from the eyes. The score represents the range of accommodation in diopters, and is equivalent to the reciprocal of the near point at which blurring occurs, expressed in cm $\times$ 100. If the near point is 33 cm, the range of accommodation is 3 diopters, or if 20 cm it is 5 diopters.

Colour vision. Simple checks on colour vision are needed, for example to ensure that people to be trained for jobs involving discrimination between signal lights do not have grossly defective vision.

Pseudoisochromatic plates, of which the best known series is that of Ishihara, consist of displays of coloured spots in which a pattern is clearly visible to the normal eye, but not to those with particular types of colour defect.

Anomaloscopes are instruments specifically designed to diagnose protanomaly and deuteranomaly, the two most common red–green colour defects.

Multiphasic vision screening. Commercially available instruments have been designed with standardized systems, so that visual acuity, accommodation power, colour vision, depth perception, etc. can be tested with the same instrument. They are in general handy, portable and inexpensive apparatuses. The results are reliable, they are easy to operate and may be usefully applied in population surveys. Vision screening tests are described in detail in standard text books of ophthalmology.

References

1. **Salonen, J.T. et al.** Physical activity and risk of myocardial infarction, cerebral stroke and death. *American journal of epidemiology,* **115**: 526–537 (1982).
2. **Carlsten, A. & Grimby, G.** *The circulatory response to muscular exercise in man.* Springfield, IL, Thomas, 1966.
3. **Johnson, R.E. et al.** A test of physical fitness for strenuous exercise. *Revue canadienne de biologie,* **1**: 491–503 (1942).
4. **Lange Andersen, K. & Elvig, A.** The resting arterial blood pressure in athletes. *Acta medica scandinavica,* **153**: 367–371 (1956).
5. **Ilmarinen, J. et al.** Prävalenz von Risikofaktoren für Herz- und Kreislaufkrankheiten in Gruppen mit unterschiedlicher habitueller körperlicher Aktivität. *International archives of occupational health,* **45**: 15–33 (1980).
6. **Rutenfranz, J. et al.** Maximum aerobic power and body composition during the puberty growth period: similarities and differences between children of two European countries. *European journal of pediatrics,* **136**: 122–133 (1981).
7. **Lange Andersen, K. et al.** *Fundamentals of exercise testing.* Geneva, World Health Organization, 1971.

8. **Hollmann, W, & Hettinger, T.** *Sportmedizin-, Arbeits- und Trainingsgrundlagen.* Stuttgart, F.K. Schattauer Verlag, 1976.
9. **Astrand, P.O. & Rodahl, K.** *Textbook of work physiology.* New York, McGraw-Hill, 1977.
10. **Consolazio, C.F. et al.** *Physiological measurements of metabolic functions in man.* New York, McGraw-Hill, 1963.
11. **Naughton, J.P. et al.** *Exercise testing and exercise training in coronary heart disease.* New York, Academic Press, 1973.
12. **Brouha, L. et al.** The step test. A simple method of measuring physical fitness for hard muscular work in adult man. *Revue canadienne de biologie,* **2**: 86–91 (1943).
13. **Astrand, P.O. & Rhyming, I.** A nomogram for calculation of aerobic capacity from pulse rate during submaximal work. *Journal of applied physiology,* **7**: 218–221 (1954).
14. **Ilmarinen, J. et al.** Die Wirkung von körperlichen Aktivitäten im Beruf bzw. in der Freizeit auf die kardiopulmonale Leistungsfähigkeit. *International archives of occupational health,* **49**: 1–12 (1981).
15. **Wahlund, H.** Determination of the physical working capacity. A physiological and clinical study with special reference to standardization of cardio-pulmonary functional tests. *Acta medica scandinavica* (Suppl.), **132**: 215 (1948).
16. **Seliger, V.** *Physical fitness.* Prague, Charles University, 1973.
17. **Lange Andersen, K. et al.** *Habitual physical activity and health.* Copenhagen, WHO Regional Office for Europe, 1978 (WHO Regional Publications, European Series, No. 6).
18. **Amsterdam, E.A. et al.** *Exercise in cardiovascular health and disease.* New York, Yorke Medical Books, 1977.
19. *The AAHPER fitness test manual.* Washington, DC, American Association for Health, Physical Education and Recreation, 1965.
20. **Larson, L.A.** *Fitness, health and work capacity. International standards for assessments.* New York, MacMillan, 1974.
21. **Cooper, K.A.** A means of assessing maximal oxygen intake. *Journal of the American Medical Association,* **203**: 135–138 (1968).
22. **Sparling, P.B. & Cureton, K.J.** Biological determinants of the sex differences in 12-min run performance. *Medicine and science in sports and exercise,* **15**: 218–223 (1983).
23. **Schilling, R.S.F.** *Occupational health practice,* 2nd ed. London, Butterworth, 1981.

7.3 Assessment of psychosocial status: measures of subjective wellbeing, social adjustment and psychiatric symptoms[a] — *K. John, G.D. Gammon & M.M. Weissman*

The psychosocial status of the general population can be assessed by using three distinct types of measurement. These are: (*a*) *measures of subjective wellbeing*, which assess happiness and/or satisfaction with life and which have been used to provide subjective social indicators in research into the quality of life *(1)*; (*b*) *social adjustment scales*, which assess social adjustment or functioning, and which have been used to measure social impairment in clinical and community psychiatry research *(2)*; (*c*) *psychiatric screening instruments*, which assess psychiatric symptoms, and which have been used to detect or estimate psychiatric disturbance in population and clinical studies *(3)*.

Measures of subjective or perceived wellbeing assess a person's relative happiness or satisfaction with life as a whole or with various aspects of life, such as work, family, income or health. Such measures do not directly assess psychological health or illness, but rather a person's attitudes and feelings about the quality of his or her life. Social adjustment scales typically assess a person's instrumental and affective functioning within major adult roles, i.e. his or her behaviour and attitudes in work, family and community roles. Such scales assume that specific ways of behaving are commonly accepted as appropriate, and the individual's role and overall social functioning are measured in terms of either the ideal or actual norms of his or her referrent group *(2)*. Psychiatric screening instruments assess the presence, absence, intensity or frequency of moods, feelings, sensations and behaviour that may constitute an episode of psychiatric illness *(3)*. Such instruments do not diagnose specific psychiatric disorders, but do indicate whether a disorder is likely to be present.

In this chapter measures of subjective wellbeing, social adjustment and psychiatric symptoms will be briefly described and illustrated. Each of these measurement techniques has been found to generate useful information about important components of psychosocial wellbeing.

Before proceeding, however, another relevant area of measurement should be mentioned. The diagnostic interview schedules *(4–8)* that have resulted from greater precision in diagnostic classification in psychiatry may be the instruments of choice in certain studies concerned with the psychosocial wellbeing of community members. Although they will not be described further, these interviews and the diagnostic systems that they use

---

[a] This work was supported by the Yale Mental Health Clinical Research Center, New Haven, Connecticut (grant MH 30929) and the John P. and Catherine T. MacArthur Foundation on Risk and Protective Factors in the Major Mental Disorders. In addition, G.D. Gammon received support from grant MH 14235 for research training in psychosocial epidemiology.

can provide precise and valid estimates of the incidence and prevalence of *specific* psychiatric disorders. Such information is sometimes necessary in planning treatment facilities and strategies or outreach and preventive intervention.

Measurement of Subjective Wellbeing

Subjective or perceived wellbeing refers to how people themselves evaluate their lives or various aspects of their lives *(1)*. As a method of measurement, it is a direct and relatively unbiased way of determining the psychosocial wellbeing of large segments of the population. An interviewer asks a respondent to rate how happy or satisfied he or she is with life as a whole and/or with specific aspects of life. It is important to note, however, that the measures to be described here are not standardized questionnaires, but rather *item formats* with specified *response scales*. Work with these formats and scales has indicated that they are valid methods with which to inquire about nearly any aspect of a person's life.

Early measures of happiness and life satisfaction

Collecting data in the spring of 1957, Gurin et al. *(9)* were the first to conduct a major study of psychological wellbeing that used a probability sample of the American population and that investigated happiness with life in addition to symptoms of psychological and social disturbance. The study used a three-alternative scale. Subjects were asked: "Taking all things together, how would you say things are these days — would you say you're *very* happy, *pretty* happy or *not too* happy these days?" Persons who said they were *not too* happy were much more likely to have psychiatric symptoms, be divorced or widowed, to be in the lowest income group, to have less education, and to be black (particularly if they lived outside the southern states).

Four years later, Bradburn & Caplovitz *(10)* used the Gurin et al. happiness question in their cross-sectional study of four small towns (population 3000–10 000) in the state of Illinois in the United States. Two of the towns were classified as economically depressed and the other two as relatively well-off economically. The position on the three-alternative measure was found by them to be related to the "relative balance of two independent conditions: positive and negative affective feelings". The findings of Bradburn & Caplovitz regarding correlations between happiness and sex, the marital status, income and education of respondents were similar to the Gurin et al. results. However, more people in general, more single and divorced men, more divorced and widowed women, and more people who had attended college (especially those in the lowest income group) were found to be *not too happy* in the later study.

The Gurin et al. happiness question has remained the most commonly used item to assess happiness with life as a whole *(1)*, and in a recent follow-up study of the quality of life among a representative sample of Canadians, in which the scale was used, people in general were found to be more unhappy than they had been two years earlier, even when their life conditions were reported by them to have improved *(11)*.

Attempting to take into account the varying needs, expectations, aspirations, and consequently satisfactions that people experience, Cantril *(12)* devised a ladder of life or self-anchoring striving scale on which respondents in his massive 13-nation study were asked to express variations between their ideal situation and their actual conditions. These variations were assessed on a scale ranging from 0 for the worst to 10 for the best actualization in a number of life areas and in life as a whole. Table 1 displays Cantril's ladder with a sample question from his study. Although Cantril tended to use the terms "happiness" and "satisfaction" interchangeably in his report, his emphasis was primarily on the concerns and satisfaction levels that adults from different societies express. Family economic situation, personal health and family wellbeing were factors mentioned spontaneously as leading to personal satisfaction by at least 50% of respondents in the study. Furthermore, in all nations, people of higher social status and those living in rural rather than urban areas were found to report significantly higher levels of satisfaction, and some of the largest differences in ratings on the 11-point scale were due to race, with blacks scoring an average of 1.4 ladder steps below whites. Cantril's ladder of life scale has been one of the most widely studied methods in life satisfaction research, probably because it is readily acceptable to and understood by individuals from diverse backgrounds and cultures *(13)*.

Subjective measures of quality of life

Early indicators of the quality of life were derived from measures of pollution, crowding, food, and other material standards of living. As Campbell & Converse *(14)* observed, however, discontent with objective or physical conditions in the United States had increased over a period of time when by most criteria those conditions had improved. It was because of such observations that interest in the assessment of subjective or perceived wellbeing increased dramatically in the 1970s.

Andrews & Withey *(1)* completed perhaps the most comprehensive and theoretically broadest investigation into the measurement and meaning of subjective wellbeing. For their study they devised a seven-point satisfaction scale, the extreme ends of which represent affectively rich descriptions of satisfactions and dissatisfactions. Their delighted–terrible scale, which is illustrated in Fig. 1, was designed to combine a cognitive evaluation with some degree of positive and/or negative feelings, i.e. "affect". Seeking to determine which aspects of life contribute to a person's satisfaction or dissatisfaction with life as a whole, Andrews & Withey administered a total of 123 "concern-level" items (items inquiring about specific aspects of life, each of which was rated on the seven-point delighted–terrible scale) and 68 global measures of the perceived quality of life (measures of satisfaction or happiness with life as a whole, many of which had been used in previously conducted studies and some of which are illustrated in Fig. 2) to a representative sample of over 5000 demographically well described adult Americans (18 years and older).

The findings of Andrews & Withey provide useful guidelines to anyone wishing to study the subjective wellbeing of well defined social groups. They

Table 1. Cantril's ladder of life with sample question

Here is a picture of a ladder. Suppose that a person who is entirely satisfied with his life would be at the top of the ladder, and a person who is extremely dissatisfied with his life would be at the bottom of the ladder.	
10	Best life I could expect to have
9	
8	
7	
6	
5	
4	
3	
2	
1	
0	Worst life I could expect to have
Where would you put yourself on the ladder at the present stage of your life in terms of how satisfied you are with your own personal life?	

Source: **Cantril, H.** *(12).*

recommended various combinations of concern-level items that might be included in questionnaires for use in future studies (see Table 2 for the selected 12 concerns that they found predicted 50–62% of the variance in evaluations of life as a whole as measured by various global items) but they stressed the importance of study-specific considerations in the selection of items: the concerns relevant to the population(s) to be studied; the substantive interests of the information users; the resources available for data collection; the desired precision of the measures to be used; and the method of data collection.

Measurement of Social Adjustment

Social adjustment is neither a unitary nor a global concept. Broadly defined it is the interplay between the individual and the social environment. In practice the concept primarily involves the evaluation of an individual's functioning in different roles, which are commonly accepted as appropriate. Normally an adult will function in most of the following roles: occupational,

Fig. 1. Delighted–terrible stage

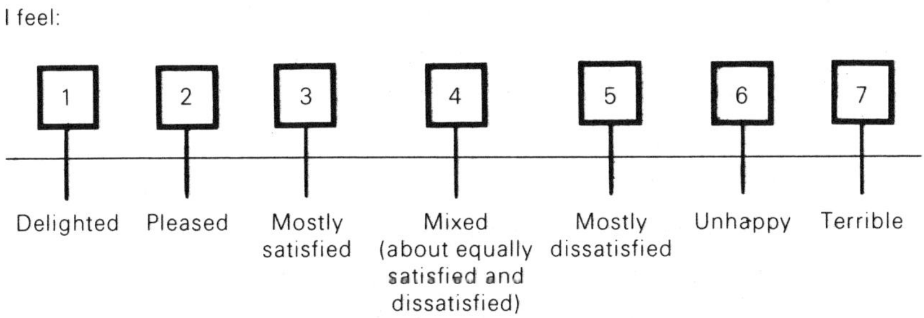

Source: **Andrews, F.M. & Withey, S.B.** *(1).*

Fig. 2. Some measures of life satisfaction

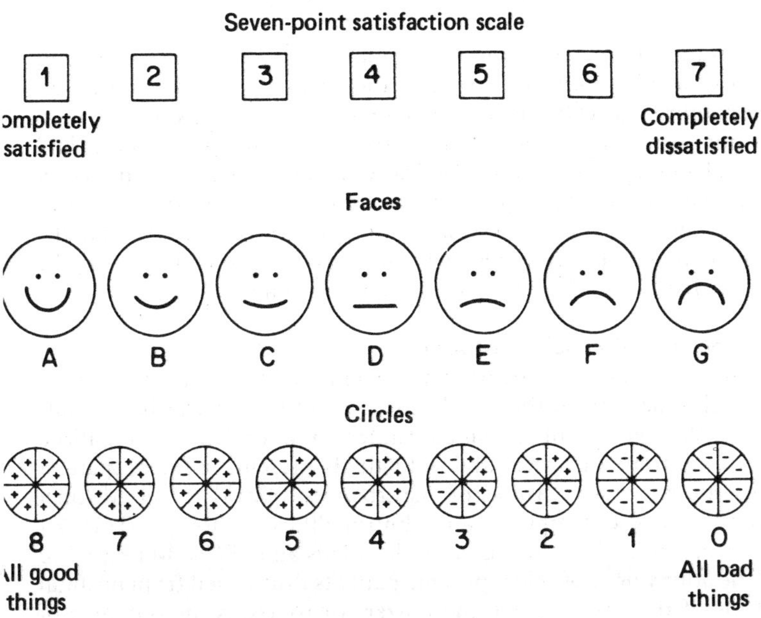

Source: **Andrews, F.M. & Withey, S.B.** *(1).*

Table 2. Selected 12 concerns

21	Yourself: what you are accomplishing and how you handle problems
4	Your own family life: your wife/husband, your marriage
83	The income you (and your family) have
28	The amount of fun and enjoyment you have
87	Your house/apartment
6	The things you and your family do together
38	The amount of time you have to do things you want to do
30	The way you spend your spare time, your non-working activities
106	What our national government is doing
101	The goods and services you get when you buy in this area: things such as food, appliances, clothes
7	Your own health and physical condition
75	Your job

Source: **Andrews, F.M. & Withey, S.B.** *(1)*.

as a paid employee or within the home; marital as a spouse and parent; within an extended family with parents, siblings and other close relatives; and in the community, with friends, acquaintances and groups. Within each role, functioning may be further divided into instrumental performance and affect, or behaviour and attitude. Typically the individual is evaluated in terms of the way his or her role performance conforms to the norms of his or her referrent group *(2)*. A discrepancy in the way the person and the environment fit together may result from a disability on the side of the individual or from disturbances in the social environment *(15)*.

Historical overview of social adjustment

In psychiatry, interest in patients' adjustment to the community was a natural development from the trend in treatment from custodial to outpatient care. Problems in the social adjustment of both deinstitutionalized patients with chronic disorders and individuals presenting for outpatient treatment required new measures of disturbances, ones that were distinct from those that assess symptoms and abnormalities of thought. The first scales in psychiatry, which appeared in the 1950s and 1960s, were used to evaluate the adjustment of schizophrenic patients discharged from hospital on regimens of the new major tranquillizers or to assess the outcome of psychotherapy in selected outpatient populations. In the 1970s, the systematic assessment of patients' social functioning became a routine part of the evaluation of their initial state as well as of the outcome of their treatment. More recently, new scales have been developed or adapted to assess the social adjustment of physically ill patients in recognition of the potential importance of this dimension in treatment and its outcome. By 1984, at least 31 published social adjustment scales had been found and reviewed *(2,15–17)*.

Typically two or three conceptual areas are measured with varying emphasis depending on the scale, but some scales concentrate on only one area. Scales can be roughly grouped into those that broadly measure functioning in a variety of roles, those that comprehensively measure functioning in only one or two roles, and those that measure social supports, networks or relationships *(17)*. A problem with many of the scales that provide comprehensive coverage of social adjustment is that symptoms of psychopathology are often contained in them, since certain symptoms are often additional aspects of the burden a person represents to his or her family and community. Even when symptoms *per se* are not included in a scale, however, behaviour that reflects psychopathology such as social withdrawal, friction with others or dissatisfaction are often reflected in one's social adjustment.

Social adjustment scales suitable for population studies

The authors selected two social adjustment scales that broadly measure social functioning in a variety of roles that do not include symptoms of psychopathology *per se*, and that have been found to be suitable for community studies of social adjustment. Each scale has an interview and a self-administered report version, with administration and scoring materials readily available. The self-administered report versions are the least expensive to administer, but there are disadvantages to them, e.g. illiterate informants need someone to read the inventory since some subjects may falsify their responses. Interviews in person cost more because of training and employing skilled interviewers, but they provide the most complete information because both respondent and interviewer ratings are made. Further, subjects need not be literate, and interviewers are likely to detect underreporting or falsification of responses *(2)*.

Inter-rater, inter-informant, and test–retest reliability has been demonstrated for both versions of the scales to be described, and good agreement between the self-administered and interview versions of each scale has been shown *(18–21)*. The scales have been found to discriminate between the adjustment scores of psychologically disturbed individuals and those with no disturbance, to be sensitive to change in functioning over time, and to distinguish the adjustment of people with different psychiatric diagnoses *(18–20,22–25)*. Further, the scales have been adapted and/or translated for use in clinical and community studies in the United Kingdom, the United States and a number of European countries.

Social adjustment scale (SAS) and social adjustment scale — self report (SAS-SR) (18,19,22–25)

Instrumental and affective performance in work (by worker, housewife or student), social and leisure activities, relationships with extended family, marital and parental adjustment and economic independence are assessed. Global evaluations are made for each role area by the interviewer when the interview is used. Each role area includes assessments of performance at tasks, interpersonal relations, friction, and satisfaction in roles. Adjustment is rated against an ideal norm for each item. Table 3 summarizes the structure and content of the SAS and SAS-SR, and for illustrative purposes mean scores for the social and leisure activities role and for overall adjustment among four populations in a single United States community are also included.

Forty-eight items in the interview and 42 in the self report are operationally defined and are rated on a five-point scale with higher scores indicating poorer adjustment. It takes 45–60 minutes to obtain information through a semi-structured interview and the self report takes 15–20 minutes. No less than two weeks and no more than two months is recommended as the time period to be assessed, to establish an adequate basis for assessment and to optimize recall and accurate reporting. Both the scoring sheet for the interview and the self-administered report are precoded for computer entry and analysis. Norms are available from United States studies on the SAS-SR for nonpatient community populations, acutely ill and recovered depressed outpatients, schizophrenics, alcoholics and methadone-maintained opiate addicts *(25)*. As can be seen in Table 3, the comparison of some SAS-SR scores among a community sample and three diagnostic groups indicates that depressives show poorer social adjustment in the role area shown, and overall, than all of the other groups.

Social maladjustment schedule (SMS) and social problem questionnaire (SPQ) (20,21)

The domains of marital and family relationships, other social relationships and activities, housing, occupation, leisure and income are assessed. Three general categories that are relevant to and cut across all domains are measured: (*a*) material conditions, which serve as an objective means with which to gauge functioning and satisfaction, include the assessment of the adequacy of finances, physical status, housing, available leisure and social activities, occupational and residential stability, opportunities for interpersonal interaction, and child management circumstances; (*b*) social management corresponds closely to instrumental role performance or how one behaves in the various domains; and (*c*) satisfaction is composed of ratings intended to measure the individual's attitudes towards various aspects of his or her life domains. Table 4 summarizes the structure and content of the SMS and SPQ, and provides an example of how different populations can produce different patterns or profiles of social maladjustment.

Forty-one ratings are made on both the interview schedule and self-administered report, but material conditions are not covered as comprehensively in the latter. A four-point scale indicates the absence or severity of each problem, and ratings of 0–3 are operationally defined in the interview, with higher ratings indicating more serious problems in both the interview and the self report. The interview is administered in about one hour and the self report takes about 5–10 minutes to complete. The time

Table 3. Social adjustment scale (SAS) and social adjustment scale — self report (SAS-SR)

Informant Patient — Subject
Significant other

Method SAS — Interview (45–60 minutes)
SAS-SR — Self-administered report (15–20 minutes)

Contents

Role areas	Qualitative aspects
Work (of worker, student, housewife)	Performance of tasks
Social and leisure	Interpersonal relations
Extended family	Friction
Marriage	Satisfaction
Parent	
Economic independence	

Sample SAS-SR item

How much time have you spent on hobbies or spare time interests during the last two weeks? For example, bowling, sewing, gardening, sports, reading?

1 ☐ I spent most of my spare time on hobbies almost every day.

2 ☐ I spent some spare time on hobbies some of the days.

3 ☐ I spent a little spare time on hobbies.

4 ☐ I usually did not spend any time on hobbies but did watch television.

5 ☐ I did not spend any spare time on hobbies or watching television.

Sample findings

SAS-SR mean role area scores[a] for social and leisure activities and for overall adjustment among four populations in a single United States community *(25)*

Population	*Social and leisure*	*Overall adjustment*
Community sample (N = 399)	1.83	1.59
Acute depressives (N = 172)	2.85	2.53
Alcoholics (N = 26)	2.50	2.23
Schizophrenics (N = 39)	2.40	1.96

[a] Mean score range from 1 to 5 with higher scores indicating greater impairment.

Table 4. Social maladjustment schedule (SMS) and social problem questionnaire (SPQ)

Informant	Patient — Subject Significant other	
Method	SMS — Interview (60 minutes) SPQ — Self-administered report (5–10 minutes)	
Contents	Housing conditions Occupation/social role Economic situation Leisure/social activities Family and domestic relationships Marital and sexual	Material conditions Social management Satisfaction

Sample SPQ item

How satisfied are you with the way you spend your leisure time?

0 ☐ Satisfied.

1 ☐ Slightly dissatisfied.

2 ☐ Moderately dissatisfied.

3 ☐ Severely dissatisfied.

Sample findings

Percentage reporting moderate or severe difficulties or dissatisfaction on selected SMS items among three United Kingdom populations studied *(20)*

Item	*Persons selected for social adversity* (N = 48)	*Women with pre-menstrual complaint* (N = 104)	*Chronic neurotic patients* (N = 221)
Satisfaction with occupation	27%	19%	43%
Management of income	19%	2%	10%
Satisfaction with income	21%	11%	29%
Opportunities for leisure activity	67%	20%	32%
Extent of leisure activity	60%	15%	44%
Satisfaction with leisure activity	33%	6%	31%

period assessed in both the interview and self-administered report is not specified, but the focus is on long-term functioning, including the present.

The comparison of three populations studied by Clare & Cairns *(20)* on the percentage of people reporting moderate or severe difficulties or dissatisfactions on selected items of the SMS, as shown in Table 4, demonstrate one way that SMS data can be summarized and subpopulations compared. People who were selected specifically because their physicians judged their social circumstances to be adverse, were found to be experiencing more difficulties and dissatisfactions than the other two groups as measured by five of the selected items. On two items, however, the chronic neurotic patients reported more dissatisfaction. The women with premenstrual complaints reported far fewer difficulties and dissatisfactions than the other groups.

Measurement of Psychiatric Symptoms

As mentioned before, the distinction between symptoms of psychopathology and impaired social functioning is not always clear. However, symptoms are primarily a reflection of internal psychological and physical states that may affect social relations, while social adjustment is a reflection of a person's interactions with others and of his or her performance and attitudes in roles. Some people may function reasonably well although symptomatic, and others may function poorly although asymptomatic *(18)*. A number of self-administered report scales have been developed to assess the absence, presence, intensity or frequency of the moods, feelings, sensations and behaviours that may constitute an episode of psychiatric illness *(3)*. In the clinic, the use of these symptom scales or screening instruments is considered to be a first stage, which sorts subjects into probable categories, leading to more extensive investigation of the probable cases at a second stage. For purposes of estimating psychiatric disturbance in the community, the symptom scales have been found to be a valid means of detecting depressive and anxiety states among respondents, but generally to be marginally useful for the identification of other forms of psychopathology in which depression and/or anxiety may not be prominent, or may be absent (such as schizophrenia) *(3)*. It has been suggested that these symptom scales may be seen as measuring demoralization rather than specific psychiatric disorders *(26)*.

Murphy *(3)* recently made an in-depth review of seven psychiatric screening instruments in which she identified five problems that arise when such instruments are used. These problems are: (*a*) "caseness"/severity or whether the instrument can measure how severe a condition is, as well as whether the condition represents a psychiatric illness or case; (*b*) psychiatric/medical or whether the instrument inadvertently identifies a medical illness rather than a psychiatric illness, since most contain a number of somatic symptoms; (*c*) chronic/acute or whether the instrument can distinguish between chronic and acute illnesses; (*d*) total/factor or whether the instrument, in addition to providing a total score, makes use of a factorial tructure from which more refined interpretations of scores can be made; and (*e*) validity or how criterion validity has been established, and which levels of *sensitivity* (ability to identify cases accurately) and *specificity* (ability to identify non-cases) have been found *(3)*. None of the seven scales reviewed by Murphy was found to overcome all of the five problems that she identified. However, all the scales were found to detect at least 80% of confirmed cases of depression and/or anxiety — states considered to represent the lowest common denominator in psychiatrically significant conditions.

Psychiatric symptom scales suitable for population studies

Two instruments that were reviewed by Murphy, both of which have been extensively studied in clinical and population studies in many countries, will be briefly described. Each was found to: (*a*) both detect cases *and* measure levels of severity; (*b*) avoid the identification of physically ill rather than psychiatrically ill patients (although psychiatrically ill people were often found to be physically ill); (*c*) identify acute rather than chronic conditions, but to detect long-standing conditions quite reliably; (*d*) make use of a factorial structure; and (*e*) show acceptable, though variable, standards of validity.

It is important to note that these instruments can be used in three ways in epidemiological surveys: as screening instruments, as estimators of psychopathology and as indicators of psychopathology. It is usually necessary to recalibrate such scales on representative samples of the population on whom they will be used, because validity coefficients obtained in one community do not necessarily hold in another. The validity coefficients should also be adjusted for the proportion of positive high scale scores that are expected in the survey and for the expected prevalence of cases, since sensitivity and specificity depend on the former and predictive values depend on the latter *(27)*.

Hopkins symptom checklist (HSCL) (28–30)

There are several versions of the HSCL, ranging from 25 to 90 items. The 90-item version, known as the SCL-90, goes beyond the original focus on neurotic symptoms and includes items selected to indicate paranoid ideation and psychoticism. The 25-item version consists of factors for depression and anxiety only. Other versions consist of 31, 35, 58, 64 and 71 items.

The time period assessed is the past week including today, and symptoms on the SCL-90 are rated on a five-point scale. The instructions clearly indicate that a symptom must have bothered or distressed the subject to be rated present, and response categories appear in order of severity from 0 (not at all) to 4 (extremely). The simplicity of the language is a major asset for minimizing any distortion of response. The items appear in most versions to follow a random order, which probably reduces the possibility that the respondent will give ratings befitting his or her interpretation of the order. Further, the random order ensures that the factors discerned have assembled items based on correlations that are not influenced by a preconceived notion of a dimension conveyed in the order of the items. Table 5 shows the factors and sample items from the HSCL, and provides a comparison of the percentage of symptomatic psychiatric outpatients and symptomatic nonpatients who were bothered by symptoms "at least a little bit" when they were studied by Derogatis using the SCL-90-R (SCR-90 revised) *(30)*.

General health questionnaire (GHQ) (31–33)
The GHQ, like the HSCL, is a self-administered report. The standard version (GHQ-60) consists of 60 items; there are 30 items in the most commonly used version, and 28 items in the "scaled" or factor analysed version. Its time period is defined as the past few weeks. It uses a four-category response pattern that directs the respondent to report symptoms in terms of whether he or she has been experiencing them the same or more than usual. One third of the items in the GHQ have been formulated so that a response that conveys the meaning of "no" is a pathological indicator, while for the remaining items a "yes" response indicates illness. Items are ordered from general health questions to psychiatric items and from less severe to more severe items. It contains many indicators of impaired function, which are generally not covered so well in other instruments. Table 6 shows the factors and sample items from the GHQ, and the effect of marital status on GHQ-60 total scores among community respondents in England and Australia, where about 90% of people with scores over 12 were found to have diagnosable psychopathology *(33)*.

Conclusion

Three types of measurement have been described that can be used to assess the psychosocial status of the general population. While each method assesses a different aspect of psychological or social wellbeing, there is some overlap in what each measures. For example, measuring people's satisfaction with various areas of their lives, which is a major component in the assessment of subjective wellbeing, is the most common way for social adjustment scales to assess people's "attitude" or "affect" in their roles. Despite such overlaps, the focus of each area is quite distinct. Studies of subjective wellbeing can reveal the areas of life that are most essential to a population's attitudes and feelings about life as a whole, as well as the characteristics and concerns of those who are unhappy or dissatisfied with their lives. Studies of social adjustment in the community can provide data on subjective and objective features of the social functioning or malfunctioning of a community's members in a number of important spheres. Studies of psychiatric symptoms can identify people in the community who may be suffering from a potentially significant psychiatric disorder, as well as estimate the number of people who are psychologically disturbed or demoralized.

Table 5. Hopkins symptom checklist (HSCL)

HSCL factors

Somatization
Obsessive compulsive
Interpersonal sensitivity
Depression
Anxiety

Hostility
Paranoid ideation
Psychoticism
} SCL-90 only

Sample instructions and items with rating scale

Listed below are symptoms or problems that people sometimes have. Please read each one carefully and decide how much the complaint bothered or distressed you during the past week, including today. Then put a check mark (✓) in any of the five boxes to show this.

How much were you bothered by:

	0 Not at all	1 A little bit	2 Moderately	3 Quite a bit	4 Extremely
Headaches	☐	☐	☐	☐	☐
Nervousness	☐	☐	☐	☐	☐

Sample findings

Psychiatric outpatients and symptomatic nonpatients bothered by selected SCL-90 symptoms at least "a little bit" *(30)*

Symptom	*Psychiatric outpatients* (N = 1002)	*Nonpatients* (N = 974)
Feeling low in energy or slowed down	82%	52%
Hot or cold spells	40%	18%
Feeling blue	88%	33%
Feeling easily annoyed or irritated	86%	57%
Crying easily	61%	16%
Feeling tense or keyed up	89%	48%
Feeling hopeless about the future	78%	18%
Feeling fearful	70%	15%
Headaches	67%	55%
Nervousness or shakiness inside	90%	40%

Table 6. General health questionnaire (GHQ)

GHQ factors

Somatic symptoms
Anxiety insomnia
Social dysfunction
Severe depression

Sample items with rating scale

Have you recently:

— been afraid you were going to collapse in a public place?	Not at all	No more than usual	Rather more than usual	Much more than usual
— felt on the whole you were doing things well?	Better than usual	Same as usual	Less than usual	Much less than usual

Sample findings

Effect of marital status on GHQ-60 score *(33)*

Study location, sample, sample size, etc.	Marital status		
	Single	Married and living together	Married but living apart/ separated/divorced
South Manchester, England Random community sample (N = 308)	(N = 60)	(N = 120)	(N = 28)
Mean GHQ score	5.00	6.29	8.40
Proportion with scores >12[a]	15%	22%	36%

	Single	Married	Separated/ divorced	Widowed
Perth, Australia Random community sample (N = 2314)				
Males (N = 1089)	(N = 282)	(N = 779)	(N = 14)	(N = 14)
Proportion with scores >12[a]	15%	13%	29%	14%
Females (N = 1225)	(N = 230)	(N = 896)	(N = 34)	(N = 65)
Proportion with scores >12[a]	21%	18%	29%	19%

[a] GHQ scores greater than 12 were on average found to identify correctly 90% of persons with psychiatric problems, and scores of 12 and under were found to classify correctly on average 90% of persons without psychiatric problems.

Which approach is selected will depend on the information needs of the investigators, but if a comprehensive assessment of the psychosocial status of a population is desired, employing a combination of the three methods would appear to be most useful. People who are unhappy or dissatisfied with their lives are not necessarily socially maladjusted nor psychologically disturbed; those who are found to be psychologically disturbed will not always claim to be dissatisfied with life, etc. Empirical evidence suggests that a multidimensional approach to the assessment of psychosocial status is both useful and desirable in community studies *(27)*. Such an approach has the advantage of supplying information users with a more meaningful view of the psychosocial status of the population *(34)*.

References

1. **Andrews, F.M. & Withey, S.B.** *Social indicators of well-being.* New York, Plenum Press, 1976.
2. **Weissman, M.M.** The assessment of social adjustment: a review of techniques. *Archives of general psychiatry,* **32**: 357–365 (1975).
3. **Murphy, J.M.** *Psychiatric instrument development for primary care research: patient self-report questionnaire.* Rockville, MD, Division of Biometry and Epidemiology, National Institute of Mental Health, 1981 (NIMH Contract No. 80M014280101D).
4. **Endicott, J. & Spitzer, R.L.** A diagnostic interview: the schedule for affective disorders and schizophrenia. *Archives of general psychiatry,* **35**: 837–844 (1978).
5. **Spitzer, R.L. et al.** Research diagnostic criteria: rationale and reliability. *Archives of general psychiatry,* **35**: 773–782 (1978).
6. **Wing, J.K. et al.** *The measurement and classification of psychiatric symptoms.* London, Cambridge University Press, 1974.
7. **Wing, J.K. et al.** Reliability of the PSE (ninth edition) used in a population study. *Psychological medicine,* **7**: 505–516 (1977).
8. **Robins, L.N. et al.** National Institute of Mental Health diagnostic interview schedule: its history, characteristics, and validity. *Archives of general psychiatry,* **38**: 381–389 (1981).
9. **Gurin, G. et al.** *Americans view their mental health.* New York, Basic Books, 1960.
10. **Bradburn, N. & Caplovitz, D.** *Reports on happiness.* Chicago, IL, Aldine, 1965.
11. **Atkinson, T.** The stability and validity of quality of life measures. *Social indicators research,* **10**: 113–132 (1982).
12. **Cantril, H.** *The pattern of human concerns.* New Brunswick, NJ, Rutgers University Press, 1965.
13. **Carley, M.** *Social measurement and social indicators: issues of policy and theory.* London, George Allen & Unwin, 1965.
14. **Campbell, A. & Converse, P.E., ed.** *The human meaning of social change.* New York, Russell Sage Foundation, 1972.

15. **Katchnig, H.** Methods for measuring social adjustment. *In:* Helgason, T., ed. *Methodology in evaluation of psychiatric treatment.* London, Cambridge University Press, 1983, pp. 205–218.
16. **Weissman, M.M. et al.** The assessment of social adjustment: an update. *Archives of general psychiatry,* **38**: 1250–1258 (1981).
17. **John, K. & Weissman, M.M.** The measurement of psychosocial and familial aspects of depression. *In:* Hirschfeld, R.M.A. & Marsella, A.J., ed. *The measurement of depression: clinical, biological, psychological and psychosocial perspectives.* New York, Guilford Press (in press).
18. **Weissman, M.M. et al.** The social role performance of depressed women: comparisons with a normal group. *American journal of orthopsychiatry,* **41**: 390–405 (1971).
19. **Bothwell, S. & Weissman, M.M.** Social impairment four years after an acute depressive episode. *American journal of orthopsychiatry,* **47**: 231–237 (1977).
20. **Clare, A.W. & Cairns, V.E.** Design, development and use of a standardized interview to assess social maladjustment and dysfunction in community studies. *Psychological medicine,* **8**: 589–604 (1978).
21. **Corney, R.H. et al.** The development of a self-report questionnaire to identify social problems — a pilot study. *Psychological medicine,* **2**: 903–909 (1982).
22. **Paykel, E.S. et al.** Dimensions of social adjustment in depressed women. *Journal of nervous and mental disease,* **152**: 158–172 (1971).
23. **Weissman, M.M. & Paykel, E.S.** *The depressed woman: a study of social relationships.* Chicago, Chicago University Press, 1974.
24. **Weissman, M.M. & Bothwell, S.** Assessment of social adjustment by patient self-report. *Archives of general psychiatry,* **33**: 1111–1115 (1976).
25. **Weissman, M.M. et al.** Social adjustment by self-report in a community sample and in psychiatric outpatients. *Journal of nervous and mental disease,* **166**: 317–326 (1978).
26. **Dohrenwend, B.P. et al.** Nonspecific psychological distress and other dimensions of psychopathology. *Archives of general psychiatry,* **37**: 1229–1239 (1980).
27. **Williams, P. et al.** Case definition and case identification in psychiatric epidemiology: review and assessment. *Psychological medicine,* **10**: 101–114 (1980).
28. **Parloff, M.B. et al.** Comfort, effectiveness and self-awareness as criteria of improvement in psychotherapy. *American journal of psychiatry,* **3**: 343–351 (1954).
29. **Derogatis, L.R. et al.** SCL-90: an outpatient psychiatric rating scale. Preliminary report. *Psychopharmacology bulletin,* **9**: 13–28 (1973).
30. **Derogatis, L.R.** *SCL-90-R (revised) version manual I.* Baltimore, MD, Johns Hopkins University School of Medicine, 1977.
31. **Goldberg, D.P.** *The detection of psychiatric illness by questionnaire.* London, Oxford University Press, 1972.
32. **Goldberg, D.P. & Hiller, V.F.** A scaled version of the General Health Questionnaire. *Psychological medicine,* **9**: 139–145 (1979).

33. **Goldberg, D.** *Manual of the general health questionnaire.* London, NFER Publishing Company, 1979.
34. **Mechanic, D.** The epidemiology of illness behavior and its relationship to physical and psychological distress. *In:* Mechanic, D., ed. *Symptoms, illness behavior and help-seeking.* New York, Prodist, 1982, pp. 1–24.

7.4 Measures of wellbeing in the elderly[a] — *G.G. Fillenbaum*

Populations are aging worldwide *(1)*. The problems of these older populations are not purely medical and their disorders are rarely curable; rather they require continuing care to facilitate their independence and personal wellbeing in the least restrictive setting feasible. The measurement of wellbeing in older adults should be comprehensive, covering not only their functional health but also their financial wellbeing and social support. Fortunately, multidimensional functional assessment strategies have been developed that facilitate comprehensive assessment, assist in evaluating alternatives in the allocation of available resources in an effective manner, and provide a means for monitoring changes in the wellbeing of the elderly.

Aging tends to be accompanied by social loss as well as personal decline. Couples become widowed; children may be scattered and may themselves be growing infirm; friends, siblings and relatives die. People retire from the labour force, which often entails both a drop in income and a reduced ability to maintain financial status in the face of inflation. The illnesses of later life are more likely to be chronic than acute and to be multiple rather than single. Hospital stays, when they occur, tend to last longer than is the case for younger people. Some age-related conditions, such as decline in vision and hearing, manifest themselves in obvious ways. Changes in mental functioning, sometimes subtle, also occur. While neither serious nor markedly disabling for most people, the progressive deterioration in cognitive function that afflicts a minority of older adults severely disrupts personal and family life. Depression, an affective disorder that afflicts a larger proportion of older people, may also be disabling.

Since such losses and declines rarely occur in isolation, the assessment of people in later life needs to take into account both the individual and the setting in which the person lives. While medical and psychiatric diagnoses are necessary to determine etiology, in the elderly full evaluation must focus on the capacity for independent living, a concept that encompasses both personal performance and personal circumstances, and thus requires a multidimensional approach.

Basic Characteristics and Preferred Attributes of Multidimensional Assessment Procedures

The procedures that have been developed to provide a multidimensional assessment strive to be comprehensive and take into account the multiple aspects of individual functioning and the characteristics of the individual's broader environment. They should meet the same scientific standards

[a] This chapter was prepared with the partial support of the Sandoz Foundation and draws on "Assessing the well-being of the elderly: why and how functional assessment is being done in the United States and abroad" which appeared in *Advances in research*, **8**(1) (1984).

expected of any well designed test *(2)*. If the information obtained is to be considered seriously and not to lend itself readily to out-of-hand dismissal, the assessment must be shown to be valid for each dimension considered (measure what it claims to measure), reliable (the same circumstances should yield the same response and the same interpretation), and sensitive (able to identify change). The multidimensional assessments considered here provide information on one or more of these criteria.

To ensure that all relevant information is obtained a structured or semi-structured standardized approach is recommended. Standardization helps ensure that information remains meaningful, regardless of where or when collected, as long as it is gathered by suitably trained people. While a structured, standardized approach to assessment is to some extent restricting, the advantage it affords of comparability of information and speed of administration and data handling outweighs the disadvantages.

Assessment procedures should also be easy to administer, unobjectionable to those asked to respond, and readily interpretable. Time is important to many investigators and clinicians. It is necessary to weigh the time and costs involved in administration, interpretation and data handling against respondent fatigue and the value of the information obtained. While it is expensive to gather information that is not needed, it may be even more expensive in the long term not to gather needed information.

All multidimensional assessment procedures must provide some means of summarizing information to facilitate its understanding, interpretation and use by practitioners and decision-makers. Available assessment procedures continue to be relatively weak in this regard. Accordingly, broadly applicable summarization procedures, that are relevant at an individual level and can be aggregated to a population level, will be described.

Basic Dimensions of Assessment: Emerging Consensus

A review of the major English language multidimensional assessment procedures indicates that there is an important core of agreement on seven dimensions that should be examined: (*a*) activities of daily living; (*b*) physical health; (*c*) mental health/cognitive functioning; (*d*) social resources; (*e*) economic resources; (*f*) environmental matters; and (*g*) level of strain on the care giver.

The first three dimensions — activities of daily living, physical health and mental health — are areas of personal functioning. The fourth and fifth dimensions, social and economic resources, are of concern to the broader society to which the individual belongs, as well as to the older adult. The final two dimensions, environmental matters and strain on the care giver, are factors that may influence the continued capacity to live in the community or within a particular environment. Each of these seven topics is itself multidimensional.

Activities of daily living (ADL)

Two major aspects of ADL should be considered: physical activities and instrumental activities.

Physical ADL (PADL) refers to self-care tasks such as feeding, transferring, dressing, continence and care of self at the toilet, and bathing. Walking (mobility) is sometimes included here although it should more properly be considered a separate type of activity *(3)*. Most of the physical ADL scales included in multidimensional assessments are derived from measures developed by Katz and his colleagues *(3–5)*. Some assessments use the original Katz scale. The items of that scale reflect the order of mastery in infancy. The illustrated items are presented in this order. As capacity deteriorates, loss is typically in the reverse direction.

Aside from problems with walking, which makes getting around difficult, few older people living at home have problems with basic physical activities as can be seen from the upper section of Table 1. Only among the very old, those aged 85 and over, does a substantial percentage need help.

Table 1. Number of persons per 1000 needing help with selected activities of daily living, in the United States in 1979

Activities of daily living	People of both sexes aged:			
	55–64 years	65–74 years	75–84 years	85+ years
Physical activities of daily living				
Bathing	11.1	20.4	50.7	172.9
Dressing	8.8	14.4	32.9	116.6
Using toilet	6.0	11.6	28.4	104.9
Getting in or out of bed or chair	6.0	9.0	25.8	72.5
Eating	2.8	3.9	8.4	37.6
Instrumental activities of daily living				
Shopping	21.6	43.6	118.5	354.9
Chores	24.8	41.2	98.3	293.4
Handling money	7.3	15.2	51.1	175.5
Meals	14.6	25.3	65.4	224.7
Needs help with one or more physical activities[a]	28.6	52.6	114.0	348.4
Needs help with one or more instrumental activities	31.9	57.3	141.8	399.0

[a] In addition to the five items listed includes walking and going outside.

Source: **Feller, B.A.** *(6)*.

Instrumental ADL (IADL) refers to those activities needed for continued residence in the community. Consequently attempts have been made to measure the capacity to perform activities important in particular cultural settings. For instance, IADL measures used in New Zealand may include gardening, in the Netherlands bed-making, and in the United Kingdom making tea. Cultural specificity unfortunately restricts the generalizability of use. It is therefore important to note that a validated modification of the original Lawton & Brody *(7)* IADL scale, broadly used because of its adaptation for the Older Americans Resources and Services (OARS) questionnaire *(8)* and for the 1979 US National Health Interview Survey *(6)*, consists of only five hierarchical items, each of which seem to be acceptable across the more developed nations. In ascending order of difficulty these items are: handling personal finances, preparing meals, shopping, getting to places beyond walking distance (transportation being available) and cleaning the house *(9)*. Information on four of these areas is given in the middle of Table 1. As can be seen, elderly community residents experience difficulty more frequently with instrumental than with physical ADL tasks. Family and friends generally help with such activities, but should none be available non-professionals would be adequate for the task. It is the capacity to perform instrumental tasks that, in the first instance, determines whether or not the individual can live independently.

Physical health

To determine whether personal physical health (rather than, say, mental health) has an impact on functional capacity, information is often sought on some combination of the following topics:

— self-assessment of health;

— presence of physical symptoms;

— diagnosed illnesses or conditions, and medications;

— level of activity;

— use of medical services;

— measures of incapacity (number of days spent disabled or in bed).

In measuring these topics, there may be problems of definition, interpretation and recall. Each may also be affected by cultural expectations and practices, and by such structural matters as access to and use of the formal medical care system. Multidimensional assessments typically include a self-assessment of health and a report of days incapacitated. Some also inquire into symptoms (in one case, the Comprehensive Assessment Referral and Evaluation (CARE), in sufficient depth that diagnosis is possible *(10)*) and others into diagnosed conditions, the emphasis being not on the condition but on the extent to which the condition hinders activities. Available procedures rarely use indicators of the quality of physical functioning (e.g. capacity for exercise, or stamina) although they could be included. The questionnaire used in the World Health Organization 11-country study *(11)* includes items concerned with intensive activity, for example:

> 51. Do you practise physical exercise, such as brisk walking, jogging or swimming, etc. now? . . . *If yes*, . . . (*b*) . . . how many hours a day . . . ? . . . (*c*) . . . do you usually do it: slowly? briskly? strenuously?
>
> 52. How many kilometres do you usually walk to improve your physical fitness?

In question 53 usual activity level can be graded from heavy activity (such as work done by a miner) to none (e.g. bedbound, housebound). The Duke-UNC Health Profile (DUHP) *(12)*, an adult health status instrument for use in ambulatory primary health care settings, emphasizes wellness rather than illness. For instance, it inquires about the ability to run 5 miles (8 km) since the ability to do that is considered to indicate an optimal state of physical function.

Mental health

Assessment of the mental health of the elderly is typically concerned with:

- the level of cognitive functioning;
- the presence of symptoms indicative of psychiatric disorder;
- a personal assessment of emotional wellbeing; and
- indicators of the quality of mental health functioning.

Although the proportion of elderly people whose cognitive functioning deteriorates to such an extent that they become a danger to themselves and to others is small (overall less than 4% among those aged 65 and over) they are nevertheless a group in need of extensive services, which are costly both in terms of money and of anguish to their families. For these reasons multidimensional assessments invariably include a measure intended to provide information on the level of cognitive functioning. A number of short instruments exist, e.g. the Mental Status Questionnaire *(13)*, the Mini-Mental State Examination *(14)* and the Short Portable Mental Status Questionnaire *(15)*. It should be noted that these do not necessarily accurately identify dementia *(16,17)*.

While there is general agreement about the necessity to ascertain the likely presence (or absence) of cognitive impairment, there is less agreement about the desirable extent of detailed enquiry into other areas of psychiatric functioning and mental health. Some instruments examine the sense of wellbeing or morale and try to determine whether any other psychiatric disorder is present (e.g. the DUHP *(12)*, the Multilevel Assessment Instrumental (MAI) *(18)* and OARS *(8)*). So in assessing mental wellbeing they try to determine the attitude to life (OARS) or focus on morale (MAI, DUHP). Examples of questions asked are given in Table 2. Other instruments try to determine the class of psychiatric disorder present (e.g. neurosis or psychosis, see the Survey Psychiatric Assessment Schedule *(19)*). Yet others try

Table 2. Representative questions on mental wellbeing from selected multidimensional instruments

OARS Questionnaire. Questions from mental health section *(8)*

31. How often would you say you worry about things — very often (0), fairly often (1) or hardly ever (2)?

32. In general, do you find life exciting (2), pretty routine (1) or dull (0)?

33. Taking everything into consideration how would you describe your satisfaction with life in general at the present time — good (2), fair (1) or poor (0)?

35. How would you rate your mental or emotional health at the present time — excellent (3), good (2), fair (1) or poor (0)?

MAI. Questions from morale section of personal adjustment domain *(17)*

59. Do things keep getting worse as you get older?	Yes	No
65. Do you have a lot to be sad about?	Yes	No
66. Do you take things hard?	Yes	No

Duke-UNC Health Profile. Questions from emotional status section *(11)*

	Yes, describes me exactly		*Somewhat describes me*		*No, doesn't describe me at all*
43. I don't feel useful.	0	1	2	3	4
45. I like who I am.	4	3	2	1	0
46. I feel hopeful about the future.	4	3	2	1	0
47. I try to look my best.	4	3	2	1	0
48. I am a clumsy person.	0	1	2	3	4
50. I like meeting new people.	4	3	2	1	0

to obtain a formal psychiatric diagnosis. CARE *(10)* now provides scales that are powerful discriminators of, among other problems, depression and dementia *(20,21)*. These instruments share a common property in that they are simple to administer and to score.

Where functional assessment is concerned, it may be neither necessary nor appropriate to obtain a precise diagnosis, because what one needs to know is whether the individual's cognitive and emotional condition facilitates or hinders personal and social functioning.

Measures of excellence in mental health are difficult to find and have not yet been incorporated into most assessments of mental health. While such measures do appear to be feasible, multidimensional approaches presently tend to rely on interviewer assessments of the quality of mental health functioning rather than on structured evaluations. The desirability of incorporating measures of excellence in mental health is demonstrated by recent findings. Based on longitudinal (rather than the more usual cross-sectional) data, Haug et al. *(22)* determined that in an older population resident in the community self-assessed mental health and psychiatric symptoms were more likely to remain stable, or to improve, than to decline (see Table 3). The findings were influenced by the manner in which mental health was measured. While psychological symptoms tended to remain stable, somatic symptoms of the type used to assess psychiatric status were distinctly more variable. Physical health status helped to explain the variance in the check list of somatic symptoms, and also helped to explain the change in self-assessed mental health, but contributed little to explaining the changes that occurred in psychological symptoms. Haug et al. *(22)* point out that many somatic symptoms included in mental health scales may indeed indicate that something is wrong, but where the elderly are concerned such indicators may reflect physiological not psychological difficulties. Misinterpreting these responses may result in an overestimate of mental health difficulties.

Social resources

Where older people are concerned, the assessment of social resources typically focuses on:

— the extent and adequacy of their contacts with family and friends, and

— the extent to which family and friends provide help or are likely to do so in time of need.

Table 3. Percentage change[a] in the mental health of a random sample of elderly people resident in the community over a one-year period

Mental health measures	Decline	No change	Improvement
Self-assessed health	31.9	36.3	31.5
Psychiatric symptom scale	33.7	26.7	39.7
Psychological symptom scale	14.4	66.9	18.6
Somatic symptom scale	25.2	50.4	24.6

[a] For details of statistical testing of these data consult Haug et al. *(22)*. Percentages do not always total 100 because of rounding.

Personally satisfying contact with others is considered an important aspect of the quality of life, and may protect against deterioration. Detailed inquiry is usually unnecessary since research indicates that maximum satisfaction is attained if there is a single confidant and at least four satisfying social relationships *(23)*.

Economic resources
The underlying concern of inquiry in this area is to determine whether income is adequate. The definition of "adequate" income, however, is rather difficult. Not only are practical issues involved, such as determining the basic amount of income needed for maintenance in society and the extent to which needs may be met from non-income sources (e.g. growing one's own food, sharing housing with others), but also matters of equity and policy (how should the standard of living of the elderly compare with their own earlier standard and with that of those currently working; to what extent is society prepared to support those who cannot support themselves?). Such issues are considered at length by Townsend *(24)*. Questions may range from very specific inquiry into precise sources and amounts of income and outlay, to the very general, such as an approximate idea of annual income and "in-kind" services, and subjective assessments of income adequacy. Because of wide variations among countries inquiry in this area must be tailored to local circumstances.

Environmental matters
Although there is increasing recognition that the architectural aspects of living environments and the social milieu of housing can facilitate or hinder continued personal independence, adequate brief structured assessments have not yet been developed. Several multidimensional assessments direct some inquiry into certain environmental aspects (e.g. CARE. MAI, Kilsyth *(25)*). Adequate environmental assessment should include information on the adequacy of housing in terms of shelter, privacy and cost; the safety of the surroundings from both a structural and personal point of view; the availability of and convenient access to services; and personal preferences about living arrangements. Environmental assessment procedures should have a high priority in future research on functional assessment.

Level of strain on care givers
It has been estimated that 5–10% of older community residents have an impairment level comparable with that of those residing in institutions. Many impaired people remain at home only because of the support they receive from family, as well as from friends and community agency sources. We can expect to see in the near future the development of better measures to assess the strain on care givers.

Overview of Selected Multidimensional Assessment Instruments for Use among Older Residents

Many multidimensional functional assessments are available *(26)*. Here the focus will be on three English-language instruments, selected because they are intended for use with all older community residents; they assess health, social and environmental issues; they appear to meet basic requirements of reliability, validity and sensitivity; and they can be administered by non-clinicians. Details of content, administration and population samples are summarized in Table 4. Each instrument will be described very briefly here.

CARE *(10,20,27–29)*

The original CARE consists of some 1500 items, primarily derived from a variety of well validated sources, designed to examine psychiatric, physical and social/environmental problems and their etiology and impact, the resources the individual can bring to bear on these problems, and the likely effect of these problems on the individual and those providing support. Information is summarized in a number of ways: primary among these are 10-point rating scales of positive and negative functioning. The 10-point physical assets scale, for instance, ranges from a score of 9 (abundance of assets: vigour, resilience, endurance, strength) to a score of 0 (no significant assets); no guide is given for intermediate ratings and assessments seem to be mainly interviewer-based. On the negative functioning scale, the 10 rating points are extensively and explicitly described. The medical symptom severity scale, for instance, shades from a rating of 0 (no significant symptoms) through minor (mild symptoms, ratings can range from 1 to 5), major symptoms (with an overlapping rating range of 4 to 8) to crucial (severe symptoms, with an overlapping range of 7 to 9).

The full questionnaire was used on random samples of elderly community residents in New York (N = 445) and London (N = 396) *(30)*. Based on the data obtained, the questionnaire was considerably refined. From the original 50 topics, 22 homogeneous scales were developed based on 314 items. These constitute CORE-CARE, a very efficient, comprehensive assessment. For increased specificity, when the focus is on depression, dementia and functional disability, a briefer instrument, SHORT-CARE, is available. Table 5 lists the 22 homogeneous indicator scales, and indicates the number of items in each scale. The activity limitations scale, which is probably the most relevant here, includes a combination of PADL, IADL and health items inquiring, for instance, about the ability to use the toilet, bath or shower, dress and cut toenails; the ability to prepare meals, go shopping and get to the doctor; and problems doing chores, carrying packages, and getting around because of health. Reliability (Cronbach's alpha, inter-rater reliability) and validity (face validity, convergent, discriminant, concurrent and predictive validity) have been carefully examined and reported.

No classification system is yet available that would take into account concomitant status on all scales. However, a "personal time dependency" measure has been developed. This is a 5-level measure on which is rated the extent to which an individual is personally dependent on another. It is based on type of physical incapacity, severity of dementia, and receipt of service intended to address a specific handicap. Investigation indicates that as personal time dependency increases, the amount of time for which help is needed and the level of skill demanded of the provider also increase *(31)*.

Table 4. Overview of content, samples and administration of three English-language multidimensional functional assessment questionnaires of established validity and reliability

	CARE[a]	MAI	OARS
Activities of daily living			
Instrumental	++	++	++
Physical	++	++	++
Physical health			
Self-assessment	+	+	+
Symptomatology	++	0	0
Diagnoses, medications	+	+	++
Medical services	+	+	+
Level of activity	+	++	++
Social impairment (bed days)	++	++	++
Mental health			
Cognitive functioning	++	++	++
Symptomatology/diagnosis	++	+	+
Self-assessment	+	+	+
Excellence of functioning	+	0	+
Social resources			
Contacts with family, friends	++	++	++
Availability of help	++	+	++
Economic			
Income	+	+	++
Environmental			
Environmental matters	++	++	0
Care giver			
Level of strain	++	0	0
Other areas examined			
Nutrition	++	+	+
Time use	0	++	0
Services	+	+	++
Main samples			
Type	Random	Purposive	Random
Main location	New York/London	Philadelphia	State, local
Approximate number	900	600	10 000
Age	≧65	≧65	≧55
Setting appropriateness			
Community	+	+	+
Institution	+	+	+
Type of questionnaire			
Structured	+	+	+
Semistructured			
Administration			
Interviewer (nonprofessional)	+	+	+
Professional			
Self			+
Average administration time	90 min	45 min	45 min
Summary scores	++	++	++

[a] Information applies to the original CARE instrument. For recent modified versions consult references.

0 = absent or essentially so, or not applicable.
\+ = present, minimal or type.
++ = present, adequate.

Table 5. CORE-CARE: 22 homogeneous indicator scales

Type of problem	Scale name	No. of items
Psychiatric problems	Cognitive impairment	10
	Depression/demoralization	29
	Subjective memory problems	9
Physical problems	Somatic symptoms	34
	Heart disorder	15
	Stroke effects	9
	Cancer	6
	Respiratory symptoms	6
	Arthritis	9
	Leg problems	9
	Sleep disorder	8
	Hearing disorder	14
	Vision disorder	11
	Hypertension	4
	Ambulation problems	27
	Activity limitation	39
Service needs	Service utilization	15
Environmental/social problems	Financial hardship	8
	Dissatisfaction with neighbourhood	8
	Fear of crime	18
	Social isolation	34
	Retirement dissatisfaction	7

MAI

The MAI *(18)* is the only questionnaire discussed here that is specifically designed to put into operation a conceptual model of the wellbeing of older people. It is a structured questionnaire, administered by an interviewer, covering all areas (except strain on the care giver) and designed so that a full-, medium- or short-length assessment may be made depending on the assessor's intentions and constraints.

The seven major domains examined in the MAI and their sub-indices are listed in Table 6. The domain of activities of daily living, for instance, has two sub-indices: personal self-maintenance (PADL) and instrumental ADL. There are seven PADL items: feeding oneself, dressing, grooming, getting around, getting in and out of bed, bathing oneself, and frequency of incontinence. All items but the last are scored so that a code of 3 means the item can be performed unaided, 2 that some help is needed, and 1 that the item cannot be done even with help. Incontinence, which is recorded on a 4-point scale (4 = never incontinent; 3 = less than once a week; 2 = once or twice a week; 1 = more than twice a week) is recoded, with 4 given a value

Table 6. MAI: major domains and domain sub-indices

Domain	Sub-indices	No. of items
Physical health	Self-rated health	4
	Health behaviour	3
	Health conditions	25
	Health aid	1
Cognitive	Mental status	11
	Cognitive symptoms	4
Activities of daily living	Personal self-maintenance	7
	Instrumental ADL	9
Time use	Activities	19
Personal adjustment	Morale	9
	Psychiatric symptoms	5
Social interaction	Interaction with friends	5
	Interaction with family	3
	Additional items	8
Perceived environment	Housing quality	9
	Neighbourhood quality	12
	Personal security	3

of 3, and 3 a value of 2. The scores are then added up. The possible range of scores is 7–21. The same applies to IADL. The items here inquire about use of the telephone, travel, shopping, meal preparation, housework, handyman work, laundry, taking medicine and managing personal finances. Each item is scored on a 3-point scale (3 = can perform unaided; 2 = can perform only with help; 1 = cannot perform even with help). The score on each IADL item is added. The possible range is 9–27. To obtain the domain index score, the scores on the two sub-indices (PADL and IADL) are added together. The higher the scores, the better the status. Cut-off scores, e.g. to determine eligibility for institutional purposes, can be selected as appropriate. Standardization data indicate that there are differences in level of PADL and IADL functioning among community residents capable of self-maintenance, those receiving in-home services, and those waiting to enter an institution (see Table 7).

Summary scores for each of the 17 sub-indices are obtained in the same way, i.e. by adding up the raw scores (or occasionally the standardized scores). These summary scores are then added together to obtain domain

Table 7. MAI: group means and standard deviations in the activities of daily living domain

Domain and sub-indices	Community residents		Public housing		In-home services		Institution waiting list	
	$\bar{x}$	SD	$\bar{x}$	SD	$\bar{x}$	SD	$\bar{x}$	SD
Activities of daily living								
Personal self-maintenance	20.61	1.18	20.77	0.64	19.26	2.49	18.51	2.81
Instrumental ADL	24.51	3.66	25.15	2.72	19.86	3.98	18.15	4.91
Domain index (sum of sub-indices)	45.12	4.57	45.92	3.07	39.12	6.03	36.66	6.97

scores. Interviewers can also make domain summary ratings on a 5-point scale. The descriptors for the points of the scale vary from domain to domain, but in general a rating of 5 represents good functioning, 4 mildly, 3 moderately, 2 severely and 1 totally impaired functioning. Although these are subjective assessments, inter-rater agreement has been found to be high (around 95%). Users should note that the manner of administration of the mental status examination differs from the usual approach, subjects being allowed to use memory aids. This should result in a lower prevalence of cognitive impairment than when assessed more conventionally.

OARS multidimensional functional assessment questionnaire *(8,32,33)*
The Duke OARS questionnaire is the only functional assessment questionnaire of those discussed that examines in detail both overall functional status and service use. It does not, however, include an assessment of environmental factors or of the strain on care givers.

For each of the five areas considered (social, economic, mental health, physical health, ADL) information can be summarized on a 6-point rating scale (in contrast with the MAI 5-point rating scale). The rating points are uniform across scales, with 1 representing excellent, 2 good, 3 mildly impaired, 4 moderately impaired, 5 severely impaired and 6 totally impaired functioning. In addition factor analysis of the OARS questionnaire has produced a number of factorially pure scales (Table 8). This structured questionnaire can be self- or interviewer-administered. It has been used for clinical assessment, epidemiological surveys, programme evaluation and service planning. A variety of applications has generated information on the functional status of over 10 000 older adults. An institutional adaptation is available. OARS is at present the most widely used functional assessment questionnaire in the United States. Its psychometric properties have been examined and reported.

Table 8. OARS: factorial structure of functional areas

Area	Factorially derived scales	No. of items
Social resources (9 items, plus additional subparts)	Social support — interaction	3
	Social support — dependability	2
	Social support — affective	2
Economic resources (16 items, plus additional subparts)	Perceived economic status	6
Mental health (6 items, plus additional subparts)	Satisfaction	6
	Sleep disturbance	2
	Energy vs. lethargy	6
	Paranoia	3
Physical health (14 items, plus additional subparts)	Subjective assessment	2
Activities of daily living (14 items)	Instrumental ADL	7
	Physical ADL	6

Summarizing Information and Developing Individual and Population Profiles

While summarization of information is not crucial at a clinical level (where detailed information is desirable), a summary overall view is essential to understand population status, assess service impact and for programme planning and evaluation.

Summarization techniques based on measures of mortality and morbidity have been reviewed by Goldberg & Dab in Chapter 7.5, and by Balinsky & Berger *(34)*. The interest here lies in considering alternative approaches to summarizing a broad array of information using methods relevant at an individual level and aggregatable to a population level. Because most of the work in this area has been done using the OARS questionnaire, data from that questionnaire will be used in illustration. The approaches discussed, however, have general applicability.

Summarizing information within areas of functioning

Within a functional area (such as physical health), sets of items may be grouped together into a limited number of unidimensional subscales using appropriate statistical techniques (e.g. factor analysis) or, where this is not feasible, by combining items that share a common conceptual basis (e.g. number of impairments). Such unidimensional measures are available in CARE, MAI and OARS. The availability of such information is important when trying to identify specific problems in functioning, targeting services or assessing the impact of specific service interventions. If an overall assessment of functional status in a particular area is desired, a single summary rating may be used. MAI uses 5-point, OARS 6-point and the original CARE 10-point rating scales.

Aggregation across areas: an overall view

Multidimensional assessments have been developed because of the importance of considering the whole person. How, then, can the mass of individual pieces of information be combined to provide the overall view desired?

Two approaches are described: that of the OARS model, based on summary ratings scales, and that of the US Government Accounting Office (US GAO), based on selected questionnaire items.

The OARS model was specifically developed to examine the impact of alternative service packages on population outcomes *(35)*. To do this it was necessary to determine functional status before and after intervention, to classify the population into functionally equivalent groups and, using a transition matrix, to note the impact on later functional state of the receipt of identified packages of services. Some of these terms may sound forbidding, but the concepts are easy to understand. OARS assesses functioning in five areas (social, economic, mental, physical, ADL), the information in each area being summarized on a 6-point rating scale where values range from excellent to totally impaired. Thus overall functional status can be portrayed by five values which provide a profile of functioning similar, for instance, to MMPI profiles. To obtain profiles relevant at a population level, the summary scales can be condensed. There are alternative ways of doing this. For instance each scale can be divided to permit comparison of those functioning adequately (ratings of 1–3) with those functioning inadequately (ratings of 4–6); or to allow comparison of those totally unimpaired (ratings of 1–2) with the rest (ratings of 3–6). Dividing the scales yields 32 profiles. Table 9, column (*a*) provides information on the functional profile of a random sample of community residents aged 65 and over based on divided (1–3/4–6) rating scales. Capitals represent adequate functioning and lower case letters represent inadequate functioning. It is worth noting that the majority of these elderly (59%) were functioning adequately (SEMPA) in all areas. Less than 0.5% were impaired in all areas (sempa). Admittedly this sample does not include that 5% of the elderly who were in institutions, but they add less than 5% to the totally impaired group because the institutionalized are not impaired in all areas.

Should 32 profiles be more than desired, or than available data can justify, the data may be aggregated according to number of areas impaired (see Table 9, columns headed (*b*)). The classification can be further reduced by considering only a few of the available areas. The information in column (*a*) is important to a clinician, since it provides more specific details, while the more condensed information in column (*b*) may be of greater relevance to policy-makers.

Table 9. Alternative summary profiles:
(*a*) including information on all dimensions;
(*b*) considering only the number of dimensions impaired

(*a*) Profile based on all information	Frequency (%)	(*b*) Profile based on dimensions impaired only: No.	Frequency (%)
SEMPA[a]	59	0	59
SEMPa	2		
SEMpA	6		
SEmPA	1	1	17
SeMPA	5		
sEMPA	3		
SEMpa	6		
SEmPa	*b*		
SEmpA	1		
SeMPa	*b*		
SeMpA	2	2	13
semPA	*b*		
sEMPa	*b*		
sEMpA	1		
sEmPA	*b*		
seMPA	1		
SEmpa	5		
SeMpa	1		
SemPa	1		
SempA	1		
sEMpa	1	3	11
sEmPa	*b*		
sEmpA	*c*		
seMPa	*c*		
seMpA	*b*		
semPA	1		
Sempa	1		
sEmpa	1		
seMpa	*b*	4	4
semPa	*b*		
sempA	1		
sempa	*b*	5	*b*
N	998		998

[a] S = Social; E = Economic; M = Mental health; P = Physical health; A = ADL. Lower case letters indicate impaired functioning, upper case letters unimpaired functioning.

[b] Less than 0.5%.

[c] None observed.

Another alternative is to add the summary ratings. With a possible range of 5–30, the substantial majority of institutional residents have scores above the midpoint (i.e. scores of 18–30), while the substantial majority of community residents have scores below it (i.e. scores of 5–17). Thus summed scores can rapidly indicate appropriateness of placement.

The full value of a functional classification system, however, becomes evident in the presence of longitudinal information. Two examples will be considered. One, based on the OARS model and on clinical practice, shows the relevance of a functional classification system for describing population or sample characteristics, assessing client outcome and evaluating the clinic itself. The second, using the US GAO approach and based on longitudinal information from a sample of urban residents, shows the importance of receiving appropriate services in an adequate amount, and estimates the national impact of appropriate service provision.

Use of functional classification in a clinic

The Geriatric Evaluation and Treatment Clinic at Duke University Medical Center focuses on the treatment of older people. When these data were gathered, the OARS questionnaire was administered to clients on intake and then every succeeding six months. Table 10 provides illustrative information on 37 clients, using the same classification system as in Table 9. The final column shows the initial distribution of the 37 clients. Only 15 of the 30 functional states represented in the community at large (Table 9) are represented initially by the clinic clients. On average the clients are sicker: only 27%, less than half the percentage in the community at large, function adequately in all areas. The bottom row shows client status six months later. After treatment 41% function adequately, although the same percentage as initially (5%) remains impaired in all areas. The body of the table indicates the proportion of people in a given initial state that remain in that state (the italicized values) and the proportion shifting to each of the other states. This permits us to see, for instance, that of the three clients judged to have only a physical health impairment (SEMpA), two improved (to SEMPA) and one remained stable, while of the three persons judged to have only a mental health impairment (SEmPA), the condition of two remained unchanged, while the mental health status of the third improved and his (or her) economic status declined (SeMPA).

At the client level such data provide information on the type of impact treatment has had and indicate the areas to which attention should be paid. At the clinic level, the clinic can judge whether it is attracting appropriate clientele, and whether its approach is having the desired effect. The clinic can also use such aggregated data for self-monitoring purposes, for such data permit the clinic to check its impact regularly and to determine whether it meets desired standards; indicate which functional states it treats successfully and which not; and provide an objective measure of where improvement is needed.

Use of functional classification for population planning

In 1975 the US Government Accounting Office used the OARS questionnaire to obtain information from a random sample of 1609 residents

Table 10. Initial functional state of selected clients, and functional state six months later

Initial state	State six months later												Initial distribution of 37 clients	
	SEMPA	SEMpA	SEmPA	SeMPA	sEMPA	SEmPa	sEMpA	SEmpa	SemPa	SempA	sEmPa	sempa	No.	%
SEMPA[a]	*0.80*		0.20										10	27
SEMpA	0.67	*0.33*											3	8
SEmPA			*0.67*	0.33									3	8
SeMPA					1.00								1	3
SEmPa						*0.50*	0.50						2	5
SEmpA	0.67					0.33							3	8
sEmPA	0.67										0.33		3	8
SEmpa								*1.00*					1	3
SemPa									*1.00*				1	3
SempA									0.50	*0.50*			2	5
sEmPa											*0.67*	0.33	3	8
Sempa	1.00												1	3
sEmpa								1.00					1	3
semPa				1.00									1	3
sempa								0.50				*0.50*	2	5
Distribution of 37 clients after six months														
No.	15	1	4	2	1	2	1	3	2	1	3	2		
%	41	3	11	5	3	5	3	8	5	3	8	5		

[a] S = Social; E = Economic; M = Mental health; P = Physical health; A = ADL. Lower case letters indicate impaired functioning, upper case letters unimpaired functioning.

Note. Figures in italics indicate proportion remaining in their initial functional state.

Source: **Fillenbaum, G.G. & Blazer, D.G.** *(36)*. Material used by permission of Aspen Systems Corporation.

aged 65 and over of Cleveland, Ohio. Of these, 1311 were reinterviewed a year later. Death, institutionalization, relocation and refusals account for the attrition *(37,38)*. The US GAO ignored the summary ratings in each area, preferring to use the responses to selected questions to determine status in four areas: health (measured by capacity to perform activities of daily living, interference by illness); security (financial status, the availability of a care giver); loneliness (defined by amount of social contact); and outlook on life (whether life is exciting and the subject feels useful). Status on each condition was summarized on a 3-point scale, indicating whether the position was best, marginal or worst. For instance, in assessing health condition a three-level classification categorizing ADL performance was developed, as follows.

1. Can do all 13 ADL tasks without help.
2. Needs help with one or more ADL tasks but can do all with help.
3. Cannot do any even with help.

The same three-level classification can be used for categorizing health.

1. No illness that interferes greatly with activities.
2. One illness that interferes greatly with activities.
3. Two or more illnesses that interfere greatly with activities.

The ADL and health categorization were then cross-tabulated. The box below shows final group assignment in the health area.

		Health 1	Health 2	Health 3
ADL	1	Best	Marginal	Worst
ADL	2	Marginal	Marginal	Worst
ADL	3	Worst	Worst	Worst

The four conditions combined indicated overall condition, which was also summarized on the same 3-point scale. Of the sample, 32% were in the best overall condition, 47% were in a marginal condition and 21% in the worst condition.

This is an alternative aggregation scheme. But what is important here is not the scheme *per se* but the questions it permitted the US GAO to ask and to answer. The US GAO wished to know which circumstances resulted in the "best" condition, the extent to which the population could be raised to that level, and the cost of doing so.

For example, consider the health condition. The US GAO assumed, reasonably, that inability to perform self-care and instrumental activities is due to severely limiting illnesses. They therefore checked whether incapacity due to illness can be reduced by medical treatment. Using their longitudinal data and controlling for adequacy of medical services received initially, they found that when adequate services are provided the illness improves, but when services are inadequate the illness deteriorates. Based on the figures so obtained they then did two things: they estimated how many people would have been in an improved situation had all their illnesses been adequately treated during the year (the estimate was an additional 9.2%); and they projected the health conditions of the 65–69 year age group over the next 20 years under alternate provisions of medical services. The results indicated that not only would a larger percentage enjoy a better state of health if medical services were expanded (state of health would be improved for an additional 1%, 14%, 14% and 12% at 5, 10, 15 and 20 years hence) but that the cost of expanded medical services was estimated to be less than the cost under the current inadequate approach because of improvements in health. Not everyone would benefit by expanded health care; for each person helped an average of 2.1 persons would have to be served.

Projections were also made for the other three conditions. To improve the overall condition, the US GAO estimated that national expenditure on the elderly would have to increase by roughly 24%, an amount that could be markedly reduced if family and friends, who already offer considerable assistance, could offer even more.

Conclusion

A variety of comprehensive, valid and reliable multidimensional functional assessments, and alternative ways of using the information they provide, is available. The measures available can be refined and accurate information on the status of the elderly obtained. It needs to be ensured, as Haug et al. *(22)* did, that the measures used are sound, for otherwise the prevalence of impairment may be incorrectly estimated, resulting in an inappropriate allocation of services. The impact of services also needs to be assessed accurately, for, as illustrated, appropriate services in adequate amounts can not only improve the functional status of the elderly, but in the long run may be less costly than an inadequate approach.

References

1. **Skeet, M.** *Protecting the health of the elderly.* Copenhagen, WHO Regional Office for Europe, 1983 (Public Health in Europe, No. 18).
2. **Green, B.F.** A primer of testing. *American psychologist,* **36**: 1001–1011 (1981).
3. **Katz, S.** Assessing self-maintenance: activities of daily living, mobility, and instrumental activities of daily living. *Journal of the American Geriatrics Society,* **31**: 721–727 (1983).
4. **Katz, S. et al.** Studies of illness in the aged. The index of ADL: a standardized measure of biological and psychosocial function. *Journal of the American Medical Association,* **185**: 914–919 (1963).
5. **Katz, S. & Akpom, C.A.** A measure of primary sociobiological functions. *International journal of health services,* **6**: 493–508 (1976).
6. **Feller, B.** Americans needing help to function at home. *NCHS advance data*, No. 92, 14 September 1983.
7. **Lawton, M.P. & Brody, E.M.** Assessment of older people: self-maintaining and instrumental activities of daily living. *Gerontologist,* **9**: 179–186 (1969).
8. *Multidimensional functional assessment: the OARS methodology,* 2nd ed. Durham, NC, Center for the Study of Aging and Human Development, Duke University, 1978.
9. **Fillenbaum, G.G.** Screening the elderly: a brief instrumental ADL measure. *Journal of the American Geriatrics Society,* **33**: 698–706 (1985).
10. **Gurland, B. et al.** The Comprehensive Assessment and Referral Evaluation (CARE) — rationale, development and reliability. *International journal of aging and human development,* **8**: 9–42 (1977).
11. **Heikkinen, E. et al., ed.** *The elderly in eleven countries: a sociomedical survey.* Copenhagen, WHO Regional Office for Europe, 1983 (Public Health in Europe, No. 21).
12. **Parkerson, G.R. et al.** The Duke-UNC health profile: an adult health status instrument for primary care. *Medical care,* **19**: 806–823 (1981).
13. **Kahn, R.L. et al.** Brief objective measures for the determination of mental status in the aged. *American journal of psychiatry,* **117**: 326–328 (1960).
14. **Folstein, M.F. et al.** Mini-mental state: a practical method for grading the cognitive state of patients for the clinician. *Journal of psychiatric research,* **12**: 189–198 (1975).
15. **Pfeiffer, E.** A short portable mental status questionnaire for the assessment of organic brain deficit in elderly patients. *Journal of the American Geriatric Society,* **23**: 433–441 (1975).
16. **Fillenbaum, G.G.** Comparison of two brief tests of organic brain impairment, the MSQ and the SPMSQ. *Journal of the American Geriatrics Society,* **28**: 381–384 (1980).
17. **Pfeffer, R.I. et al.** A survey diagnostic tool for senile dementia. *American journal of epidemiology,* **114**: 515–527 (1981).
18. **Lawton, M.P. et al.** A research and service oriented multilevel assessment instrument. *Journal of gerontology,* **37**: 91–99 (1982).

19. **Bond, J. et al.** The reliability of a survey psychiatric assessment schedule for the elderly. *British journal of psychiatry,* **137**: 148–162 (1980).
20. **Golden, R.R. et al.** Development of indicator scales for the Comprehensive Assessment and Referral Evaluation (CARE) interview schedule. *Journal of gerontology,* **39**: 138–146 (1984).
21. **Gurland, B. et al.** Criteria for the diagnosis of dementia in the community elderly. *Gerontologist,* **22**: 180–186 (1982).
22. **Haug, M. et al.** Mental health and the elderly: factors in stability and change over time. *Journal of health and social behavior,* **25**: 100–115 (1984).
23. **Donald, C.A. et al.** *Conceptualization and measurement of health for adults in the health insurance study. Vol. IV. Social health.* Santa Monica, CA, Rand Corporation, 1978 (R-1987/4-HEW).
24. **Townsend, P.** *Poverty in the United Kingdom.* Harmondsworth, Penguin Books, 1979.
25. **Powell, C. & Crombie, A.** The Kilsyth questionnaire: a method of screening elderly people at home. *Age and aging,* **3**: 23–28 (1974).
26. **Israel, L. & Kozarevic, D.** *Source book of geriatric assessment. Vol. 1. Techniques for the evaluation of mental functioning in the elderly. Vol. 2. Review of analyzed instruments.* Basle, Karger, 1984.
27. **Gurland, B.J. et al.** The SHORT-CARE: an efficient instrument for the assessment of depression, dementia and disability. *Journal of gerontology,* **39**: 166–169 (1984).
28. **Gurland, B.J. & Wilder, D.E.** The CARE interview revisited: development of an efficient, systematic clinical assessment. *Journal of gerontology,* **39**: 129–137 (1984).
29. **Teresi, J.A. et al.** Construct validity of indicator-scales developed from the Comprehensive Assessment and Referral Evaluation interview schedule. *Journal of gerontology,* **39**: 147–157 (1984).
30. **Gurland, B.J. et al.** *The mind and mood of aging.* New York, Haworth Press, 1983.
31. **Gurland, B. et al.** Personal time dependency in the elderly of New York City: findings from the US-UK cross-national geriatric community study. *In:* Ferleger, B., ed. *Dependency in the elderly of New York City.* New York, Community Council of Greater New York, 1978.
32. **Fillenbaum, G.G. & Smyer, M.A.** The development, validity and reliability of the OARS multidimensional functional assessment questionnaire. *Journal of gerontology,* **36**: 428–434 (1981).
33. **George, L.K. et al.** *Developing measures of functional status and service utilisation: refining and extending the OARS methodology.* Final report to NRTA-AARP Andrus Foundation, 1982.
34. **Balinsky, W. & Berger, R.** A review of the research on general health status indexes. *Medical care,* **13**: 283–292 (1975).
35. **Fillenbaum, G.G. et al.** Assessment of individual functional status in a program evaluation and resource allocation model. *In: Multidimensional functional assessment: the OARS methodology.* Durham, NC, Center for the Study of Aging and Human Development, Duke University, 1978.

36. **Fillenbaum, G.G. & Blazer, D.G.** The living textbook of geriatric care. *In:* Whanger, A.D. et al. *Mental health assessment and therapeutic intervention with older adults.* Aspen, MD, 1984.
37. **Comptroller General.** *The well-being of older people in Cleveland, Ohio.* Report to Congress. US Government Accounting Office, 1977 (HRD-77-70).
38. **Comptroller General.** *Conditions of older people: national information system needed.* Report to Congress. US Government Accounting Office, 1979 (HRD-79-95).

7.5 Complex indexes for measuring a complex phenomenon[a] — *M. Goldberg & W. Dab*

Justification of Complex Measurements of Health Status

Afifi et al. *(1)* have defined the terms indicator and index as descriptors of the activity or the state of a system. Indexes are aggregated quantitative measurements intended to describe the overall activity of the system, whereas indicators may or may not be quantitative and normally reflect only limited aspects of the system. In this chapter these terms will be used in their accepted sense, adopting in addition Berg's recommendations *(2)* that the term indicator should be reserved for specific measurements and the term index for composite measurements combining several indicators.

For purposes of measurement health has to be regarded as a "system" consisting of partial elements which, taken together, yield a characteristic product of the system, in this case the entity "health", whether that of an individual or a population. Indicators which only reflect a partial aspect and only measure an isolated phenomenon give only an imperfect picture of the complexity of the system as a whole.

Mortality rates, for example, or the prevalence of a particular disease do not alone provide an adequate picture of the general health of the population or a basis for comparison of different pathological states. For assessing the magnitude of health problems, deciding on the allocation of resources and evaluating health activities, a method of measurement which integrates different phenomena in a system with a single frame of reference is needed.

This is the aim pursued by all those who attempt to construct complex health status indexes. In this chapter the main approaches which have been followed will be described, restricting the discussion to the health status indexes of a *population*, leaving aside the very large number of individual health status indexes (even though some of the population indexes include a stage in which the health status of individuals is assessed).

Concepts of Health

The measurement of a phenomenon as complex as health status necessitates a number of specific stages, mainly the elaboration of an operational definition of health, the choice of elementary phenomena capable of reflecting the health status, the determination of the information to be collected and

[a] This chapter reproduces broadly and in summary form some of the authors' earlier papers *(36,38–40)* to which the interested reader is referred for a more detailed presentation. These contain, in particular, a more comprehensive bibliography.

the choice of a method of combining the separate elements. The primary concerns here will be the first two, very complementary stages, the discussion being restricted to what is strictly necessary for understanding the procedure for developing complex indicators.

As is clear from the classical definition adopted by the World Health Organization and indeed has been suggested by a number of other definitions, health is not merely the absence of disease. Only recently, however, have attempts been made to measure the "positive" aspect of health, this "something more" than the absence of disease.

Until the end of the nineteenth century measurement of the state of health of a population was based solely on mortality statistics. During the twentieth century, as Siegmann *(3)* has pointed out, health indicators have been developed to meet the changes which have occurred in health problems in the industrialized countries. The mortality indicators were thus joined by morbidity indicators. The latter in the form of incidence or prevalence rates were used initially for infectious diseases before being applied to acute or chronic conditions in general. These "classical" measurements of the state of health of a population have three common characteristics.

1. Being based on the concepts of mortality and morbidity, they do not measure health but rather the state of bad health, what one may call "negative" health. In other words, the health of the group is being measured on the basis of the minority of the population who fall ill or die during the year.

2. The phenomena recorded (in this case death or disease) are recorded in binary form, the presence or absence of a phenomenon, all or nothing.

3. The person responsible for the measurement is the doctor.

Many authors have listed the shortcomings of these "classical" indicators and emphasized their unsuitability as criteria of current health problems in the industrialized countries. That is why so much work has been done on devising and confirming the validity of complex indicators.

To remedy the defects of indicators based solely on the concepts of morbidity and mortality, research workers in this field have proposed two major conceptual changes, the first relating to the concept of morbidity, which has been extended and interpreted in different ways depending on the type of observer (coding) and the second relating to the concept of global health.

Extension of the concept of morbidity

Many authors have set themselves the task of obtaining a measurement of morbidity which is not based on the concept of the presence or absence of disease but rather on the *consequences* of the disease. The work of Wood is pre-eminent in this field. In the ninth revision of the *International classification of diseases*, Wood proposed a threefold conceptual distinction: deficiency, incapacity and handicap.

This classification was intended as a basis for a system of measuring states of ill health in a population which was not exclusively linked to disease statistics but took into account also the personal and social consequences of the disease.

The concepts of positive health and global health

Efforts to extend the concept of morbidity, although intended to eliminate some of the shortcomings of classical indicators of the health of a population, still only provide a negative measurement of health. Some workers have, however, made a clean break with the concept of disease and attempted to measure a state of global health. The fundamental basis of this line of research is the existence in the individuals making up a population of a continuum of states of health ranging from perfect health to death *(4,5)*. When defining levels of health, account is taken not only of the consequences of ill health (i.e. the "extended" morbidity) but also — and this is the characteristic feature of the new approach — of phenomena which reflect "positive" health (i.e. capacity, potential, performance, etc.). This approach is clearly influenced by the definition of health as a global phenomenon. Without discussing here the ample literature devoted to possible definitions of health, it is possible to indicate in general terms the three main approaches adopted by the different authors.

1. The perceptual approach, as in the definition put forward by WHO and followed by authors such as Sigerist *(6)* and Hoyman *(7)*.

2. The functional approach in which the accent is placed on the ability of the individual to perform his tasks and the role he is required to play *(8–10)*.

3. An approach based on the concept of adaptation to the environment *(11–14)*.

Many authors have, of course, combined these approaches.

Apart from the lack of precision and some arguable features in the majority of the quoted definitions, there are two problems common to all of them.

In the first place, irrespective of the definition adopted, it is impossible to avoid introducing *standards* into the definition as a means of measuring health. This is suggested indirectly by the use of adjectives such as "optimal", "appropriate", "reasonable", etc. The various problems involved in the standardization approach have been discussed by many of the authors who have brought out clearly the difficulties arising from the variation in what is regarded as socially normal. A health problem in a particular cultural, ideological or professional context is not necessarily so regarded elsewhere. How can one then decide that one state of health is better than another? As the proverb says, "the tallest dwarf is as tall as the smallest giant".

The second point to be emphasized is that all the morbidity measurements which have been described here have one common characteristic: they are based on individual observations, these observations being subsequently combined to provide a measurement of the health of a group or of a population. Many authors, in particular in the field of sociology, have made it amply clear, however, that the health of a population is not merely the sum of the states of health of individuals forming that population. Lerner *(15)*, for example, has emphasized the specific contribution to the health problems of a community of social, institutional, geographical, etc. factors, while Kelman *(16)* has demonstrated the social nature of the definition of health problems.

In spite of their essential differences, the three approaches to a definition of health listed above agree in not being based on the concept of disease, although the latter possesses, of course, the undeniable practical advantage of providing a convenient frame of reference for a classification of the different forms of ill health. Once this stage has been reached, new frames of reference have to be established, incorporating categories of what has come to be known as "states of health" (the adjectives "good" or "bad" being coupled with them as appropriate so as to distinguish clearly the pathological phenomena responsible for those states of health).

It is immediately apparent that this is a more abstract procedure than the classification of individual disorders, organic, functional or relational, such as Wood's classification of deficiencies, incapacities and handicaps referred to above. What has been done here is to define global states of health, these global states of health being based, of course, on known disorders which, either alone or in combination, make up a continuum ranging from the best to the worst and enabling graduated lists of states of health to be drawn up.

Some such procedure appears to be necessary in order to obtain an operational criterion of global health levels, although nothing prevents us from distinguishing, among these global states of health, one or more specific states above a limit threshold in which individuals are free from any apparent morbidity. In addition to the theoretical possibility of grasping the general idea of positive health, one essential advantage of the state of health concept is its global nature which combines all the characteristic features of the health of an individual.

The establishment of a classification of global states of health will depend in the first place on the definition of health adopted for purposes of the classification. One would, therefore, expect to find three different types of classification of global states of health, based on the functional, perceptual and "adaptational" approaches referred to above. The situation is not as clear cut as this in practice; classification systems do not in principle fall into homogeneous groups from this point of view, but combine the perceptual and functional aspects with particular emphasis on one or other depending on the author's views. It is curious to find, in spite of the important position occupied by the "adaptational" approach in a large number of definitions of health, that no studies have been made (to the authors' knowledge) on the measurement of states of health based on adaptation phenomena. A great deal of research has, of course, been done on adaptation, especially in the fields of ergonomics and psychology, but so far as is known no health indicator has been proposed based on the measurement of adaptation capacities, although Terris *(17)*, for example, believes that it will only be possible to develop an "epidemiology of health" by means of studies on the related concepts of performance, performance capacity and impediments to performance.

Principal distinctions between conventional and complex indicators
A twofold classification has therefore been retained at the conceptual level: on the one hand global health and on the other negative health, with a triple subdivision depending on whether the measured parameter is the mortality, the morbidity or what the authors have called the "extended morbidity".

On the practical level a measure of health, which is independent of the precise nature of the pathological symptoms, permits an assessment of complex situations to be made. For example, taking the case of a patient who has just recovered from tuberculosis, how can one assess the possible "gain in health" after the secondary occurrence of a duodenal ulcer, using only diagnostic criteria to describe his health status? A measure based on appreciation of the global health status does not run into the same difficulties, although clearly other problems will arise in the latter case in regard to quantification of his condition (how can one say whether a patient with a duodenal ulcer is in better or worse health than when he was suffering from pulmonary tuberculosis?). The principle generally adopted is to specify a unit of measurement making use of the measured phenomenon in order to determine the repercussions of a problem or of a state of health. Three types of unit have been used:

(*a*) the functional unit based on actions which have been carried out;

(*b*) a chronological unit based on the duration of an incapacity;

(*c*) an economic unit relating to the costs incurred, which is only used very rarely as an element in a complex indicator.

Table 1 shows the principal differences between complex and conventional indicators.

Quantitative Expression for Measuring the Health Level of a Population which is not Based on the Concepts of Mortality and Morbidity

The health status indices of a population proposed in the literature, which are not based solely on the concepts of mortality and "conventional" morbidity may be divided broadly speaking into three groups.

1. Those which make use of normal diagnostic categories but add to them weighting elements so as to arrive at a single index which provides a general measure of health.

2. Those which propose a single measure of health based both on the mortality and "extended" morbidity, i.e. expressed in terms of incapacity

Table 1. Principal differences between conventional and complex indicators

	Conventional indicators	Complex indicators
Reference concept	Mortality or morbidity	Extended morbidity or global health
Number of phenomena measured	1	>1
Use of a weighting coefficient	No	Yes
Unit of measurement	The specific case	Functional, chronological or economic (rare)

and handicap, irrespective of any diagnostic category. This type of measure is well represented by healthy life expectancy, which makes use of a chronological unit.

3. Indices grouped together under the generic term "global health status index", which are based on an attempted overall assessment of the level of health of individuals.

This breakdown into three groups does not represent a genuine attempt at classifying health status indices, since it is based on only one criterion, the nature of the measured phenomena. It will become clear later on that no classification of indices is possible unless several criteria are taken into account simultaneously. The only reason for dividing indices into three groups at this stage is to mark out the boundaries between them. In the present section, however, only the third group of indices will be dealt with.

The procedure used by authors who have drawn up global health status indices is to prepare a list of activities and/or situations and/or judgements which may be positive or negative, and compare each individual with this list. In some cases the list is graduated from the best to the worst state of health and each section represents a state of health determined by the corresponding activities (or situations or judgements); in other cases the list is not a graduated one, but the individual is scored under each head and classified in a group corresponding to his health status on the basis of the total score obtained.

The above description has, of course, been given in very general terms and a wide range of variants will be found in the literature with regard to the method of preparing the reference list of activities, etc., the content of the list, the method of allocating each patient to a category and relating the category to each element on the list, etc. A few typical examples of different approaches to the problem will be given later. It is clear that this procedure is extremely arbitrary, since each author imposes, implicitly or explicitly, his own concept of health and his own choice of the observable phenomena which reflect the state of health. This does not condemn the method out of hand provided that one consciously accepts its limitations, which are in principle linked with the aspect of standardization involved in any measurement of health. There is at present no general agreement on what form a satisfactory classification of health status should take and there is really no reason to suppose that there ever will be, since it would be necessary first of all to agree on a definition of health. It has already been seen that such agreement is not feasible, and possibly not desirable, in view of the uncertainties inherent in such a definition. Accepting this weakness, it is still possible, within the framework of an explicit specific definition, for a method which consists of establishing a classification of health status to do useful service at the operational level, especially when attempting to express the level of health of a population in quantitative terms.

Some of the most representative of these indicators derived from the main schools of thought will be described below, after which the principal problems which they raise will be examined.

A distinction will be made during this description between models of health status index relating to individuals and those relating to the health of the population, built up either by combining individual indices of global states of health or based on non-global individual measurements, which can again be combined so as to define the global health status of the population as a whole.

Models of individual global health status indexes

Individual indexes can be classified in general terms in three categories depending on their authors' concept of global health, of the phenomena which reflect a patient's state of health and of the methods used to measure these phenomena:

(*a*) indexes based on "objective" physiological measurements;

(*b*) indexes based on measurements of functional incapacity;

(*c*) indexes based in principle on a perceptual approach.

Indexes based on physiological measurements

Chen's "H" index *(18)* is a theoretical model designed to measure the physiological state of health of an individual belonging to a clearly defined homogeneous population group. It is justified by the relationship found between the results of physiological measurements on members of the group to which the individual belongs. The proposed model takes into account the results obtained on the group as a whole and enables the individual results to be expressed as a combined value, weighted in relation to the group results and in relation to the size of the reference group. As proposed by Chen, the H index is a form of response to the standardization problem referred to above. Nevertheless, it is only a very partial response, since it relates only to the standards to be applied to the measurement results and not to the conceptual standards of a definition of health.

Indexes based on measurements of functional incapacity

One of the best known indexes in this group is the Grogono & Woodgate index *(19)*; it has the further advantage of being both simple in conceptual terms and simple to implement, which explains why it has been used as a base model by many other authors. Ten activities or aspects of daily life have been selected in such a way as to be reasonably exhaustive without including any obvious redundancy: work, leisure, physical suffering, mental suffering, communication, sleep, dependence on others, nutrition, excretion and sexual activity. A trained observer allocates under each of these heads a score which may be 1 (normal), 0.5 (inconvenience) or 0 (incapacity). The total of these partial scores, divided by 10, is the global health status index. It has been used on an experimental basis to classify in order of severity a number of hospitalized patients suffering from various conditions.

Skinner & Yett *(20)* designed their debility index to meet a specific requirement, namely the management of health care institutions for chronic patients. This is one of the earliest uses of global health status indexes, for which a number of different types of index have been developed based on daily life activities; these indexes, the principle of which was established by Katz *(21)* are known in the Anglo-American literature under the generic term "ADL indexes" (activities of daily living indexes). The Skinner & Yett debility index is a particularly interesting example in this category, both because it is the most sophisticated and also because the methodological problems involved in the development and validation of the method have been given serious consideration. It covers five types of activity, for each of which different assessments are listed so as to yield a Gutman scale (a cumulative scale in which a positive response to a possible activity implies a positive response in regard to all subsequent activities also). The different combinations of responses are grouped together to define a number of "classes of debility" which are at the same time states of global health, so that the index can be immediately regarded as a global measurement. It is not strictly speaking an index, however, since it does not provide a global quantitative expression for each individual who is merely allocated to a class; each class has then to be given a score which will constitute the required health status index.

This is, in fact, what Bush has suggested. In his first paper with Fanshel *(22)* he indicated the principles governing the measurement of global health status, applicable at the individual level but intended to form the basic element in a population index. The individual component in the index will not be described here, although its application as a population index will be covered later.

The central element in the individual index is in this case as in Skinner & Yett's debility index a graduated scale of functional states built up by combining elementary activities. These elementary activities have been selected so as to apply in theory to any type of population and in particular a population "in good health". The first version of the index *(22)* covered 11 separate functional states; the number was subsequently increased to 30 *(23)*.

Each patient may be allocated to one of these states, thus indicating his functional health status. All that is then required is a method of quantifying these functional states so as to calculate the global health status index. This is based on the concept of "social preference" in which each of the functional states is given a weighting (weightings being known as "utilities" in the language of decision theory). To make this weighting operation genuinely realistic, a matrix has been established in which the functional states are distributed between five age groups and 42 "symptom/problem complexes" selected for their liability to cause functional disorders. The different techniques, drawn from the methods of decision theory, which are used to measure "levels of well-being", i.e. to allocate the utilities expressing the global level of health corresponding to each category, have been described in detail previously *(24)*. An example of this will be given later.

Indexes based essentially on a perceptual approach

Included in this category are global health status indexes based on the replies given by individuals to questions on their state of health. Some of these questions may relate to factual phenomena which do not easily lend themselves to a "subjective" interpretation by the subject, but a series of items is always included, in some cases the predominant group, which enables the individual to express his "feeling", his personal appreciation of his level of wellbeing.

The widest range of variation is certainly found in this group of indexes, since the perceptual approach easily lends itself to very different ideas of the nature of health. Three indexes of this type will be described, each representative of a specific approach to the measurement of global health; they have been selected both because they give a general picture of the main schools of thought and also because each system has been tried out on the ground on a fairly extensive scale.

Breslow *(25)*, taking as a basis the experience gained at the Human Population Laboratory (where a study has been made of the population of a Californian county as a whole), has developed an index intended to provide a quantitative approach based on the World Health Organization definition of health. It is based on a questionnaire comprising three categories of items corresponding to physical health, mental health and social health. In the physical health category, the questions cover incapacitating conditions, chronic states, symptoms experienced and the "energy level". Mental health is the subject of a group of questions designed to elicit negative and positive sentiments, while the social aspect of health is examined on the basis of items dealing with professional life, marital satisfaction, sociability and activities within the community.

An index is then calculated by means of a Ridits (Relative to an Identified Distribution) analysis in which, as its name indicates, a value is obtained for each subject as a function of the distribution of the results obtained in the complete group to which the subject belongs. It therefore combines an individual index, giving each subject an overall score for his level of health, and a population index; such scores can be calculated for groups defined on the basis of different criteria. The method has been used, for example, to compare the global health indices of groups defined on the basis of age, sex, income, ethnic origin, etc.

Some results obtained in the measurement of physical health, for example, are shown in Table 2. They provide a prototype of the information which global health indicators are capable of supplying. The state of physical health of the population is distributed over a continuum ranging from severe incapacity to a high "energetic" state. One way of expressing the result is to indicate the proportion of the population which corresponds to each state of health. These are the percentages which are shown inside the continuum. It is evident that 7% of the population are in a state of severe incapacity, while 6% enjoy a state of optimal health. Another method of presenting these results, taking into account the respective weight of each state of health, is to calculate an indicator by the Ridits method, which is a useful technique both because it is easy to calculate and because it allows a summary presentation of the results. The indices thus obtained are shown above the continuum. They are found by taking the proportion of individuals who enjoy a better state of health and adding to them half of those in the state of health under examination. For example, persons in a state of minor incapacity have a state of health of 0.89, a value which is obtained by adding 0.04 (i.e. half the percentage of persons in this state of health) to 0.85 (since 85% enjoy a better state of health). Under these conditions, the mean value of the health status of the population is 0.5. Higher values indicate a lower health status.

The Sickness Impact Profile is an index developed by Bergner et al. *(27)*, designed to measure the perceptual and behavioural dimensions of the state of health. The questionnaire has been divided into 14 categories (social activity, locomotion, sleep, nutrition, household activities, mobility, body movement, intellectual functions, family life, personal hygiene, leisure, emotion, communication, work) representing a total of 235 possible responses. Each of these is given a weighting by a group of 25 experts. The sum of the values corresponding to the subject's responses to the questions provides his global health status index. This index has been tried out on a very large scale in the United States and self-administered questionnaires have been perfected and widely used. An abridged version of the Sickness Impact Profile, consisting of only 85 items, has been developed at the University of Nottingham by Martini et al. *(28)* and tried out in the United Kingdom on 14 500 patients aged between 18 and 60. The aim pursued by both the American and the British teams was to develop an index capable of producing a quantitative picture of the effect of medical care on the overall health status of patients.

Ware et al. *(29)*, on the other hand, have endeavoured to develop "a perceptual measure of health status", i.e. a measure of how individuals perceive their level of health. This has been done by drawing up a "scale of measures of perception regarding health status" comprising six dimensions each covered by a specific index: indices of current health status, previous

Table 2. State of physical health of a population measured by means of a self-administered questionnaire and calculated by the Ridits method

	States of health						
	Incapacity		Chronic conditions		Presence of symptoms	No complaints	
	Severe	Slight	More than one	One only		Low energy level	High energy level
Global indicator	0.97	0.89		0.67	0.43	0.18	0.03
Distribution of the population N = 6928 (100%)	0.07	0.08	0.09	0.28	0.28	0.23	0.06

Source: **Belloc, N.D. et al.** *(26).*

health status, future health status, anxiety with regard to health status, susceptibility and resistance to disease, and acceptance or rejection of the disease. A series of judgements in respect of each of the dimensions are put to the subjects, on which they are required to give their opinion, the result being scored from 1 to 5 according to the extent of their agreement with each statement on the list. The scores attributed to each dimension are totalled up by a fairly simple method of calculation and combined to form a single index expressing, in the authors' view, the patients' global health level as perceived by them.

This research has been taken up, supplemented and confirmed in a study carried out on behalf of Rand's Health Insurance which assesses the impact on health of different forms of medical protection *(30).*

Model of global health status indexes of a population

All individual health status indexes can, of course, provide the basic building blocks for the construction of population indexes for measuring the global health status of the population to which the individuals belong. In some cases, population indexes corresponding to the individual index model are built up directly, either by simple addition of the individual values followed by division of the total number of individuals or by a simple transfer in cases where the individual index has been based on values for the population as a whole, as in the case of the Breslow index described above. The aggregation method provides a more sophisticated approach, so as to take into account phenomena which only appear at the population level or again the heterogeneity of a large population. The Ridits method is one example of this, but there are many others.

Chen, for example, in his paper referred to above *(18)* has proposed a population index T calculated from the individual index H. Since the heterogeneity of a large population does not permit direct aggregation of the H indices, built up on the basis of the homogeneous subpopulations, the author has defined the T index as a weighted mean of the measurements carried out in all the subpopulations, the weighting factors being the numbers included in these subpopulations.

Bush and co-workers *(31)* have built up a population index on the basis of the individual index in the following way. First of all, the individual indices were directly combined to form an index W which they designated the "functional health status index".[a]

They then introduced the prognostic factor, i.e. the probability of the transition from one functional state to another during the course of time (the mortality rate being regarded as the probability of passing into the state of death from a different state). A Markov model was used to calculate the "functional state expectancy" Y, which is in fact the distribution of life expectancy among different functional states.

The final state, the index Q, which is designated the "value-adjusted life expectancy" is obtained on the basis of the values for the functional state expectancy (Y_j) and the utilities (weightings) allocated to these states (W_j):

$$Q = \sum_j W_j Y_j$$

in which Q is the required global health status index. This index has proved to be a very effective criterion in two major cost-effect studies, one a phenylketonuria screening programme *(32)* and the other a tuberculosis screening programme *(33)*.

Table 3 gives a general summary of the principal phenomena measured by means of five complex indicators representative of this type of analytical tool.

The main problems involved in global health status indexes

A group of American experts met in 1972 to assess the situation with regard to global health status indexes. The conclusions of this meeting were issued in the form of recommendations for future research *(6)*. Although more than ten years have passed, these conclusions appear to have retained their validity;

---

[a]

$$W = \frac{\sum_j N_j W_j}{N} \text{ with } 0 \leqq W \leqq 1$$

where N = number in the population as a whole

N_j = number in the functional state j

W_j = utility allocated to the functional state j

j = index of the functional state 0, 1, 2, . . ., m

Table 3. Phenomena measured by five complex indicators

	Author				
	Grogono, Woodgate	Bush, Fanshel	Breslow	Bergner, Martini	Ware, Brook
Designation of indicator	—	Index of wellbeing	Human population laboratory index	Sickness Impact Profile	—
Observer	Health professional	Health professional and the individual	The individual	The individual	The individual
Phenomenon measured					
Duration of incapacity	—	X	—	—	X
Activities of daily living	X	X	X	X	X
Social roles	X	X	X	X	X
Mental function	X	X	X	X	X
Pathogenic risk factors	—	X	—	—	—
Symptoms experienced	—	X	X	—	X
Vitality	—	—	X	X	X

therefore those relating to conceptual problems are summarized, pending a fully satisfactory solution and disregarding the purely technical aspects.

The first and undoubtedly the most important problem to solve is clearly the selection of components for a global health status index which are valid and feasible to collect under real conditions especially from the economic point of view. This point, which has already been largely covered above, is not gone into in further detail, except to repeat that in this field the definition of a universally accepted index is a Utopian dream; there is nothing wrong in defining an index of one's own choice, provided that it reflects a precise and operational concept of health and meets the requirements of validity and feasibility.

Once the stage of selecting the components of a global health status index has been successfully completed, another fundamental problem immediately arises: is there a need for weighting the different components and if so how is it to be done? Some authors, whose arguments have been summarized by Grogono *(34)*, are opposed in principle to any form of weighting. Others, however, believe it to be essential for any valid comparison of situations, individual or collective, in which the states of health and the nature of the problems are different. A choice has to be made in this case with regard to the procedure to be followed. Which weighting criterion or criteria should be selected (an economic criterion, prosperity for example)? Who will be responsible for determining the weightings (doctors, patients, potential health service users, etc.) and on what basis? Is it justifiable to combine weightings determined by different individuals or groups and how should it be done? Should a decreasing scale ("discount" in the language of economists) be applied to the weightings as a function of time and how can one determine the rates to be applied? These questions raise numerous problems, both of a methodological and practical nature. The accumulation of experience in this field is particularly important, since it is very closely concerned with the problem of standardization which is fundamental in the context of health indexes. One thing is certain, that the score given by an index has no absolute value. It will always vary according to the groups studied and the observers making the study. The variation between the individals studied can be verified by means of standardization techniques (for example the Ridits method). The variation between different observers raises once again the question of the weighting of different states of health. Once a finite list of the various possible states of health has been drawn up, each state has to be given a value. In many cases experts are brought in to do this assessment. Table 4 gives a very good example of this procedure, in which 30 states of health are defined on the basis of three parameters: mobility, difficulties in the performance of physical activity and limitations on social activity. The authors then asked 62 graduate students or nurses to score these states of health at equal intervals on a scale from 0 to 1. The figures in the right-hand column are the means scores allocated by the "experts" to each state. The authors also compared the scores allocated by different groups of experts *(23)*.

When the components of an index have been selected and the corresponding weightings defined (or not, as the case may be) a model of a

Table 4. Function level classification and measured values

Level number	Mobility (step)	Physical activity (step)	Social activity (step)	Measured values
L30	Travelled freely (5) (no symptom/problem complex)	Walked freely (4)	Performed major and other activities (5)	1.000
L29	Travelled freely (5) (symptom/problem complex present)	Walked freely (4)	Performed major and other activities (5)	0.804
L28	Travelled freely (5)	Walked freely (4)	Performed major but limited in other activities (4)	0.689
L27	Travelled freely (5)	Walked freely (4)	Performed major activity with limitations (3)	0.694
L26	Travelled freely (5)	Walked freely (4)	Did not perform major but performed self-care activities	0.646
L25	Travelled with difficulty (4)	Walked freely (4)	Performed major but limited in other activities (4)	0.516
L24	Travelled with difficulty (4)	Walked freely (4)	Performed major activity with limitations (3)	0.536
L23	Travelled with difficulty (4)	Walked freely (4)	Did not perform major but performed self-care activities (2)	0.495
L22	Travelled with difficulty (4)	Walked with limitations (3)	Performed major but limited in other activities (4)	0.519
L21	Travelled with difficulty (4)	Walked with limitations (3)	Performed major activity with limitations (3)	0.522
L20	Travelled with difficulty (4)	Walked with limitations (3)	Did not perform major but performed self-care activities (2)	0.469
L19	Travelled with difficulty (4)	Moved independently in wheelchair (2)	Performed major activity with limitations (3)	0.503
L18	Travelled with difficulty (4)	Moved independently in wheelchair (2)	Did not perform major but performed self-care activities (2)	0.458
L17	In house (3)	Walked freely (4)	Did not perform major but performed self-care activities (2)	0.594

L16	In house (3)	Walked freely (4)	Required assistance with self-care activities (1)	0.505
L15	In house (3)	Walked with limitations (3)	Did not perform major but performed self-care activities (2)	0.519
L14	In house (3)	Walked with limitations (3)	Required assistance with self-care activities (1)	0.436
L13	In house (3)	Moved independently in wheelchair (2)	Did not perform major but performed self-care activities (2)	0.491
L12	In house (3)	Moved independently in wheelchair (2)	Required assistance with self-care activities (1)	0.444
L11	In house (3)	In bed or chair (1)	Did not perform major but performed self-care activities (2)	0.534
L10	In house (3)	In bed or chair (1)	Required assistance with self-care activities (1)	0.436
L9	In hospital (2)	Walked freely (4)	Did not perform major but performed self-care activities (2)	0.528
L8	In hospital (2)	Walked freely (4)	Required assistance with self-care activities (1)	0.440
L7	In hospital (2)	Walked with limitations (3)	Did not perform major but performed self-care activities (2)	0.440
L6	In hospital (2)	Walked with limitations (3)	Required assistance with self-care activities (1)	0.388
L5	In hospital (2)	Moved independently in wheelchair (2)	Did not perform major but performed self-care activities (2)	0.445
L4	In hospital (2)	Moved independently in wheelchair (2)	Required assistance with self-care activities (1)	0.397
L3	In hospital (2)	In bed or chair (1)	Did not perform major but performed self-care activities (2)	0.428
L2	In hospital (2)	In bed or chair (1)	Required assistance with self-care activities (1)	0.343
L1	In special unit (1)	In bed or chair (1)	Required assistance with self-care activities (1)	0.267
L0	Death (0)	Death (0)	Death (0)	0.000

Source: **Chen, M.M. et al.** *(31).*

global index has to be constructed. The problem here is to obtain an index which is suitable for use in practice, i.e. an index which can be easily understood and interpreted by a layman and which inspires confidence. It is by no means obvious that all the indexes described satisfy this criterion.

The final question to be dealt with is the collection of data. An ideal global health status index would be of little use if the necessary data could not be collected correctly for reasons of feasibility and/or cost.

Conclusions: The Value of a Multi-criterion Approach

A number of general comments may be made on the basis of this review of current research trends on measurement of the health status of a population.

In the first place, the limitations of conventional indexes have led virtually all health statisticians to advocate the development of methods of health measurement which are more sensitive to changes in factors affecting health, mainly the economic and social environment and also the activities of the health care system. It is clear that we have now moved on from the age of medical pre-eminence in which it was generally accepted that "more medical care produces a proportional improvement in the level of health". We are entering a period of critical evaluation when the challenge has to be met of demonstrating that there really is a positive relationship between the level of health of the population and the utilization of health services.

What pointers have been given by the studies discussed above? There is no doubt whatever that they have substantially widened the field of health, introducing new dimensions and suggesting methods of measuring health phenomena which had been overlooked in previous methods. One may therefore hope to see a possible quantitative improvement in various aspects of the "quality of life" which will in turn bring the population to make wider use of the health care system. A great deal of research will be required to verify this working hypothesis.

One specific result of the research quoted above has been to do away with the monopoly of the medical profession in the assessment of health problems; at the same time the individual has emerged as a credible source of opinion, either on his own or in a group. The need to obtain his personal opinion on a wide range of phenomena, where he alone is capable of supplying pertinent information, has also had very important methodological and practical consequences: surveys based on personal interviews or self-administered questionnaires now play a fundamental part in the work of "health epidemiologists". As a result, the conventional epidemiological approach is now accompanied by a "psycho-sociological approach" to health *(35)*.

Another fairly obvious point is the simultaneous development of health status indexes in two opposite but complementary directions; in the first place towards very general indexes applicable to very large populations, for example the "healthy life expectancy" index, and secondly towards "micro-indexes" designed to measure widely varying phenomena often in very small groups. These opposing trends are perfectly feasible bearing in mind the limits imposed on the application of general indexes and the multiplicity of health problems which arise depending on the target population, problems which may have to be defined in relation to different criteria (age, geographical location, profession, income level, specific pathological condition, observation hospital, etc.). Under these conditions, the diversity of the phenomena to be covered and the measuring instruments required will necessitate the timely use of "batteries" of indicators and indexes as recommended in particular by Levy et al. *(5)*. The underlying reason for this, whether explicitly recognized or not, is that any measurement only provides a partial and distorted picture of the phenomenon under examination, namely "health". Health is a multiple and variable concept, which can be studied by widely different approaches. From this point of view it is not unreasonable to say that in objective terms health is an abstract entity which only exists as a convenient unifying concept.

What is of concern at the practical level is the value of this tool in public health and the use to which it can be put. In a previous paper *(36)* the authors identified three different major functions in which health indicators, in particular complex indicators, could play a part. These were the determination of priorities, decisions on resource allocation and the appraisal of individual measures and of the performance of the health care system as a whole.

The authors believe that an indicator should always be selected in relation to the type of use to which it is intended to be put, assuming the availability of a multi-criterion tool for the description and analysis of health indicators. The tool selected for this purpose was a grid, the main headings of which are presented below (the interested reader may refer to *(36)* for a full explanation of the grid):

(*a*) reference concept;

(*b*) phenomena covered by the indicator;

(*c*) method of construction: weighting, scales aggregation;

(*d*) reliability, validity, ease of interpretation;

(*e*) possible uses.

The conventional indicators, mortality and morbidity, still have an important part to play in the determination of priorities. More recent indicators such as the Loss Rate of Potential Years of Life provide useful improvements but remain within the framework of conventional indicators. Indexes based on incapacity are also potentially valuable when defining public health priorities. They give an idea of the weight to be assigned to health problems for the group as a whole which complements the picture obtained from the traditional indicators, morbidity and mortality, thus widening the range of choice at the decision-making level.

Various complex indicators have been proposed in connection with allocation of resources, in particular those developed by Bush, but the obvious complexity of this indicator makes it difficult to interpret. It is uncertain whether the use of complex indicators for this purpose really contributes to the transparence of the decisions made. In addition, there is no hiding the essentially political and controversial character of decisions in this field. There is a danger of an *a posteriori* technocratic legitimation of decisions. Judgement should therefore be reserved concerning the value of complex indicators, the exact significance of which can often be recognized only by a minority of the decision-making group.

The appraisal/evaluation field is certainly the one in which complex indicators can make their most important contribution. Indicators which are simple to understand and even more easy to compare from one country to another, such as healthy life expectancy, appear to be already in operational use (although they depend on the availability of data on functional incapacities in the population, data which have to be collected from representative samples during major health surveys). An example of this is provided by a recent publication from the Ministry of Social Affairs of Quebec, setting out the changes which have occurred in healthy life expectancy in Canada and the United States *(37)*. This shows, for example, that whereas life expectancy for males in the United States increased by two years between 1962 and 1976, healthy life expectancy increased by less than six months during the same period. This is a very illuminating item of information for the public health authorities, especially if it is compared with the very substantial increase in the availability and technical sophistication of medical care during this period.

Not all complex indicators are as valuable as healthy life expectancy. Complex indicators using an aggregated unit of the functional rather than the chronological type appear to be better suited to assessing the impact of health care on the individual than on the complete population. This may reflect the concentration on the duration of life in western society rather than on the quality of life, which has only recently come to the fore.

Since, to paraphrase Einstein, a discipline is as old as its measuring instruments, it is clear that public health must concentrate on the further development of indicators enabling the public health authorities to get to grips with the complex phenomenon of health. Complex indicators are a necessary step forward, provided that they do not monopolize research resources and the attention paid to the decision-making process in public health.

References

1. **Afifi, A.A. et al.** Some terminology revisited. *In:* Bailey, N.T.J. & Thompson, M., ed. *Systems aspects of health planning.* Amsterdam, North-Holland, 1974.
2. **Berg, R.L., ed.** *Health status indexes.* Chicago, Hospital Research and Educational Trust, 1973.
3. **Siegmann, A.E.** A classification of socio-health indicators: perspectives for health administrators and health planners. *In:* Elinson, J. & Siegmann, A.E., ed. *Socio-medical health indicators.* New York, Baywood, 1979, pp. 197–213.

4. **Reed, L.J.** Principles applying to the collection of information on health as related to socio-environmental factors. *In: Background of social medicine.* New York, Milbank Memorial Fund, 1969, pp. 24–32.
5. **Chiang, C.L. & Cohen, R.D.** How to measure health. A stochastic model for an index of health. *International journal of epidemiology,* **2**: 7–13 (1973).
6. **Sigerist, H.E.** *Medicine and human welfare.* New Haven, Yale University Press, 1941.
7. **Hoyman, H.S.** *Our modern concept of health.* Communication to the American Public Health Association, **16**: 1, Detroit, MI, 1961.
8. **Lifson, M.W.** *Definitions and terminology.* Los Angeles, California Center for Health Services Research, 1969.
9. *Organisation de coopération et de développement économique: mesure du bien-être social.* Progrès accomplis dans l'élaboration des indicateurs sociaux. Paris, OECD, 1976.
10. **Parsons, T.** *In:* Garthy Jaco, E., ed. *Patients, physicians and illness.* New York, Free Press, 1972, pp. 107–127.
11. **Bonnevie, P.** The concept of health. A sociomedical approach. *Scandinavian journal of social medicine,* **1**(2): 41–43 (1973).
12. **Ganguilhem, G.** *Le normal et le pathologique.* Paris, PUF, 1966.
13. **Rossdale, M.** Health in a sick society. *New left review,* **34**: 82–90 (1965).
14. **Wylie, C.M.** The definition and measurement of health and disease. *Public health reports,* **85**: 101–104 (1970).
15. **Lerner, M.** Conceptualization of health and social well being. *In:* Berg, R.L., ed. *Health status indexes.* Chicago, Hospital Research and Educational Trust, 1973.
16. **Kelman, S.** The social nature of the definition problem in health. *International journal of health services,* **5**: 625–642 (1975).
17. **Terris, M.** Approaches to an epidemiology of health. *American journal of public health,* **65**: 1037–1045 (1975).
18. **Chen, M.K.** Aggregated physiological measures of individual and group health status. *International journal of epidemiology,* **4**: 87–92 (1975).
19. **Grogono, A.W. & Woodgate, D.J.** Index for measuring health. *Lancet,* **2**: 1024–1026 (1971).
20. **Skinner, D.E. & Yett, D.E.** Debility, index for longterm care patients. *In:* Berg, R.L., ed. *Health status indexes.* Chicago, Hospital Research and Educational Trust, 1973.
21. **Katz, S. et al.** The ADL index: a standardized measure of biological and psychological function. *Journal of the American Medical Association,* **184**: 914–921 (1963).
22. **Fanshel, S. & Bush, J.W.** A health status index and its application to health services outcome. *Operations research,* **18**: 1021–1066 (1970).
23. **Patrick, D.L. et al.** Methods for measuring levels of well being for a health status index. *Health services research,* **8**: 228–245 (1973).
24. **Blischke, W.R. et al.** Successive intervals analysis for preference measures in a health status index. *Health services research,* **10**: 181–198 (1975).

25. **Breslow, L.** A quantitative approach to the World Health Organization definition of health: physical, mental and social well-being. *International journal of epidemiology,* **1**: 347–355 (1972).
26. **Belloc, N.D. et al.** Measurement of physical health in a general population survey. *American journal of epidemiology,* **23**: 328–336 (1971).
27. **Bergner, M. et al.** The Sickness Impact Profile: conceptual formulation and methodology for the development of a health status measure. *International journal of health services,* **6**: 417 (1976).
28. **Martini, C.J.M. et al.** Health indexes sensitive to medical care variation. *International journal of health services,* **7**: 292–309 (1977).
29. **Ware, J.E. et al.** *Measures of perceptions regarding status: preliminary findings as to scale reliability, validity and administration procedures.* Carbondale, Southern Illinois University School of Medicine (Technical Report MHC, 74-13).
30. **Brook, R.H. et al.** Overview of adult health status measures fielded in Rand's Health Insurance Study. *Medical care,* **17**(Suppl.): 7 (1979).
31. **Chen, M.M. et al.** Social indicators for health planning and policy analysis. *Policy sciences,* **6**: 71–89 (1975).
32. **Bush, J.W. et al.** Cost effectiveness using a health status index. Analysis of the New York State PKU screening program. *In:* Berg, R.L., ed. *Health status indexes.* Chicago, Hospital Research and Educational Trust, 1973, pp. 172–208.
33. **Bush, J.W. et al.** Analysis of a tuberculin testing program using a health status index. *Socio-economic planning sciences,* **6**: 49–68 (1972).
34. **Grogono, A.W.** Measurement of ill health: a comment. *International journal of epidemiology,* **2**: 5–6 (1973).
35. **Pineault, R.** Eléments et étapes d'un programme de santé communautaire. *Union médicale du Canada,* **105**: 1208–1224 (1976).
36. **Dab, W. et al.** Un outil multicritères d'analyse des indicateurs d'état de santé d'une population. *Revue d'épidémiologie et de santé publique,* **30**: 325–342 (1982).
37. *Collection : la santé des Québecois. Durée ou qualité de vie?* Quebec, Conseil des affaires sociales et de la famille, 1983.
38. **Goldberg, M. et al.** Indicateurs de santé et "sanométrie" : les aspects conceptuels des recherches récentes sur la mesure de l'état de santé d'une population. *Revue d'épidémiologie et de santé publique,* **27**: 51–68; 133–152 (1979).
39. **Goldberg, M. et al.** Mesure de la santé individuelle et mesure de la santé d'une population. *In:* Grémy, F. et al., ed. *Medical informatics Europe 81.* Springer-Verlag, 1981.
40. **Dab, W.** *La mesure de la santé d'une population: étude critique à partir d'une typologie des indicateurs de santé.* Paris, INSERM, 1980 (Miméo-GERSS-INSERM U 88).

7.6 Monitoring progress and failure: sentinel health events (unnecessary diseases, disabilities and untimely deaths) — *D.D. Rutstein*

The lack of reliable measuring sticks has made it difficult to determine the level of health of the population or to evaluate the quality of medical care necessary for the maintenance and improvement of health and for the prevention and treatment of disease.

Criteria for Monitoring Progress and Failure

The following criteria are proposed for a satisfactory method to monitor progress and failure in health status and in the measurement of the quality of medical care. The method must:

- be relevant to the health problems affecting any single country or combination of countries of the world and the particular area under investigation;
- be based on up-to-date epidemiological and clinical scientific knowledge about the maintenance and improvement of health, and the prevention and treatment of disease;
- have an immediate alerting function indicating that an undesirable health event exists and needs to be rectified; and
- yield useful data to define health deficiencies in individuals and population groups in specified geographical areas; measure the quality of medical care in its broadest sense; recognize limitations including those of financial, educational and technological resources; and provide guidance for the maintenance and improvement of individual and community health as well as aid in arriving at practical solutions to specific preventive and therapeutic problems.

Background

Routinely, analyses of death certificates are depended upon for mortality evaluation, and hospital discharge or ambulatory care diagnoses for morbidity appraisals. Established methods of presentation do not serve well for determining the state of health of a particular population or the quality of medical care it receives because they do not separate those deaths and diseases that are preventable or manageable from those conditions for which little specific can be done. Thus, the identification and recording of those events has not automatically alerted the physician or the health or hospital administrator to realize that something: may be amiss; has to be looked into immediately; or may require specific action to maintain or improve the health of a population or to prevent or treat disease.

Similarly, the kinds of data routinely collected during the course of hospital or ambulatory medical care are not designed to identify those deviations from optimum medical care that may result in undesirable patient outcomes. This statement is often documented, for example in the *Morbidity and mortality weekly reports* of the Centers for Disease Control in the United States. Repeatedly, preventable or manageable conditions are either unsuspected or unrecognized and not finally identified until a local catastrophe or a general outbreak of illness occurs.

The Model of Infant and Maternal Mortality Control

In sharp contrast to the data usually collected from death certificates and hospital discharge records, routinely collected infant and maternal mortality data do have an immediate alerting function. Those indices are quantitative counts of individual maternal or infant deaths that are used as a screening device to identify gaps or deficiencies in the medical care of mothers and babies. The use of the maternal mortality rate and the infant mortality rate has been fruitful in saving many lives *(1)*. But these two classical quantitative indices do have a serious limitation. They apply only to mothers and babies and not to the state of health of, or to the quality of medical care provided to, the general population. In order to extend the immediate alerting function of the maternal mortality rate and the infant mortality rate to the general population, a new method has been devised.

New Method

With the assistance of specialists in many fields of medicine the Working Group on Preventable and Manageable Diseases selected a new set of indices based on *all* unnecessary diseases, unnecessary disabilities and unnecessary untimely deaths in both sexes at all ages *(2)*. The conditions in Tables 1 and 2 have an alerting function similar to that of infant and maternal mortality. The occurrence of an unnecessary disease, unnecessary disability or unnecessary untimely death is a sentinel health event about which something can be done. It has been assumed that if everything had gone well, the conditions would have been prevented or managed. Moreover, if an unnecessary disease, unnecessary disability or unnecessary untimely death is screened out by use of the method, one may ask the question "Why did it happen?" and then institute a carefully controlled scientific search to identify remediable underlying causes.

The conditions in Tables 1 and 2 were selected on a worldwide basis to have international applicability. Every effort was made to include conditions that are directly relevant to the health and medical care in national and local geographical areas and to hospital populations throughout the world. Although the method has been applied mostly in developed countries, the sentinel health event tables were compiled originally with the developing countries in mind. To keep the list up to date with medical science and to allow for changes from the eighth revision of the *International classification of diseases (3)* to the ninth revision (ICD9) *(4)*, the original tables were revised in 1977 *(5)* and again in 1980 *(6)*. To maintain their medical validity they must be kept up to date in the future.

In the application of the method to a specific problem the term medical care is used in its broadest sense. This includes the application of all relevant medical knowledge; basic and applied research to increase that knowledge and make it more precise; the services of all medical and allied health personnel, institutions and laboratories; the financial, educational and administrative resources of governmental, voluntary and social agencies; and the cooperative responsibilities of the individual himself. Thus, the physician alone cannot be responsible for every sentinel health event.

The chain of responsibility to prevent the occurrence of any unnecessary disease, disability or untimely death may be long and complex. The failure of any single link may precipitate a sentinel health event. The unnecessary case of diphtheria, measles or poliomyelitis may be due to lack of funds available for medical care, the limited resources of a developing country, the failure of government to appropriate needed funds, the health officer who did not implement the programme, the physician who did not immunize his patient, the religious views of the family, the lack of effective public health education, inadequate transport facilities or the mother who did not bring her baby for immunization. Permanent blindness from chronic simple glaucoma may result from inadequate funds, lack of a screening programme for older people in health institutions such as hospitals, medical personnel who are not educated or interested in preventive medicine, or the patient who did not return for follow-up examination or who failed to follow instructions for treatment. Death from cancer of the lung may be due to the patient's unwillingness or inability to give up cigarette smoking, the reassuring statements put out by advertisers or manufacturers of cigarettes, the absence of an effective health information programme in schools and in the community, or more rarely from an error in diagnosis or from poor surgical care. It is clear that the occurrence of any sentinel health event has to be related to the reason for the failure and to whether appropriate resources could possibly be made available to prevent its recurrence in the future.

The method provides for gradations in the sensitivity of sentinel health events. Thus, the conditions shown in Table 1 are single case indices, where the occurrence of a single case of unnecessary disease, e.g. cholera, unnecessary disability, e.g. silicosis, or an unnecessary untimely death, e.g. beriberi heart disease[a] in an infant, is adequate to pose the question "Why did it happen?".

In Table 2 the indices are based on rates. Conditions are listed when prevention or management is highly effective, but when more than a single case of disease or disability or a single death is required to initiate an

[a] Beriberi heart disease (No. 265.0 in ICD9) is included in Table 1 within Nos. 260–269, nutritional deficiencies (including avitaminoses).

Table 1. Unnecessary disease, disability and untimely death — single case indexes

No. (ICD9)	Condition	Unnecessary disease	Unnecessary disability[a]	Unecessary untimely death	Notes[b]
001	Cholera	P[c]		P,T[d]	
002.0	Typhoid fever	P		P,T	
003.0, 003.1	Salmonella gastroenteritis and septicaemia	P		P	
005.0	Staphylococcal food poisoning	P		P,T	
005.1	Botulism	P		P	
010–018, 137	Tuberculosis (all forms)	P	P,T	P,T	P — Contact spread prevented by frequent tuberculin testing and treatment of converters
013	Tuberculosis of meninges and central nervous system	P		P,T	Sensitive index, TBC testing of maternity hospital personnel and persons from high risk groups
020	Plague	P		P,T	P — Urban — domestic rat control
021	Tularaemia			T	
022	Anthrax	P		P,T	P — Occupational exposure
026	Rat-bite fever	P		P,T	
032	Diphtheria	P		P,T	
033	Whooping cough	P		P	
034	Streptococcal sore throat and scarlatina			T	
036	Meningococcal infection:				
	Type A and Type C	P		P	P — Limit epidemics and household outbreaks by immunization or prophylactic treatment
	Type B	P		P	P — Limit household outbreaks by prophylactic treatment
036.2, 038.2, 038.8M[e]	Overwhelming septicaemia following splenectomy (s)[f]	P,T		P,T	P — Prophylaxis against infection with pneuomococcus, *Haemophilus influenzae*, and meningococcus
037, 771.3	Tetanus	P		P	Including neonatal tetanus

045	Acute poliomyelitis	P	P	P	
050	Smallpox	P		P	
055	Measles	P		P	
056, 771.0	Rubella	P	P	P	Congenital rubella syndrome and disability in offspring
060	Yellow fever	P		P	
070.2, 070.3	Viral hepatitis B (serum hepatitis)	P	P	P	P — Via transfusion of blood and blood components (see Table 2)
071	Rabies	P		P	
072	Mumps	P	P	P	
073	Ornithosis	P		P,T	
080	Louse-borne [epidemic] typhus			T	
081.0	Murine [endemic] typhus (flea-borne)			T	
082.0	Spotted fevers			T	
090.0, 090.1, 090.2	Early congenital syphilis	P	P	P,T	Age under 2 years
091	Early syphilis, symptomatic	P	P	P,T	P — Prevent disease in case contacts
093–094	Major complications of syphilis(s)	P,T	P,T	P,T	
098	Gonococcal infections	P	P,T	P,T	P — Prevent disease in case contacts
102	Yaws	P		P,T	
124	Trichinosis	P		P	
126	Ancylostomiasis and necatoriasis (hookworm disease)	P		P,T	
127.0	Ascariasis	P		P,T	
140	Malignant neoplasm of lip	P		P,T	P — Pipe smokers and sun exposure
141.1, 141.2, 141.3, 144, 145.0	Malignant neoplasm of dorsal and ventral surfaces, borders and tip (not base) of tongue, floor of mouth, or buccal mucosa	P		P,T	P — Tobacco smokers and cud and betel-nut chewers
160.0	Malignant neoplasm of nasal cavities	P		P	P — Occupational — chromium industry and wood workers
161	Malignant neoplasm of larynx	P		P,T	P — Cigar and cigarette smokers
162	Malignant neoplasm of trachea, bronchus and lung	P		P	P — Cigarette smoking, asbestos and occupational exposure

Table 1 (contd)

No. (ICD9)	Condition	Unnecessary disease	Unnecessary disability[a]	Unnecessary untimely death	Notes[b]
163	Malignant neoplasm of pleura	P		P	P — Asbestos exposure — "mesothelioma"
172	Malignant melanoma of skin			T	T — Diagnosis and treatment in early stages of disease
173	Other malignant neoplasm of skin	P		P,T	P — Radiation and sun exposure
180	Malignant neoplasm of cervix uteri			T	
182	Malignant neoplasm of body of uterus			T	
184.0	Malignant neoplasm of vagina	P	P	P	In offspring of mothers treated with diethylstilbestrol early in pregnancy
188	Malignant neoplasm of bladder	P		P	P — Aniline dyes and cigarette smoking
189.0M	Malignant neoplasm of kidney, except pelvis — Wilms' tumour (during infancy and childhood)			T	Early recognition and treatment
190.5	Malignant neoplasm of retina — retinoblastoma (under age 5)		T	T	Genetic — screening and treatment
NIC[g]	Neuroblastoma			T	Under 1 year of age and early stage at any age
193	Malignant neoplasm of thyroid gland	P		P,T	P,T — Papillary and follicular carcinoma following radiation exposure treated early P — Medullary carcinoma diagnosed early in patient and family contacts by plasma calcitonin test
201	Hodgkin's disease			T	Lower stages of malignancy
205.1	Myeloid leukaemia, chronic	P		P	P — Radiation exposure or benzene
240.0	Goitre, specified as simple	P			Iodine deficiency
242	Thyrotoxicosis with or without goitre			T	Includes excessive thyroid material ingestion
243, 246.1	Congenital hypothyroidism (cretinism) and dyshormonogenic goitre (s)		T	T	Thyroid screening test (T4 and TSH)
244	Acquired hypothyroidism (myxedema)		T	T	Including that from drugs; early diagnosis by high TSH level

260–269	Nutritional deficiencies (including avitaminoses)	P	P,T	P,T	Not associated with neoplasia or malabsorption
261	Nutritional marasmus	P	P,T	P,T	Under 1 year of age
274M	Gout — tophaceous	T	T		
275.1	Hepatolenticular degeneration (Wilson's disease)		T	T	T — Early recognition by testing patient, screening siblings and treating positives with penicillamine
278.2	Hypervitaminosis A	P	P	P	
278.4	Hypervitaminosis D	P	P	P	
280	Iron deficiency anaemias	P	P,T	P,T	Good public health index for malnutrition
281.0	Pernicious anaemia		T	T	
281.1	Other Vitamin-B_{12}-deficiency anaemias	P,T	P,T		
281.2	Folate-deficiency anaemia		P,T	P,T	
284	Aplastic anaemia	P	P	P	P — Benzene exposure, drugs including chloramphenicol, and radiation
320.0	Haemophilus meningitis (*Haemophilus influenzae* Type B)			T	Early recognition and prompt treatment
362.2	Retrolental fibroplasia (s)	P	P		P — Excessive oxygen therapy in premature babies
365.1M	Blindness — glaucoma, chronic (simple)		T		
382, 383	Otitis media (suppurative) or mastoiditis (s)		T	T	
390–392	Acute rheumatic fever		P	P	P — Prevent recurrences
416M	Chronic pulmonary heart disease secondary to chronic pulmonary disease	P	P	P	P — Occupational and environmental exposure
460–466, 480–483, 485, 486, 490	Acute respiratory infections, pneumonia, and bronchitis			T	Deaths less than age 50 unless associated with immunologic defects or neoplasms
487	Influenza	P		P,T	P — Vaccine immunization to targeted poplations defined by virulence of particular strain T — Deaths less than age 50 unless associated with immuno ogic defects or neoplasms

Table 1 (contd)

No. (ICD9)	Condition	Unnecessary disease	Unnecessary disability[a]	Unnecessary untimely death	Notes[b]
492, 496	Emphysema or chronic obstructive lung disease (s)	P	P	P	P — Cigarettes and other environmental risks
493	Asthma			T	T — Self-inhalation therapy deaths under age 50
495, 500–505, 506, 507.1 508.0, 508.1	Extrinsic allergic alveolitis, pneumonoconioses, chemical fumes and vapours, lipid inhalation, and radiation effects (s)	P	P	P	
531M	Ulcer, gastric (stress)	P		P	P — From severe trauma including major surgery and burns — antacid prophylaxis
550–553	Inguinal or other hernia of abdominal cavity with or without obstruction (s)			T	Deaths under age 65
574, 575.0, 575.1	Acute or chronic cholecystitis and/or cholelithiasis (s)			T	Deaths under age 65
633	Ectopic pregnancy			T	
680–686	Infections of skin and subcutaneous tissue			T	
692, 693	Dermatitis from contact and substances taken internally (s)	P	P	P	P — Environmental and occupational exposure to specific agents
711.0	Pyogenic arthritis	P	P,T	P,T	P — Secondary to pyogenic infection
714.32	Blindness — pauciarthritis (s)		T		Repeated slit-lamp examination and, if positive, local steroids
730.0	Acute osteomyelitis	P	P,T	P,T	P — Secondary to pyogenic infection
730.1	Chronic osteomyelitis		T	T	
630–675	All maternal deaths (including abortion) (s)			P	
760–772, 774–779	Infant mortality, general (s)			P	Plus all other deaths less than 1 year of age regardless of cause

773.0, 773.3, 773.4	Haemolytic disease due to Rh isoimmunization	P	P,T	P,T	Immune globulin
NIC	Iatrogenic prematurity	P	P	P	P — From too early induction or Caesarian section
NIC	Neural tube defects	P	P	P	P — Alpha fetaprotein measurement
758.0	Down's syndrome	P	P	P	P — Amniocentesis — mothers over age 35, or previous baby with Down's syndrome
317M–319M	Mental retardation induced by:				
	Maternal nutritional deficiency		P		
	Tay-Sachs disease		P		Genetic counselling and screening
	Lead intoxication	P	P	P	
NIC	Man-made (including occupational and environmental) diseases induced by (with examples): 1. *Toxic agents*, including direct chemical hazards (carbon tetrachloride); carcinogens (vinyl chloride); mutagens (lead); teratogens (thalidomide); pesticides (cholinesterase inhibitors); contact irritants (occupational dermatoses); dusts (pneumonoconioses with and without tuberculosis); contact sensitizers (nickel); water contaminants (polychlorinated biphenyls); air pollutants (sulfur dioxide). 2. *Physical hazards*, including radiant energy (medical, industrial and war); noise (rock and roll); and vibration (jack hammers). 3. *Artificial environments*, including space travel, aeroplanes, caissons, air conditioned sealed buildings, and intensive-care units.				

Table 1 (contd)

No. (ICD9)	Condition	Unnecessary disease	Unnecessary disability[a]	Unnecessary untimely death	Notes[b]
	4. *Accidents* (manifold varieties inducing injury).				
	5. *Biological hazards*, including laboratory accidents, antiobiotic-resistant microorganisms, and contact allergic dermatitis (plants and wood).				
780–789, 799	Symptoms and ill defined conditions				Unless specified as "cause unknown" frequent diagnoses consisting only of symptoms or ill defined conditions are evidence of poor quality

No.[h] (ICD9)	Operative procedure	Unnecessary untimely death[i]	Notes
28.2, 28.3	Tonsillectomy with or without adenoidectomy	P	Indications for tonsillectomy are TB, tumour, post-peritonsillar abscess, recurrent infections not responsive to adequate therapy (seldom) and obstructive hypertrophy (rare)
47.0	Appendectomy for appendicitis	P	Normal appendices should be a relatively small proportion of those removed, i.e. the result of unavoidable false positive diagnoses
68.3–68.8	Hysterectomy (s)	P	Each hysterectomy must be justified by sufficient pathologic findings in the removed uterus or by extenuating circumstances documented by consultation

66.2, 66.3, 66.5, 66.63	Tubal sterilization (s)	P
74.0–74.9	Elective Caesarian section (s)	P

[a] This refers to the unnecessary ongoing disability characteristic of the specific disease and not to general disability that may be associated with acute or debilitating illness.

[b] The symbol P or T in the notes indicates that the prevention or treatment is limited to the circumstances described by the phrase that follows.

[c] P = prevention.

[d] T = treatment.

[e] M = scope not congruent with ICD definition.

[f] (s) = summary statement.

[g] NIC = the condition is not identifiable as such in the ICD code.

[h] Code numbers refer to the Operative and Diagnostic and Non-Surgical Procedures Classification within the ICD code.

[i] A death from tonsillectomy, appendectomy for appendicitis, hysterectomy, tubal sterilization or elective Caesarian section is a sentinel health event.

Table 2. Unnecessary disease, disability and untimely death — indexes based on rates

No. (ICD9)	Condition	Unnecessary disease	Unnecessary disability[a]	Unnecessary untimely death	Notes[b]
004	Shigellosis	P[c]		P,T[d]	
005.2–005.9	Food poisoning (bacterial) other than salmonellosis, shigellosis, staphylococcal, and botulism (see Table 1) (s)[e]			T	
070.0, 070.1	Viral hepatitis A	P	P	P	
070.2, 070.3	Viral hepatitis B (serum hepatitis)	P	P	P	Transmission other than by transfusion of blood and blood components (see Table 1)
070.4, 070.5 070.6, 070.9	Viral hepatitis non-A-non-B	P	P	P	P — Avoid commercial paid blood donors
084	Malaria	P?[f]	P?	P?,T	Early treatment of falciparum infection
153–154	Malignant neoplasm of colon, rectum, rectosigmoid junction and anus			T	
204.0	Lymphoid leukaemia, acute			T	"Favourable form" (ages 2–9 and WBC under 20 000)
250.1, 250.2, 250.3(CM)[g]	Diabetes mellitus w/mention of acidosis or coma			T	Above specified death rate and hypo-glycaemic death due to overtreatment
286.0, 286.1	Congenital factor VIII disorder (haemophilia) and congenital factor IX disorder (Christmas disease)	P	P,T	P,T	P — Prenatal diagnosis
345.1	Epilepsy, generalized convulsive		T	T	
401–405	Hypertensive disease		T	T	Above specified rates
410, 411, 413, 430–436 w/codes 401–405 above	Vascular complications of heart or brain associated with hypertensive disease (s)	P	P	P	Relates to excess of complications due to the hypertension
521.0	Dental caries	P			P — Adequate fluorides and reduced sugar intake
531–532	Ulcer of stomach or duodenum with or without haemorrhage or perforation			T	Deaths less than age 65

714	Rheumatoid arthritis and other inflammatory polyarthropathies		P		P — Incapacitating deformity from inadequate treatment
737	Curvature of spine		T	T?[h]	
745–747.3	Congenital anomalies of heart and great arteries			T	Early recognition and referral
317M–319M[i]	Mental retardation associated with:				
	Blood-group incompatibilities other than Rh		T	T	
	Phenylketonuria			T	
	Neonatal sepsis			T	
	Herpes simplex infection			T	
E850–E858, E930–E949, 960–979	Accidental poisoning and adverse effects by drugs and medicaments, including all contraceptives (s)	P	P	P	Includes iatrogenic disease and deserves special study
E870–E876, E878, E879, 996–999	Surgical and medical complications and misadventures	P	P	P	Includes many varieties of iatrogenic and deserves special study
NIC[j]	Nosocomial infections	P	P	P	
NIC	Iatrogenic disease — a category of the man-made diseases (not eligible for Table 1)				

[a] This refers to unnecessary ongoing disability characteristic of the specific disease and not to general disability that may be associated with acute or debilitating illness.

[b] The symbol P or T in the notes indicates that the prevention or treatment is limited to the circumstances described by the phrase that follows.

[c] P = prevention.

[d] T = treatment.

[e] (s) = summary statement.

[f] P? = prevention controversial.

[g] CM = clinical modification, code used for hospital tabulations.

[h] T? = treatment controversial.

[i] M = scope not congruent with ICD definition.

[j] NIC = the condition is not identifiable as such in the ICD code.

immediate inquiry. Examples are: unnecessary disease, e.g. an epidemic of hepatitis A; unnecessary disability, e.g. nosocomial infections due to inadequate control of disease spread in hospitals; and unnecessary untimely deaths, e.g. from surgical and medical complications and misadventures.

Specialized tables to meet specific needs are also being prepared. Thus, from the general category in Table 1 of "man-made (including occupational) diseases", a new table was compiled for sentinel health events in the occupational sphere as a basis for physician recognition and public health surveillance *(7)*. It was put together in collaboration with the National Institute for Occupational Safety and Health (NIOSH) of the US Centers for Disease Control. The sentinel health event (occupational) (SHE(O)) subtable has had an immediate success. It is a reference point for the occupational disease surveillance programe of NIOSH working with individual states. It has been recommended as a focal point in medical education in occupational disease in the United States by the Committee on Government Operations of the US House of Representatives *(8)*. In medical education, the table should be helpful in guiding the medical student to include specific occupational illnesses in his pattern of differential diagnosis as he learns to identify specific diseases. For the physician, it should improve the quality of medical care by alerting him to the occurrence of unnecessary disease, unnecessary disability and unnecessary untimely death in his patients. The success of the (SHE(O)) subtable should justify exploration of the compilation of new subtables including one to focus on the sentinel health events of the developing countries.

Application of the method

It should be clear that if a particular question is under study, the screening stage will not require the simultaneous use of all of the sentinel health events in the tables. Instead, those sentinel health events that are directly relevant to the questions posed should be selected from the tables for the particular study. If, for example, one were concerned with evaluating the effectiveness of preventive care for children in a defined population, relevant sentinel health events might include among others: the categories of infectious diseases that are controlled by immunization, e.g. cases of diphtheria or deaths from measles in a developing country; and conditions in children caused by toxic agents, e.g. lead poisoning. In contrast, if the study were concerned with the efficacy of certain therapeutic measures, one might select from the tables a list of unnecessary untimely deaths from such manageable conditions as Hodgkin's disease or vascular complications of the heart or brain associated with hypertension.

There are two steps in the application of the method to the solution of a specific problem:

— screening of aggregations of diagnostic data such as from death certificates, hospital discharge summaries, and research studies for identification of the occurrence of sentinel health events; and

— a careful scientific search for remediable underlying causes for the identifed sentinel health events.

Screening

Screening as the first stage of application of the method will provide useful information by identifying unnecessary untimely deaths among death certificate diagnoses in a particular population group. For example, screening might reveal the number, names and location of women dying unnecessary untimely deaths owing to carcinoma of the cervix. A number of such deaths, particularly in younger women, would warrant an in-depth study to identify underlying etiological factors.

In the same way the occurrence of unnecessary disease, unnecessary disability and unnecessary untimely death due to particular sentinel health events could be identified among hospital discharge diagnoses by computer matching at specified intervals against the list of conditions in the tables. A careful review of such events could raise interesting and important questions concerning patient care. Thus, the occurrence of cases of hepatitis B in a particular hospital over a period of months would require examination of the blood transfusion service. Also, screening for fatal or other undesirable outcomes from drug reactions or from late admissions of bacterial meningitis due to *Haemophilus influenzae* Group B, pneumococcus or streptococcus Group A would identify an appropriate focus for postgraduate medical education for the hospital staff, the referring physicians or for both groups.

The screening step of the method, therefore, can reveal what happened to a particular population, but not provide an answer to the question "Why did it happen?".

Search for remediable underlying causes

The identification of an unnecessary disease, disability or untimely death by this screening method often requires a careful scientific search for remediable underlying causes. Once again, advantage may be taken of previous experience with maternal and infant mortality rates. In the classic maternal mortality studies in New York City in the early 1930s *(9)*, when a maternal death was reported the relevant facts were collected and reviewed by expert clinicians to determine "Why did it happen?". Information so collected was studied to determine how similar events could be prevented in the future. The lessons so learned were publicized in postgraduate medical education and in programmes to improve obstetrical practice. There followed an immediate and continuing sharp drop in the maternal mortality rate.

A similar study of infant deaths in 1967–1968 in Massachusetts *(10)*, followed by the institution of a regionalized programme for the management of premature babies, resulted in a sharp decrease in the infant mortality rate *(11)*.

The search for the underlying preventive or therapeutic inadequacies is an essential step in the complete application of the method. Returning to the example of deaths from carcinoma of the cervix, it can now be seen why a complete study would require not only the screening step to identify the cases, but also a thorough inquiry into the occurrence of possible remediable underlying causes that could then be eradicated in much the same way as has been successful in the past for decreasing infant and maternal mortality.

Examples of the use of the method
Ways in which the method has been used included the following.

Monitoring therapy detected the distribution by health area of unnecessary untimely deaths due to selected sentinel health events resulting from inadequate therapy in England & Wales *(12)*. This therapy is now being expanded to the European Community.

Combined morbidity and mortality surveillance established the distribution of unnecessary disease, disability or untimely death (including occupational diseases) on death certificates and among discharge diagnoses in hospitals in Rhode Island in the United States *(13–16)*.

Racial differences in death rates were found by comparisons of age-specific death rates among Blacks and Whites in the United States. A set of sentinel health events was identified that is responsible for a significant proportion of the increased death rates among Blacks *(17)*.

Future Trends

Likely applications of the method to current health problems include the following.

Emergency monitoring. In this period of worldwide poverty and increasing financial pressure in many countries, there is an acute need to monitor various population groups to identify sudden deterioration in health status precipitated by economic and political factors. For example, in the United States the Child Health Outcome Project is instituting a programme to detect sudden worsening in the health of infants and children by the use of indicators, including sentinel health events *(18)*.

Hospital costs of sentinel health events. A beginning has been made in measuring the increases in the cost of medical care that are due to the occurrence of sentinel health events. For example, an analysis has been made in the state of Missouri calculating the cost of the number of unnecessary hospital days resulting from the occurrence of sentinel health events.[a]

Occupational disease control. As already noted, NIOSH is collaborating with individual states in the creation of a uniform surveillance programme in occupational disease throughout the country. NIOSH is testing the SHE(O) method *(7)* for: routine monitoring of occupationally related morbidity and mortality; selected epidemiological studies of unusual SHE(O) patterns; case studies of specific SHE(O) conditions; and its guidance to practising physicians caring for patients with occupational

---

[a] **McEvoy, L.** Unpublished data.

illness. State-based data resources (e.g. vital statistics, workers' compensation claims and hospital discharge abstracts) are the focal point for these activities.

All of these examples are from the developed countries. A major effort, including the creation of a new subtable on sentinel health events in developing countries, is needed to see how the method can be used to help control the great burden of unnecessary disease, unnecessary disability and unnecessary untimely death in the developing countries.

References

1. **Department of Health and Social Security.** *Report on confidential enquiries into maternal deaths in England and Wales 1976–1978.* London, H.M. Stationery Office, 1982 (Report on Health & Social Subjects, No. 26).
2. **Rutstein, D.D. et al.** Measuring the quality of medical care, a clinical method. *New England journal of medicine,* **294**: 582–588 (1976).
3. *International classification of diseases*, eighth revision. Geneva, World Health Organization, 1969.
4. *International classification of diseases*, ninth revision. Geneva, World Health Organization, 1977.
5. **Rutstein, D.D. et al.** Measuring the quality of medical care: revision of tables of indexes. Letter to the editor. *New England journal of medicine,* **297**: 508 (1977).
6. **Rutstein, D.D. et al.** Measuring the quality of medical care: second revision of tables of indexes. Letter to the editor. *New England journal of medicine,* **302**: 1146 (1980).
7. **Rutstein, D.D. et al.** Sentinel health events (occupational): a basis for physician recognition and public health surveillance. *American journal of public health,* **73**: 1054–1062 (1983).
8. **Committee on Government Relations, 60th Report, US House of Representatives.** *Occupational illness data collection: fragmented, unreliable, and seventy years behind communicable disease surveillance.* Washington, DC, US Government Printing Office, 1984 (House Report 98-1144. Union Calendar No. 641).
9. **New York Academy of Medicine, Committee on Public Health Relations.** *Maternal mortality in New York City: a study of all puerperal deaths 1930–1932.* New York, Commonwealth Fund, 1933.
10. **Perinatal Welfare Committee.** *Report on perinatal and infant mortality in Massachusetts, 1967 and 1968.* Boston, Massachusetts Medical Society, 1971.
11. **Ryan, G.M. et al.** Regionalizing perinatal health services in Massachusetts. *New England journal of medicine,* **296**: 228–230 (1977).
12. **Charlton, J.R.H. et al.** Geographical variation in mortality from conditions amenable to medical intervention in England and Wales. *Lancet,* **1**: 691–696 (1983).

13. **Kelley, B.C. & Gute, D.M.** *The development of occupational disease surveillance tool, based on available health data sources in Rhode Island.* Presented at the Annual Meeting of the American Public Health Association, Los Angeles, 3 November 1981.
14. **Kelley, B.C.** *Sentinel health events: occupational disease in Rhode Island.* Presented at the Annual Meeting of the American Public Health Association, Montreal, 15 November 1982.
15. **Gute, D.M. & Kelley, B.C.** *Using death certificate data to contribute to a statewide occupational health surveillance system: the Rhode Island experience.* Presented at the Public Health Conference on Records and Statistics held on 22 August 1983, Washington, DC.
16. **Kelley, B.C. et al.** Using existing data systems to estimate the burden of selected preventable or manageable conditions and possible etiologic factors in Rhode Island (1974–1978). *Morbidity and mortality weekly report.*
17. **Woolhandler, S. et al.** Racial differences in preventable deaths in Alameda County, California. *International journal of health services,* **15**: 1–22 (1985).
18. **Schorr, L.B. et al.** *Overview and context of current monitoring efforts using child health outcome measures.* Presented at the Workshop on Indicators for Monitoring Child Health Outcomes held on 24 January 1983, Cambridge, MA.

7.7 Alternative ways of presenting statistics on sickness, disability and death — *E. Schach*

The demonstration of health improvement for populations requires concise aggregate measures at the country level, because only such measures summarize the information for the desired purpose. In particular, such measures should be generally understood and appropriate for comparisons in time and location. Thus, measures to describe health and health improvement of populations should be relevant, concise, constructed on the basis of widely available statistics, reasonably accurate, timely and suitable for comparisons in and among countries.

When such requirements are demanded, analyses may be based on life table and mortality data. In most European countries, for example, such data have been available for the major part of this century and in some countries even for a substantial portion of the last. Standardized documentation, production and analysis of data, and uniform dissemination policies make comparisons of these data among countries possible. Data about sickness and disability do not currently exist for many countries. If they do, they have neither been collected with uniform methodology, nor for extended periods in the past. Thus, comparisons of the development of sickness within European countries over time are difficult to carry out and international comparisons based on routinely available data are almost impossible *(1)*. For reasons of accessibility of data, analyses will be based on life tables of European populations. However, the approaches demonstrated may obviously be applied to other countries if the data described below are available or attainable there as well. These approaches are also applicable to national analyses if data are available for subregions and for several years in a row.

This volume focuses on ways to present the health of populations and its improvement, not on disease and death, as has been the case for a long time. It is the specific task of this section to concentrate on alternative approaches to achieve this goal. Due to a relatively small common data base among countries and the lack of established indicators of positive health of populations, such approaches have to restrict themselves to working with data bases on mortality and morbidity. In the framework of this section alternative ways of presenting data implies that alternative ways of analysis and of combining available data sets will have to be investigated or developed. This chapter takes up the challenge by:

— analysing the time trend in age- and sex-specific mortality, thereby showing differences in the improvement of the mortality rates by these population characteristics;

— estimating the maximal age of population members and showing how the development toward this maximum occurred in a specific population;

- examining variabilities of life expectancies in selected European countries to study the hypothesis of a north–south trend in life expectancies;
- investigating the time trend of disability-free life expectancy in order to examine whether the reduction and/or compression of mortality is accompanied by a compression of morbidity as well;
- investigating the shape and development of the survival function in time, thereby showing the survival pattern of populations in this and in the last century;
- studying the potential for further improvement of these functions by comparison with one of the more favourable survival functions in Europe; and
- estimating the average relationship between the reduction in mortality and the increase in life expectancy to ascertain the average effect on life expectancy of the population of a small change in the mortality rate.

Data

Data for construction of life tables originate from various sources. Deaths are recorded in the death registration system by age and sex. Numerators for computed rates are derived from estimates of the mid-year population. These latter quantities are ascertained in censuses or extrapolations thereof between census years.

Data for construction of life tables for time lived free of disability use the above data and estimates of lifetime in the state of disability, usually originating from interview surveys.

Methods

As the construction of current life tables has been well documented *(2)*, only methods specific to this chapter will be described here. It may be noted that the methods described require a minimal population size in order to keep the random variability of the estimated statistics within predictable bounds.

Life tables are usually computed around census years, and often more frequently in developed countries, to describe the mortality experience of the population of a country at a particular time. The tables are based on the population distribution by age and sex obtained in the census, and they are the result of applying mortality rates to the population at a particular time. They display expected numbers of additional years of life for each age and sex group and the pattern of survival prevailing in a particular population during one year (or during several years around census time). These statistics may be compared in time and across countries. The paper is based on the entries in the column labelled number alive at age x (usually labelled l_x) in the life table. This column usually starts with 100 000 persons. If the mortality conditions prevalent at a specific time and place operate on the population, the survivors for the different ages and sex groups displayed there are obtained. These survivors for different points in time by age and sex are plotted in Fig. 1 and 2. They are also the l_x in the formula of the entropy, where x stands for the different age groups. Furthermore, they also form the basis for the estimates in Tables 1 and 3.

Life expectancy (the mean number of additional years of life expected by persons in the respective age and sex group) is computed by averaging the mean number of years experienced by persons in the respective age/sex groups in the years observed *(2)*. Such estimates for different time periods are presented in Fig. 3 and 4 and in the section on the variability of life expectancies within Europe.

By analogy, life expectancy free of disability may be estimated on the basis of life tables by subtracting the respective average duration of disability for the corresponding age and sex groups from the life expectancies in life tables *(3)*. In addition, the lengths of disability may be differentiated by the severity of disability.

The concept of years of life lost or gained offers another approach to the use of mortality information.

One method of estimating the years of life lost for a population consists of multiplying the category of number of deaths by age, sex and disease category by the life expectancy of the respective age/sex category. When average years of life lost are then computed by dividing the total years of life lost in a cause of death category by the number of deaths, it is implied that the dead would have survived as long as the living had they not died of that particular cause. For reasons of successive further risks of dying this assumption is, of course, not realistic for all diseases. Another approach consists of setting a maximum age for a population and adding up all years lost by age, sex and disease categories that the dead would have lived through up to that chosen age, had they not died of the particular cause. The problem here is that a maximum age limit has to be set. As both approaches have methodological limitations, results of a procedure drawing on both approaches developed by Geissler *(4)* are presented below. It consists of arbitrarily setting 90 years as the maximum for a population's age and adding up years of life lost up to that age by age and sex for the observed cause of death and successive hypothetical causes, had the person survived the first and been exposed to further ones up to the maximum age. This way, the allocation of years of life lost to specific categories of causes is more accurate than in the first approach to the years of life lost. Geissler separates between directly and indirectly lost years of life and displays them through cause of death group. (Selected data are given in Table 3.)

Life Expectancy

The most widely used measure of life expectancy is the life expectancy of a newborn. It is a "summary measure of the total mortality experience of a population which is little affected by any pattern of the age and sex pyramid, by the pattern of the birth rate or the history of migration" *(2)*. Life expectancy of a newborn is one of the specific life expectancies contained in a life table.

Fig. 1. Survivors among 100 000 females at age x: Germany, 1871–1880 to (Federal Republic of Germany) 1977–1979

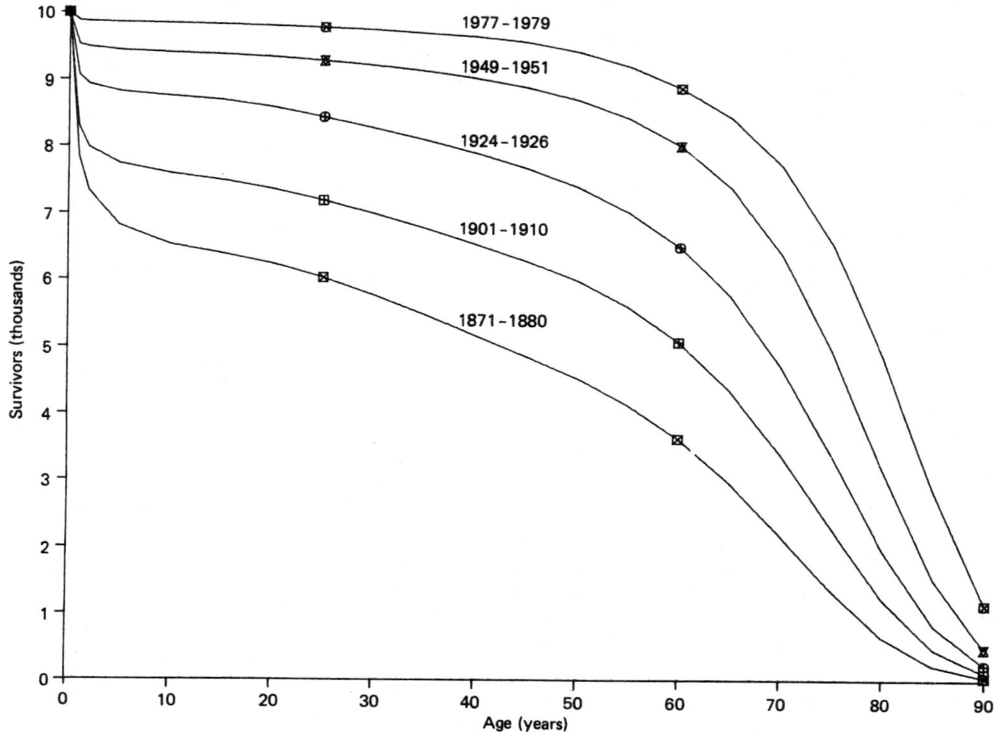

Fig. 2. Survivors among 100 000 males at age x: Germany, 1871–1880 to (Federal Republic of Germany) 1977–1979

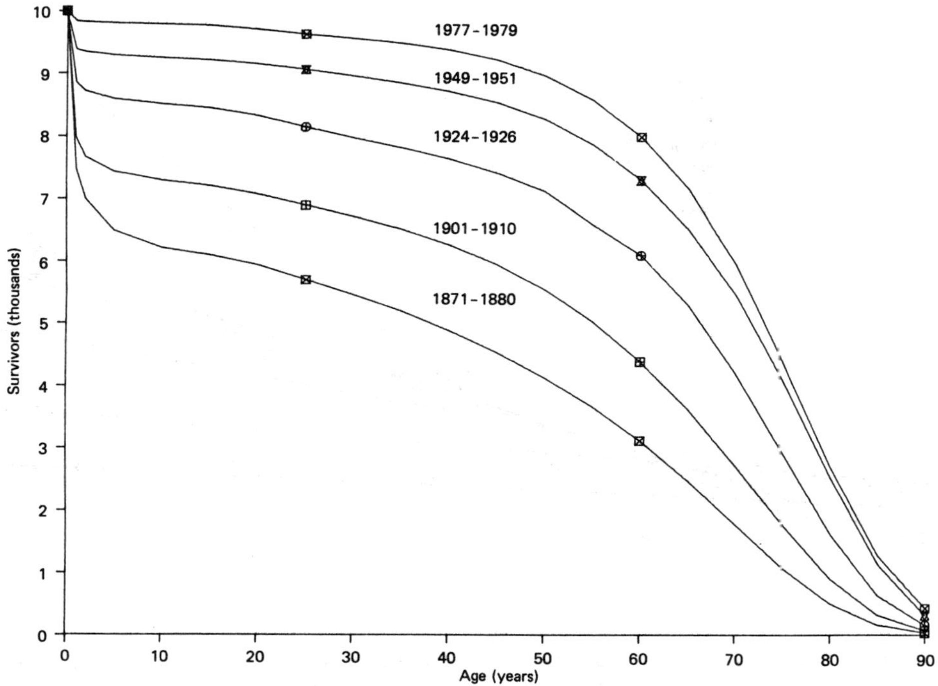

Fig. 3. Life expectancy for females by age: Germany, 1871–1880 to (Federal Republic of Germany) 1977–1979 and a projection to 2100

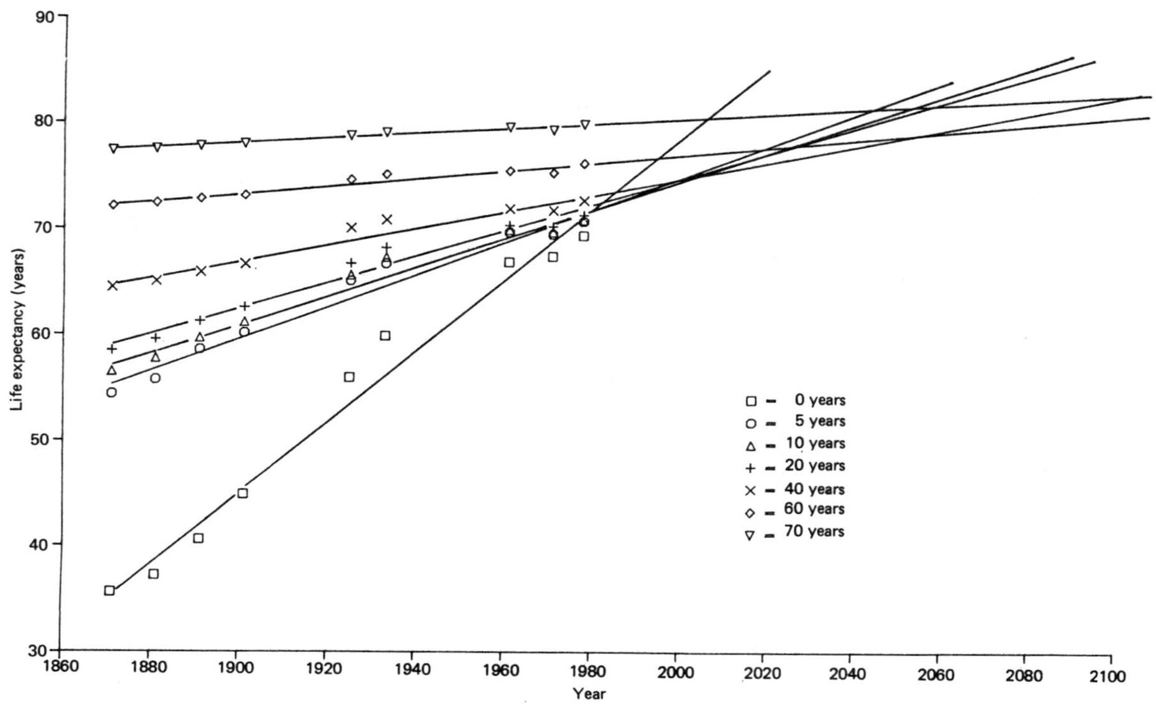

Fig. 4. Life expectancy for males by age: Germany, 1871–1880 to (Federal Republic of Germany) 1977–1979 and a projection to 2100

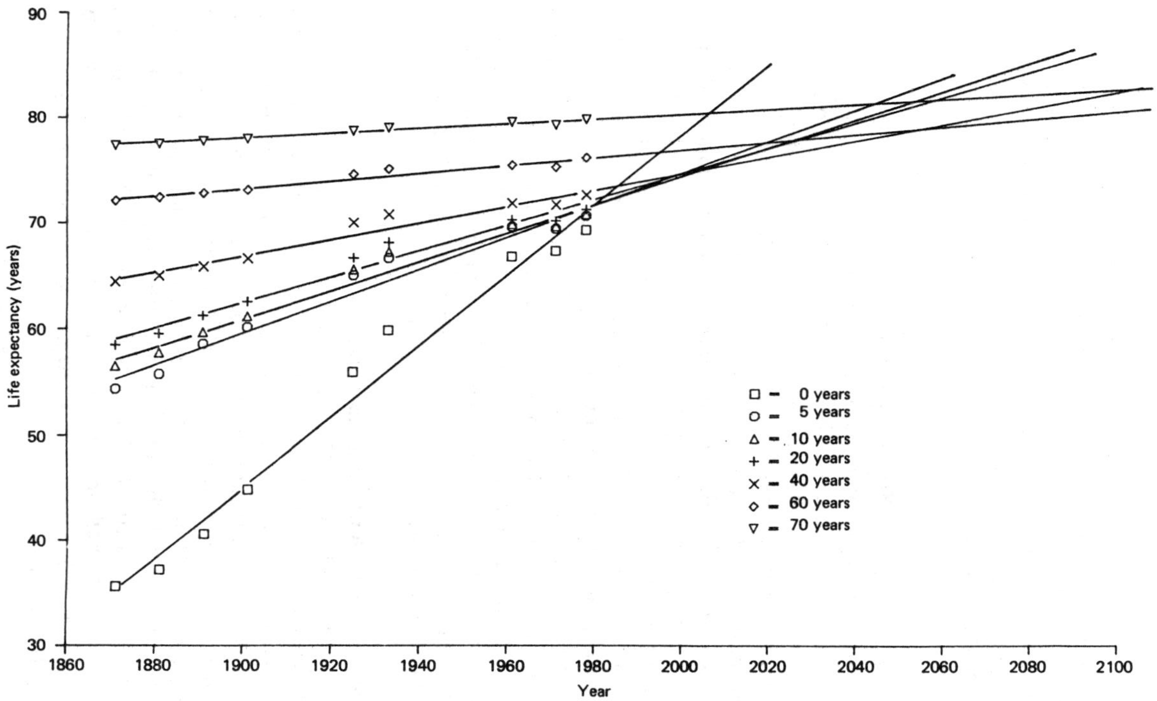

However, like any summary statistic, the life expectancy of the newborn represents only a portion of the total mortality information of a population. This limitation has to be taken into consideration with comparisons. The most important aspect to watch out for in these comparisons is the variation of life expectancies between the sexes and ages. The life expectancy of the newborn shows a different development over time than the life expectancy of other age groups. Thus, the ratio of the life expectancies of the newborn and that of other age groups is not constant in a population at different times and it differs across countries. Therefore, the examination of the life expectancy of the newborn has to be supplemented by estimates of this statistic for higher age groups (such as people of 5, 10, 20, 40, 65, 70 or 85 years of age).

Life expectancy in different age groups

The expected total length of life of a person increases with age. However, life expectancy is not necessarily greatest at birth; in only 7 out of 22 European countries between 1974 and 1977 was the life expectancy of newborn males greater than that for one-year-old males. These countries were those with low infant mortality rates, namely Denmark, Finland, France, the Netherlands, Norway, Sweden and Switzerland *(5)*. For females, 10 out of 22 countries showed a higher or equal life expectancy for newborns as compared to life expectancies for one-year-olds *(5)*. These 10 countries were those listed above for males plus Belgium, the German Democratic Republic and the Federal Republic of Germany. At the beginning of the 1980s more than half of the countries of the Region reported higher or equal life expectancies for newborns as compared to one-year-old males, and more than three quarters showed higher or equal life expectancies for newborns compared with one-year-old females. Thus, when reporting life expectancies by age, it is of interest to point out the relationship between these figures for the newborn and one-year-olds.

Life expectancy for females and males

Fig. 3 (females) and 4 (males) present the development of life expectancies for Germany by age, from 1871–1880 to 1977–1979 (Federal Republic of Germany) *(6, 7)*. They contain the life table estimates of life expectancies and fitted lines for each age group under the simplified assumption that life expectancies by age and sex increased by a constant percentage in each of the last 100 years. While this seems to be an adequate assumption for the age groups beyond 60, the time series of life expectancies for the middle and young ages may better be described by parabolas. This is because the relative yearly improvement in life expectancies for these latter age groups slowed down after 1950. With respect to life expectancies for females and males these figures show:

- that for all ages female average length of life exceeded male length of life in 1977–1979;
- that the development for both sexes differed over time, with the discrepancies in life expectancy widening between the two groups

(the slopes of the fitted lines are greater for all female age groups than those for the corresponding male age groups); and

— that absolute differences in male/female life expectancy decrease with increasing age.

Variability of life expectancy across Europe

When the life expectancy of the newborn in European countries is examined, it is found that countries differ substantially with respect to this statistic. The figures ranged from 72.8 (Sweden, 1977) to 66.7 (Hungary, 1975) *(5)*. In the framework of this investigation it is of interest to examine whether there are any explanations for this observed variability. One hypothesis that may be examined on the basis of these data is whether there exists a north–south gradient of life expectancies in Europe. One possible explanation for such a gradient might be differences in climate or geographic location of countries. To follow up on this hypothesis data from Ewert & Marcusson *(5)*, who divided 22 European countries (1974–1977) into three groups by order of magnitude of life expectancy of the newborn, may be used. Countries with high life expectancy at birth for males were Denmark, Greece, the Netherlands, Norway, Sweden and Switzerland. Countries occupying intermediate positions were Austria, Belgium, Bulgaria, England & Wales, France, the German Democratic Republic, the Federal Republic of Germany, Italy and Spain, and countries with low values were Czechoslovakia, Finland, Portugal, Romania and Yugoslavia. Most northern European countries are found in the high group and, conversely, proportionately more central and southern European countries occupy the low group. In order to examine whether this ordering is only valid for the 1970s, the life expectancies of selected countries of Europe around 1870 were checked. The life expectancies of newborn males averaged 41.4 years for the Netherlands, Sweden and Switzerland, and 38 years for England & Wales, France, the German Democratic Republic and the Federal Republic of Germany; life expectancy was 32.7 years for males in Czechoslovakia. On the basis of these data it appears that the gradient between life expectancies of selected European countries today could already be observed in the last century and these seven countries would have occupied almost the same positions in 1870 as they do today, had they been ranked by magnitude of life expectancy of the newborn. The absolute difference of life expectancies of newborn males for countries in the high and intermediate life expectancy groups was almost identical in 1871–1880 and 1977–1979. In the latter period Czechoslovakia, a country in the low life expectancy group, reduced the difference to the mean newborn male life expectancy of countries in the high group by about two thirds, still maintaining its lowest position in life expectancy among the seven countries compared in 1975. However, if the gradient between life expectancies existed and if it was due to climate and/or location, then developments in life expectancy of a particular country should be compared with countries of the same climate group when descriptions of health improvement and improvement potential are desired. In particular, it would be important to learn which portion of the variability of life expectancy was attributable to climate and geography.

Life expectancy by socioeconomic variable

It has been suggested that life expectancy differs with socioeconomic variables. In particular, mortality rates have been shown to vary with income *(8)* or social class *(9)*, thus it is expected that life expectancy will vary correspondingly. Fox & Goldblatt *(10)* recently found that mortality rates differ with socioeconomic variables, such as ownership of a house or the availability of cars. As these differences imply that higher mortality rates are associated with lower income and lower values of socioeconomic variables, it might follow that within a country the differences in mortality should diminish as income increases and as the differences in income among citizens is reduced. Consequently, mortality rates are expected to be lowest in the countries with a relatively high level of income and, among these, lowest in those with relatively high income homogeneity. If the mortality patterns of a country are affected by the general level of wealth and its distribution among the citizens, life expectancy improvements within one country should be studied as they relate to the distribution of income and wealth in that population.

Life expectancy free of disability

Life expectancy free of disability is obtained by extending methods of obtaining the life expectancy of the population on the basis of life tables to years lived without disability. Estimates of disability and its duration are obtained from population health surveys. Life expectancy free of disability is a further method of deriving an indicator of the health of the total population. While the concept of years of life lost elucidates the relative importance of certain diseases to the mortality of a country, years of life lived with disability does the same for the relative importance of disease categories in the total disease spectrum. By deducting the years spent in a state of disability from the expected years of life by age and sex the expected average years of life free of disability for a population by age and sex is obtained.

Colvez & Blanchet *(3)*, by applying the concept to the United States between 1966 and 1976, found that while life expectancy at birth increased by 2.7 years (from 70 in 1966 to 72.7 years in 1976), life expectancy free of disability was 56.5 in 1966 and 56:0 years in 1976. The total loss was higher in 1976 (16.7 years) than in 1966 (13.5 years). About one third of the loss of life expectancy free of disability for the United States was attributed to severe limitation of activity in the time period between 1966 and 1976 *(3)*. A prerequisite for comparisons of disability over time within one country or across countries is that the comparison be based on the same concept of disability. In particular, the fact that the extension of social and health insurance and of specific health services for the elderly may change the concept of disability over time or across nations should be taken into account. Thus, an extension of such services might imply more use of them and might consequently result in an increase of measured disability.

Survival

In addition to studying life expectancies for different population groups and across countries, the survival function constructed as part of the life table provides further information about the health of populations. The survival curve is a functional representation of the survival rates of 100 000 persons from a population at a particular time. Survival functions seem to describe characteristic aspects of certain species. Whereas most animal species have been reported to be associated with convex (oysters, most plants and animals) or diagonal survival functions (birds and the hydra), survival functions of humans seem always to have been concave in shape, if the number of survivors is represented on a log-scale *(11)*. This means that humans seem to have been more successful than other species in stretching the lives of a major portion of its members. In addition to examining the overall shape of the curves, learning about the specific parameters of these curves for specific populations at specific times is interesting.

Survival functions of European populations in the late 1970s are shaped like the upper curves in Fig. 1 and 2. These curves show how a population of 100 000 persons would diminish if it were subjected to the mortality experience of a particular year or group of years. Starting at 100 000, there is a small drop between the ages of 0 and 1. Subsequently the curve falls very slowly up to the age of about 50, then it drops sharply to the age of 90 years. Female functions (Fig. 1) are located at a higher level than male functions (Fig. 2), and the functions are not parallel for the two sexes, because the ratio of female to male death rates is not constant across the ages. It tends to be closer to 1 in the older age groups than to the young and middle age groups. When comparing survival functions for European countries, it is found, for example, that Sweden's survival curves exceed those of the Federal Republic of Germany for both males and females in the late 1970s *(12)*, with the absolute differences between the curves being larger for males than for females.

Summarizing this information, the area under the curve may be chosen as a description of the shape of the survival function. The area under the curve might also be described as a percentage of the total area of the rectangle defined by 100 000 persons living up to 90 years of age. In this case the area would be 100%. Thus, the difference[a] between the curve area and 100% represents the gap between the possible ideal survival curve and the situation represented by the curve. This difference describes the order of improvement ideally possible. Relating the area above the survival curve to the area under the curve amounts to relating years of premature deaths to the survival years of the life table population. The maximum age for this analysis may, of course, be chosen arbitrarily.

---

[a] The difference may be expressed in mathematical notation for life tables as follows:

$$1 - \frac{T_0 - T_x}{x} \cdot l_0,$$

where $l_0 = 100\,000$ and x is the age at which any death is considered premature. It is 90 years in the example above.

In order to make this indicator more realistic, one may want to relate the area under the curve for a particular country to that country's curve with a survival function close to the 100% line at that particular time (Sweden in 1975–1979 was chosen in this case).

The relative difference between these respective areas could serve as a description of the potential for improvement in the survival pattern for that population. Performing these analyses, the results given in Table 1 *(12)* are obtained.

While the survival function for females of the Federal Republic of Germany for 1977–1979 covers 84% of the total area of the rectangle, the curve for males covers only 77% of that area. The corresponding figures for Sweden are 85% and 80%, respectively. Comparing the figures for the Federal Republic of Germany and Sweden, the percentage difference in area is only about 1.2% (1/84) for females in Sweden, as compared with those in the Federal Republic of Germany, while for Swedish males, as compared with males in the Federal Republic of Germany, it is 3.9% (3/77). Taking Swedish survival curves from 1975–1979 as implementable standards for Europe, the potential improvement in survival functions (total years lived by a population) would be about 1% for females and about 4% for males of the Federal Republic of Germany in 1977–1979.

Keyfitz suggests yet another measure for the description of the survival curves, the entropy H,[a] and he remarks that it is around 0.2 for males and around 0.15 for females in Europe and the United States *(13)*. This measure is small if nearly all of the population survives to a high age and it will be large (close to 0.5) when people die early. This statistic may be used for quantifying the elasticity of life expectancies in conjunction with an average reduction of mortality. If $H = 0.2$, then a reduction of the overall mortality rate by 10% will result in an average increase at all ages of 2% ($0.2 \times 10\%$) in the expectation of life. Another use of H would be: if H and the expectation of life were given for two countries, then the excess mortality of one over the other can be computed *(13)*. Thus, the entropy is a concise measure of the survival patterns characteristic of a country at a particular time.

Months of Life Gained

The concept of life gained is an approach to displaying the effect of early deaths, due to certain diseases on life expectancy. (As these analyses are based upon disease information in death certificates, the inaccuracies of this data source must be taken into consideration when interpreting the results.) Expressed in months of life gained, this statistic shows how many months of life expectancy could be gained at most, if all deaths due to a particular disease group could be eliminated. Table 2 shows months of life gained due to the elimination of deaths of selected causes for a newborn in 1952 and in 1975 for the Federal Republic of Germany *(4)*. If all causes of death could

[a] $H = -(\Sigma \ln l_x \times l_x)/\Sigma l_x$, where l_x are the life table probabilities of survival in the different age groups.

Table 1. Areas under survival curves of the Federal Republic of Germany, based on Fig. 1 and 2

Country	Year	Females	Males
Percentage of total area defined by 100 000 persons living for 90 years			
Germany, Federal Republic of	1977-1979	84	77
Sweden	1975-1979	85	80
Percentage of area defined by survival curve of Sweden in 1975-1979			
Germany, Federal Republic of	1977-1979	99	96

Table 2. Months of life gained for a newborn when eliminating selected causes of death in the Federal Republic of Germany, 1952 and 1975

Cause of death	Months of life gained by newborn		Difference of months of life gained (1952-1975) as a percentage of time gained in 1952[a]
	1952	1975	
All causes	166.29	142.92	14.1
Diseases of the circulatory system	40.49	46.74	15.4
Neoplasms	25.92	29.95	15.5
Accidents, such as poisoning	15.64	17.75	13.5
Infectious and parasitic diseases	8.93	2.18	-75.6
Diseases of the respiratory system	13.56	7.98	-41.2
Certain causes of perinatal mortality	25.97	9.27	-64.3

[a] Column 3 is 100 times the value obtained by subtracting column 2 from column 1, and dividing the result by the value given in column 1.

Source: **Geissler, U.** *(4).*

have been eliminated in 1952, the life expectancy of a newborn would have been increased by 13.9 years (166.29 months). The corresponding figure for 1975 was 11.9 years (142.92 months). Examining one particular disease group, it is found that if deaths due to diseases of the circulatory system could have been eliminated totally, the life expectancy of a newborn would have been increased by 40.49 months in 1952 and by 46.74 months in 1975. Quantifying this for selected causes of death, Table 2 shows that the effect on life expectancy of eliminating diseases of the circulatory system, accidents and neoplasms would have been greater in 1975 than in 1952 (columns 1 and 2 of Table 2). Total elimination of deaths due to infectious and parasitic diseases, diseases of the respiratory system and certain causes of perinatal mortality would have had less effect on the life expectancy of a newborn in 1975 than in 1952.

Furthermore, Table 2 shows that for this latter group of causes of death a major portion of potential gains in life expectancy had already been achieved by 1975, namely a reduction of 75% of the potential gains in 1952 of infectious and parasitic diseases (see column 3 of Table 2). Projecting the developments between 1952 and 1975 of these three causes into the future (35 years from 1975), it is expected that their role will be so reduced that their total elimination would have only a very minor effect on the lengthening of life. Consequently, if these causes of death are reduced to minor importance, the role of the first three causes in life expectancy will be more prominent. However, as the portion of premature deaths in these groups is relatively small and prevention seems to be more difficult than with the former deaths, reducing them will be difficult, thus the potential for their total or partial elimination rather limited.

Health Improvement of Populations

When searching for measures of health improvement of populations, time series of the above statistics may be studied. Life expectancy of the newborn increased substantially over time. It was reported as being 18 years by Graunt in 1662, around 28 years in 1693 as given by Halley and estimated at 31 years around 1700 from data by Cruclai *(14)*. Between 1974 and 1977 it ranged from 66.7 (Hungary, 1975) to 72.8 years (Sweden, 1977) in Europe *(5)*.

When fitting straight lines to selected age-specific life expectancies in Germany between 1871–1880 and 1977–1979 (Federal Republic of Germany), it was discovered that the average improvements in life expectancy for the female and male newborn per year were 0.37 and 0.34 years respectively (Fig. 3 and 4). On the other hand, the corresponding improvement for 70-year-olds was 0.04 years for females and 0.02 years for males. As Fries *(15)* suggests, projecting this experience into the future enables us to estimate the ideal life span and the year when a particular country may reach it, assuming conditions are similar to today. When attempting to locate the approximate respective years and ages, the upper right-hand corners of Fig. 3 and 4 were examined for those points farthest removed from the origin where at least three fitted (to age groups in time) lines intersect. Performing this analysis for Germany and the Federal Republic of Germany, it was observed that the estimate for females would be 85 years and might be reached in 2035. For males the ideal life span for that same country is estimated at about 81 years and it might be reached by 2060. As Fries *(15)* remarks for the United States, the trends will probably be better described by fitting parabolas to the data points of the young age groups, as their improvement in life expectancy has been slower than proportional since 1950. This holds true for Germany (Federal Republic of Germany after 1955) as well. Thus, the ideal life expectancy provides an estimate for the improvement to be expected, if past trends are projected into the future. The estimate of the year when the ideal life expectancy may be reached provides another view of this statistic, namely the number of years required to reach that goal for persons of that age. Pursuing this aspect for one country and comparing the estimates and discrepancies between actual and ideal life expectancy across nations will show the variability of ideal life expectancies and the possible improvements in years to come.

Due to early deaths, the ideal life span of a population will always be lower than the maximal life expectancy for selected individuals. However, maximal life expectancy sets the absolute upper limit on the improvement of population life expectancies. Nevertheless, it may not have changed substantially in absolute terms in time, as Fries *(15)* implies. The expectation of life for 85-year-old French males varied between 3.8 (1817–1831) *(16)* and 4.29 years for 1973–1977 *(17)*. However, this age-specific life expectancy did not increase continuously from 1817. A value for French males of 4.2 years was observed for the period 1877–1881 *(16)* and one of 3.1 years for the years 1920–1923 *(16)*. For French females a value of 3.8 years was observed in 1817–1831 *(16)* and one of 5.19 years in 1973–1977 *(17)*. Again, as with the corresponding statistics for males, the increase in life expectancy showed some variability around an upward trend. For example, a life expectancy of 3.6 years was found for 85-year-old French women in 1920–1923 and in 1928–1933 *(16)*. As these improvements will partly be due to the fact that more persons reach higher ages now than in the last century, a study of the maximal observed lengths of life within and across countries would be required in order to examine whether the maximum life span of humans underwent an increase in time.

Life expectancy without disability may currently be estimated for only a few nations. However, as actuarial methods may readily be used for its estimation, once disability duration information becomes available for more countries, the relationship between mortality and morbidity time trends may be studied more intensively.

In addition to the years of life gained in time, health improvement may be expressed in terms of changes in the shape and level of survival curves. Examining Fig. 1 (females) and 2 (males) for the Federal Republic of Germany as an example, the survival curves flattened with time and have moved up since 1871–1880. This change may be expressed in terms of area under the survival curve divided by the area of the rectangle defined by 100 000 persons living for 90 years. The figures for Germany were 43% for females and 40% for males in 1871–1880 *(12)*. Up to 1977–1979 in the Federal Republic of Germany, they had improved to 84% for females and 77% for males. This means that in the course of one century the total number of years of survival had almost doubled for the population.

The entropy, i.e. the curve development in time, is shown in Table 3.

This means that in 1871–1880 a reduction of the overall mortality by 1% would have resulted in an average increase of life expectancy, for all ages, of 0.564% for females and of 0.608% for males. On the other hand, that same relative reduction in mortality would be expected to result in an increase of life expectancy of 0.117% for females and 0.151% for males in 1977–1979.

Improvement in the health of populations may further be described in terms of the median age of life table populations, that is the age at which 50% of the population have died. These figures were 60.15 (72.97) years for males in 1901–1910 in Germany (1977–1979, Federal Republic of Germany) and 60.54 (79.59) years for German females in 1901–1910 (in the Federal Republic of Germany, 1977–1979). The upward movement of the median life table age is associated with a steepening of the downward sloping portion of the survival function, a phenomenon Fries *(15)* calls the compression of mortality. He states that it is also associated with a compression of morbidity. Unfortunately, because of the lack of data it is difficult to describe such a possible compression of morbidity empirically for many countries. Colvez & Blanchet *(3)* seem to show that a compression of mortality in the United States may be associated with an extension of the average disability period. Therefore, years of life gained through the successful reduction of premature mortality and years of life free of disability gained through the successful reduction of disease or of disease severity may be negatively associated in a population. Further study of this subject is required.

So far, the focus has been on indicators of health improvement in populations by relying on changes in life expectancy, survival and derivatives thereof. Most of these measures were measures of location of these statistics. However, indicators of the variability of these statistics should be used increasingly to allow the monitoring of the changes in variability of

Table 3. Entropy (average improvement of life expectancy in percentage at each age when mortality rate is decreased by 1%) by sex: Germany, 1871–1880 to (Federal Republic of Germany) 1977–1979

Year	Females	Males
1871–1880	0.564	0.608
1901–1910	0.422	0.463
1924–1926	0.280	0.310
1949–1951	0.178	0.211
1977–1979	0.117	0.151

Table 4. Aggregate measures to describe life expectancy, survival and their improvement

Statistic	Indicator of status	Indicator of improvement
Life expectancy		
— of a newborn — of a 1-year-old — for males and females, most recent year	Estimate in number of years	Number of years gained since 1945
		Percentage difference between newborn and 1-year-old life expectancy for males and females
		Sign of that difference
		Average gain in life expectancy since 1870 per year for both sexes for 0- and 1-year-olds
		Male/female ratio in life expectancy for newborns
— free of disability	Estimate in number of years	Average gain in 10-year period
— of persons aged 5, 10, 20, 40, 65, 70 and 85 for males and females	Estimate in number of years by age and sex	Number of years gained since 1945
		Average gain in life expectancy within 100 years per year by age and sex
		Ratio of male/female life expectancy for most recent life table
Survival		
Survival curve for males and females, most recent life table	Area under the curves; curve area as percentage of area for 100 000 persons living for 90 years	Development of areas under survival curves in time, expressed as percentage of 100 000 persons living for 90 years
Survival curves (males, females) of country with best survival function in region, most recent life table	Curve areas as percentage of area delineated by country with best survival curve	Development of relative difference of area under survival curve of investigated country and country with best survival function at the time
	Entropy	Development of entropy for one country by sex over time
		Development of entropies for countries of one region over time
Months of life gained by eliminating early deaths	For total population in months	Relative gain/loss in months in a 10-year period
	For specific causes of death in months	Relative gains/losses in months by cause for a 10-year period

these statistics. Fries *(15)* further points out that, in order to understand the aging process more thoroughly, analyses should increasingly focus on the variability between individuals in order to find out which factors determine aging, disability and death.

Table 4 summarizes some of the measures discussed above that may be suitable to describe concisely the health status, and its improvement, of populations. When applied within one country in time and computed for one region, indicators will emerge that can show:

— the improvements in health status that have been reached;

— the improvements in the health of populations that may be possible in the future and how long it might take to achieve them; and

— the improvements in health status of populations that may be possible when countries of the same region are compared.

References

1. **Schach, E. & Pflanz, M.** *Von Gesundheitsstatistiken zum Gesundheitsinformationssystem.* Dortmund, Manuskript, 1981.
2. *Manual of mortality analysis.* Geneva, World Health Organization, 1977.
3. **Colvez, A. & Blanchet, M.** Potential gains in life expectancy free of disability. *International journal of epidemiology,* **12**: 224–229 (1983).
4. **Geissler, U.** *Verlust an Lebensjahren. Wido-Materialien 5.* Bonn, Wissenschaftliches Institut der Ortskrankenkassen, 1979.
5. **Ewert, G. & Marcussen, H., ed.** *Sterblichkeit und Lebenserwartung.* Berlin, VEB Verlag Volk und Gesundheit, 1981.
6. **Statistisches Bundesamt.** *Statistisches Jahrbuch für die Bundesrepublik Deutschland.* Wiesbaden, Kohlhammer, 1952.
7. **Statistisches Bundesamt.** *Statistisches Jahrbuch für die Bundesrepublik Deutschland.* Wiesbaden, Kohlhammer, 1981.
8. **Hadley, J. & Osei, A.** Does income effect mortality? An analysis of the effects of different types of income on age/sex/race-specific mortality rates in the United States. *Medical care,* **20**: 901–914 (1982).
9. **Office of Population Censuses and Surveys.** *Occupational mortality 1970–72 for England and Wales.* London, H.M. Stationery Office, 1978.
10. **Fox, A.J. & Goldblatt, P.O.** *1971–1975 longitudinal study of socio-demographic mortality differentials.* Series LS, No. 1. Office of Population Censuses and Surveys. London, H.M. Stationary Office, 1982.
11. **Thomlinson, R.** *Population dynamics.* New York, 1976.
12. **Schach, E.** *Einige Analysen zur Gesamtmortalität in der Bundesrepublik Deutschland.* Paper given at the 1982 Annual Meeting of the German Society for Social Medicine, Heidelberg, 1982.
13. **Keyfitz, N.** *Applied mathematical demography.* New York, Wiley, 1977.
14. **Smith, D. & Keyfitz, N.** *Mathematical demography.* New York, Springer, 1977.

15. **Fries, J.F.** Aging, natural death, and the compression of morbidity. *New England journal of medicine,* **303**: 130–135 (1980).
16. **Institut national de la statistique et des études économiques (INSEE).** *Annuaire statistique de la France.* Paris, Ministère de l'économie et des finances, 1966.
17. **Institut national de la statistique et des études économiques (INSEE).** *Annuaire statistique de la France.* Paris, Ministère de l'économie et des finances, 1982.

8. Measurement in health promotion and protection

8.1 Personal protection — *Z.J. Brzeziński & V.H. des Fontaines*

The health promotive and/or protective technologies used vary widely in kind and scope of application. They also differ with regard to the level at which the intervention is delivered. Many of them are applied at community level, such as control of air, water or food pollutants and do not require the direct involvement of the individual. Certainly, some of the interventions applied at community level have in view personal participation, especially if they aim at changes in the individual's health behaviour, such as educational programmes which encourage healthy eating or non-smoking practices. However, these are dealt with elsewhere. This chapter concerns interventions physically delivered to a person with a specific purpose: personal protection of the recipient against more or less specific hazards.

Accordingly, the measurements in the field of personal protection considered in this chapter relate to immunization, breastfeeding, prenatal care and family planning, and personal protection in traffic and occupational safety. Each of these illustrates different aspects of the problems associated with measurement. For example, immunization is an activity aimed at both individual and community protection; breastfeeding demonstrates the contribution of a physiological function to health promotion; prenatal care exemplifies the earliest contribution of preventive measures for health enhancement; in family planning, the emphasis is on the balance of risk limitations for mother and child; and, finally, personal protection in traffic and occupational safety shows the possibilities of reducing the adverse effects of hazards that cannot be totally eliminated.

Scope of Measurements in Personal Protection

The detailed list of measurements used in personal protection depends upon the specific area in question. However, certain aspects are common to all fields in which personal intervention is applied.

Enabling conditions

The provision of personal protection requires certain conditions that limit the effective delivery of intervention technology. The basic condition is the consciousness of people concerned and the existence of appropriate legislation allowing and/or enforcing the application of a given measure. At the same time, it defines the potential beneficiaries. With regard to the existence of an appropriate law, the measurement is reduced to simple yes/no reading. However, if the law specifies to whom or where and when the protective device should be delivered or used, one can count the number of potential recipients or calculate the proportions of persons potentially protected out of all those at risk. For example, legislation can specify the requirements for the use of protective devices, such as headgear or seat-belts. Similarly occupational safety regulations may indicate the conditions under which a given kind of personal protection is to be enforced.

Enabling conditions also include the availability of resources, physical and organizational infrastructures or health education that could be measured in terms of their volumes or in relation to potential beneficiaries. The measurements used in this area are frequently referred to as measurements of availability, accessibility and acceptability of a service.

Efficacy measurements

Efficacy measurements tell to what extent the applied intervention achieves what was intended. In the case of personal protection, it gives the answer to the question whether, and to which degree, a given protective measure protects an individual from an adverse health effect from a hazard against which it is applied.

Process measurements

Process measurements are the basic tools to monitor the implementation of any programme promoting and protecting health. The two most important categories in the field of personal protection are measurements of coverage and compliance. The first reflects the proportion of the target population to which the intervention was delivered and the second the proportion of population that actually took advantage of the intervention, or actually complied with the advice to use the given protective device or technology.

Outcome measurement

Outcome measurements express the health benefits resulting from the implementation of the personal protection programme. The health benefits can be shown by a reduction in adverse health effects of the hazards against which protection was used, such as the reduction of the number of deaths, diseases, injuries or disabilities. Certainly, the effect of a protective programme depends on several factors. The most important ones are the coverage of the target population and the efficacy of the delivered intervention.

Immunization

The progress made in control and prevention of infectious and parasitic diseases is the result of a variety of changes in many fields; environmental sanitation, personal hygiene and improved nutrition, especially in the more developed parts of the world, were of primary importance. However, one should not underestimate the role of immunization in past achievements and future prospects in this respect. A spectacular example is the successful eradication of smallpox. The existing vaccines of proven efficacy (Table 1) as well as the ones of the immediate future (Table 2), if effectively used, may substantially contribute to the improvement of health in the world either independently or with other preventive measures.

The possible directions of the use of immunization range from protection of an individual against a disease for which there is no treatment (rabies) to the protection of all individuals from a disease to which all have a high chance of being exposed (poliomyelitis), with intermediate situations in which a specific group is given protection against a disease to which the group has an abnormally high chance of being exposed (hepatitis among hospital workers), or for which it has a higher chance of developing complications (influenza among the elderly).

Table 1. Important existing vaccines

Period	Vaccine
1798–1950	Smallpox
	Rabies
	Yellow fever
	Viral influenza
	Epidemic and murine typhus
	Japanese encephalitis
	Russian spring–summer encephalitis
	Cholera
	Typhoid fever
	Diphtheria
	Tuberculosis
	Pertussis
	Tetanus
1950–1980	Measles
	Mumps
	Rubella
	Poliomyelitis
	Adenovirus
	Pneumococcus — 14 types
	Meningococcus A and C
	Improved rabies

Source: **Hilleman, M.R.** *(1)*.

Table 2. Vaccines for the 1980s and beyond

Viral hepatitis B
Viral hepatitis A
Viral hepatitis non-A, non-B
Herpesvirus family
Herpes simplex 1 and 2
Infectious mononucleosis (EB virus)
Varicella-zoster
Cytomegalovirus
Respiratory viruses
Respiratory syncytial
Parainfluenza 1, 2, 3
Gastroenteritis
Rotavirus
Norwalk agent
Pneumococcus polysaccharides (more types, more antigenic)
Meningitis-septicaemia
Meningococcus
Haemophilus influenzae B
Streptococcus B
Gram-negative bacilli
Gonorrhoea
Dental caries

Source: **Hilleman, M.R.** *(1).*

The most important immunization activity that is being carried out on a global scale is the Expanded Programme on Immunization (EPI) initiated and implemented by WHO. Its goal is to immunize all newborn in the world against diphtheria, whooping cough, tetanus, measles, poliomyelitis and tuberculosis by the year 1990. At the moment only about 20% of all children born into the developing world every year are being immunized (Fig. 1). The potential gain from successful implementation of EPI represents some 5 million lives saved every year (Fig. 2).

Basic information needed

In planning and implementing the immunization programmes, numerous factors should be taken into account. These include:

— characteristics related to the population, such as age in the case of influenza vaccination among the elderly, or sex in the case of vaccination against rubella;

— characteristics related to the environment, such as aerosol dispersion in the case of droplet infections, or the level of sanitation in the case of enteric and waterborne diseases;

— characteristics related to season, such as influenza and enteric disorders;

— characteristics related to geographical location of the disease, such as yellow fever, or to population distribution; and

— characteristics related to sociopolitical factors or to natural disasters.

In addition to the general background data one should also consider specific information, such as vaccine cost and availability, and staff and equipment to perform the immunizations and to support the vaccination programme (transport, accommodation, cold chain and statistical support). The important epidemiological aspects of planning immunization programmes first relate to the assessment of the expected outcome (Table 3) and secondly to the monitoring of progress (Fig. 3) and the incidence of the relevant diseases (Fig. 4).

Selection of immunization strategies

The main criteria on which decisions concerning immunization strategies are based come from knowledge of the natural history of the disease concerned: its frequency, persons affected, and factors involved both in its causation and spread. If there are alternatives in the approaches of control and prevention, a cost–benefit analysis should be done to compare immunization with other programmes such as environmental sanitation or standardized therapy. This argument is often raised in the case of the salmonelloses, for which existing vaccines are neither very effective (40–70%) nor well tolerated. It is also valid in other instances and has been studied with particular attention in the case of cholera in the South Asian subcontinent.

Knowledge of the disease assists in selecting the target population. The target groups to be vaccinated are assessed by identifying individuals receptive or exposed to infection. The target group may be defined more narrowly by expected optimal immunological response. Age may be a limiting factor. For example, measles vaccine has maximal efficacy when administered to children between 12 and 15 months old although maximal incidence of the disease can occur at an earlier age. Another limiting factor may be the age at which complications are more severe. Sex can also be a limiting factor, as in the case of rubella vaccination where the group at risk is the fetuses of pregnant women, and the question arises of whether immunization should be limited to females or cover the whole population. Finally, the choice of a target population may be linked to occupation, with diseases such as brucellosis and rabies, or travel, with such diseases as yellow fever.

Various logistic problems should be considered in selecting immunization strategies and require appropriate measurements. These include:

— vaccine production and availability, including quantity and quality of available vaccines, stock management, shelf-life and costs; and

— problems linked to vaccine use and delivery, such as transport, the cold chain, packaging and feasibility of administration.

Fig. 1. Percentage of children immunized in the first year of life

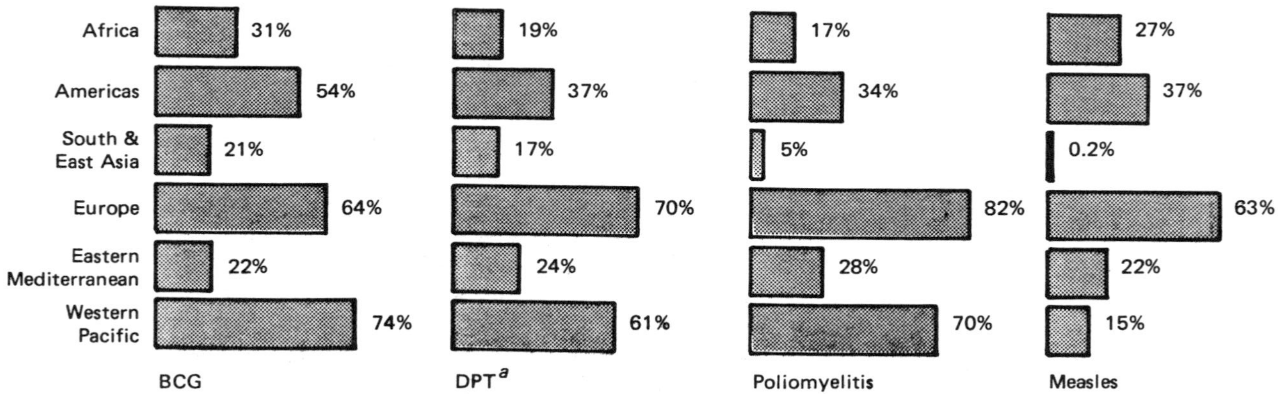

[a] Diphtheria, pertussis (whooping cough) and tetanus.

Source: **Henderson, R.** *(2).*

Fig. 2. Total child deaths from immunizable diseases, 1980

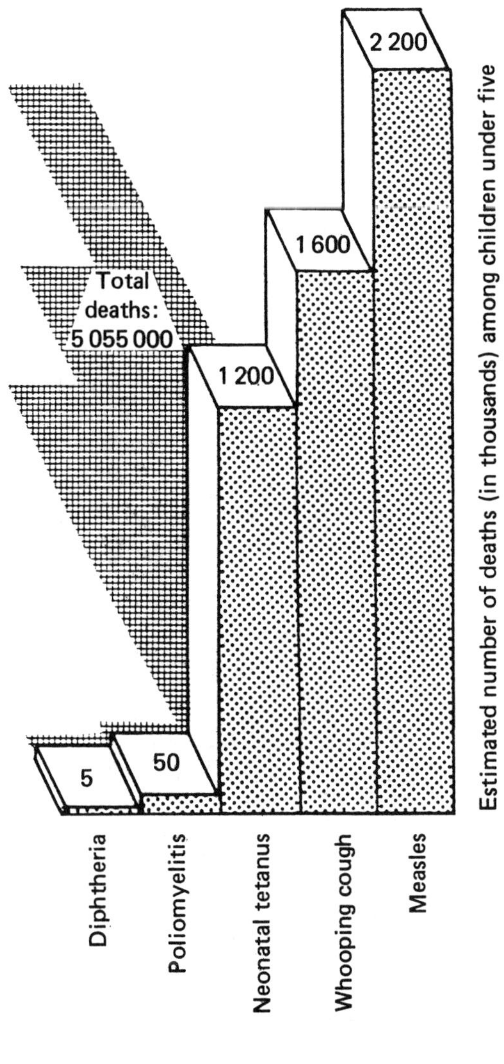

Note: No reliable estimates available for tuberculosis.

Source: **Henderson, R.** *(2).*

Table 3. Poliomyelitis: expected incidence rate in relation to birth rate and immunization coverage

(1)	(2)	(3)	(4)	(5)	(6)	(7)
Birth rate (births/100 000 population)	Poliomyelitis incidence rate expected with no immunization programme (cases/100 000 population)[a]	Efficacy of three doses of oral trivalent poliomyelitis vaccine given at interval of at least four weeks	Immunization coverage	Children protected by immunization programme (children/100 000 population)[b]	Poliomyelitis incidence rate expected with immunization programme (cases/100 000 population)[c]	Percentage reduction in poliomyelitis incidence expected from immunization programme[d]
2900	19	95%	70%	1929	6.4	67%
1580	10	95%	70%	1051	3.5	67%
2900	19	95%	75%	2066	5.5	71%
1580	10	95%	75%	1126	3.0	71%
2900	19	95%	80%	2204	4.6	76%
1580	10	95%	80%	1201	2.5	76%
2900	19	95%	85%	2342	3.7	81%
1580	10	95%	85%	1276	2.0	81%
2900	19	95%	90%	2480	2.8	86%
1580	10	95%	90%	1351	1.5	86%

[a] Column (1) × 0.0066. Note that factor of 0.0066 can be highly variable in different countries and in different outbreaks within countries.

[b] Column (1) × column (3) × column (4).

[c] (Column (1) – column (5)) × 0.0066.

[d] Column (3) × column (4) or (column (2) – column (6)) ÷ column (2).

Source: *Indicators and targets for the Expanded Programme on Immunization*, WHO document EPI/GEN/81/2.

Fig. 3. Proportion of children under 1 year of age in countries where immunization coverage in this age group is at least 50%, 20 Latin American countries, 1978 and 1983

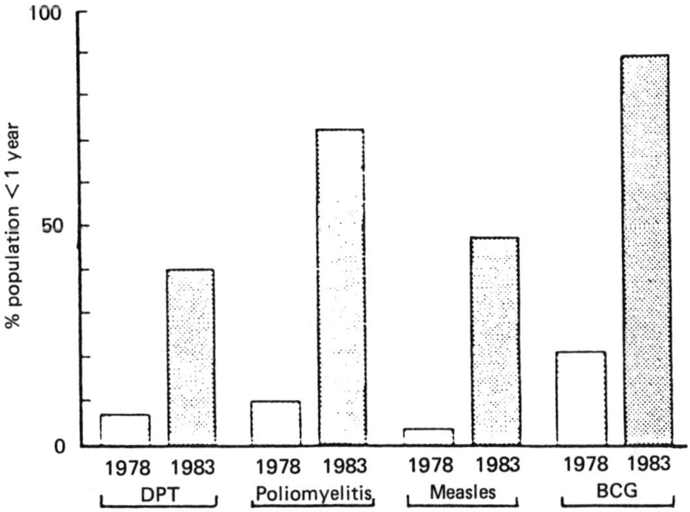

Source: *EPI newsletter*, Vol. VI, No. 2, April 1984.

There are other constraints, such as problems linked to vaccine contraindications and adverse effects. This may, for instance, imply decisions on whether to respect or adapt classical contraindications, whether these are temporary (prematurity or steroid therapy) or permanent (congenital disorders, a contraindication to the administration of some live vaccines). In cases where emergency immunization is undertaken during an epidemic, for instance, it is recommended not to administer multiple vaccines.

The risk of adverse reactions after immunization must be weighed and compared with the complication rates following natural diseases as done in the EPI (Tables 4 and 5) *(2)*. However, if the immunization programme is carried out in areas lacking health infrastructure (deprived, remote, or difficult to get to) the contraindications should be kept to a minimum.

The adverse effects may influence the public, who may not be well informed, and affect the compliance rate of the target population. This can be measured by the proportion of the target population that accepted the service (immunization) offered.

Evaluation

The evaluation of an immunization programme is a complex exercise covering all stages and aspects, going from planning through implementation to monitoring. In this respect it should follow the procedure applicable to any

Fig. 4. Incidence of five vaccine-preventable diseases, Region of the Americas,[a] 1970–1983 (provisional data)

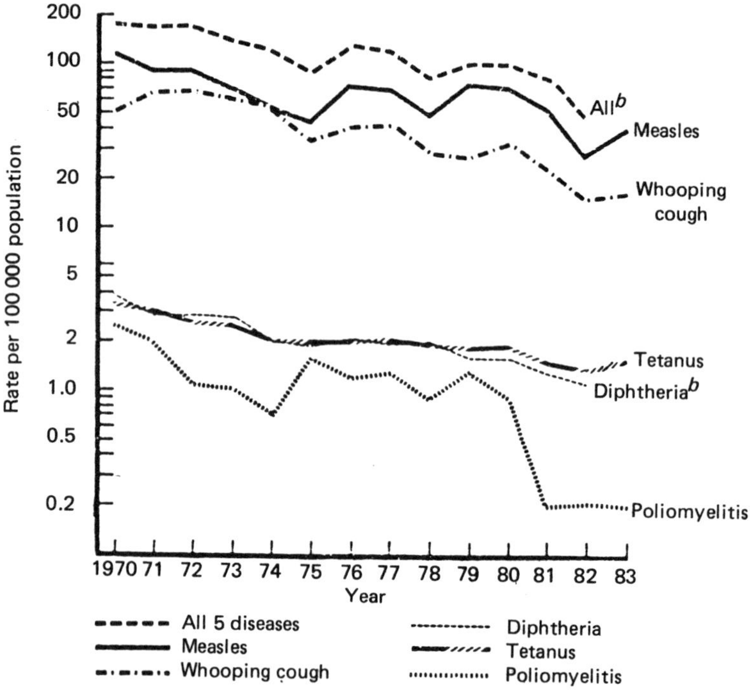

[a] Excluding Bermuda, Canada and the United States.

[b] Data for 1983 incomplete.

Source: *EPI newsletter*, Vol. VI, No. 2, April 1984.

health programme. The most specific features of an evaluation of immunization programmes relate to measurements of the efficacy of the vaccines and the ultimate effectiveness of the programme. The assessment of vaccine efficacy is carried out throughout the development of a new vaccine and is a routine procedure during its production. It includes in its advanced stages the response of the organisms to the vaccine, which indicates increased immunity (Fig. 5), as well as field trials in which the attack rate of the disease in people who received the vaccine is compared with the attack rate in those who did not or received another kind of a vaccine (Fig. 6). Usually the efficacy of a vaccine is well known before its mass application and manufacturers are expected to provide proof when they develop and sell the vaccine. However, the efficacy of a vaccine under field conditions may be modified by environmental influences, such as the nutritional status of the

Table 4. Estimated rates of adverse reactions following DPT immunization compared to complications of natural whooping cough

Adverse reaction	Whooping cough complication rates/ 100 000 cases	DPT vaccine adverse reaction rates/ 100 000 immunizations
Permanent brain damage	600–2000 (0.6–2.0%)	0.2–0.6
Death	100–4000 (0.1–4.0%)	0.2
Encephalopathy encephalitis[a]	90–4000 (0.09–4.0%)	0.1–3.0
Convulsions	600–8000 (0.6–8.0%)	0.3–90
Shock	—	0.5–30

[a] Including seizures, focal neurological signs, coma and Reye's syndrome.

Source: **Galazka, A.M. et al.** *(3).*

Table 5. Estimated rates of serious adverse reactions following measles immunization compared to complications of natural measles infection and background rate of illness

Adverse reaction	Measles complication rates/100 000 cases	Measles vaccine adverse reaction rates/100 000 vaccinees	Background illness rate/100 000 persons
Encephalitis/ encephalopathy	50–400 (0.05–0.4%)	0.1	0.1–0.3
Subacute sclerosing panencephalitis	0.5–2.0	0.05–0.1	—
Pneumonia	3800–7300 (3.8–7.3%)	—	—
Convulsions	500–1000 (0.5–1.0%)	0.02–190	30
Death	10–10 000 (0.01–10%)	0.02–0.3	—

Source: **Galazka, A.M. et al.** *(3).*

Fig. 5. Seroconversion rates in adult human subjects given lot 751 human hepatitis B vaccine in graded doses in alum formulation

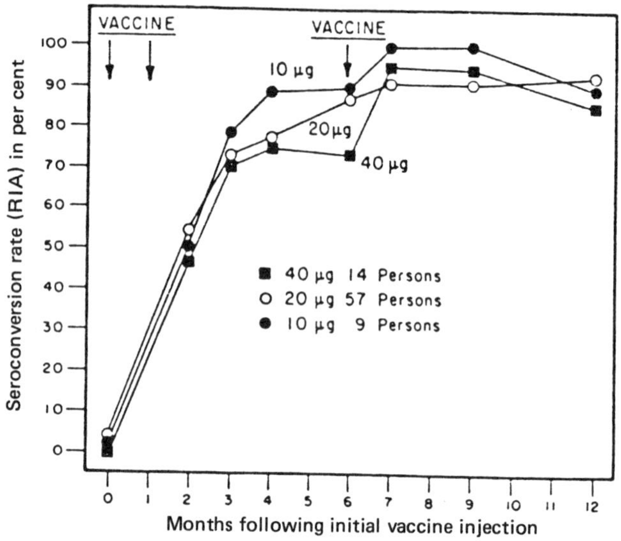

Source: **Hilleman, M.R.** *(1)*.

target population *(4)*. Therefore the efficacy and safety of the vaccine used in any immunization programme must be monitored.

The evaluation of an immunization programme in the community should be based on the time trend in the occurrence of the disease and the relation of this trend to the annual or cumulated number (by proportion) of people subjected to the vaccination programme in the community.

The effectiveness of vaccination programmes against many communicable diseases on the population level relies on the phenomenon of herd immunity. This implies that a minimum percentage of the population must be effectively vaccinated so that the spread of the disease may be arrested. This is generally estimated to be about 80% or more of the target population. In order to ensure the control or elimination of a communicable disease, the coverage need not necessarily be much higher, as demonstrated in the eradication of smallpox, but vaccination must be complemented by surveillance activities and the containment of epidemic foci, including systematic investigation of suspected cases. However, in the control of some infectious diseases, such as tetanus and rabies, herd immunity plays a less important role.

Fig. 6. Cumulative hepatitis B attack rates (clinical and subclinical) by life table method

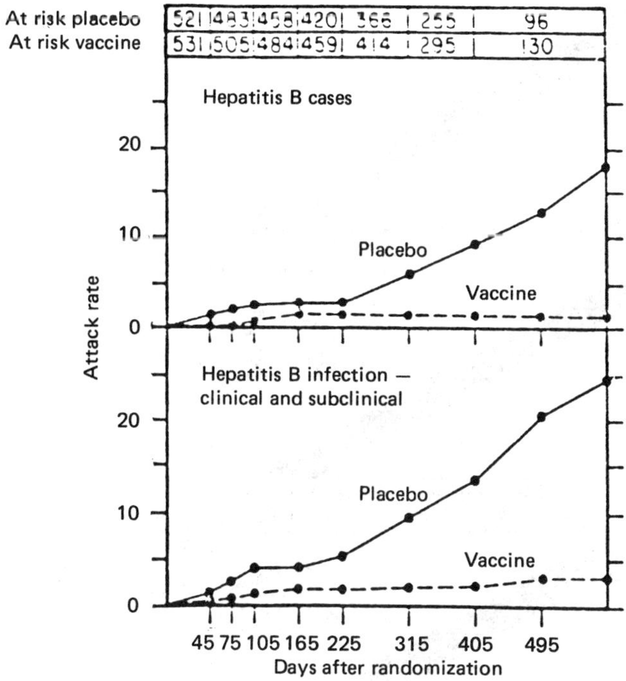

Source: **Hilleman, M.R.** *(1).*

Breastfeeding

Breastfeeding appears naturally superior to any alternative. However, breastfeeding has decreased as opposed to bottle-feeding in all socio-economic classes and areas in recent decades, throughout the industrialized countries and, increasingly, in the developing world, with horrendous consequences for the health of small children (Fig. 7). Two main lines of argument have been advanced against this physiological feeding: from sociology on the one hand, and from the profit motive on the other. The sociological arguments are based on factors that include changes in the child's upbringing (for instance, the practice of wet-nursing became increasingly common in France in the eighteenth and nineteenth centuries) and on the supposedly adverse effects of breastfeeding on aesthetic aspects of the breast. The profit motive arguments have been linked to the availability of commercially produced milk apparently very close in composition to human milk. This was found not to be so apparent as soon as investigations

Fig. 7. Breastfeeding and child survival

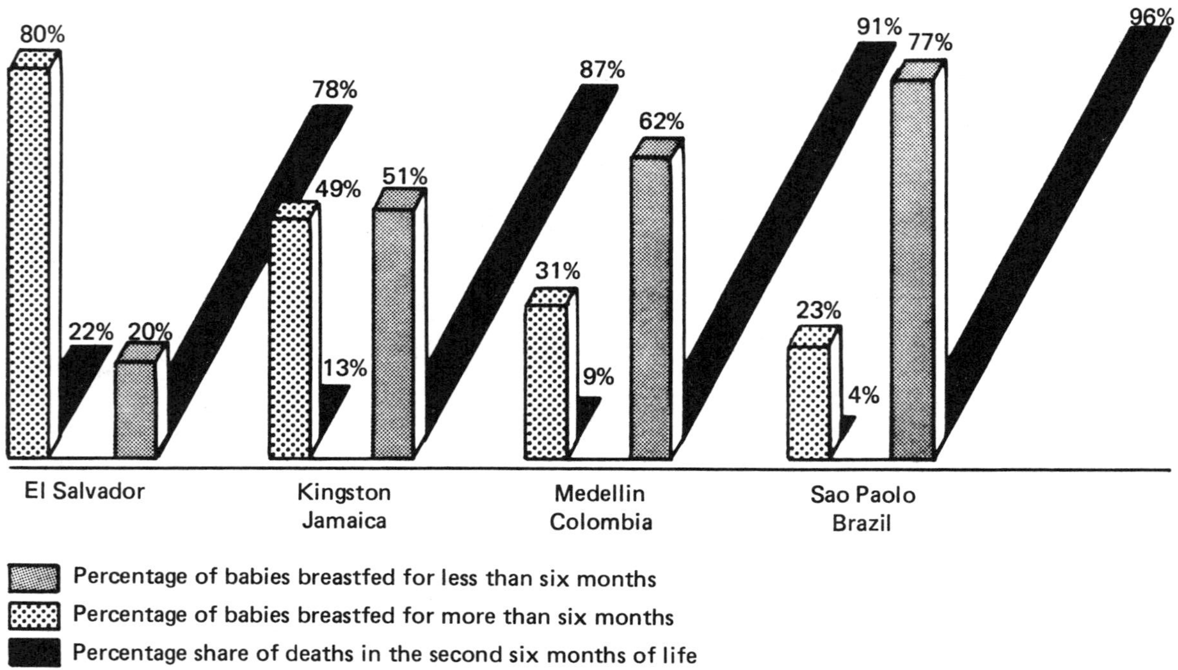

Source: **Henderson, R.** *(2).*

took into account not only nutritional equilibrium, but also the immunological and allergic implications of breastfeeding and bottle-feeding.

In a recent review *(5)*, 17 out of 22 studies indicated that breastfeeding protects infants against a variety of problems, including respiratory diseases, otitis media, enteric infections and allergies. In some communities, breastfeeding has been shown to ensure considerable protection against infectious diseases, as measured both by hospital admissions and the number of days in hospital. The protective effect was independent of family size, overcrowding in the house, family income and education of the parents *(6)*. Similar findings were reported for a rural community. Significant differences were found in the number of office visits for illness in the first months of life between infants who had been breastfed and those who had been bottle-fed from birth. During the first six months of life, breastfed infants had significantly fewer months of illness than bottle-fed infants *(7)*. In the study mentioned above *(6)*, the protective effect lasted even after breastfeeding was discontinued.

An analysis of data from health visitors on 238 000 infants born during the period 1941–1972 in Copenhagen showed that breastfed infants had a lower overall morbidity than infants exclusively bottle-fed. The largest difference was found for gastroenteritis and dyspepsia. The difference in morbidity was still visible in the second and third years of life *(8)*. Breastfeeding also has a positive effect on early milk production and infant weight gain *(9)*.

In some communities breastfeeding alone is continued for more than a year and a recent study on breastfeeding and growth of infants has shown that no impairment was found up to the age of around six months *(10)*.

In conclusion, there seems to be little doubt that breastfeeding has a positive effect on the health and growth of infants. Furthermore, it is especially recommended for the social groups that experience more problems with infant mortality, morbidity and infant growth.

Knowledge of the beneficial effects of breastfeeding prompted promotion programmes that resulted in a reversal of the trends (Fig. 8). However, in many countries that could benefit most there is a need for improvement. Even if initial breastfeeding is relatively high, for a large proportion of babies it lasts for a relatively short period (Fig. 9). There are also differences according to social stratification: breastfeeding is becoming more fashionable among mothers in the more privileged social groups. Mothers in the lower social classes, who again could benefit most, breastfeed their babies less frequently and for shorter periods *(11)*. Accordingly, in programmes promoting breastfeeding, mothers who require special attention should be identified. In some communities even simple scores can be a useful tool to predict those who are more or less likely to adopt breastfeeding (Fig. 10 and 11).

In planning intervention technologies in breastfeeding promotion it is important that, in addition to improvements in knowledge and changes in attitudes, other factors should not be forgotten, such as the timing of the first breastfeed and rooming-in facilities (Fig. 12). Appropriate provisions to facilitate the continuation of breastfeeding by working mothers should also be remembered.

Fig. 8. Breastfeeding in Oslo, Norway, 1950–1980

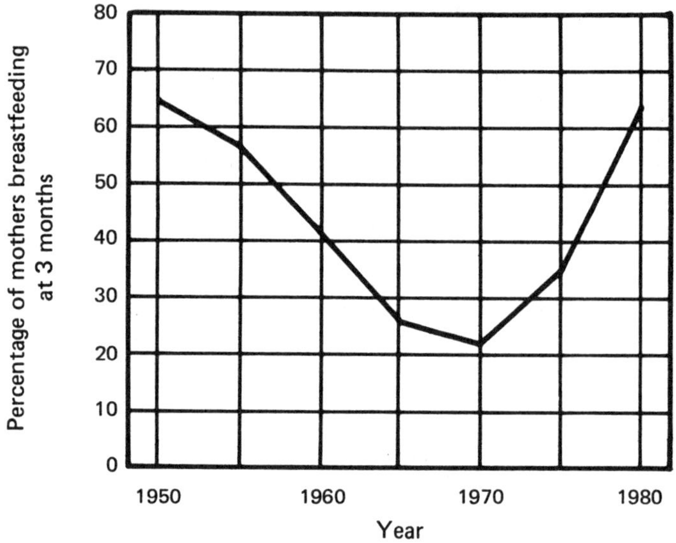

Source: **Henderson, R.** *(2).*

Evaluation of effectiveness of breastfeeding promotion programmes requires two kinds of measurements: process (trends in the number of breastfed children, the duration of breastfeeding, the proportion of children breastfed by a given age and the quality of weaning, which is linked to the quality of the breastfeeding) and outcome (physical and mental development, dental health, and the occurrence of respiratory and gastroenteric infections).

The efficiency of programmes in the promotion of breastfeeding can be assessed by relating the process and outcome measurements to the amount of resources and efforts put into alternative interventions through health education campaigns, individual counselling schemes and environmental manipulation (rooming-in).

Prenatal Care

Prenatal care aims at producing a healthy child through personal protection of its mother. The interventions are delivered before birth and are directed against maternal factors that may be removed or modified during pregnancy. Therefore, the programming of prenatal care should be based on knowledge of, first, the characteristics and/or factors influencing the survival and health of the newborn and, second, the conditions present and/or events occurring during pregnancy that are responsible for these characteristics and factors.

Fig. 9. Prevalence and duration of breastfeeding

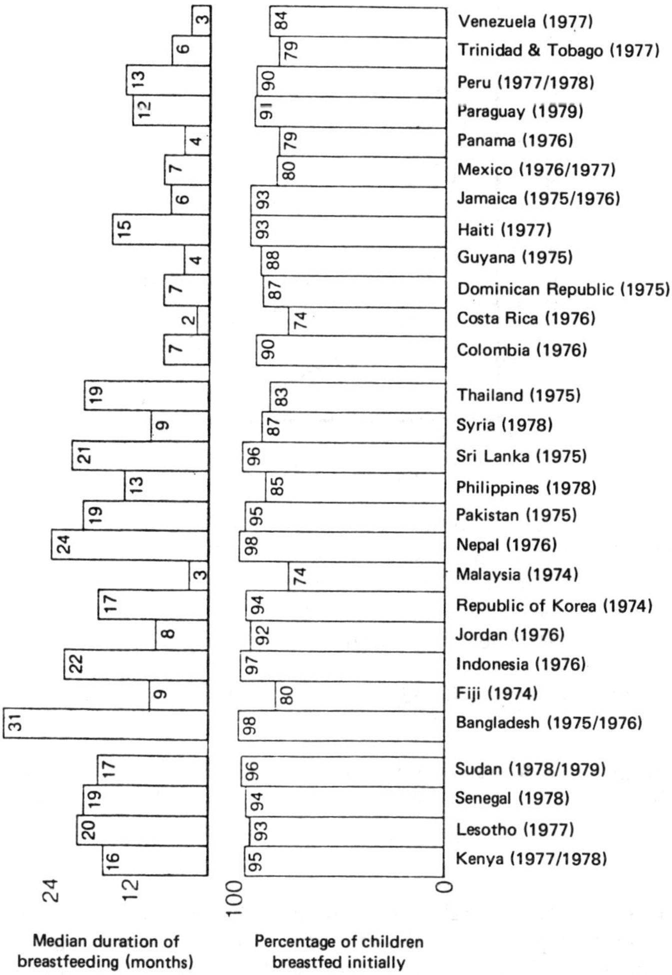

Source: **Henderson, R.** *(2).*

Fig. 10. Percentages of mothers still breastfeeding at different stages by age of mother at confinement and age at leaving school

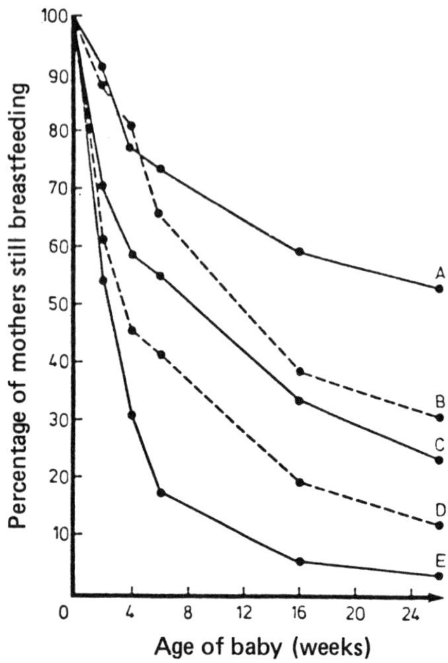

A = aged 25 or over; left school at 17 or over (n = 79).
B = aged 20-24; left school at 17 or over (n = 26).
C = aged 25 or over; left school at 15 or 16 (n = 89).
D = aged 20-24; left school at 15 or 16 (n = 123).
E = aged under 20; left school at 15 or 16 (n = 53).

Note: Only three mothers aged under 20 who left school at 17 or over attempted breastfeeding.

Source: **Wright, H.J. & Walker, P.C.** Prediction of duration of breast feeding in primiparas. *Journal of epidemiology and community health,* **37**: 89-94 (1983).

The most important single determinant of the survival of a newborn is the birth weight. Depending on the level of neonatal mortality some 60–80% of all perineonatal deaths are in infants with a birth weight of less than 2500 g. In terms of rates of perineonatal death, the mortality rate among the newborn with low birth weights may be over 20 times higher than corresponding rates among babies of over 2500 g *(12)*.

The magnitude of the problem is well illustrated by the frequency of occurrence of low birth weight, which is estimated at 7% in developed and 18% in developing parts of the world (Fig. 13).

Fig. 11. A tool for the predictive identification of bottle-feeding primiparae

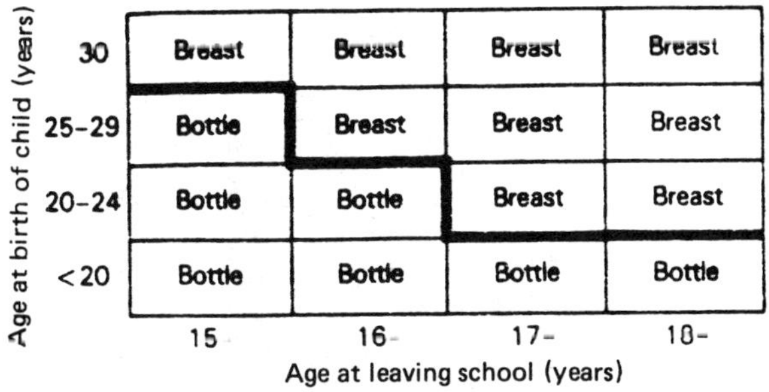

Source: **Wright, H.J. et al.** The prediction of choice in infant feeding: a study of primiparae. *Journal of the Royal College of General Practitioners*, **33**: 493–497 (1983).

Fig. 12. Infant deaths, Baguio General Hospital, 1973–1977

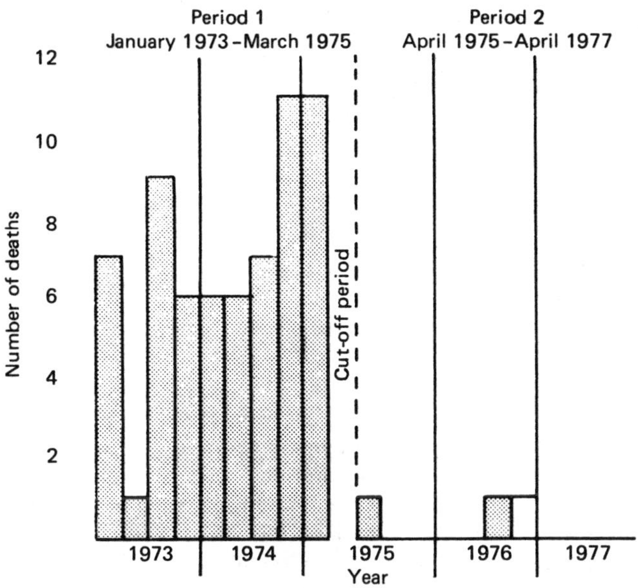

Period 1. 4 720 live births. Babies in nursery. Almost all babies bottle-fed.

Period 2. 5 166 live births. Babies in bed with mothers. Almost all babies breastfed.

Source: **Henderson, R.** *(2).*

Fig. 13. Global incidence of low birth weights

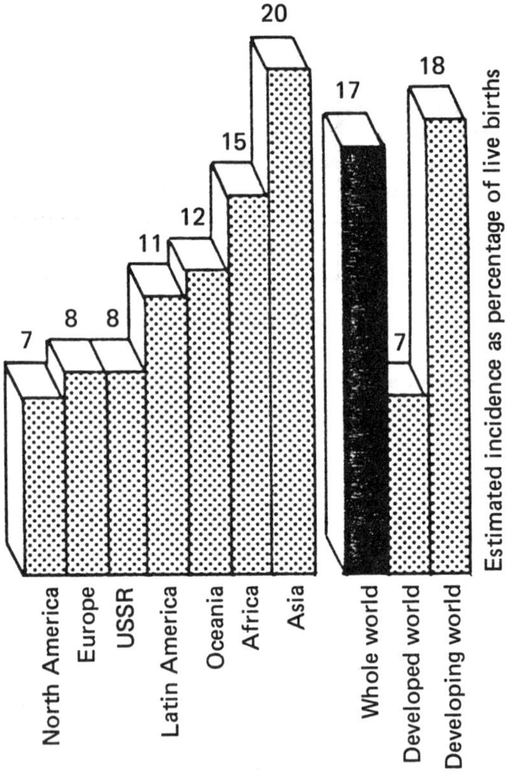

Note: Low birth weight = infants weighing 2500 g or less at birth.

Source: **Henderson, R.** *(2).*

Several factors are associated with low birth weight. Some of them, such as nutrition, smoking or alcohol consumption, could be the aim of intervention within prenatal care programmes. Others, such as maternal age, parity or social class, lie outside the immediate reach of prenatal care.

Mothers who smoke have smaller babies than those who do not, and on average their babies weigh about 200 g less. This relationship is independent of all other factors that influence birth weight *(13)*. Infants whose mothers stop smoking show increased birth weight *(14)*. Smoking influences not only intra-uterine growth, but also growth after birth as measured by weight gain, and, to a lesser degree, body length and head circumference *(15)*. There are indications that tobacco smoking by other family members in the home of a mother who does not smoke also exposes the fetus to a measurable increase in at least some metabolic by-products of tobacco smoke *(16)*.

It has been shown that smoking in pregnancy clusters with social variables, such as marital status and education, as well as with age *(17)*. In another study it was found that although smoking was much more frequent among women in lower social classes, there was little difference across social classes in the birth weight decrement associated with smoking. Perinatal mortality, however, was increased only among smokers in the lower social classes *(18)*.

Similarly, birth weight is affected by alcohol consumption. It was found that with adjustment for social class and cigarette smoking, women drinking more than 100 g alcohol a week had more than double the risk of delivering a baby at or below the tenth centile, compared with women drinking less than 50 g a week. The effect of alcohol was synergistic with that of smoking. Drinking habits about the time of conception seems to be important for this effect *(19)*.

Health education should be directed at stopping smoking and reducing alcohol consumption both before and during pregnancy. Attempts are being made to develop methods of screening for alcohol abuse in pregnancy *(20)* and treatment of pregnant women who were problem drinkers demonstrated benefits to offspring when heavy drinking ceased before the third trimester *(21)*.

In communities with nutritional problems, the use of dietary supplements may produce spectacular results. A recent study in Gambia showed that this kind of intervention reduced low birth weight from 28% to 5% of all births (Table 6). Although such extreme circumstances do not exist in developed regions, certain underprivileged population groups may benefit from dietary supplementation.

The next group of factors presenting pregnancy outcome risk that may be reduced by prenatal care are maternal diseases such as essential hypertension, diabetes, pre-eclampsia, antepartum haemorrhage and early gestational bleeding.

Prenatal advice may also concern the mother's work since certain hazards in the workplace affect pregnancy outcome and infant mortality. However, work may influence the overall social conditions of women and become a positive rather than a negative factor *(22)*. Improvement in working and living conditions may also eliminate or reduce health hazards. Work and fetal risk should therefore be considered in a broad framework of social policies affecting the overall situation of women in contemporary societies.

The measurements used in surveillance and evaluation of prenatal care may concern the process or the outcome. Process measurements concern mostly the frequency of contacts with prenatal services during pregnancy. Less frequently, they are aimed at the content of care and its quality.

The main outcome indicators include: perinatal mortality rate (also linked to improved care at delivery and immediate postnatal care); birth weight (which includes a large variety of environmental, behavioural and genetic influences); and gestational age at birth as a measure of maturity (also resulting from a large group of determinants).

The evaluation of prenatal care is, therefore, a complex issue. Research undertaken in several countries does not provide simple, straightforward answers. For example, in France, a recent investigation has not been able to

Table 6. Effect of supplementation on birth weight distribution (percentage of total births)

Birth weight (g)	Dry season	Wet season	Combined
Pre-supplementation			
>3500	5.4	2.2	3.8
3001-3500	40.4	25.8	33.3
2501-3000	42.5	43.8	43.2
<2500	11.7	28.2	19.7
Post-supplementation			
>3500	8.0	11.6	9.7
3001-3500	42.0	37.2	39.8
2501-3000	42.0	46.5	44.1
<2500	8.0	4.7	6.4
χ^2 test	NS	$P<0.01$	$P<0.01$

Source: **Prentice, A.G. et al.,** Prenatal dietary supplementation of African women and birth-weight. *Lancet,* **1**: 490-492 (1983).

state more than an improvement in infant health concurrent with increased prenatal surveillance (Table 7) since other factors have also intervened. The percentage of children of birth rank three or more has decreased and the age distribution of pregnant mothers has also changed. These factors are sufficient to explain 40% of the decrease in prematurity rates. The undoubted inverse links between parity and compliance with prenatal care complicate the picture still further. Further research is needed to identify more precisely the influence of different factors involved and elucidate the role of confounding variables. Some analytical approaches are presented in Part III.

Family Planning

Where family planning programmes are undertaken mainly for demographic reasons, such as to balance population and resources and the relation between population growth and overall development, demographic indices such as modifications in birth rate, fertility rate and gross or net rates of population increase can serve as a basis for measurement of the achievement of population control.

From a health promotion point of view, the personal protection provided by the family planning services is aimed at improving the quality of life through preventing stressful events due to unwanted pregnancy as well as reducing adverse effects on health linked with uncontrolled reproduction.

Table 7. Modifications in some indicators of prenatal care and outcome, France, 1972–1981 (random samples of 5000 in each year)

	1972	1976	1981
Prematurity rate (less than 37 weeks)	8.2%	6.8%	5.6%
Birth weight less than 2500 g	6.2%	6.5%	5.3%
Breastfeeding on fifth day	31.7%		47.5%
Perinatal deaths (stillbirths + deaths at less than one week) per 1000 births	21.3		12.3
Maternal mortality rate/100 000	25.0	17.3	15.5
Less than 4 prenatal contacts	15.3%	10.6%	3.9%
More than 7 prenatal contacts	22.2%	33.9%	54.9%
First contact before third month of pregnancy		96.4%	97.6%
Less than one contact with specialist	72.9%		8.8%
More than 6 weeks leave		34%	62%
Not working in last term of pregnancy		13%	25%

Several groups of measurements can quantify the above aspects. They relate to the assessment of the need for family planning, potential gain resulting from controlled reproduction, evaluation of efficacy of interventions, monitoring of process and assessment of the outcome of relevant services.

The assessment of the need can be obtained through population surveys on people's aspirations for family size or attitudes towards future pregnancies (Fig. 14). The data on legal abortions can also be used as an indirect measure of the need for family planning services. However, these statistics underestimate the actual number of induced abortions, especially in countries where such procedures are restricted.

The potential benefits to health of controlled reproduction can be illustrated by several measurements showing the relationship between infant deaths and such variables as parity or age of the mother (Fig. 15). The most important factor that could be controlled through family planning practices is the length of the interval between births; the shorter the interval the higher the infant mortality (Fig. 16).

The efficacy of methods used in family planning, in a narrow sense, relates to the power of a given contraceptive technique in preventing pregnancy. In a broader perspective, it is concerned with the evaluation of alternative strategies and approaches tried to promote family planning practices.

The process measures should in turn cover such aspects as availability, accessibility and acceptability of services. Measurements in this particular

Fig. 1.4. Percentage of women with three living children who want no more pregnancies

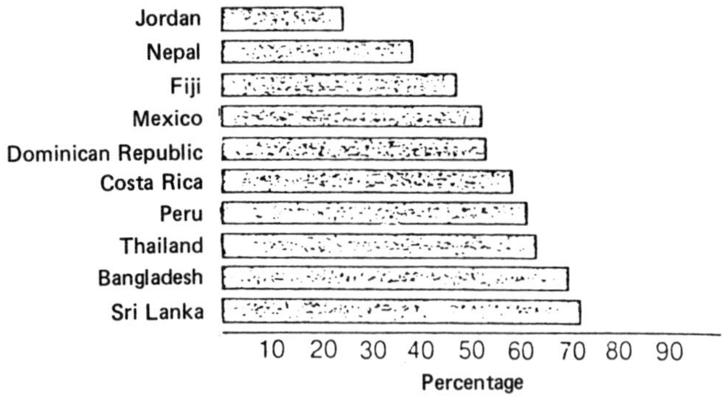

Source: **Henderson, R.** *(2)*.

Fig. 15. Deaths by age of mother:
fetal deaths during the last two months of pregnancy and deaths during first week after birth, by age of mother

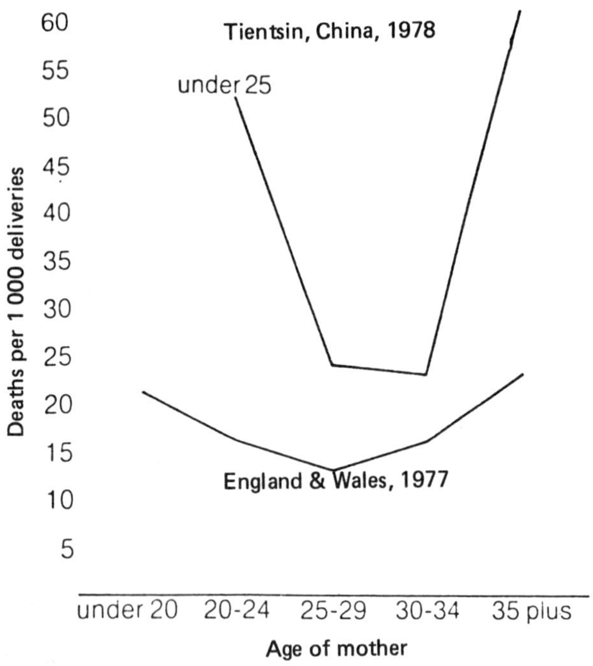

Source: **Henderson, R.** *(2)*.

Fig. 16. Birth spacing and infant mortality

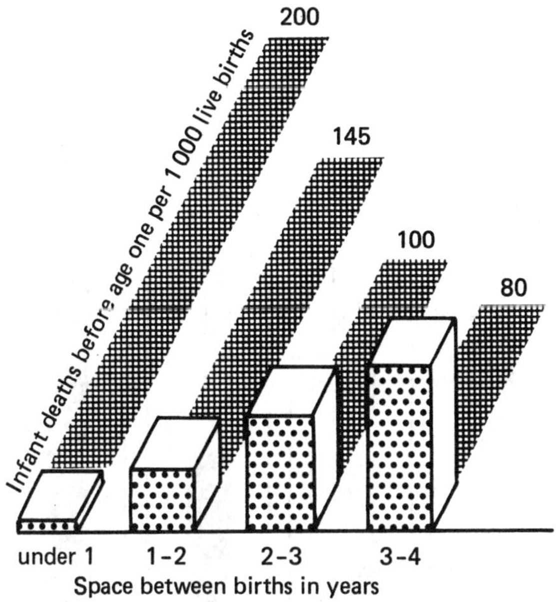

Note: Space between births is the interval between the termination of the preceding pregnancy and the birth of the infant.

Source: **Omran, A.R. & Standley, C.C., ed.** *Family formation patterns and health.* Geneva, World Health Organization, 1976, p.215 (data from South India sample, 1971–1975, 6541 women).

field will be largely based on surveys among the relevant population and should also include monitoring of the adequacy and effectiveness of the various functions of such services in the use of various family planning methods (Fig. 17).

Measurements of various health outcomes related to family planning practices are obviously of central importance in assessing the effectiveness and impact of family planning programmes. Some of them, such as reducing infant deaths or induced abortions, have already been mentioned. The elimination of these negative aspects must be balanced against the complications linked to the prolonged use of contraception. These are themselves influenced by factors such as age, smoking, parity and the existence of certain disorders.

More refined measurements, especially concerned with the quality of life of the family and its members, are not so readily available. Furthermore, their interpretation, in the presence of many confounding variables, both personal and social, is a difficult task.

Fig. 17. Family planning: access and use — percentage of women aged 25-34 who have ever heard of a place to obtain contraceptive advice or supplies, and who have used a method of contraception, by years of education, Kenya, 1977-1979

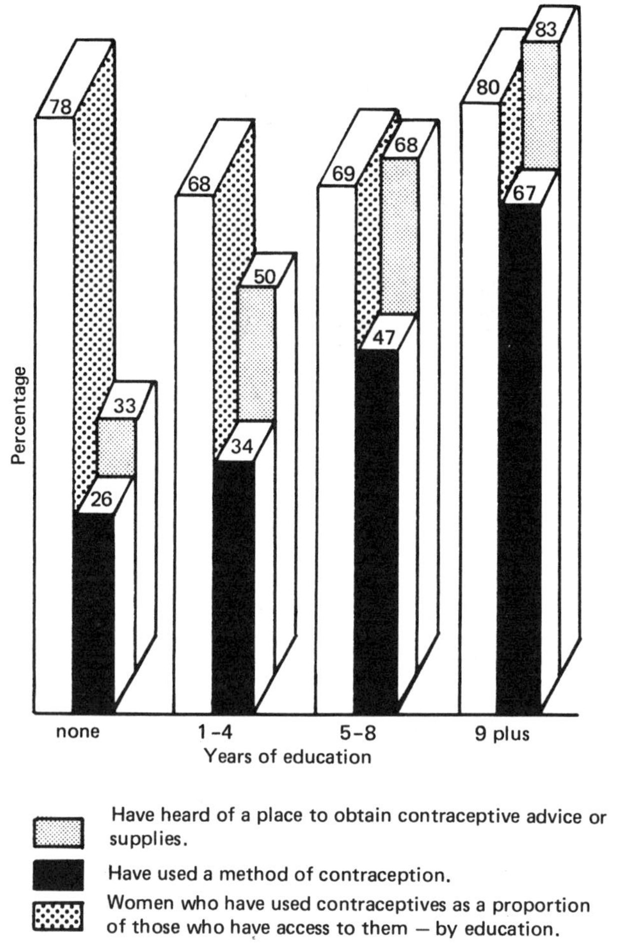

Note: Excludes never married women.

Source: **Central Bureau of Statistics.** *Kenya Fertility Survey, 1977-1978.* First Report Volume 1. Nairobi, Ministry of Economic Planning and Development, 1980.

Personal Protection in Road Safety

Motor vehicle accidents represent the largest group among all deaths due to external causes (accidents, suicide, violence), accounting for up to one third of all such deaths in people under 65 years of age. For every death in road accidents there are about 15 cases of severe injuries and at least twice as many cases of slight injuries.

Motor vehicle accidents result from a variety of personal and environmental factors. Of the factors that significantly increase the risk of road traffic accidents, alcohol and drugs are of particular importance. This applies to all categories of road users. It has been shown that in the adult population the relative risk and the severity of an injury increase with an increase in alcohol concentration *(23,24)*. Furthermore, it appears that a hangover the morning after excess drinking may also diminish driving ability by as much as 20%, even when the blood alcohol concentration is at zero level *(25)*.

There are several environmental factors involved in the causation of road traffic accidents: roads, traffic signs, speed limits and other traffic regulations, as well as car design. A level of education of all users of the roads (drivers, motorcyclists, cyclists and pedestrians) is also of great importance.

Primary prevention, or prevention of occurrence, aims at the individual and the community or at the environment. The first group of measures include education (highway code), surveillance (highway police), regulations (speed limits) and punishment (withholding of driving licence), while the second involves abolition of risk (car-free areas), avoidance of risk (separate passages for bicycles or pedestrians), limitation of risk (improved road surfaces) or notification of risk (highway signs).

The goal of secondary prevention is a reduction of the adverse effects of an accident, such as death, injury or disability, if primary prevention fails. It may be directed towards a vehicle or towards an individual in providing protection devices.

Measurements, in road safety, present many difficulties because the available data are either not always relevant or fragmentary. For example, no valid information exists on exposure, population at risk, or total volume of accidents or injuries. Similar difficulties are encountered when dealing with such particular aspects of road safety as personal protection. The three main kinds of measurements needed in this field relate to the efficacy of the given personal protection device, their use and their effectiveness at population level.

According to the evidence available at present the most cost—beneficial appear to be seat belts. In all countries in which appropriate legislation was introduced and enforced, it resulted in a noticeable reduction (about 25%) of deaths and serious injuries. The experience of Switzerland is very informative in this respect. Fig. 18 shows the relationship between legislation, compliance and deaths. More recently impressive effects of seat belt legislation on injuries in road traffic accidents were reported in the United Kingdom (Table 8).

Fig. 18. Switzerland: occupants killed in cars and the frequency of use of seat belts

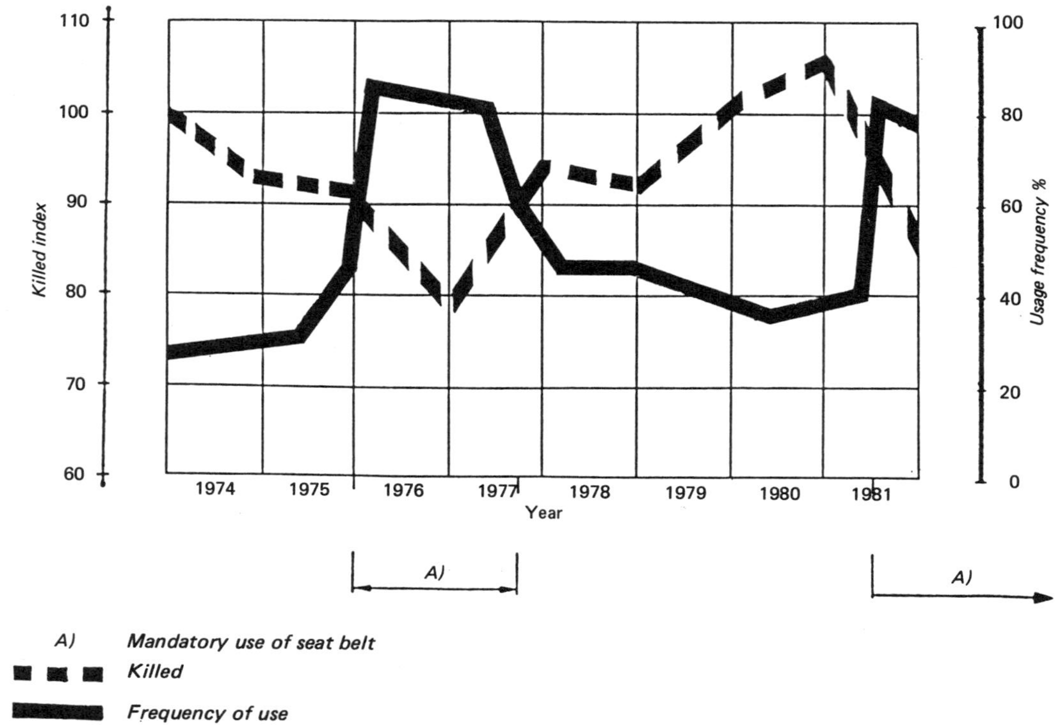

Source: *Journal of traffic medicine,* **11**(2): 25–26 (1983).

Table 8. Non-fatal injuries sustained by car drivers and passengers in road traffic accidents in Nottingham before and after seat belt legislation

Severity of injuries[a]	No. of injuries		Fall (%)	Significance[b]
	Nov.-Jan.	Feb.-April		
	Facial injuries			
Mild	72	24	67	$P<0.001$
Moderate	11	2	81	$P<0.025$
Severe	10	0	100	$P<0.01$
Total	93	26	72	$P<0.001$
	Head injuries			
Mild	66	30	55	$P<0.001$
Moderate	17	0	100	$P<0.001$
Severe	6	3	50	NS
Total	89	33	63	$P<0.001$
	Neck injuries			
Mild	38	23	39	NS
Moderate	3	0	100	NS
Severe	7	1	86	$P<0.05$
Total	48	24	50	$P<0.01$
	Chest injuries			
Mild	19	27		NS
Moderate	4	1	75	NS
Severe	8	1	88	$P<0.025$
Total	31	29	6	NS
	All injuries			
Mild	245	133	46	$P<0.001$
Moderate	29	7	76	$P<0.001$
Severe	21	2	90	$P<0.001$
Total	295	142	52	$P<0.001$

[a] Assessed with injury severity score.

[b] Using χ^2 test.

Source: **Pye, Q. & Waters, E.A.** *British medical journal,* **288**: 756–757 (1984).

In addition to seat belts, other personal protective devices can reduce injuries from traffic accidents *(26)*. However, the information on their use and effectiveness is scanty.

Personal Protection in Occupational Safety

Personal protection in occupational health practice includes protective clothing and equipment to safeguard workers from more or less specific occupational hazards and keep the users healthy and safe. Certainly, the elimination and control of the source of the hazard is preferable to relying on personal protection, which should be regarded as the last line of defence when all other possibilities are exploited *(27)*.

Protective clothing is used to protect people from dirty conditions, atmospheric influences, cold, or thermal or other radiation. Protective equipment is often required to supplement environmental control measures and has more specific applications, such as protection from dust or noise. Protection of the skin is also a special problem *(28)*.

The three main kinds of measurements used in the evaluation of personal protection are: measurements of the degree of protection, measurements of use (compliance), and measurements of effectiveness (outcome).

The degree of protection from noise is measured by the reduction in sound level provided by a hearing protector. This is called the attenuation of the sound level and depends upon the noise in which it is worn (Fig. 19) *(27)*.

With regard to respiratory protection the degree of protection is defined by the nominal protection factor (npf), expressed as the ratio of the concentration of the contaminant present in the ambient atmosphere to the calculated concentration within the facepiece when respiratory protection is being worn *(27)*:

$$\text{npf} = \frac{\text{concentration of contaminant in atmosphere}}{\text{concentration of contaminant in facepiece}}$$

The nominal protection factor depends upon the kind of respiratory protection equipment (Table 9).

The effectiveness of the personal protection of workers is measured by outcome indicators that provide information on the degree of the reduction in adverse health effects among the exposed workers. This would require special epidemiological studies with the use of appropriate control groups. Information on the outcome indications derived from routine statistics on the occurrence of certain occupational diseases should be interpreted with caution because of the influence of confounding factors, such as the actual use of the protectors (compliance).

Conclusions

Personal protection plays an important role in health protection and promotion. In addition to the specific interventions or measures applied against specific hazards presented in this chapter, there are procedures of a more

Fig. 19. Comparisons of the attenuation data for four hearing protectors

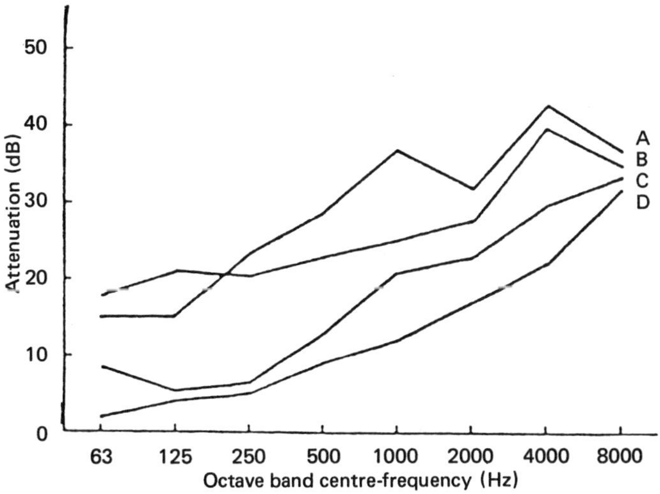

A = high attenuation earmuff.

B = disposable expanding polyurethane foam earplugs.

C = low attenuation earmuff.

D = disposable earplugs.

Source: **Else, D.** Personal protection. *In:* Schilling, R.S.F., ed. *Occupational health practice.* London, Butterworths, 1981.

general character, such as personal hygiene and other health practices. These include healthy eating habits, oral hygiene, non-smoking, physical exercise, etc. Health benefits resulting from some of them are well documented. For example, nonsmoking leads to a substantial reduction of lung cancer and other tobacco-related malignancies. Measurements of effects of other less specific health practices present more difficulties. Nevertheless, it was shown that even such simple means as handwashing produce a measurable reduction of enteric infections. Further discussion of issues of measurement related to individual behaviour can be found in Chapter 8.2. The question of participation in health promotion is also relevant in this connection and is covered in Chapter 8.3.

There is no doubt that personal protection technologies effectively applied on a mass scale could significantly improve the global health situation. However, the difficulties involved in shaping human behaviour present a problem. The oversimplified traditional health education or victim-blaming approaches failed. Comprehensive strategies based on national health policies that make proper health behaviour an easy and attractive one may promote wider use of available personal protection technologies.

Table 9. Approximate nominal protection factors for respiratory protection equipment

Type of respiratory protection equipment	Nominal protection factor
Respirators	
single use filtering facepiece respirator	5
half-mask (cartridge) respirator	10
full facepiece (canister) respirator	500–1000
powered air-purifying respirator	500
powered visor respirator	10–20
Breathing apparatus	
fresh air hose apparatus	50
compressed airline apparatus	1000–2000
self-contained breathing apparatus	2000

Source: **Else, D.** Personal protection. *In:* Schilling, R.S.F., ed. *Occupational health practice*. London, Butterworths, 1981.

References

1. **Hilleman, M.R.** Vaccines for the decade of the 1980s and beyond. *South African medical journal,* **61**: 691–698 (1982).
2. **Henderson, R.** Expanded immunization. *The state of the world's children 1984.* UNICEF, Oxford University Press, 1984, pp. 82–85.
3. **Galazka. A.M. et al.** Indications and contraindications for vaccines used in the Expanded Programme on Immunization. *Bulletin of the World Health Organization,* **62**(3): 357–366 (1984).
4. **Katz, S.P.** Effects of malnutrition and parasitic infections on the immune response to vaccines. Evaluation of the risks associated with administering vaccines to malnourished children. *In: Recent advances in immunization.* 1983, pp. 81–89 (PAHO Scientific Publication, No. 451).
5. **Evensen, S.** *Relationship between infant morbidity and breast-feeding versus artificial feeding in industrialized countries: a review of the literature.* Copenhagen, WHO Regional Office for Europe, 1982 (unpublished document ICP/NUT 010/6 Rev.1).
6. **Ellestad-Sayed, J. et al.** Breast-feeding protects against infection in Indian infants. *Canadian Medical Association journal,* **120**: 295–298 (1979).
7. **Paine, R. & Coble, R.J.** Breast-feeding and infant health in a rural U.S. community. *American journal of diseases in children,* **136**(1): 36–38 (1982).

8. **Biering-Sørensen, F. et al.** Breast-feeding and infant health in Copenhagen 1941–1972. *Danish medical bulletin,* **30**(1): 36–41 (1983).
9. **de Carvalho, M. et al.** Effect of frequent breast-feeding on early milk production and infant weight gain. *Pediatrics,* **72**: 307–310 (1982).
10. **Visweswavo, R.K. & Parvati, R.** Appropriate age for introduction of supplementary food for infants. *Courrier,* **32**(4,5,6): 307–310 (1982).
11. **Durnin, J.V. & McKillop, F.M.** Infant nutrition in Glasgow. *Health bulletin (Edinburgh),* **41**(3): 165–171 (1983).
12. **Edouard, L.** Regional variations in perineonatal mortality. *Public health,* **95**(3): 148–151 (1981).
13. **United States Department of Health and Human Services.** *The health consequences of smoking for women: a report of the Surgeon General.* Washington, DC, United States Government Printing Office, 1980.
14. **Wainright, R.L.** Change in observed birth weight associated with change in maternal cigarette smoking. *American journal of epidemiology,* **117**(6): 668–675 (1983).
15. **Luke, B. et al.** Influence of smoking, weight gain and pregravid weight for height on intrauterine growth. *American journal of clinical nutrition,* **34**: 1410–1417 (1981).
16. **Bottoms, S.F. et al.** Maternal passive smoking and foetal serum thiocyanate levels. *American journal of obstetrics and gynecology,* **144**(7): 787–791 (1982).
17. **Dalaker, K. et al.** Some social background variables among smoking and non-smoking primiparae. *Scandinavian journal of social medicine,* **11**(1): 23–26 (1983).
18. **Rush, D. & Cassano, P.** Relationship of cigarette smoking and social class to birth weight and perinatal mortality among all births in Britain, 5–11 April 1970. *Journal of epidemiology and community health,* **37**: 249–255 (1983).
19. **Wright, J.T. et al.** Alcohol consumption, pregnancy and low birth weight. *Lancet,* **1**: 663–665 (1983).
20. **Barrison, J.G. et al.** Screening for alcohol abuse in pregnancy. *British medical journal,* **285**: 1318 (1982).
21. **Rosett, H.L. et al.** Treatment experience with pregnant problem drinkers. *Journal of the American Medical Association,* **249**(15): 2029–2033 (1983).
22. **Saurel, M.J. & Kaninski, M.** Pregnant women at work. *Lancet,* **1**: 475 (1983).
23. **Irwin, S.T. et al.** Association between alcohol consumption and adult pedestrians who sustain injuries in road traffic accidents. *British medical journal,* **286**: 522 (1983).
24. **Jacobsen, B. et al.** Alcohol and drugs in road traffic accident victims. *Journal of traffic medicine,* **11**(2): 28–32 (1983).
25. **Franck, D.H.** "If you drink, don't drive" motto now applies to hangovers as well. *Journal of the American Medical Association,* **250**(13): 1657–1658 (1983).

26. *Seat belts and other devices to reduce injuries from traffic accidents:* report on a WHO Technical Group. Copenhagen, WHO Regional Office for Europe, 1979 (EURO Reports and Studies, No. 40).
27. **Else, D.** Personal protection. *In:* Schilling, R.S.F., ed. *Occupational health practice.* London, Butterworths, 1981.
28. **Schilling, R.S.F.** Prevention of occupational disease and ill health. *In:* Schilling, R.S.F., ed. *Occupational health practice.* London, Butterworths, 1981.

8.2 Indicators of behaviour conducive to health promotion — *S.B. Kar & E. Berkanovic*

This chapter discusses issues in measuring health-promoting behaviour. For this purpose, health promotion is defined as the advancement of wellbeing and the avoidance of health risks by achieving and maintaining optimal levels of the behavioural, societal, environmental and biomedical determinants of health.[a] This definition is basically similar to that given in Chapter 1. Since health is defined as physical, social and mental wellbeing, all behaviour conducive to the achievement of physical, mental and social wellbeing as well as disease prevention is defined as health-promoting behaviour. Health-promoting behaviour can be performed by individuals (abstinence from or cessation of cigarette smoking) and by societies (legislation banning cigarette sales to minors). Thus health-promoting behaviour needs to be measured at both individual and societal levels.

Although conventional health promotion is most frequently discussed as specific acts of individuals, actions may be taken either by individuals or by societies that may promote the physical, psychological or social wellbeing of individuals. Consistent with the definition presented above, therefore, health promotion encompasses a wider range of behaviour than is usually discussed under the rubric of prevention. A complete enumeration of indicators and instruments for each health-promoting behaviour would be an impossible task; some examples, however, are provided. The objective is to present an analytical framework that could assist decision-makers, researchers and practitioners to answer the following questions.

1. What kinds of indicator should be used to measure health-promoting behaviour?

2. Are there valid measures readily available for key health-promoting behaviour?

3. Where should efforts be focused in developing additional measures of health promotion?

Health-promoting behaviour may be conceived as final actions that result in desired health outcomes and that are necessarily preceded by a preliminary sequence of actions. Thus, health promotion is the product of certain stages of behaviour. This point will be discussed in detail below. Although this system addresses behavioural processes believed to be related to health outcomes, it does not speak to the epidemiological concerns of morbidity

---

[a] This definition is formulated jointly by the senior author and the members of the Long-Range Planning Committee, School of Public Health, University of California, Los Angeles, USA.

and mortality. Nevertheless, to the extent that scientifically valid measurement of health-promoting behaviour occurs and to the extent that scientifically valid research designs are used to obtain these measurements, the testing of epidemiological hypotheses will be facilitated. Indeed, one difficulty with the testing of many epidemiological hypotheses linking health-promoting behaviour to morbidity or mortality is in demonstrating that health promotion has an invariant relationship with its hypothesized outcome.

This is a review of the actual measures of health-promoting behaviour that have appeared in the recent research literature. Two observations can be made about this literature. First, few measures are comprehensive with respect to health-promoting behaviour. Thus, although many measures seek information about one or another health-promoting activity such as cigarette smoking, diet or the use of preventive services, well developed scales that attempt to measure a wide range of such activities are rare. Indeed, no measures deal with the entire spectrum of the behaviour promoting physical health that is discussed in this paper.

A second observation that can be made about the measures of health-promoting behaviour currently in research literature is that it depends heavily upon self reports. This is especially true of measures of health-promoting behaviour at the individual level. As will be discussed subsequently, such measures rely heavily on unbiased memory in situations in which the phrasing of the question affects the response. Thus, one cannot discuss such measures without discussing their validity.

A Conceptual Scheme for Analysing Health-promoting Behaviour

Health promotion can be conceptualized as a dynamic process involving various stages of behaviour that range from the performance of essential initial actions to the achievement of health outcomes that indicate the effective performance of the final actions needed to achieve each health outcome. Table 1 presents an analytical framework for identifying indicators at each stage of behaviour (initial, intermediate and final action). These affect both proximal and distal outcomes. Exogenous factors affecting the likelihood that both actions and outcomes will occur are also identified.

A researcher may choose to measure the proximal outcome, the actual behaviour itself, or both. The choice would depend upon several considerations. One consideration is the strength of the relationship between the actual behaviour and its proximal outcome. For instance, recently both Breslow *(1,2)* and Reed *(3)* demonstrated that much healthy behaviour is directly related to mortality and physical health status. Research by Breslow and his colleagues in the Human Population Laboratory, in Alameda County, California, demonstrated an association between seven health habits and the health status of an adult population measured in terms of age-adjusted mortality rates *(1,2)*. Data presented from this longitudinal study also suggested that these seven healthy habits had an additive effect on health status, that is, those who followed all seven habits had better health

Table 1. Stages of behaviour and corresponding indicators: a methodological framework

Initial action	Intermediate action	Final action	Outcome		
			Physical	Mental	Social
Seek/obtain knowledge about preventive behaviour	Subjective cost–benefit evaluation of preventive behaviour	Effective preventive behaviour	Reduced risk of illness	Mental satisfaction derived from self-control	Increased opportunities for social, economic, interpersonal role performance
Seek/obtain social support for preventive behaviour	Formation of intention to engage in preventive behaviour	Subjective evaluation of results of preventive behaviour			
Communication and consultation regarding prevention	Seek/obtain access to services/supplies required to carry out preventive behaviour	Maintain intention, social support, access relevant to preventive behaviour			
		Structural support requirements			
Availability/accessi-bility/acceptability of source of knowledge, communication, consultation	Physical ability to engage in preventive behaviour		Social norms and opportunities for achieving these outcomes		
Social norms promotive of knowledge-seeking	Adequate intellectual and decision-making skills				
Social networks capable of producing support	Availability/accessibility/accept-ability of services/supplies				
	Social norms promotive of continued preventive behaviour				

than those who followed six; those who followed six habits were better off than those who followed five, and so on. These seven habits were: eating moderately, eating regularly, eating breakfast, no cigarette smoking, moderate use of alcohol, at least moderate exercise, and 7–8 hours of sleep per night *(1)*. Health promotion programmes often justify activities aimed at changing behaviour because of such epidemiological evidence. If the primary objective of the researcher is to test the relationship between health status and these specific actions, then the strength of the relationship between the final actions and the outcome becomes an issue of critical importance requiring measurement of each. If, on the other hand, a strong relationship between the action and an outcome has already been established (such as taking antibiotics and controlling a bacterial infection), then the researcher may focus on measuring either the action or the outcome. Finally, if the action increases the probability of an outcome, but does not result in that outcome in almost all of the cases (cigarette smoking and lung cancer), then the researcher interested in determining whether the behaviour occurred (smoking cessation) must measure the action itself. Thus, both the purposes of the researcher and the nature of the link between the action and the outcome must be taken into account in selecting indicators.

The second consideration is the extent to which measures are reliable, valid and feasible. For instance, observation of contraceptive use is a reliable and valid measure of the actual behaviour, but it is not feasible. Similarly, verbal reports on contraceptive use may be feasible but may not be valid. Research shows that when saliva samples are obtained along with verbal reports on smoking habits respondents report a higher level of smoking than when only verbal reports are obtained *(4)*. Presumably, the respondents expect saliva tests to detect smoking; hence, the simple act of seeking validation increases the reported frequency of the behaviour.

The issue of the validity of self-reports of health-promoting behaviour involves several questions. First, if the purpose of such measures is to make comparisons between groups about the extent to which they engage in such behaviour, then any differences in either the ability or the willingness of each group to report these will result in bias that invalidates the comparison. Second, certain behaviour may be more sensitive than other behaviour in one or another group. This may result in underreporting of this behaviour in relation to others. For example, both sexual behaviour and drug use may not be reported accurately among individuals who feel their actions in these areas are not socially acceptable. Third, both the context within which questions about healthy behaviour are asked and the phrasing of the questions will affect the results. For example, Harris & Guten *(5)*, using an open-ended question that was not time-bound but that expressed the assumption that the respondent actively engaged in health-promoting behaviour, found that 97% of a sample of urban Americans reported such behaviour. Berkanovic *(6)*, on the other hand, using an open-ended question that was time-bound and that expressed no expectations about whether health-promoting behaviour actually was undertaken, found that only 51% said they engaged in such behaviour. The difference between these results is due to the implications of Harris & Guten's question, that the researcher expected the respondent to report behaviour that promoted health. This interpretation is confirmed by the fact that Kurz & Wolinsky *(7)*, using the same questions as Berkanovic, found results similar to his in a different sample of urban Americans.

Other issues that affect the validity of measurement are the specificity of the behaviour and corresponding attitudes, and the intensity of intention in performing that behaviour. Research on consistency between health attitude and behaviour shows that questions that measure very specific attitudes and corresponding specific behaviour reveal a greater consistency between health attitudes and behaviour. Conversely, measures of general attitudes are weakly related to specific activities *(8–12)*. In a cross-cultural study Kar and others *(10–12)* found that verbal reports suggesting general attitudes are poor predictors of specific contraceptive practices while specific intentions for contraception had a strong relationship with corresponding behaviour. In addition, the stronger the intention (intensity), the greater the likelihood of action. Behavioural outcome measures, such as fertility histories, validated this trend. It is critical, therefore, that any attempt to interpret self-reports of health-promoting behaviour evaluate these threats to validity.

A third consideration is the extent to which all the stages of health-promoting behaviour should be measured. For example, if the final action is the use of contraceptives, this cannot take place in the absence of certain antecedent actions. If the research objective is simply to describe whether the behaviour occurred, then measurement could be confined to that. If, on the other hand, the objective is to analyse and to facilitate the process leading to the behaviour, then measures of the earlier stages of behaviour, such as use of services, are also required. Furthermore, analytical research into health-promoting behaviour should also identify the social, structural and environmental factors that affect individual behaviour, such as the extent of social support or access to acceptable services. The lower half of Table 1 presents indicators of structural conditions that may facilitate or inhibit actions by individuals.

A final consideration is the extent to which the theories and models identify indicators that are appropriate at the various stages of behaviour preceding a final action. For instance, Kar's model of the psychosocial determinants of health behaviour *(10–13)* holds that, given that the exogenous variables are homogeneous, (socioeconomic status, age, sex), the final action is a function of direct, additive and interacting effects of behavioural intention, social support, accessibility of information and services, personal autonomy, and action situation. These independent variables, some of which are within the psyche and others outside it, are the initial and intermediate stages (preconditions) leading to the desired health-promoting behaviour, such as the use of contraception. Also, relevant knowledge is a necessary but not sufficient condition for behaviour; a combination of positive knowledge and positive behavioural intention is a much better predictor of the final action. In addition, consistent with numerous other studies, it was found that specific behavioural intention is a better predictor of future actions than generalized attitudes towards such actions. Furthermore, the relative weights of the five predictors of the model used varied significantly by culture and sociodemographic status *(10–12)*. Models such as this can be quite useful in identifying indicators to be included in studies in which health-promoting behaviour is to be analysed.

A Matrix of Health-promoting Behaviour

Table 2 presents a 3 × 2 matrix of physical, psychological and social health-promoting behaviour at the individual and social levels. The indicators of physical, psychological and social health behaviour presented here are chosen because they have appeared in recent empirical research. However, the inclusion of particular indicators and instruments does not imply that the validity of each measure has been well established.

The distinctions between physical, psychological and social health behaviour are not mutually discrete or exclusive; one mode of behaviour may have effects on all three levels. Furthermore, physical, psychological and social health have mutual interactions and circular relationships. This implies that the measurement of health-promoting behaviour can seldom be restricted to one level. Due to these synergistic effects, indicators of health behaviour must often extend beyond and measure more than one category of the matrix.

Health status is a function of factors both internal to individuals and external in their environment. These factors may have direct, interacting and additive effects *(9–12)*. Any measurement that focuses only on personal behaviour, although useful for specific research objectives, is of limited value in understanding the overall determinants of the health-promotion status of the individual. Behaviour at the individual, group and societal levels interacts with biological and physical or environmental factors to determine the overall health status of people. It is thus imperative that a systems approach encompassing individual, societal and environmental subsystems be used in studying the determinants of health behaviour and its results.

Physical Health-promoting Measures

In Table 2, 12 physical health-promoting activities by individuals are listed. The selection of these indicators is heavily influenced by the Institute of Medicine's compilation of health behaviour research, which lists several behavioural risks to health *(1,2)*, the behavioural risk factors expounded by Breslow and his colleagues *(1–3,14)*. Physical health-promoting behaviour at the individual level includes: moderation with alcohol, exercise, abstinence from or cessation of cigarette smoking, recommended dietary practices, and adequate sleep and rest. The Institute of Medicine's volume also includes activities preventing disease or risk in addition to those enumerated above. These are: medical check-ups, hazard or accident prevention, and preventive measures against specific communicable diseases *(13)*. While the latter expands the list of health-promoting behaviour proposed by Breslow and his colleagues, it still does not deal fully with responsible sexual behaviour as a category of health-promoting behaviour. Health behaviour,

Table 2. A proposed matrix of health-promoting behaviour: individual and social level indicators

Level	Physical health	Psychological health	Social health
Individual	Cigarette smoking	Stress management and coping	Adequacy of role set
	Alcohol and substance abuse	Psychological distress	Life satisfaction
	Recommended dietary habits	Psychological wellbeing	Adequacy of role performance
	Physical exercise	Self-esteem	Adequacy of social network, social support, social participation
	Rest/sleep	Substance dependence	
	Safety or accident prevention	Antisocial behaviour	
	Use of preventive health services		
	Contraception		
	Prevention of sexually transmitted diseases		
	Maternal and child health care		
	Early seeking of diagnosis		
	Social support/coping behaviour affecting physical health		
Social	Availability/accessibility/acceptability of effective health-promoting programmes and services	Availability/accessibility/acceptability of mental health resources and services	Availability/accessibility/acceptability of opportunities for social participation (e.g. political, religious, occupational, interpersonal, aesthetic)
	Norms governing health-related behaviour	Norms governing deviance and help-seeking	Levels of alienation/anomie
	Institutional support (e.g. legislation, community organization) for health promotion	Institutional support (e.g. police and political, religious, educational), recognition of and referral for psychological problems	Adequacy of status and reward system

undertaken to prevent the adverse effects of communicable and noncommunicable diseases, sexually transmitted diseases, and unwanted pregnancy, and action to seek and offer social support for coping with stress and health risks, are important categories of health-promoting behaviour. Thus, the following means of behaviour are added: use of preventive services or contraception, prevention and treatment of sexually transmitted diseases, accident prevention and safety, early seeking of health care, maternal and child health care, and social interactions and coping behaviour that affect an individual's health. This expanded list contains health-promoting behaviour aimed at the prevention of a specific disease or hazard, as well as the promotion of overall wellbeing.

There are several approaches to the measurement of these indicators; none is comprehensive. One approach has been to develop detailed measures of specific actions, such as frequency and dose of cigarette smoking by an individual; a second has been to design summated indicators of healthy behaviour, such as the number of activities performed out of a recommended list. A third has been the development of health risk appraisal scales. Research by Breslow *(1,2)* and Reed *(3)* shows that a summated scale is an effective approach for measuring overall physical health-promoting behaviour. Thus, their studies indicate that the greater the number of activities performed, the better the health status when measured by age-adjusted mortality rates. Table 3 shows the relationship between selected health practices and measures of physical health status reported by Breslow and others *(1,2)*. For example, among men with four or more health practices, only 5.7% experienced any symptoms, while among those who reported two or less positive health practices, 15.5% experienced symptoms. A similar trend is observed for women.

Several studies have shown a significant correlation between subjective health ratings and health status measured by either clinical assessments or subsequent mortality *(14,15)*. It is important to note that these measures are effective in comparing group aggregates even though they may not be useful in predicting the health of individuals. They are often used as indicators of the relative effectiveness of health-promoting programmes and practices in cross-group comparisons. Health risk appraisal scales attempt to identify factors that are associated with mortality. In most cases, these factors are added together into a set of probabilities of death at various ages.

Fig. 1 presents a scale for measuring nutritional risk developed by Wolinsky and his colleagues *(16)*. These items measure behavioural difficulties that some people encounter during eating, physical symptoms that interfere with eating and other practices that may contribute to nutritional risk. Subsequently, Wolinsky and others found that this nutritional risk index correlated with measures of perceived health, sensory functioning, activities of daily living and mental health status among a sample of American elderly people *(17)*. Measures such as this can be quite useful in identifying factors that must be overcome in order for the individual to engage in health-promoting behaviour such as appropriate nutrition. Indeed, although this measure mixes behaviour and symptoms, it illustrates the importance of structural support for health-promoting behaviour.

Table 3. Relationship between Health Practices Index and Physical Health Spectrum: age-adjusted mortality rates from all causes (per 100), men and women aged 30–69 years, 1965–1974

Number of low-risk health practices	Physical Health Spectrum									
	Disability		Chronic conditions		Symptoms		No health problems		Total	
	%	*(N)*	%	*(N)*	%	*(N)*	%	*(N)*	%	*(N)*
Men										
0, 1, 2	28.5	*(58)*	10.4	*(157)*	15.5	*(91)*	16.3	*(98)*	16.0	*(404)*
3	24.1	*(56)*	10.3	*(264)*	7.8	*(200)*	8.4	*(228)*	10.9	*(748)*
4, 5	13.8	*(48)*	6.6	*(358)*	5.7	*(254)*	3.4	*(417)*	5.8	*(1077)*
Total *(N)*	22.8	*(162)*	8.7	*(779)*	8.1	*(545)*	6.5	*(743)*	9.5	*(2229)*
Women										
0, 1, 2	18.5	*(100)*	10.0	*(157)*	5.5	*(105)*	8.0	*(64)*	11.9	*(426)*
3	15.0	*(105)*	5.7	*(296)*	2.8	*(233)*	7.9	(175)	7.1	*(809)*
4, 5	5.7	*(87)*	4.3	*(412)*	3.9	*(410)*	2.6	*(352)*	3.9	*(1261)*
Total *(N)*	14.0	*(292)*	5.7	*(865)*	3.8	*(748)*	4.7	*(591)*	5.4	*(2496)*

Source: **Berkman, L.F. & Breslow, L.** *Health and ways of living.* Oxford, Oxford University Press, 1983, p. 98.

Fig. 1. Frequency distributions and exact wording of the 16 items comprising the nutritional risk measure

Item number	Actual item	Percentage responding "yes" (indicating risk)
5.	Do you wear dentures?	75
14.	In the past month, have you taken any medicines prescribed by a doctor?	73
11.	Have you ever had an operation on your abdomen?	59
15.	In the past month, have you taken any other medicines that were not prescribed by a doctor?	45
9.	Do you have any trouble with your bowels that makes you constipated or gives you diarrhoea?	36
4.	Are there any kinds of foods that you don't eat because they disagree with you?	35
3.	Do you have trouble biting or chewing any kind of food?	25
1.	Do you now have an illness or condition that interferes with your eating?	24
13.	Do you smoke cigarettes regularly now?	23
16.	Are you now on any kind of a special diet?	22
12.	Have you ever been told by a doctor that you were "anaemic" (had iron poor blood)?	19
6.	Have you had any spells of pain or discomfort for 3 days or more in your abdomen or stomach in the past month?	14
2.	Do you have an illness that has cut down on your appetite?	12
7.	Did you have any trouble swallowing at least 3 days in the last month?	5
8.	Did you have any vomiting at least 3 days in the last month?	5
10.	Have you gained or lost any weight in the last 30 days? (*Note:* net gain/loss must have exceeded 10 pounds)	5

Scale statistics: $M = 4.77$; $SD = 2.43$; Cronbach's alpha = 0.603

Source: **Wolinsky, F. et al.** The preliminary validation of a nutritional risk measure among the elderly. *Journal of community health,* May 1973.

Psychological Health Promotion

The part of Table 2 relating to psychological health at the individual level includes stress management and coping, psychological distress, psychological wellbeing, self-esteem, substance dependence and antisocial behaviour. While coping is a process that is linked both to physical and to psychological wellbeing *(18)*, psychological distress, substance dependence and antisocial behaviour represent maladaptive behaviour that increases the risk of morbidity *(19)*. Although many indicators have been developed for measuring stress management and coping, most are specific to a context. More general measures are difficult to locate. However, Pearlin & Schooler *(20)* and Lazarus *(21)* have developed two scales for assessing how the individual handles the stresses and strains of everyday life. Both focus on the daily problems that people encounter in their work and family lives and both attempt to examine the techniques used in dealing with these problems. Both, however, contain a large number of items.

Psychological distress has also been examined in many different ways. Indeed, the concept includes clinically defined depressions and anxiety, negative affect with no specific clinical diagnosis, and lack of self-esteem. Two measures of depressive affect that have been widely used are the CES-D *(22)* and the Hopkins Symptom Checklist *(23)*. Negative affect has also been measured through a scale of psychological wellbeing by Bradburn *(24)*. The CES-D, the Hopkins Checklist and the psychological wellbeing scale have all been associated with physical symptoms, perceived health status and the use of medical services. Finally, although there are a myriad of self-esteem scales in the literature, the Simmons scale *(25)* has been found to be quite useful in predicting responses to health threats.

In the area of substance dependence and antisocial behaviour, there is at the moment one pre-eminent instrument, the Diagnostic Interview Schedule *(26)*. This instrument has been translated into a number of languages and has been tested in China, Peru and the United States. Further, it was designed for the purpose of permitting precise clinical diagnoses of self-report data obtained through population sample surveys. In addition, Jessor & Jessor *(27)* developed the concept and a set of indicators of problem behaviour syndrome among adolescents that can be used among adults. Fig. 2 presents examples of the measures used in the Diagnostic Interview Schedule to indicate alcohol abuse.

Social Health Promotion

Social health at the individual level (see Table 2) refers to the individual's satisfaction with the various spheres of life. Three approaches have been used frequently in this issue *(28–30)*. Each examines subjective satisfaction in a facet of social life such as occupation, family, neighbourhood, and opportunities for political, religious and/or aesthetic participation. A related dimension is the adequacy of the individual's performance in each of these areas. This dimension examines how others, such as the spouse or fellow workers, view the individual's behaviour as a contribution to their

Fig. 2. Selected indicators of alcohol abuse

164. Has there ever been a period of two weeks when every day you were drinking 7 or more beers, 7 or more drinks or 7 or more glasses of wine? ___ 27

No	1	Go to question 165	
Yes	5	Ask A	

A. How long has it been since you drank that much or do you still?

	Still or within last 2 weeks	1	Go to question 166	___ 28
Code most recent time possible	Within last month	2	Go to question 165A	
	Within last 6 months	3		
	Within last year	4		
	More than 1 year ago	5		

---

167. Have *friends*, your doctor, your clergyman, or any other *professional* ever *said* you were *drinking too much* for your own good? — 1 — 5*

IF YES: Was this only because you needed to lose weight? YES = 1

Recency		
— 2 weeks	1	___ 34
— 1 month	2	
— 6 months	3	___ 35
— 1 year	4	
+ 1 years	5	

---

168. Have you ever *wanted to stop* drinking but couldn't? — 1 — 5*

Recency		
— 2 weeks	1	___ 36
— 1 month	2	
— 6 months	3	___ 37
— 1 year	4	
+ 1 years	5	

170. Did you ever need a *drink just after* you had *gotten up* (that is, before breakfast)? — 1 — 5*

Recency		
— 2 weeks	1	___ 40
— 1 month	2	
— 6 months	3	___ 41
— 1 year	4	
+ 1 years	5	

---

171. Have you ever had *job* (or school) *trouble* because of drinking — like missing too much work or drinking on the job (or at school)? — 1 — 5*

Recency		
— 2 weeks	1	___ 42
— 1 month	2	
— 6 months	3	___ 43
— 1 year	4	
+ 1 years	5	

Source: Los Angeles ECA Survey, University of California, Los Angeles, 1982.

shared activities. Unfortunately, apart from a few studies of married couples, few measures have been developed in this area. With respect to occupational roles, however, an employment history could be used to draw some inferences about the extent to which the individual is performing well.

The adequacy of social networks and social support can only be determined through the subjective responses of the individual; thus they are matters best explored through population survey samples. Cross-cultural studies have shown significant impacts of social support on health-promoting behaviour *(9–12,31)*. Although the adequacy of social participation might also be examined in the same way, scales are available that permit independent judgements about this dimension. One such scale, by Donald & Ware *(32)*, examines both the resources available to the individual and the amount of contact with each resource. Although it permits quantification of social participation, it does not address the qualitative aspect.

Health Promotion at the Social Level

Although health promotion is usually thought of as the behaviour of individuals, the fact is that behaviour at the organizational and societal levels can also promote health. As the list in Table 2 indicates, such behaviour may be viewed as structural constraints by individuals (availability/accessibility/acceptability of services). Nevertheless, they represent behaviour affecting health promotion undertaken by institutions and organizations in society. Indeed, as Table 1 indicates, it is difficult to understand or affect the health-promoting behaviour of individuals without an understanding of how the larger institutions within which the individual must carry out such behaviour act. Further, there may be some circumstances under which health promotion among individuals is blocked by behaviour at the social level. For example, it is unlikely that unwanted pregnancies will be reduced where it is difficult to gain access to contraceptives.

The social behaviour listed in Table 2 includes three classes: policy in the form both of legislation and of institutional support; administrative decisions affecting the organization of services; and the broader social processes affecting levels of satisfaction. These factors are covered elsewhere in this volume. Health promotion by individuals cannot be understood without an understanding of how the behaviour of the institutions and organizations of a society affect the ability and the willingness of the individual to pursue health promotion.

References

1. **Hamburg, D. et al., ed.** *Health behavior frontiers of research in biobehavioral science.* Washington, DC, Institute of Medicine, National Academy of Sciences, 1982.
2. **Berkman, L.F. & Breslow, L.** *Health and ways of living.* Oxford, Oxford University Press, 1983.
3. **Reed, W.L.** Physical health status as a consequence of health practices. *Journal of community health,* **8**(4): 217–228 (1983).

4. **Fisher, E.B. et al.** *Cessation of smoking: health consequences of smoking on cancer:* a report of the US Surgeon General. USDHHS PHS: 82-50179, pp. 255–304.
5. **Harris, D.M. & Guten, S.** Health-protective behavior: an exploratory note. *Journal of health and social behaviour,* **20**: 17–29 (1979).
6. **Berkanovic, E.** Who engages in health protective behavior. *International journal of community health education,* **2**: 225–237 (1982).
7. **Kurz, R. & Wolinsky, F.N.** Who engages in health protective behavior: a replication. *International journal of community health education,* **4**: 251–263 (1983/1984).
8. **Freedman, R.** *The sociology of human fertility: an annotated bibliography.* New York, Halsted Press Division, John Wiley, 1975.
9. **Kar, S.B.** Impacts of behavioural intentions, social support, and accessibility on contraception: a cross-cultural study. *Population and environment,* **7**(1) (1984).
10. **Kar, S.B.** Consistency between fertility attitudes and behaviour: a conceptual model. *Population studies,* **32**(1): 173–185 (1978).
11. **Kar, S.B. & Talbot, J.M.** Attitudinal and non-attitudinal determinants of contraception: a cross-cultural study. *Studies in family planning,* **11**(2): 51–64 (1980).
12. **Kar, S.B.** Psychosocial environment: a health promotion model. *International quarterly of community health education,* **4**(4): 311–341 (1984).
13. **Hamburg, D. et al., ed.** *Health behavior: frontiers of research in the behavioral sciences.* Washington, DC, Institute of Medicine, National Academy Press, 1982.
14. **Kaplan, G.A. & Camacho, T.** Perceived health and mortality: a nine year follow-up of the human population laboratory cohort. *American journal of epidemiology,* **117**(3): 292–304 (1983).
15. **Kisch, A. et al.** New proxy measure for health status. *Health services research,* **4**: 223–230 (1969).
16. **Wolinsky, F.D. et al.** A preliminary validation of a nutritional risk measure for the elderly. *American journal of preventive medicine,* **1/2**: 53–59 (1985).
17. **Wolinsky, F.D. et al.** Measurement of the global and functional dimensions of health status in the elderly. *Journal of gerontology,* **39**: 88–92 (1984).
18. **Cohen, F. & Lazarus, R.S.** Coping and adaptation in health and illness. *In:* Mechanic, D., ed. *Handbook of health, health care and the health profession.* New York, Free Press, 1983.
19. **Regier, D.A. et al.** The *de facto* US mental health services system. *Archives of general psychiatry,* **34**: 685–693 (1978).
20. **Pearlin, L.I. & Schooler, J.C.** The structure of coping. *Journal of health and social behavior,* **19**: 2–21 (1978).
21. **Lazarus, R.S.** The psychology of coping: issues of research and assessments. *In:* Coehlo, G.V. et al., ed. *Coping and adaptation.* New York, Basic Books, 1974.

22. **Radloff, L.S.** The CES-D Scale: a self report depression scale for research in the general population. *Applied psychological measurement,* **1**: 385–401 (1977).
23. **Derogatis, L.R. et al.** The Hopkins Symptom Checklist (HSCL): a self report symptom inventory. *Behavioral science,* **19**: 1 15 (1974).
24. **Bradburn, N.** *The structure of psychological well being.* Chicago, Aldine, 1969.
25. **Simmons, R. et al.** *The gift of life.* New York, John Wiley, 1977.
26. **Robins, L.N. et al.** National Institute of Mental Health Diagnostic Interview Schedule: its history, characteristics and validity. *Archives of general psychiatry,* **38**: 381–389 (1981).
27. **Jessor, R. & Jessor, S.** *Problem behavior and psychosocial development: a longitudinal study of youth.* New York, Academic Press, 1977.
28. *National data program for the social sciences. General social surveys, 1972–1978: cumulative codebook.* National Opinion Research Center, University of Chicago, 1978.
29. **Palmore, E. & Luikart, C.** Health and social factors related to life satisfaction. *Journal of health and social behavior,* **13**: 68–80 (1972).
30. **Gurin, G. et al.** *Americans view their mental health.* New York, Basic Books, 1960.
31. **Chrisman, N.J. & Kleinman.** Population health care, social networks and cultural meanings. *In:* Mechanic, D., ed. *Handbook of health, health care and the health profession.* New York, Free Press, 1983.
32. **Donald, C.A. & Ware, J.E.** *The quantification of social contacts and resources.* Santa Monica, Rand Corporation, 1982.

8.3 Participation in health promotion — *J.K. Davies*

In the past people have not been considered active participants in their own health care:

> In most people's minds the health field and the personal medical care system are synonymous. This has been due in large part to the powerful image projected by medicine in its role in the control of infective and parasitic diseases *(1)*.

The 1970s saw a conscious move away from this highly specialized medical care model, culminating in the Alma-Ata Declaration *(2)*, highlighting the duty and right of people individually and collectively to participate in the development of their own health. Underlying an emphasis on primary health care was the clear recognition of the role of the individual's health beliefs, and those of the community, in both the maintenance and promotion of health. This move from a traditional medical model to a more participatory model has been adequately documented elsewhere in this volume.

The relevance of the wider social structure and its influence on the lifestyle, and thereby the health, of the individual has begun to be identified *(3,4)*. Alongside the development of the social concept of health *(5)* in association with these formal developments, a tide of consumerism has emerged, claiming more direct participation by individuals in their own health care. To understand how people participate in health maintenance, comprehensive information is needed on how people think and act in relation to health, including details of their beliefs, attitudes, levels of knowledge and awareness of health matters. It has been suggested that the individual strives to maintain a health balance, an equilibrium achieved by reducing health risks and improving health resources, including health potential. Noack, elsewhere in this volume, refers to the health potential of the community as "the capacity to prevent health imbalance and to maintain or establish health balance". The health resources used by individuals begin with basic resources such as safe water and adequate nutrition and continue through to the complex features of health culture, including health beliefs and the knowledge held by individuals that may determine behaviour, lifestyles and use of services, as well as social network factors such as support and stability. Within these latter features exist more complex concepts such as coping ability, self-care and self-esteem.

The Social Concept of Health

Health is influenced by a variety of external factors based on the complex interactions between the individual and his immediate environment:

> The most important medical advance in the nineteenth century was the discovery that infectious diseases are largely attributable to environmental conditions and

> can often be prevented by control of the influences that lead to them; the most significant advance in the twentieth century is the recognition that the same is true of many non-communicable diseases *(6)*.

The social environment plays a decisive role in individuals' capacity to maintain and promote their health, and to prevent disease *(7)*. These social and structural factors need to be examined in more detail. Badura has extended this model to include the lifestyle variable *(8)*. Of central importance in understanding this extension is the analysis of psychosocial factors within the relationship between the person and the environment. He called psychosocial risks "those environmental conditions which lead to a sudden and serious or longer-lasting overload on the individual's resources, and which consequently cause maladjustment at the physical and/or emotional levels and/or in lifestyle and social behaviour" *(8)*. These psychosocial disease factors have also been highlighted elsewhere *(9)*. Researchers have tended to categorize them in three ways: threatening life events, strain at work and/or home, and major transitions in the lifecycle. In each case the dependent variable has tended to be stress reactions. Research has moved beyond examining the physiological and behavioural factors involved to attempts to identify social and emotional factors. Recently, intervening variables have been highlighted: health beliefs, self-esteem, personality factors, coping ability and social support. All of these variables relate to people's potential ability to control their own lives. Knowledge about these variables and their interrelationship is extremely scarce at present.

The Concept of Lifestyle

In attempting to understand how people manage and resolve their problems, one must look for theoretical models. In the past there has tended to be a polarization between classical epidemiology and traditional sociology; both disciplines attempt to analyse and measure health and health-related behaviour. Recently the field of social epidemiology has offered some help in the development of models to understand how individuals participate in health care, and work in this area has attempted to define the social variables conducive to good health and those that make people more susceptible to illness. The mediating concept of lifestyle has been proposed as a bridge between the individual and his social environment. Reference is then made to healthy and unhealthy lifestyles, but an analysis is needed of why some people are predisposed towards one or the other, what constitutes healthy behaviour, and why some people adopt unhealthy behaviour as a reaction to pressures in their daily lives.

Traditionally people have played little or no part in the management of their own health. This was considered the realm of the doctor or health professional. In this approach little consideration has been given to what participation individuals can have in their own health care. It is now becoming clear that people are adaptable; they can change to accommodate their physical and social environment. They have the ability to cope with daily situations, to maintain some form of psychosocial and physiological equilibrium. People adopt healthy lifestyles by avoiding the risk of breakdown and illness with the help of various health potential variables. They can also be predisposed to unhealthy lifestyles when short-term reactions to stress, such as alcohol and drug abuse, smoking, obesity or risk-taking, become long-term, firmly established patterns of behaviour. To understand the processes that influence or predispose people to healthy or unhealthy lifestyles, the new measures of positive and negative health as proposed by WHO must be adopted *(10)*. To do this, better knowledge of the influence of lifestyles on health is needed, along with examination, definition and attempts to measure the intervening variables involved. This task is complicated further when the WHO concept of health, involving physical, mental and social wellbeing, is used. Therefore more specific tools need to be designed to assess the concept of health held by different social and cultural groups in society. It is necessary to know the extent to which people link daily decisions (about what they eat, whether they exercise, what social relationships they make, for example) with choices that influence their health *(11)*. People adopt specific behavioural patterns and habits in their lives. These are developed within a social and cultural context. These patterns of behaviour can protect and promote health, but unfortunately they often take the opposite direction, with disastrous consequences for the health of the person involved.

To understand and measure how individuals and groups participate in health care, the intervening variables influencing health behaviour must be examined. They must be identified, and then measured empirically before their interaction can be studied. First, the complex concepts that are used to explore the social and psychological processes related to participation in health care should be examined. These concepts can be used to help explain how individuals cope with various forms of both psychological and emotional distress or, on the other hand, how they lead people to adopt dangerous health practices *(12)*. Lifestyles may be positively or negatively related to health: health and disease are the expressions of the relative degree of success or failure experienced by man as he tries to respond adaptively to environmental changes and also to the inner demands created in him by traditions and aspirations *(13)*.

In the practice of traditional medical epidemiology, lifestyle has been used without considering its sociopsychological context. This has usually led to blaming the victim, or saying that unhealthy lifestyles are due to people themselves without any consideration of their living conditions. The ecological paradigm stresses these environmental living conditions and considers the various sociopsychological processes involved. This follows from the health field concept *(1)* that considered health as dependent on such lifestyle and environmental factors. Recently, further emphasis has been given to the need to understand the independent and combined effects of specific behaviour on health and what determines such behaviour *(14)*. People's living conditions can affect the choices they have of various behaviour patterns. Political, social and economic conditions can be determining factors, as well as beliefs, values, attitudes, aspirations and the personality of each individual. The ways people live can be influenced both by external environmental factors and by internal factors that govern the extent to which individuals feel in charge of their own future. The interaction of these factors can produce behaviour patterns that promote or harm health. The interaction of these factors is extremely difficult to conceptualize in a model. Some of these factors must be identified and discussed.

Social Support

The relevance of social support and social support systems has recently been recognized in the study of lifestyles. Evidence has shown that morbidity is not a direct function of stress, but that social support acts as a mediating structure to filter the effects of stress *(15)*. Most of the traditional work in this area has consisted of epidemiological studies on groups of patients or general population samples. These studies have tended to concentrate on examining relationships between social variables and negative health outcomes. In particular, they have explored mental health and its relationship to various factors in the social environment *(16)*.

Other work has extended this field of study to examine where the lack of social support and/or lack of social cohesion has shown in higher incidence rates in tuberculosis *(17)*, hypertension *(18, 19)*, heart disease *(20)*, problems in pregnancy *(21)*, and road accidents *(22)*. Rocella *(23)* has examined social support in relation to health care costs. The Alameda County Study *(24)* showed that for each of four social contact variables, people with strong social ties had lower mortality rates than those without such ties. Good social support and strong social networks are essential to the maintenance and promotion of health *(3)*. There has been a relative neglect of research into the social and environmental conditions that influence health behaviour *(25)*. Recent strategies proposed under the umbrella of health promotion have seen factors in the social support network as their major targets. These factors influence the development of an individual's personality and thereby the decisions a person makes to become, and stay, healthy *(26)*.

Self-care

Lay self-care can range from individual involvement in self-care to large-scale self-help networks. The rapid growth of various health-related mutual aid groups, such as the women's health movement, has shown clearly the abilities and resources that people within the community can use to tackle health issues without professional intervention. Often these actions by the community itself have been related to people's roles as patients or receivers of health services and not to the development of policies to promote health, as in the growth of patient associations in the United Kingdom during the 1970s *(27)*. The Patient Counselling and Patient Organization Project, in Limburg in the Netherlands, has developed training programmes that focus on the improvement of the quality of patients' lives by reducing stress and anxiety and by increasing skills in self-care and relaxation. Numerous self-help groups have appeared, with various and specific structures, aims, functions and methods. These groups are organized and emphasize face-to-face social interactions, with the members assuming personal responsibility *(28,29)*. Self-help groups have tended to flourish where people suffer from chronic illnesses or handicaps by providing mutual support.

In examinations of individuals' abilities and resources for self-care, past research has tended to reveal the wide range of health-related behaviour that people practise as part of their daily lives. This behaviour includes self-treatment, self-care, self-medication and voluntary care. This work has shown that a sense of personal control helps people to cope better with a variety of stressful experiences and affects their commitment to behaviour that promotes health *(30)*. Self-care has the potential of empowering people to assume critical responsibility for the maintenance and promotion of their own health. Its limitation lies in the motivation, knowledge and competence of the individual *(31)*. Self-care has been defined as "unorganized health activities and health-related decision-making by individuals, families, neighbours, friends, colleagues at work ..." *(32)*. Estimates of the proportion of lay care within total health care now vary from 60% to 90% *(15)*. Although the research on self-care has adopted a professional view of illness, Dean *(33)* has reported that self-evaluation of symptoms and lay decisions about self-treatment and/or professional treatment are the main forms of health care in illness. Very few studies have attempted to evaluate the effectiveness of self-treatment, partly owing to methodological problems *(34)*. The validity of the data on factors governing self-care responses to illness is limited because the work was carried out on small samples and often on convenient groups of patients. There is some evidence that the majority of people who suffer from some form of non-acute illness either medicate themselves or wait for symptoms to subside; they approach professional medical help only when the problem persists or becomes more acute *(35–39)*. Therefore people are continually engaged in health care through individual decisions and expressed demands. The provision of social support may help people to cope better and more appropriately with these decisions.

Health Awareness

There is a dearth of knowledge about the concepts of health held by different groups of people. This also applies to the degree of awareness among the population about the relationship between their lifestyles and their health. For example, to what extent do people believe that the daily decisions they make influence their health? Some work has been carried out on the public's awareness of the causes of disease *(40)*, and on its health beliefs and attitudes *(41–45)*. Unfortunately these studies have tended to be small-scale and ad hoc; they do not allow large-scale trend analysis over time. Nevertheless, recent work reported shows that the public has an awareness about health that may be different from that of the medical profession. Therefore their assessment of the influences on health may be different *(46)*.

Health Beliefs and Health Behaviour

The Knowledge, Attitudes, Practice Model was used for many years as the underlying paradigm for health education intervention programmes. This rational model assumed that once people had knowledge, they would change their attitudes and then their behaviour. In reality the health choices of individuals were influenced by various social, economic and environmental factors, and by a complex system of beliefs and values. These latter components proved difficult to measure accurately. In the early 1970s Maiman & Becker *(47)* argued that behaviour was the result of a process of sociopsychological balance involving the individual's perception of the seriousness of the health problems and his own susceptibility to it. When these two factors are operating and the perceived disadvantages of recommended action are outweighed by the benefits, change will occur. Built into the model was the assumption that some trigger to action is required for the change. This latter assumption made the model extremely difficult to operate in practice.

Wallston & Wallston *(48)* reviewed evidence that showed that individuals who typically believe that their good or ill health is the result of their own doing (health internals) are more likely to seek information about health and engage in preventive health behaviour than people who feel that their health status depends on chance (health externals). The Internal Locus of Control Scale was developed by Wallston et al. *(49)*. This measure was found to be associated with weight control, family planning, preventive dental behaviour and use of seat belts in cars *(48)*. More recently, Dean *(50)* has confirmed that, in relation to smoking and preventive health behaviour, the belief variable with the greatest explanatory power was the internal locus of control measure. She also compared direct risk behaviour with both health beliefs and social network variables. She found that both variables were related to preventive health behaviour. Other studies have found that the locus of control measure is related to perceived vulnerability and self-esteem *(51–55)*.

Langlie *(54)*, when studying preventive health behaviour, found that health behaviour had two dimensions: direct risk behaviour (personal hygiene, driving) and indirect risk behaviour (exercise, nutrition, use of seat belts), the latter being related to social network variables and health beliefs. Therefore, these underlying factors may be crucial to understanding how people make decisions about health behaviour.

Coping Abilities

Factors such as health beliefs and social support networks may be crucial to understanding how people make decisions about health behaviour. People use different methods to resolve or handle various life problems. If people are in stressful situations, they may practise habits related to negative health outcomes. Relevant work has been carried out on smoking behaviour *(56)*. People's decisions and patterns of coping affect their psychological, physical and social wellbeing *(57)*.

Attempts have been made to analyse the dimensions of effective coping. Pearling & Schooler *(58)* have subdivided coping into social resources, psychological resources, and specific coping responses. Social resources consist of the social networks within which people function and from which they receive or do not receive support. Factors involved with social networks are their size, function, and the support they give, as well as the obligations and costs involved. Psychological resources consist of various personality characteristics that may help people solve problems and withstand threats, although they may reduce stress or increase it. Specific coping responses are behaviour, cognitions and perceptions used in actual problems. Folkman & Lazarus have defined coping as "the cognitive and behavioural efforts made to master, tolerate or reduce external and internal demands and conflicts" *(57)*. Coping has two main functions: the management of the relationship between the person and the environment that is the source of stress (problem-focused coping) and the regulation of stressful emotions (emotion-focused coping). Further studies are needed to determine the effect of early learning and patterns of coping on lifestyles.

The psychological resources dimension has been subdivided into the study of defensive or ego processes *(59–61)* and the study of behaviour traits *(62)*. In methodological terms, however, it has proved extremely difficult to obtain reliable measures of ego processes, and personality traits have not been good predictors of coping *(57)*. The category of specific coping responses has produced research that has been related to situations *(63–65)*. There is no cumulative research on how people with common sociopsychological characteristics respond to the problems of daily living. Nevertheless, most people develop some form of coping skills to reduce the incidence of disease, either by avoiding the direct effects of stress on the body *(66,67)* or by preventing or limiting the use of health-damaging behaviour when attempting to reduce feelings of stress *(58)*. Pearlin & Schooler showed that the most influential of the psychosocial variables on effective coping was the feeling that one is in control of the circumstances of one's life and has a high level of self-esteem. Badura *(8)* defined stress reactions as the dependent variable, and referred to the intervening variables of social resources, psychological resources and specific coping responses as the psychosocial immunity system. He concluded that more information is needed about these intervening variables for a full understanding of how some people cope with stress better than others.

Future Research Needs

Most studies of health behaviour and participation have examined how people maintain their health within a framework of medically approved services (consultation rates, immunization rates, check-ups and engaging in medically approved practices). Harris & Guten have proposed a more positive definition of health behaviour: "... any behaviour performed by a person, regardless of his or her perceived health status, in order to protect, promote or maintain his or her health, whether or not such behaviour is objectively effective towards that end" *(68)*.

Patterns of living have a profound effect on health, but research on how these patterns of living are defined, and how they influence health, is urgently required. It has been suggested that more surveys are needed to measure the extent of health problems in various social groups and categories of the population, along with comparative studies of those most at risk *(69)*. It has also been proposed that cheap and simple community surveys need to be developed *(70)*. These could involve local people themselves identifying problems, developing priorities and making recommendations for action. This process lies at the heart of the WHO strategy for health for all: "... any significant improvement in the physical, mental and social wellbeing to a large extent will depend on the individuals' and the communities' will to fend for themselves ..." *(71)*.

Encouragement should be given to the development of appropriate health indicators that concern personal lifestyles, and their determinants, to provide baseline measures to produce and evaluate strategies for the promotion of health. The WHO Regional Committee for Europe, when discussing this issue, "... acknowledge the complexity of the issue and of the difficulty of defining the concept of healthy lifestyles" *(72)*. All available resources should be devoted to help create a clearer understanding of the underlying factors influencing health-related behaviour *(73)*.

References

1. **Lalonde, M.** *New perspecitves on the health of Canadians.* Ottawa, Government of Canada, 1974, p. 11.
2. The Alma-Ata Conference on Primary Health Care. *WHO Chronicle,* **32**: 409–430 (1978).
3. *Intervention studies related to lifestyles conducive to health:* report on a WHO Workshop. Copenhagen, WHO Regional Office for Europe, 1983.
4. **Robertson, J.** *Scenarios for lifestyles and health.* Edinburgh, Scottish Health Education Group, 1984 (European Monographs in Health Education Research, No. 6).
5. **Kickbusch, I.** Involvement in health: a social concept of health education. *International journal of health education,* **24**(Suppl. 4): 1–15 (1981).
6. **McKeown, T.** *Research strategy: the role of WHO.* Geneva, World Health Organization, 1984.
7. **Dean, K.** Self-care: what people do for themselves. *In:* Hatch, S. & Kickbusch, I., ed. *Self-help and health in Europe. New approaches in health care.* Copenhagen, WHO Regional Office for Europe, 1983.
8. **Badura, B.** *Social epidemiology in theory and practice.* Edinburgh, Scottish Health Education Group, 1983 (European Monographs in Health Education Research, No. 5), pp. 27–50.
9. **Levi, L.** Psychosocial factors in preventive medicine. *In: Healthy people.* Washington, DC, US Government Printing Office, 1979.

10. *Global strategy for health for all by the year 2000.* Geneva, World Health Organization, 1981 ("Health for All" Series, No. 3).
11. *WHO regional programme in health education and lifestyles.* Copenhagen, WHO Regional Office for Europe, 1981 (unpublished document EUR/RC31/10).
12. **Badura, B.** *Lifestyles and health. The socio-ecological perspective.* Paper presented for Jornadas Internacionales sobre Estilos de Vida e Investigacion Social, Bilbao, 1984.
13. **Dubos, R.** *Man, medicine and environment.* London, Pall Mall, 1968.
14. *Targets for health for all.* Copenhagen, WHO Regional Office for Europe, 1985.
15. **Levin, L.S. & Idler, E.** *The hidden health care system: mediating structures and medicine.* Cambridge, MA, Ballinger, 1981.
16. **Andrews, G. et al.** Life event stress, social support, coping style, and risk of psychological impairment. *Journal of nervous and mental disease,* **166**: 307–316 (1978).
17. **Holmes, T.** Multidiscipline studies of tuberculosis. *In:* Sparer, P., ed. *Personality, stress and tuberculosis.* New York, International Universities Press, 1956.
18. **Harburg, E. et al.** Socioeconomic stressor areas and black-white blood pressure. *Detroit journal of chronic disease,* **26**: 595–611 (1973).
19. **Henry, J. & Cassel, J.** Psycho-social factors in essential hypertension: recent epidemiological and animal experimental evidence. *American journal of epidemiology,* **90**: 171 (1969).
20. **Syme, S. et al.** Some social and cultural factors associated with the occurrence of coronary heart disease. *Journal of chronic diseases,* **17**: 227 (1964).
21. **Nuckolls, K. et al.** Psychosocial assets, life crises and the prognosis of pregnancy. *American journal of epidemiology,* **95**: 431–441 (1972).
22. **Tillman, W. & Hobbs, G.** The accident-prone automobile driver: a study of the psychiatric and social background. *American journal of psychiatry,* **106**: 321 (1949).
23. **Rocella, E.** Potential for reducing health care costs by public and patient education. *Public health reports,* **9**(3): 223–225 (1976).
24. **Berkman, L. & Syme, S.** Social networks, host resistance and mortality: a nine-year follow-up study of Alameda County residents. *American journal of epidemiology,* **109**: 186–204 (1979).
25. **Berkman, L.F.** *The social context of health behaviours.* Copenhagen, WHO Regional Office for Europe, 1982.
26. **Deliege-Rott, D.** *Indicators of physical, mental and social wellbeing.* Geneva, World Health Organization, 1982.
27. **Fisher, B.H. & Cochran, M.** Peckham health project: raising health consciousness. *British medical journal,* **284**: 1843–1845 (1982).
28. **Richardson, A. & Goodman, M.** *Self-help and social care: mutual aid organizations in practice.* London, Policy Studies Institute, 1983.
29. **Katz, A.H. & Bender, E.** *The strength in US: self-help groups in the modern world.* New York, Franklin-Watts, 1976.

30. **Hamburg, D.A. et al., ed.** *Health and behaviour. Frontiers of research in the bio-behavioural sciences.* Washington, DC, Division of Mental Health and Behavioural Medicine, Institute of Medicine, 1982.
31. **Levin, L.S. et al.** *Self-care.* London, Croom Helm, 1977.
32. **Kickbusch, I. & Hatch, S.** A reorientation of health care? *In:* Hatch, S. & Kickbusch, I., ed. *Self-help and health in Europe.* Copenhagen, WHO Regional Office for Europe, 1983.
33. **Dean, K.** Self-care response to illness: a selected review. *Social science and medicine,* **15a**: 673 (1981).
34. **Anderson, J. et al.** Users and non-users of doctors: implications for self-care. *Journal of the Royal College of General Practitioners,* **27**: 155–159 (1977).
35. **Greve, J.** *Consumer participation and responsibility in the planning and delivering of health care.* Copenhagen, WHO Regional Office for Europe, 1980.
36. **Dunnell, K. & Cartwright, A.** *Medicine takers, prescribers and hoarders.* London, Routledge & Kegan Paul, 1972.
37. **Fry, J.** 21 years of general practice: changing patterns. *Journal of the Royal College of General Practitioners,* **22**: 521–528 (1972).
38. **Levin, L.S. et al.** *Self-care: lay initiatives in health.* New York, Prodist, 1976.
39. **Pratt, L.** The significance of the family in medication. *Journal of comparative family studies,* **4**(1) (1973).
40. **Davison, L.E.** An analysis of knowledge, beliefs and behaviour relating to the development of coronary heart disease. *Health education journal,* **39**(4): 103–109 (1980).
41. **Stott, N.C.H. & Pill, R.** *Health beliefs in an urban community.* Cardiff, Department of General Practice, Welsh National School of Medicine, 1980.
42. **Pill, R. & Stott, N.C.H.** Concepts of illness causation and responsibility: some preliminary data from a sample of working-class mothers. *Social science and medicine,* **16**(1): 43–52 (1982).
43. **Lockyer, D.** *Symptoms and illness: the cognitive organization of disorder.* London, Tavistock, 1981.
44. **Blaxter, M. & Patterson, E.** *Mothers and daughters: a three-generational study of health attitudes and behaviour.* Studies in deprivation and disadvantages. London, Heineman, 1982.
45. **Cunningham-Burley, S.** *Mothers' perceptions of their children's illnesses: changes in behaviour as problematic concerns.* Paper presented to the BSA Medical Sociology Conference, Sheffield, 1984.
46. **Anderson, R.** How have people changed their health behaviour? *Health education journal,* **42**(3) (1983).
47. **Maiman, L.A. & Becker, M.H.** The health belief model: origins and correlates in psychosocial theory. *Health education monographs,* **2**(4) (1974).
48. **Wallston, B. & Wallston, K.** Locus of control and health: a review of the literature. *Health education monographs,* **6**: 107 (1978).

49. **Wallston, K. et al.** Development of the multidimensional health locus of control (MHLC) scales. *Health education monographs,* **6**: 160–170 (1978).
50. **Dean, K.** *Influence of health beliefs on lifestyle: what do we know?* Edinburgh, Scottish Health Education Group, 1984 (European Monographs in Health Education Research, No. 6).
51. **Gochman, D.** Children's perceptions of vulnerability to illness and accidents. *Public health reports,* **85**: 69–73 (1970).
52. **Gochman, D.** The organizing role of motivation in health beliefs and intentions. *Journal of health and social behaviour,* **13**: 285–293 (1972).
53. **Hallal, J.** The relationship of health beliefs, health locus of control and self-concept to the practice of breast self-examination in adult women. *Nursing research,* **31**: 137–142 (1982).
54. **Langlie, J.** Social networks, health beliefs and preventive health behaviour. *Journal of health and social behaviour,* **18**: 244–260 (1977).
55. **Mechanic, D. & Cleary, P.** Factors associated with the maintenance of positive health. *Preventive medicine,* **9**: 805 (1980).
56. **Tompkins, S.** Psychosocial models for smoking behaviour. *American journal of public health,* **56**(Suppl.): 17–20 (1966).
57. **Folkman, S. & Lazarus, R.** An analysis of coping in a middle-aged community sample. *Journal of health and social behaviour,* **21**: 219–239 (1980).
58. **Pearlin, L. & Schooler, C.** The structure of coping. *Journal of health and social behaviour,* **19**: 2–21 (1978).
59. **Haan, N., ed.** *Coping and defending.* New York, Academic Press, 1977.
60. **Vaillant, G.** Theoretical hierarchy of adaptive ego mechanisms. *Archives of general psychiatry,* **24**: 107–118 (1971).
61. **Morrisey, R.** The Haarn model of ego-functioning: an assessment of empirical research. *In:* Haan, N., ed. *Coping and defending.* New York, Academic Press, 1977.
62. **Lazarus, R. et al.** The psychology of coping: issues of research and assessment. *In:* Coelho, G. et al., ed. *Coping and adaptation.* New York, Basic Books, 1974.
63. **Lucas, R.** *Men in crisis.* New York, Basic Books, 1969.
64. **Moos, R. & Tsu, V.** The crisis of physical illness: an overview. *In:* Moos, R., ed. *Coping with physical illness.* New York, Plenum, 1977.
65. **Parkes, C.** *Bereavement: studies of grief in adult life.* New York, International Universities Press, 1972.
66. **Cassel, J.** The contribution of the social environment to host resistance. *American journal of epidemiology,* **104**: 107–123 (1976).
67. **Dohrenwerd, B.S. & Doh, B.P., ed.** *Stressful life events: their nature and effects.* New York, John Wiley, 1976.
68. **Harris, D.M. & Guten, S.** Health protective behaviour: an exploratory study. *Journal of health and social behaviour,* **20**: 1, 17–29 (1979).
69. **Council of Europe.** *A European approach to health promotion* (two reports: Prevention and Education of health). Strasbourg, Conference of European Ministers responsible for Public Health, 1981.

70. **Catford, J.C.** Positive health indicators — towards a new information base for health promotion. *Community medicine*, **5**: 125–132 (1983).
71. **Mahler, H.** Problems of medical affluence. *WHO Chronicle*, **31**: 8–13 (1977).
72. *Lifestyles and their impact on health.* Copenhagen, WHO Regional Office for Europe, 1983 (unpublished document EUR/RC33/Tech. Disc./1).
73. **Pissarro, B.** *Notes on the document entitled targets in support of the regional strategy for health for all by the year 2000.* Copenhagen, WHO Regional Office for Europe (European Advisory Committee for Medical Research), 1984 (unpublished document ICP/RPD 103/m01/7).

8.4 Environmental protection — *Z.J. Brzeziński*

The term environment may denote many different things. In a broad sense it means "the totality of influences which infringe on man and affect his well-being" *(1)* and therefore embraces the physical environment (atmosphere, water, soil), the biological environment and the human and social environment (distribution, density and mobility of population, housing and human settlement, agricultural practices, industrial processes and hazards, diet, pollution, cultural traits).

The volume of knowledge on the relationships between health and environmental factors is impressive *(2)*. However, in spite of much evidence that environmental influences affect human health, there are still gaps and uncertainties concerning either the nature of the effect of many environmental aspects or the mechanisms involved in causation of health damage. In particular, there is a need for research and monitoring systems aimed at faster and more precise identification of environmental health hazards and at evaluation of the effects on human populations of agents whose potential harmful influence is suspected on the basis of information derived from other sources such as laboratory experiments.

Environment and Health

Environmental influences on human health can be classified in various ways. Some are due to factors that occur in nature independent of human activities. Although people can modify the effects of many of them, they have accompanied the existence of the human race for centuries and do not threaten its survival. More important are factors resulting from human life, production and consumption. These may be physical, chemical, biological or social, although only the first three categories are of concern here. Environmental factors may be viewed in regard to the medium through which they affect man (air, water, food, soil) or according to the kind of environment in which they occur (occupational or home environment, urban or rural). Health effects resulting from environmental influences depend on the properties of the agents involved. With environmental pollutants, depending on their toxicity, concentration and the duration of exposure, the effects may be acute or chronic (Fig. 1). From the public health point of view, the size and distribution of the exposed population groups is also important.

Environmental Protection

Human existence and activities have always led to changes in the environment. Population growth, and production and consumption have a particularly profound impact on the depletion of resources and the level of air,

Fig. 1. The interrelationships between man and his environment showing adverse effects on man's health by pollutants

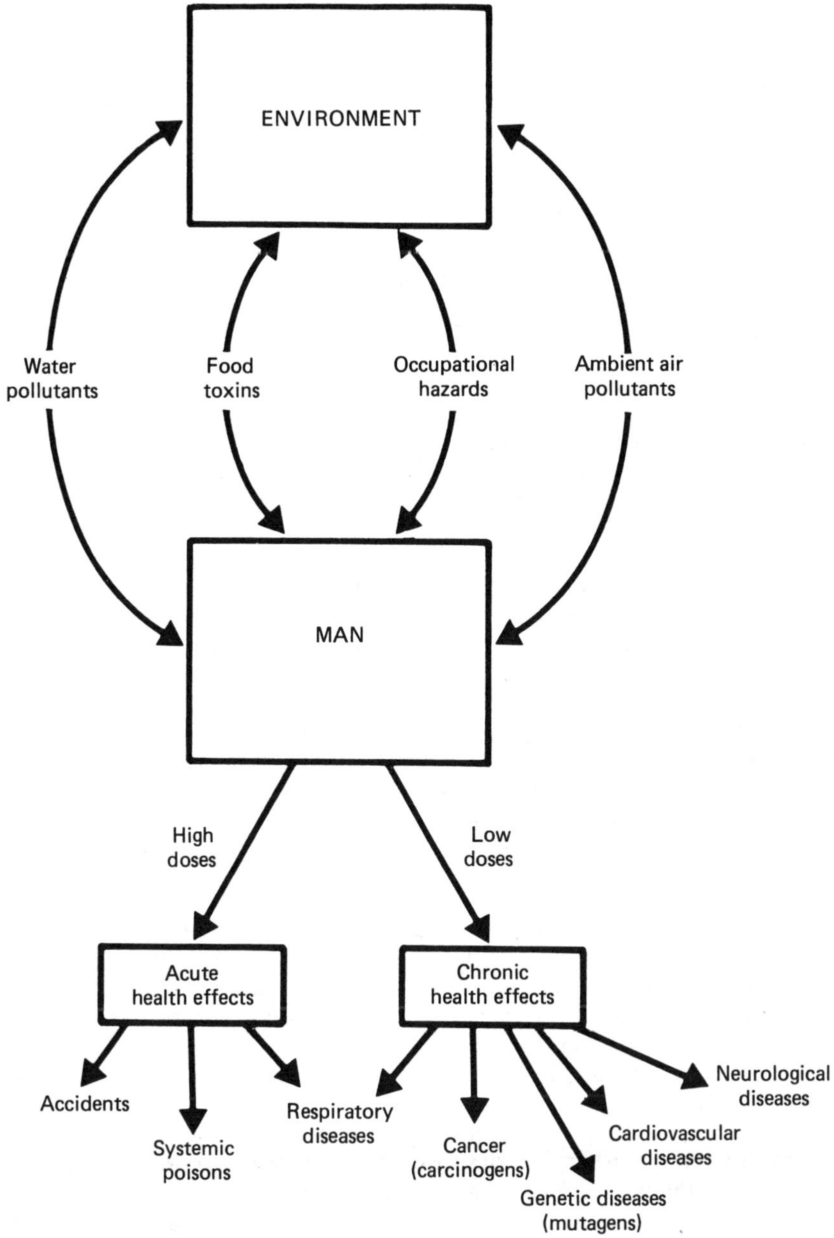

Source: Adapted from **Trieff, N.M.** *(3).*

water and soil pollution. Many who look into the future have come to rather pessimistic conclusions *(4)*, predicting a collapse sometime in the next century. Therefore, if the human race is to alter its course towards disaster, action should be taken without delay. Although it should be comprehensive and involve all the sectors of community life, environmental protection should get very high priority.

Intervention strategies for the prevention and control of environmental health hazards should be based on a thorough examination of the problem, which should involve risk assessment and the formulation of relevant programmes for risk management.

Risk Assessment

Risk assessment is an appraisal of both the kind and degree of threat posed by an environmental hazard *(5)*. It includes three elements: hazard identification, risk estimation and social evaluation (Fig. 2).

Hazard identification. Information on potential health hazards comes from various sources: toxicological research, epidemiological studies and observations of pathological changes in animals or plants. Frequently, such information requires further clarification through research, monitoring or screening. Today many of the main recognized health hazards are related to industrial and occupational exposure and present a risk to a rather limited proportion of the population. Apart from industrial and occupational exposure, pollutants in the air, water, soil and food, although not evenly distributed, pose a threat to much larger population groups (Table 1). The most important pollutants are recommended for monitoring in the Global Environmental Monitoring System (Table 2).

The International Agency for Research on Cancer carries out systematic evaluations of potential carcinogens. In addition to established human carcinogenic agents and circumstances (Table 3), it listed over 60 chemicals, groups of chemicals or industrial processes that are probably carcinogenic to humans *(7)*. Since the level and distribution of known hazards are changing, and new potential hazards will continue to appear, their identification should be a continuing process.

Risk estimation. Risk estimation is a measure of the health outcome of the influence of the environmental hazard. It provides information on the magnitude or kind of health damage, and its frequency of occurrence. In statistical terms risk can be expressed in several ways, such as a probability that an event will occur in a specified period of time. The event could be the appearance of a symptom, or the occurrence of an illness or death *(8)*. In this case it derives from morbidity or mortality rates.

Relative risk, frequently used in environmental health research, is the ratio between the risk or rate of disease or death among those exposed to a hazard and the risk among the unexposed population.

Other ways of expressing the risk are the use of life tables and the calculation of life expectancy lost due to the presence of the risk factor or of life expectancy added if the risk factor is removed (Tables 4 and 5).

Fig. 2. Risk assessment elements

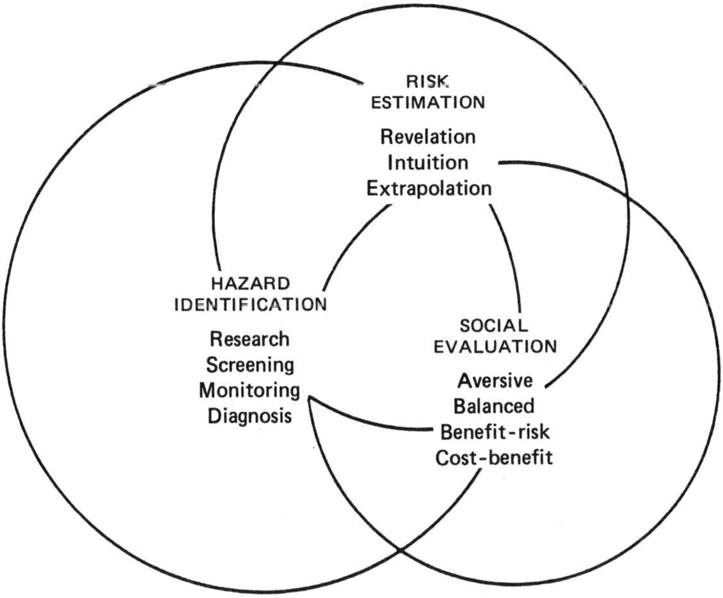

Source: **Kates, R.W.** *(5).*

Social evaluation. Social evaluation adds a new dimension to risk assessment and is probably the most difficult to measure. It comprises such aspects as priority given to health, as compared with other social values recognized by a given society such as its culture and tradition, beliefs and habits. It should take into account both the aspirations and needs of the community and its resources and capabilities.

Finally, it should weigh various risk categories, and compare the benefits of risk reduction with its costs to society *(9)*.

The ultimate outcome of social evaluation is the will and commitment to change. However, as history shows, in this struggle health is not necessarily the victor.

Risk Management

Risk management is, as are many other environmental issues, a complex problem. Generally it may aim at the elimination or reduction of risk to an acceptable level, at protection from exposure, or at improving the defensive mechanisms of the human organism. The selection of a strategy will depend on its feasibility and acceptability and on the costs involved.

In theory, certain actions are simple and do not cause excessive costs. Using seat belts markedly reduces the risk of serious injury or death in road

Table 1. Principal environmental health hazards

General category	Specific examples
Air pollutants	Particulate or dust, sulfur dioxide (SO_2), ozone (O_3), hydrocarbons, carbon monoxide (CO), nitrogen oxides (NO_x), hydrogen sulfide (H_2S), mercaptans (RSH) and sulfides, carcinogens and heavy metals
Water pollutants	Pathogenic bacteria, viruses, amoeba and other protozoa; mercury and other heavy metals; organic compounds (oxygen depleting); toxic substances — nitrite (NO_2^-), cyanide (CN^-); excess nutrients such as phosphate (PO_4^{-3}) and nitrate (NO_3^-), which cause algal blooms (eutrophication)
Industrial and occupational pollutants	*Physical:* noise, thermal, cold, radiation *Carcinogens:* absestos, **β**-naphthylamine, soot, radium, radon, nitrosamines, benzo-[α]-pyrene *Dusts:* silica, cotton, sugar cane, coal dust *Metals:* beryllium (Be), lead (Pb), cadmium (Cd); mercury (Hg); arsenic (As), nickel (Ni), manganese (Mn), copper (Cu), etc. *Gases:* halogens (chlorine (Cl_2), bromine (Br_2) and fluorine (F_2)), halogen acids (hydrogen fluoride (HF), hydrogen chloride (HCl), hydrogen bromide (HBr)), sulfur oxides (SO_x), nitrogen oxides (NO_x), ozone (O_3) *Organic toxins and solvents:* carbon tetrachloride (CCl_4), benzene (C_6H_6) and other organic solvents *Neurotoxins:* parathion and other organophosphate insecticides
Ecopoisons	Mercury, DDT, PCBs[a] and other chlorinated hydrocarbons, petroleum (in water)
Food toxins	Produced by *Clostridium botulinum, Salmonella* and *Staphylococcus*
Solid wastes	Organics, nonmetabolizable toxic substances and heavy metals

[a] Polychlorinated biphenyls.

Source: **Trieff, N.M.** *(3).*

accidents. The cessation of smoking would prevent some 30% of cancer deaths. Nevertheless, some people do not wear seat belts and far too many smoke.

Most risks are less vulnerable to intervention, especially those posed by environmental pollutants. However, in most instances appropriate technologies to manage these risks already exist and their implementation is only a question of the availability of the necessary resources.

Table 2. Substances and environmental stress indicators potentially important to their direct and indirect effects on man and the biosphere

1. Airborne sulfur dioxide and sulfates (a)
2. Suspended particulate matter (b)
3. Carbon monoxide (a)
4. Carbon dioxide and other trace gases that affect the radiative properties of the atmosphere (c)
5. Airborne oxides of nitrogen (a)
6. Ozone, photochemical oxidants and reactive hydrocarbons (a)
7. Polycyclic aromatic hydrocarbons (n)
8. Toxic metals, especially mercury, lead and cadmium (d)
9. Halogenated organic compounds, especially DDT and its metabolites, PCBs, PCT, Dieldrin and short-chained halogenated aliphatic compounds (d)
10. Asbestos (n)
11. Petroleum hydrocarbons (n)
12. Toxins of biological origin (from algae, fungi and bacteria) (n)
13. Nitrates, nitrites and nitrosamines (f)
14. Ammonia (m)
15. Selected indicators of water quality: biological oxygen demand (BOD), dissolved oxygen (DO), pH, coliform bacteria (e)
16. Selected radionuclides (g)
17. Airborne allergens (n)
18. Eutrophicators (e.g. nitrates and phosphates) (i)
19. Soluble salts of the alkali metals and alkaline earth metals (h)
20. Other substances that have caused significant local environmental problems in the past, such as arsenic, boron, elemental phosphorus, selenium and fluoride (j)
21. Noise (k)
22. Waste heat (l)

Substances and environmental stress indicators recommended for monitoring in Phase I of the Global Environmental Monitoring System (GEMS)

(a) Air	(d) Man, soil, food, biota, water	(g) All media
(b) Air, water	(e) Water	
(c) Air, oceans	(f) Water, food, soil	

Substances that should be monitored locally or regionally wherever there are specific problems

(h) Groundwater, soil	(j) Air, soil, water, food	(l) Air, water
(i) Water, soil	(k) Air	(m) Soil

Substances not recommended for GEMS Phase I (mainly because the feasibility of systematic monitoring has not yet been demonstrated) (n)

Source: **Wöhlers, H.C.** *(4).*

Table 3. Established human carcinogenic agents and circumstances[a,b]

Agent or circumstance	Exposure[c]			Site of cancer
	Occupational	Medical	Social	
Aflatoxin			+	Liver
Alcoholic drinks			+	Mouth, pharynx, larynx, oesophagus, liver
Alkylating agents:				
Cyclophosphamide		+		Bladder
Melphalan		+		Marrow
Aromatic amines:				
4-Aminodiphenyl	+			Bladder
Benzidine	+			Bladder
2-Naphthylamine	+			Bladder
Arsenic[d]	+	+		Skin, lung
Asbestos	+			Lung, pleura, peritoneum
Benzene	+			Marrow
Bis(chloromethyl) ether	+			Lung
Busulphan		+		Marrow
Cadmium[d]	+			Prostate
Chewing (betel, tobacco, lime)			+	Mouth
Chromium[d]	+			Lung
Chlornaphazine		+		Bladder
Furniture manufacture (hardwood)	+			Nasal sinuses
Immunosuppressive drugs		+		Reticuloendothelial system
Ionizing radiations[e]	+	+		Marrow and probably all other sites
Isopropyl alcohol manufacture	+			Nasal sinuses
Leather goods manufacture	+			Nasal sinuses
Mustard gas	+			Larynx, lung

Nickel[d]	+			Nasal sinuses, lung
Estrogens:				
Unopposed		+		Endometrium
Transplacental (DES)		+		Vagina
Overnutrition (causing obesity)			+	Endometrium, gallbladder
Phenacetin		+		Kidney (pelvis)
Polycyclic hydrocarbons	+	+		Skin, scrotum, lung
Reproductive history:				
Late age at first pregnancy			+	Breast
Zero or low parity			+	Ovary
Parasites:				
Schistosoma haematobium			+	Bladder
Chlonorchis sinensis			+	Liver (cholangioma)
Sexual promiscuity			+	Cervix uteri
Steroids:				
Anabolic (oxymetholone)		+		Liver
Contraceptives		+		Liver (hamartoma)
Tobacco smoking			+	Mouth, pharynx, larynx, lung, oesophagus, bladder
Ultraviolet light	+		+	Skin, lip
Vinyl chloride	+			Liver (angiosarcoma)
Virus (hepatitis B)			+	Liver (hepatoma)

[a] Expanded from IARC working group, 1980.

[b] By restricting this table to firmly established causes, some of the more important determinants of human cancer have undoubtedly been omitted. (A few borderline cases might not command uniform agreement; e.g. on balance cadmium has just been included and beryllium has just been excluded.)

[c] A plus sign indicates that evidence of carcinogenicity was obtained.

[d] Certain compounds or oxidation states only.

[e] For example, from X-rays, thorium, thorotrast, some underground mining, and other occupations.

Note. Occupational exposure to phenoxyacid/chlorophenal herbicides (or their impurities) is a reasonably well established cause of soft tissue sarcomas or perhaps lymphomas.

Source: **Doll, R. & Peto, R.** *(6).*

Table 4. Years of life expectancy lost due to various smoking patterns

Type of smoking	Men	Women
Cigarettes — average	6.2	2.2
1-9/day	4.5	0.2
10-19/day	6.2	1.7
20-39/day	6.8	3.5
over 40/day	8.6	
inhalation — none	4.5	0.6
slight	6.4	1.9
moderate	7.2	2.5
deep	8.6	4.6
began after 30	2.0	1.1
25-29	4.5	1.9
20-24	5.7	2.7
15-19	7.7	2.7
before 15	8.6	
had smoked > 20/day		
still smoking	7.6	
stopped 1-4 years	6.9	
stopped 5-9 years	3.9	
stopped 10+ years	2.3	
had smoked 1-19/day		
still smoking	5.9	
stopped 1-4 years	3.8	
stopped 5-9 years	3.8	
stopped 10+ years	0.3	
Cigars only — average	0.9	
1-4/day	0.1	
5+/day	1.2	
no inhalation	0	
inhalation	3.2	
Pipe only — average	0.6	
no inhalation	0	
inhalation	1.4	

Source: **Cohen, B.L. & Lee, Y-Sing** *(8)*.

Table 5. Days of life expectancy added by various actions

Action	Added life expectancy (days)
Using seat belts	50
Installing air bags in car	50
Buying larger cars[a]	50
Smoke alarm in home	10
Training family in resuscitation	≧100
Annual PAP test	4

[a] Standard rather than sub-compacts, or large rather than standard.

Source: **Cohen, B.L. & Lee, Y-Sing** *(8).*

Measurement of Environmental Pollution

Almost any aspect of the environment can be measured, but available measures vary in precision, specificity and applicability. The selection of the appropriate measurement depends on the kind of information needed and for what purpose it will be used.

Overall waste load. Waste can be measured in weight units, usually tons. It may also indicate the main contributors to waste production (Table 6). This measure can be used for monitoring overall time trends in a country or in a given locality. If used for comparisons, it should be expressed per unit of surface area (km^2) or per unit of population.

Emissions. Emissions are measured in units of weight of the pollutants and can be disaggregated by source and by the media into which they are emitted, such as air or water. These measures are useful indicators of the overall time trends (Fig. 3). Again, for comparison, emissions can be expressed per unit of surface area or per unit of population.

Level of pollution. The level of pollution is measured by its concentration in a given medium and is expressed by unit of weight of a pollutant per unit of volume of the medium, such as the cubic metre, the litre or the millilitre, or by unit of weight of a pollutant per unit of weight of the medium. This measurement is widely used in monitoring environmental pollution (Fig. 4), and for setting standards and norms for pollution of air, water and soil, or permissible levels of various substances in food.

Table 6. Waste by category, Netherlands

Category	Year	Tons (in thousands)
Municipal waste	1979	7400
Industrial waste	1977	2400
Building and demolishing waste	1977	6100
Agricultural waste (postassium surpluses excluded)	1980	1000
Sludge from sewage purification plants	1979	5200
Chemical waste (used oil included)	1980	1100
Ash and slags from municipal incinerators and coal-fired power plants	1980	1040
Dismissed tyres	1980	39
Waste from hospitals	1977	85
Dilapidated cars (motor-trucks included)	1980	530

Source: **Central Bureau of Statistics.** *Vademecum Gezondheidsstatistiek 1983* [Vademecum of health statistics 1983]. The Hague, Staatsuitgeverij, 1983.

Temporal variation. The level of concentration of pollutants changes over time. Fluctuations can be measured daily, weekly, monthly or at other intervals, depending on the monitoring design. Accordingly, the measurements would then be presented as appropriate averages, such as monthly averages (Fig. 5). Variations over time are of particular importance to health since exceedingly high concentrations of pollutants can produce dramatic health consequences in relatively short periods of time, as has been shown by several instances of high air pollution, such as London smog. In relation to some environmental agents, such as noise, the peak intensity may also be of relevance to health. Similarly, one may count the number of instances in which the concentration of the pollutant exceeds a defined level.

Spatial variation. Many pollutants are emitted from more or less defined locations and spread to surrounding areas. Depending on the local climatic conditions and other factors such as the location of the emittor in relation to ground level, the concentration of the pollutant will show spatial variation. An appropriate network of measurement points will allow appraisal of the variation in levels of pollution. Series of such measurements can be used for drawing maps showing spatial distribution of the pollution over an area covered by the measurement network.

Other measurements of the quality of the environment. Numerous other measurements are used for the appraisal of the quality of the environment, including: ordinal scales for the quality of surface water, the surface area of green areas in cities, the length of roads with different kinds of surface,

Fig. 3. Air pollution in the United Kingdom, by source

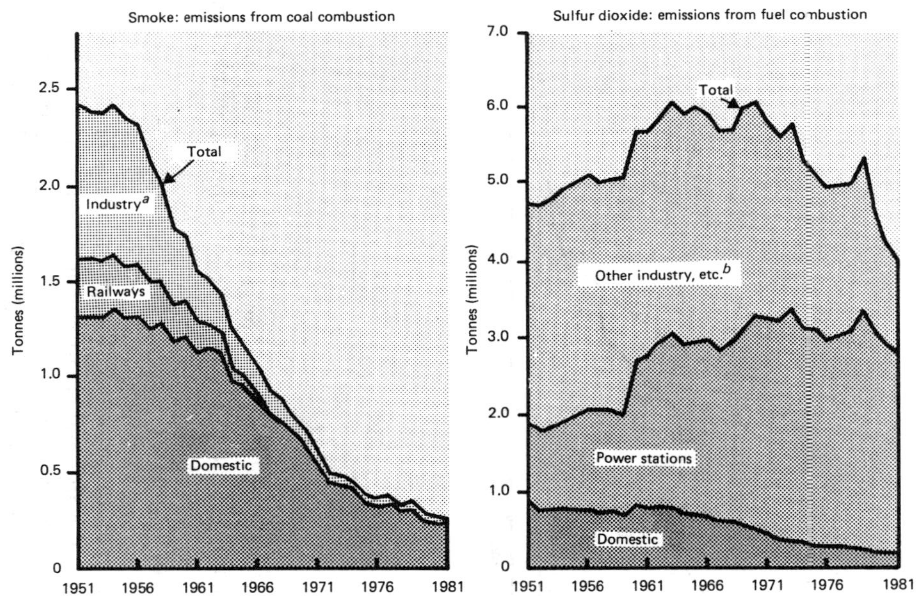

[a] Includes commercial/public services, agriculture, and miscellaneous. Excludes fuel conversion industries (e.g. power stations) where smoke emissions are relatively low.

[b] Includes commercial/public services, agriculture, and road and rail transport.

Source: **Central Statistical Office.** *Social trends 14.* London, H.M. Stationery Office, 1984.

Fig. 4. Time trend in the level of smoke and sulfur dioxide (SO_2) in Middlesborough, United Kingdom

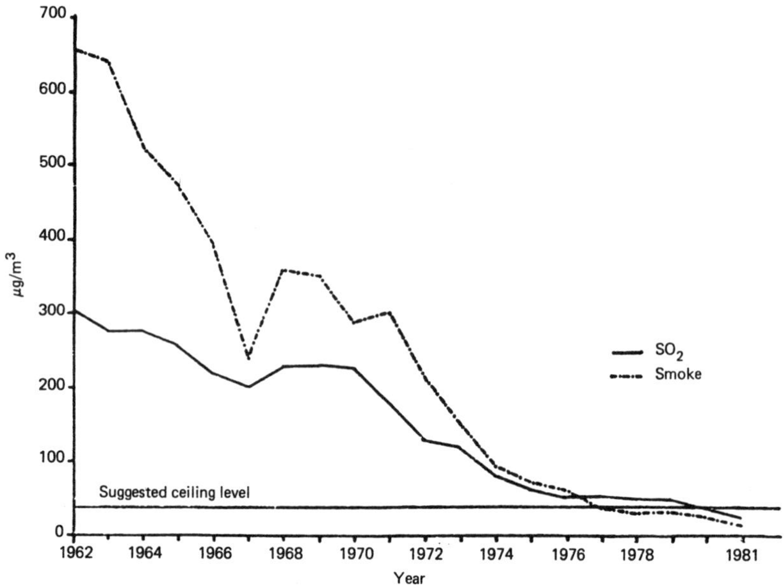

Source: **Clark, D.** *(10).*

the proportion of the population or of dwelling units with a piped water supply or with sanitary facilities and measures of crowding in dwellings.

Measurements of Exposure

Measurements of exposure are the basis for any consideration of the relationship between human health and environmental agents. There are several ways of assessing exposure. They vary in precision, moving from indicators only indirectly related to exposure, through indicators related directly to intake, to measures of actual intake and retention.

Indirect exposure indicators. Although concentrations of pollutants in soil, plants or the tissue of animals does not indicate the direct exposure of people, such measures may be used as indicators of an overall pollution burden on the environment and so indicate a potential threat to health. If measured systematically these can be useful in following trends and monitoring changes in the environment that may have implications for health.

Fig. 5. Monthly averages of air pollution with sulfur dioxide (SO_2) in the centre and in the remaining area of Cracow, 1968–1973

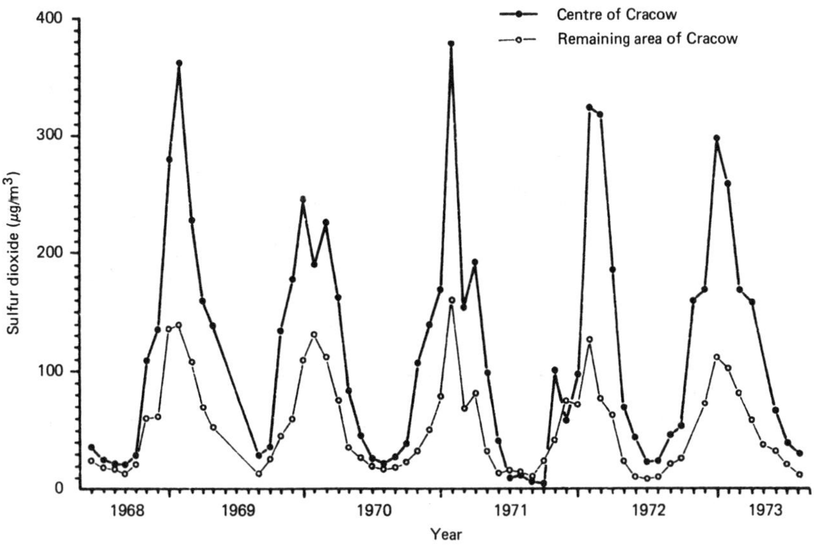

Source: **Krzyzanowski, M. & Wojtyniak, B.** *(11).*

Direct intake indicators. The concentration of pollutants in air, water and food is a much more precise indicator of exposure, since everyone breathes air, drinks water and eats food. In most countries, more or less sophisticated monitoring systems generate information on the concentrations of certain pollutants in air, water and food, as well as their temporal and spatial variations. This information can be used to estimate the exposure of the population to the monitored pollutants. Many factors, however, prevent this exposure estimate from being accurate. For example, it is known that the level of air pollution varies between urban and rural areas, and even within cities there are zones of different concentration levels. The long- and short-term mobility of the population results therefore in variations in the intake among individuals and population groups. Even the length of time one spends indoors and outdoors will result in intake differences (Fig. 6). Certain population groups are, in addition, exposed to pollutants in the workplace. Similar difficulties arise in measuring exposure to polluted water and food.

Fig. 6. Monthly mean respirable sulfate particle concentrations, expressed as averages, for six cities in the USA

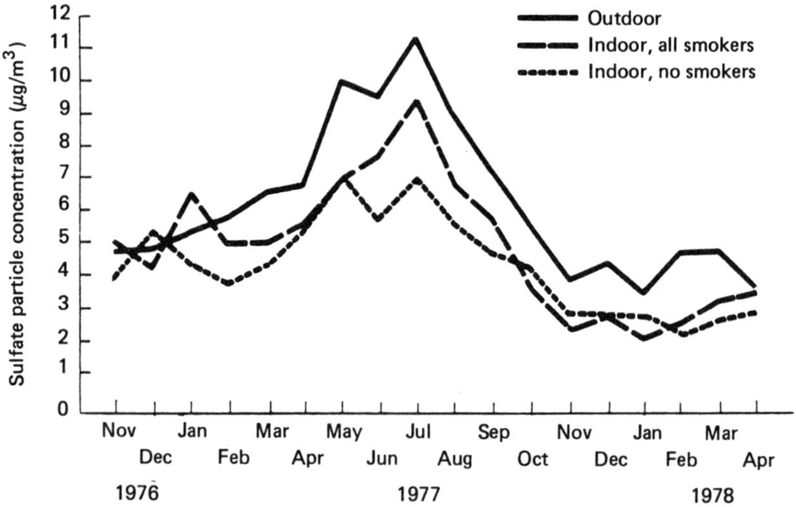

Source: **World Health Organization** *(12).*

Actual intake. Estimating exposure by measuring the actual intake is much more accurate than the other two methods although it is more difficult. In the case of air pollution, two methods are used: portable personal monitors and personal monitoring by keeping an activity diary, showing type of activity and its duration and location.

With regard to food, information on intake can be obtained by interviews with questions on the consumption of various foods and dietary habits, by the keeping of a diet diary or by weighing and analysing samples of meals consumed by individuals or families. Because of organizational problems and the resources required, all of these approaches cannot be applied on a large scale and therefore population samples studied are usually small.

Retention. Because of differences in individual characteristics, people exposed to similar concentrations of pollutants in the environment retain different amounts of them. Therefore, if there is a dose–effect relationship between the environmental agent and damage to health, the most appropriate way to measure the exposure is by measuring concentrations of the substance in human tissues. This approach, known as biological monitoring, has the advantage of allowing the measurement of the results of all sources of exposure (air, water, food) as well as individual behaviour (Fig. 7). An example of such monitoring is the United Nations Environment Programme/WHO Global Study on Exposure to Lead and Cadmium *(14)*. Biological monitoring carried out over a period of time may indicate changes in exposure or the outcome of an environmental intervention. For example, Fig. 8 shows that the level of lead in the blood decreased by approximately 37% between 1976 and 1978 and could be explained by a decline in the amount of lead in gasoline *(15)*.

Type of Environment

Environmental conditions vary from place to place with regard to health hazards, in terms of both the kind and the degree of threat. Living in an urban area, with its air pollution and noise, carries a different potential for people than life in a rural surrounding, which poses other risks, such as those related to chemicals used in modern agriculture. There are differences between countries in this respect, depending on population density, degree of industrialization and urbanization. Two types of environment deserve special attention: the workplace, since it carries the highest number of risks; and the home, because of its role in human life.

Fig. 7. Frequency distribution of CdB-levels in non-smokers and smokers in an adult population aged 60–65 years in the Federal Republic of Germany

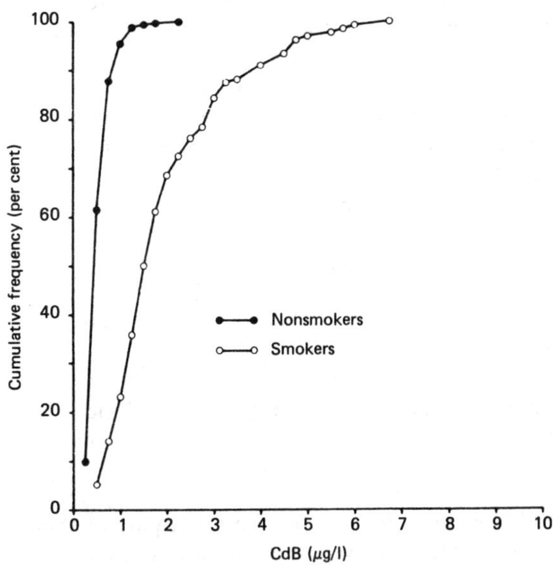

Source: **Brockhaus, A. et al.** *(13)*.

Fig. 8. Chronological trend in average blood lead levels in persons aged from 6 months to 74 years, February 1976 to February 1980, where the chronology is based on the date of examination

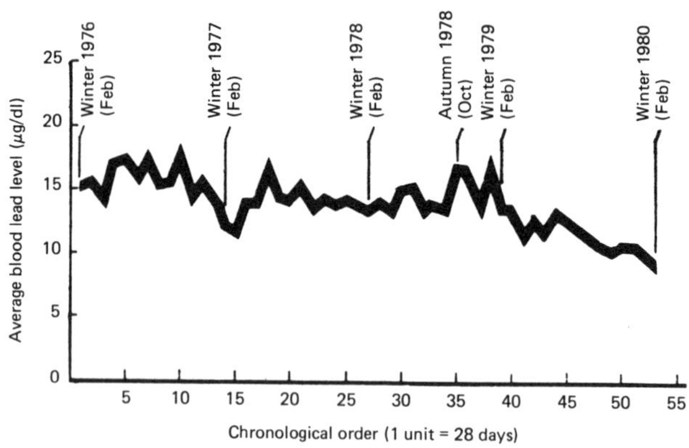

Note. Between 1970 and 1979 a 40% drop in the amount of lead in gasoline was reported.

Source: **Annest, J.L. et al.** *(15).*

Work environment. Occupational risks have long been recognized. They include all types of known environmental health hazard: physical (thermal stress, radiation, noise and dust), chemical, biological and social. Exposure to occupational risk results in various effects on health. Some, such as occupational diseases, are linked with specific agents or occupations. Others tend to be more frequent in certain occupations, but they are difficult to relate to any specific factor or factors. Although progress in occupational health and safety has led to the disappearance of some occupational diseases, at least in developed countries, technological development has brought new hazards (Table 7).

Measurements related to the work environment cover the concentration or intensity of the whole range of occupational hazards. The kind of measurement and its frequency depend on the risks present at a given workplace. In most countries measurement is done within the framework of a well defined monitoring system. Information collected in this way is used to classify workplaces according to health risk.

If required, monitoring workers' health may be carried out along with the measurement of hazards. This may include clinical examinations and laboratory tests for the early detection of pathological manifestations resulting from exposure to occupational risks.

Home environment. People spend a great part of their lives at home. However, until recently relatively little attention has been paid to its health risks. Some pollutants do come from the outdoor environment but others mainly originate indoors (Table 8). Among the more important indoor

Table 7. Some new environmental and occupational diseases

Agent	Disease(s)	Groups at risk
Vinyl chloride	Angiosarcoma, acroosteolysis, narcotic syndrome, hepatomegaly	Workers involved in the manufacture of polyvinyl chloride; exposure to vinyl chloride
Bischloromethyl ether (BCME)	Carcinoma of respiratory tract, lymphoendothelial carcinoma of nasopharynx	Workers involved in the manufacture of chloromethyl methyl ether (CMME)
Combustion of Teflon and other fluorinated polymers	Polymer fume fever	Individuals exposed to combustion of Teflon or workers smoking in Teflon fabrication plants
Methyl butyl ketone	Peripheral neuropathy	Workers who are fabricating printing ink
Methylmercuric chloride	Minamata disease	Individuals exposed to methylmercuric chloride, either directly or by eating fish from waters contaminated with mercury
Cadmium	"Itai-Itai"	Individuals exposed to high levels of cadmium from either occupational or environmental sources
Manganese	Pseudo-Parkinsonism syndrome	Manganese miners
Phosvel (leptophos) insecticide	Severe neurological symptoms, including cholinesterase inhibition and demyelination of nerve fibres	Workers in the manufacture and packaging of leptophos; consumers of grain to which compound has been added (only exported)
1,2-Dibromo-3-chloropropane (DBCP), a nematocide	Sterility and mutagenicity	Male production workers
Benzene	Aplastic anaemia and leukaemia (acute stem cell or myeloblastic; and chronic)	Workers in rotogravure, shoe manufacturing and rubber industries; also nonindustrial exposure

Source: **Trieff, N.M.** *(3).*

Table 8. Summary of indoor pollutants, emission sources, and concentrations (column 3 shows typical ranges of indoor concentrations in the presence of indoor emission sources)

Pollutant	Major emission sources	Typical indoor concentrations	Indoor/outdoor concentration ratio
	Origin: predominantly outdoors		
Sulfur oxides (gases, particles)	Fuel combustion, smelters	0–15 $\mu g/m^3$	<1
Ozone	Photochemical reactions	0–10 ppb	$\leqq 1$
Pollens	Trees, grass, weeds, plants	L.V.[a]	<1
Lead, manganese	Automobiles	L.V.	<1
Calcium, chlorine, silicon, cadmium	Suspension of soils, industrial emissions	N.A.[b]	<1
Organic substances	Petrochemical solvents, natural sources, vapourization of unburned fuels	N.A.	<1
	Origin: indoors or outdoors		
Nitric oxide, nitrogen dioxide	Fuel burning	10–120 $\mu g/m^3$[c] 200–700 $\mu g/m^3$[d]	$\geqq 1$
Carbon monoxide	Fuel burning	5–50 ppm	$\geqq 1$
Carbon dioxide	Metabolic activity, combustion	2000–3000 ppm	$\geqq 1$
Particles	Resuspension, condensation of vapours, combustion products	10–1000 $\mu g/m^3$	1
Water vapour	Biological activity, combustion evaporation	N.A.	>1

Organic substances	Volatilization, combustion, paint, metabolic action, pesticides	N.A.	≧1
Spores	Fungi, moulds	N.A.	>1
	Origin: predominantly indoors		
Radon	Building construction materials (concrete, stone), water	0.01–4 pCi/litre	≧1
Formaldehyde	Particle-board insulation, furnishings, tobacco smoke	0.01–0.5 ppm	>1
Asbestos, mineral and synthetic fibres	Fire retardant materials, insulation	0–1 fibre/ml	1
Organic substances	Adhesives, solvents, cooking, cosmetics	L.V.	>1
Ammonia	Metabolic activity, cleaning products	N.A.	>1
Polycyclic hydrocarbons, arsenic, nicotine, acrolein, and so forth	Tobacco smoke	L.V.	≧1
Mercury	Fungicides, paints, spills in dental-care facilities or laboratories, thermometer breakage	L.V.	>1
Aerosols	Consumer products	N.A.	≧1
Microorganisms	People, animals, plants	L.V.	>1
Allergens	House dust, animal dander, insect parts	L.V.	≧1

[a] L.V.: limited and variable (limited measurements, high variation).

[b] N.A.: not applicable.

[c] Annual average.

[d] One-hour average in homes with gas stoves, during cooking.

Source: **Spengler, J.D. & Sexton, K.** *(16).*

pollutants associated with health or irritative effects are: tobacco smoke, radon decay products, carbon monoxide, nitrogen dioxide, formaldehyde, asbestos fibres, microorganisms and airborne allergens *(15)*.

Too little measurement has been done to assess the magnitude of the problem and the health risks to people exposed to various kinds of pollution in the home. The changing technology of building construction and the increasing use of chemicals in building materials, finishing products and furniture calls for studies on indoor exposure and its effects on health.

Health Effects of Environmental Hazards

The effects of environmental influences cover a full range of health phenomena: overall mortality from specific causes; overall and specific morbidity; physical signs and symptoms; physical functioning; morphological changes; biochemical, physiological, neurological characteristics; and subjective, perceived psychosomatic symptoms.

The effect may appear as an acute, sudden event or as a chronic condition, frequently with increasing severity of manifestation. Some effects are very specific and can be linked with a specific environmental agent. However, most lack this specificity; several different agents can produce similar effects and several different manifestations may be observed in response to the same hazard.

Sources of Information on Health Effects

Information on health in relation to the environment may be obtained from a variety of sources. In most countries, a large volume of health data that are routinely collected for other purposes can be used for studies on the health effects of environmental influences. These include statistics on mortality, hospital admission or discharge, the occurrence of notifiable diseases, outpatient diagnosis or absence from work due to sickness. Some of the above data are occasionally presented in such a format that they may be related to certain types of environment or certain environmental hazards, such as the data on occupational mortality in England & Wales. Usually it is very difficult to relate routinely collected data to specific target population groups unless a special design is developed for a particular purpose, such as mortality and morbidity monitoring among workers exposed to a defined hazard. For the general population, disease registries in an area well stratified according to the environmental risks would be a useful tool.

Routinely collected data, however, have certain innate shortcomings, that are difficult to overcome with any design for data gathering, processing and analysis. The main, although not the only, deficiency is the lack of standardized diagnostic procedures based on well defined criteria.

In most instances, therefore, special studies are needed, based on precise protocols and employing standardized measuring and diagnostic procedures.

Measurements of Health Effects

The simplest measuring-stick is the crude count of such events as death or disease among the population at risk. If the population is stable and the count is carried out regularly and frequently, any unexpected change in the number of events may be a warning and prompt an investigation to explain the change. Otherwise this measure is of limited value.

The number of deaths and cases of disease is usually related to the population at risk, and is therefore presented as a rate: a mortality rate, i.e. the number of deaths divided by the number of persons at risk during a given period of time; an incidence rate, i.e. the number of new cases of disease divided by the number of persons at risk during a given period of time; or prevalence rate, i.e. the number of present cases divided by the number of people at risk at a certain point in time (point prevalence) or during a given period of time (period prevalence). Information on symptoms is obtained through interview surveys and presented in terms of the frequency of occurrence among the populations studied.

In addition to interviews, health examination surveys include clinical examination and, according to a study protocol, biochemical, physiological or other tests. The presentation of results depends on the characteristic in question, such as averages, concentrations or frequencies.

Relationship. In principle, the inference of a relationship between an environmental hazard and a health effect derives from comparisons of the occurrence of the effect in two populations, only one being exposed to a given hazard, as shown below.

		Hazard	
		Present	Absent
Health effect	Present	a	b
	Absent	c	d

The greater the difference in the frequency of the health effect in the exposed population $a/(a + c)$ as compared to unexposed people $b/(b + d)$, the stronger the relationship, and more likely, although not necessarily, that it is causal.

By introducing appropriate scales for both health effect and environmental hazard instead of a simple dichotomy, a dose–response model can be obtained (Fig. 9).

Multiple causation, multiple relationship. Most health effects result from multiple influences. Similarly, environmental hazards are frequently interrelated. This creates difficulties in the interpretation of results and inferences about the nature of the relationships. This is well known to everyone involved in environmental health research.

As may be seen from Fig. 10, there is a relationship between water level and blood level. However, blood level is also related to water hardness (Fig. 11). Furthermore, it was found the the level of lead in an individual's

Fig. 9. Frequency of residents "strongly" annoyed by industrial noise related to mean industrial noise

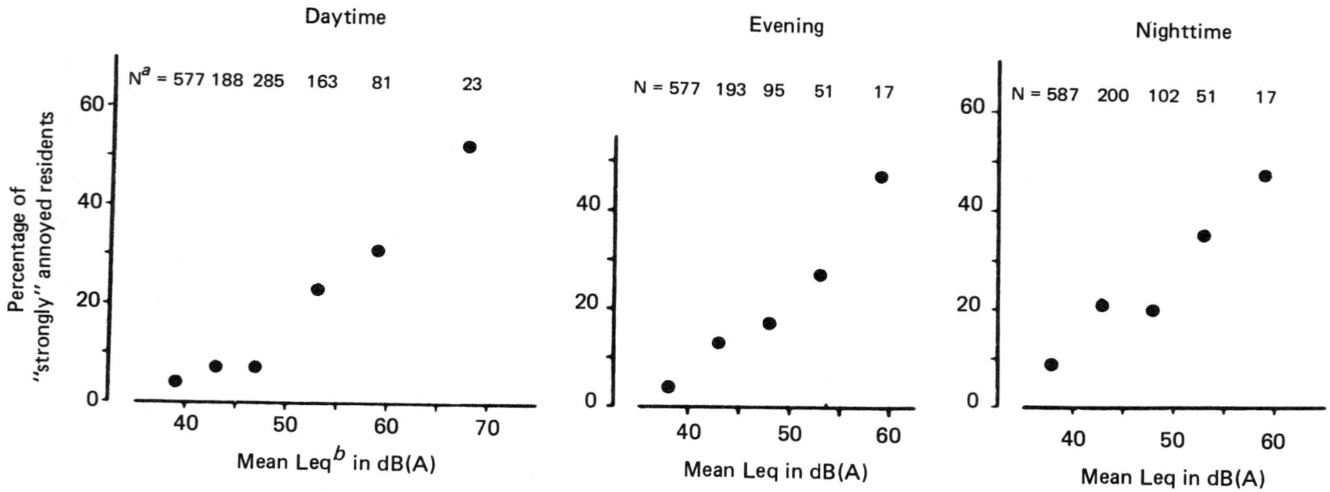

[a] N: number of answered questionnaires.

[b] Leq: equivalent continuous sound level.

Source: **Gyr, S. & Grandjean, E.** *(17).*

Fig. 10. Mean blood lead for men grouped by first draw water concentration

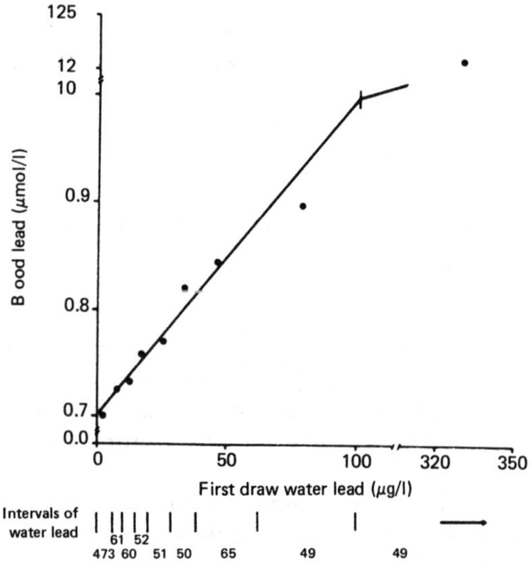

Source: **Pocock, S.J. et al.** *(18).*

Fig. 11. Mean blood lead and water hardness in 24 towns

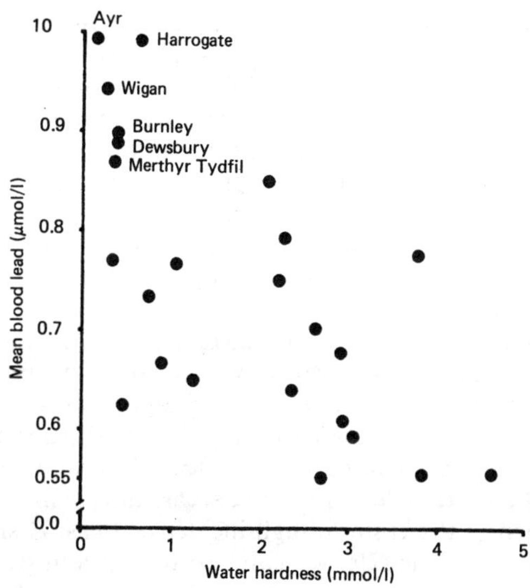

Source: **Pocock, S.J. et al.** *(18).*

blood is affected by alcohol consumption and cigarette smoking. These two habits contribute an estimated 17% to the concentration of lead in the blood of middle-aged men *(18)*.

Because of the complex nature of the relationship between environmental hazards, the personal characteristics of people exposed to them and ultimate effects on health, more or less sophisticated statistical techniques, such as multiple regression, frequently have to be used to appraise the actual influence of different agents.

Epidemiological Research on Environmental Influences on Human Health

Many disciplines are involved in studying the health effects of environmental hazards, including toxicology, physiology, clinical medicine, sociology, chemistry, engineering and ergonomics. Epidemiology, however, plays a special role as a discipline concerned with the distribution of health phenomena in the human population and factors that determine their occurrence.

There are two main epidemiological approaches in studying environmental influences on human health. The first is based on differences in the occurrence of deaths or disease from one place to another and leads to the identification of environmental factors that could eventually explain these differences. The second deals with differences from place to place in occurrence and levels of environmental agents likely to be related to health, and measures the occurrence of diseases possibly caused by the agents in question.

Differences in disease occurrence. The differences in the occurrence of disease according to place have long been recognized. Studies in this field, initially concerned with communicable diseases, were later applied to noncommunicable diseases such as cancer. The data compiled and published by the International Agency for Research on Cancer show wide variation in the incidence of malignant neoplasms. In general, the occurrence is higher in industrialized countries than in developing countries, although the pattern varies according to the site. For example, cancer of the liver, frequent in men in Africa and Asia, is comparatively rare in North America and Europe, while cancer of the breast has a high incidence in Europe, North America, Australia and New Zealand.

Differences in the distribution of cancer occur not only on a global scale, but also on a national or local scale as well. Geographical variations in the incidence of certain cancers, such as oesophageal cancer, occur in a relatively limited area of the Caspian littoral of Iran *(19)*. The age-standardized incidence rates per 100 000 lie between 13.0 and 20.1 for men and 2.3 and 6.2 for women in the western, low-incidence areas, and reach 165.5 for men and 195.3 for women in the eastern, high-incidence areas. A similar variation was found in north China *(20)*, with an average age-adjusted mortality rate of 37.4 per 100 000. There was almost a 100-fold difference between the areas with low or high incidence. High mortality rates from cancer of the oesophagus were found in Brittany, in France, ranging from 16 to 27 per 100 000 in males and reaching, in some localized areas over 50 per 100 000 *(21)*. Although the search for environmental factors responsible for these peculiar incidence patterns did not yield a complete and conclusive explanation, certain relationships were found that indicated possible causal agents. For example, investigation in Iran showed that people living in high-incidence areas had low intake of calories and total protein, vitamin A, riboflavin and vitamin C. In China, food samples from high-incidence areas showed higher quantities of nitrosamines, nitrites and secondary amines in comparison with low-incidence regions. Animal experiments showed that a certain fungus contaminating pickled cabbage eaten in high-incidence areas might be cocarcinogenic. In Brittany the findings are consistent with the hypothesis about the role of alcohol.

The incidence of cancer of the colon and rectum, one of the the major causes of morbidity in most industrialized countries, also shows marked geographical variation. An international study in two areas of Denmark and Finland found that the four-fold variation in colon cancer may be multifactorial and is not associated in a simple manner with dietary fat, neutral steroids or their bacterial metabolites. However, meat consumption was greater in high-incidence areas. It was also suggested that higher intakes of dietary fibre and milk in the low-incidence area may have a possible protective effect *(22)*.

Investigations on the high incidence of laryngeal cancer in Torino, Italy *(23)*, suggested an increase in the environmental carcinogenic load as an explanatory factor.

A survey of oral cancer in the United States revealed elevated rates of incidence among males in urban areas and among females in the rural south *(24)*. Indirect evidence suggested that the urban gradient in males resulted largely from the consumption of alcohol and from smoking, while the southern gradient in females related primarily to the oral use of snuff.

The geographical approach to examining the causes of disease is still not totally exploited. According to estimates based on geographical variations, and supported by other studies, most cancers are related to the environment and thus theoretically preventable (Table 9). Geographical analyses may also be useful in many other problem areas of health, disease, and environment.

Differences in environmental factors. Differences in environmental factors and their relation to the occurrence of disease may be considered from various points of view, according to the media in which a given factor or factors occur (air, water, soil, food), the type of environment in which people are more or less specifically exposed to health hazards (workplace, home, urban or rural areas), or the kind of particular factor or factors (pollutants, climatic conditions, natural physiochemical and biological factors, pyschosocial factors).

All of these conditions vary in place and time, and their relationship to health and disease has been investigated. For example, numerous studies were conducted on the adverse health effects of various categories of air pollutants, such as the sulfur oxide/particulate complex, photochemical

Table 9. Proportions of cancer deaths attributed to various factors

Factor or class of factors	Percentage of all cancer deaths	
	Best estimate	Range of acceptable estimates
Tobacco	30	25-40
Alcohol	3	2-4
Diet	35	10-70
Food additives	<1	-5[a]-2
Reproductive and sexual behaviour	7	1-13
Occupation	4	2-8
Pollution	2	<1-5
Industrial products	<1	<1-2
Medicines and medical procedures	1	0.5-3
Geophysical factors[b]	3	2-4
Infection	10?	1-?
Unknown	?	?

[a] Allowing for a possibly protective effect of antioxidants and other preservatives.

[b] Only about 1%, not 3% could reasonably be described as "avoidable". Geophysical factors also cause a much greater proportion of non-fatal cancers (up to 30% of all cancers, depending on ethnic mix and latitude) because of the importance of ultraviolet light in causing the relatively non-fatal basal cell and squamous cell carcinomas of sunlight-exposed skin.

Source: **Doll, R. & Peto, R.** *(6)*.

oxidants, nitrogen dioxide, carbon monoxide and others. They showed the association of air pollution with mortality, acute and chronic respiratory disease morbidity, ventilatory function, cancer of the lung, and cardiovascular disease, as well as with sensory, neurological and behavioural symptoms.

There are also numerous studies on factors related to other media, such as water and food, and their relationship to health. These include studies of water hardness or certain elements in water and ischaemic heart disease, of nitrates in drinking-water and hyptertension, and of surface water supply and mortality from malignant neoplasms.

An interesting example is a recent study on the incidence of cancer and reuse of drinking-water *(24)*. Areas supplied with water of different degrees of reuse (Fig. 12) were correlated with cancer incidence (Fig. 13). Positive associations were found between the average percentage of domestic sewage

Fig. 12. Sources of water supply, south London, England, 1926–1975 (broken line: Greater London boundary; solid lines: boundaries of boroughs and districts)

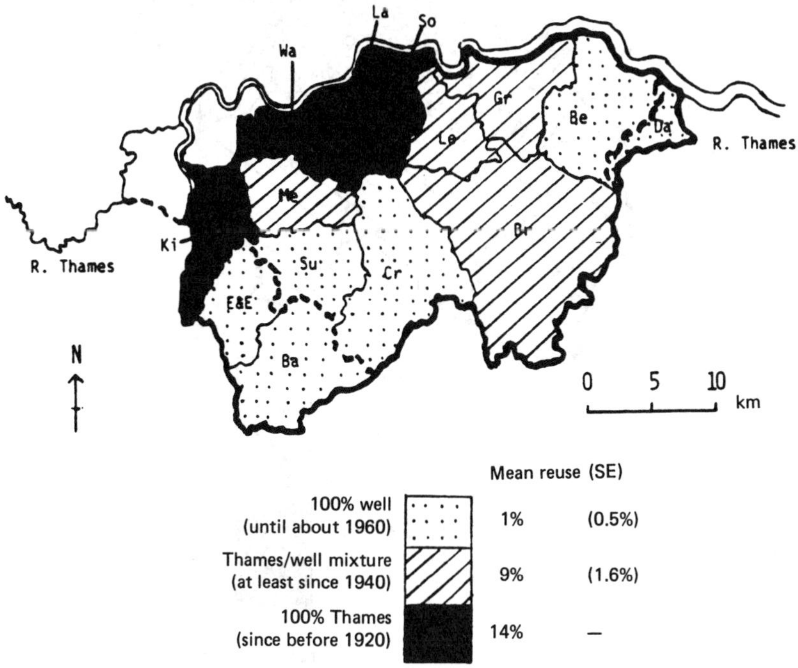

Note. Abbreviations of boroughs: Ba, Banstead; Be, Bexley; Br, Bromley; Cr, Croydon; Da, Dartford; E&E, Epsom and Ewell; Gr, Greenwich; Ki, Kingston; La, Lambeth; Le, Lewisham; Me, Merton; So, Southwark; Su, Sutton; Wa, Wandsworth. (SE = standard error.)

Source: **Beresford, S.A.A.** *(24).*

in the water supplied to an area and the incidence of stomach and urinary cancers in females. However, there was also an association between these two variables and socioeconomic characteristics (Fig. 14). Although the associations between water reuse and cancer were reduced when social factors and variations in area size were taken into account, the study provides evidence of a small health risk associated with the reuse of drinking-water.

In another study on the relationship between the main foodstuff and nutrient intakes and the chief causes of mortality in 20 different countries, complex patterns of food consumption were identified and related both to geographical latitude and to levels of affluence. These, in turn, were related to complex patterns of mortality. Some findings suggested causal

Fig. 13. Mean socioeconomic rank, south London, England, 1971

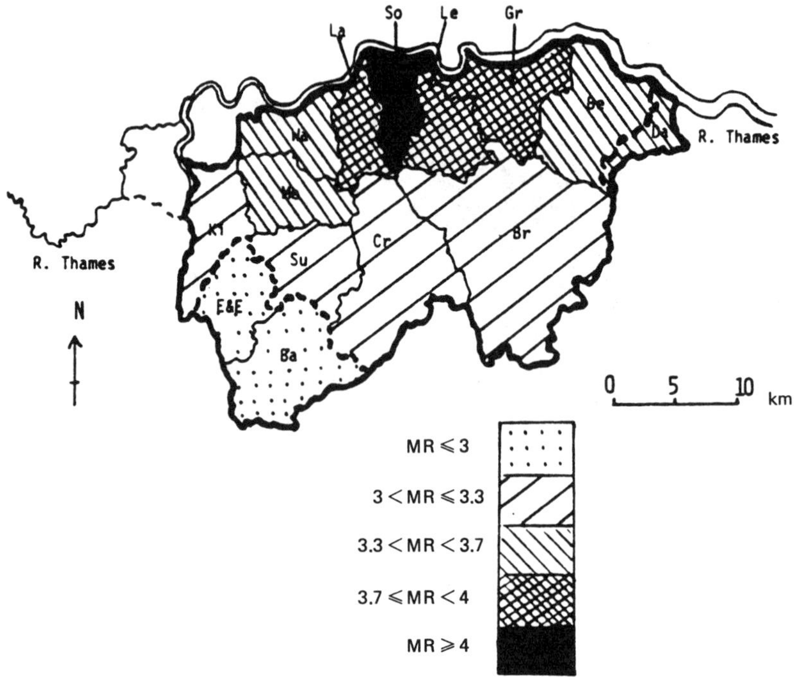

Note. For key to boundaries and definition of borough abbreviations, see Fig. 12. Mean socioeconomic rank (MR) is the mean score for a borough where the economically active males are scored as follows: 1 — professional (socioeconomic group (SEG) (Registrar General's classification of occupations) 3, 4); 2 — employers and managers (SEG 1, 2, 13); 3 — intermediate and junior non-manual (SEG 5, 6); 4 — skilled manual (SEG, 8, 9, 12, 14); 5 — semi-skilled manual and personal service (SEG 7, 10, 15); 6 — unskilled manual (SEG 11).

Source: **Beresford, S.A.A.** *(24).*

relationships between consumption and disease in the cases of: alcohol intake and cirrhosis of the liver, cancer of the mouth and cancer of the larynx; total fat intake and multiple sclerosis, cancer of the large intestine, and cancer of the breast; and beer and cancer of the rectum *(25).*

In regard to variations related to the type of environment, the working environment offers a unique opportunity for environmental health research since both the population at risk and exposure can be estimated with much greater precision than can be done with other population groups or types of environment. Occupational health research may be focused on particular groups of workers, types of industry, specific occupational hazards, or diseases. Although the volume of knowledge on occupational epidemiology

Fig. 14. Stomach cancer incidence in females, south London, England, 1968–1974

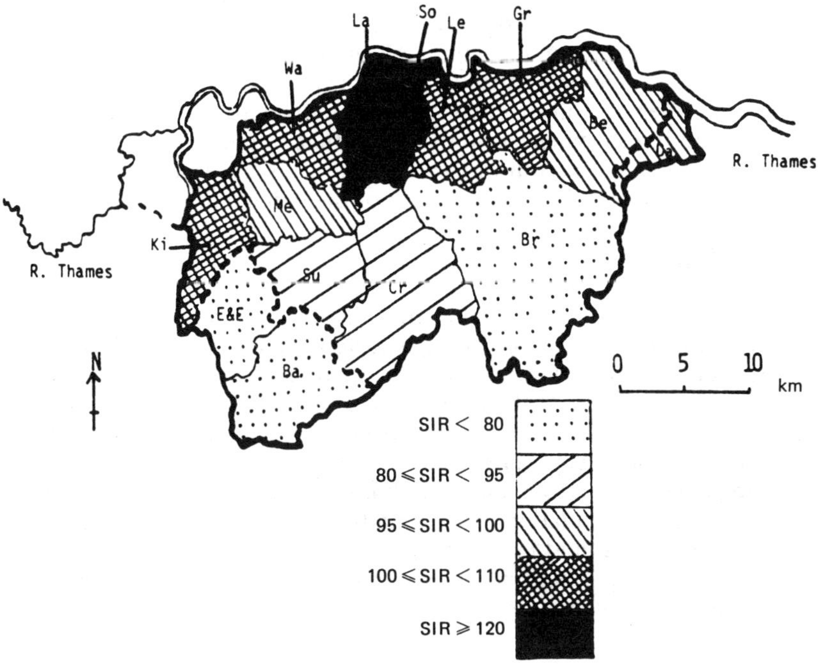

Note. For key to boundaries and definitions of borough abbreviations, see Fig. 12. SIR = standardized incidence ratio (%).

Source: **Beresford, S.A.A.** *(24).*

is growing rapidly, many problems remain unsolved. as in other fields of epidemiological research, it is often difficult to differentiate between occupational and other environmental influences. For instance, variations in cancer mortality by site, from one country to another, suggest that most cancers may be attributed to environmental factors. What proportion of cancer rates, however, is related to the occupational environment? To interpret the importance of even a single well documented factor such as the effects of smoking in occupational cancer is difficult because of the lack of sound epidemiological data on the joint action of occupational carcinogens and tobacco smoke.

Causal inferences in epidemiological studies on urban and rural or housing environments, in which the researcher deals with the combined influences of biological, environmental, social, economic and cultural factors, are far more difficult to make.

If future epidemiological studies on the relationship between variations in environmental factors and health are to yield a better understanding of the causation of disease to aid in the prevention and control of disease, they should employ sharper investigative tools, be more detailed, and take into account both host characteristics and environmental factors. What is needed, first, is an improvement in the information available on exposures of communities and individuals to potentially hazardous factors and, secondly, an improvement in study design that would make it possible to relate variations in exposure to variations in disease frequency in communities and to the effect on the health of the individual exposed.

Conclusion

Measurements in environmental protection are a complex issue. Environmental hazards affect people through various kinds of media. They vary according to types of environment and individuals' ways of life. In addition to this wide variation in the occurrence and intensity of environmental hazards, there is also wide variation in the response of the human organism to environmental agents. Present knowledge of the actual threat of the changing environment to human health is still limited, although enough is known to protect populations from already identified risks. To do so, more research based on sound methodology is also needed. Recently published guidelines and studies in environmental epidemiology offer valuable assistance in this development *(26)*.

References

1. *The role of geographical factors in the planning of health programmes:* report on a working group. Copenhagen, WHO Regional Office for Europe, 1975.
2. *Health hazards of the human environment.* Geneva, World Health Organization, 1973.
3. **Trieff, N.M.** Introduction: environment and health. *In:* Trieff, N.M., ed. *Environment and health.* Ann Arbor, Ann Arbor Science, 1980.
4. **Wöhlers, H.C.** Worldwide environmental problems. *In:* Trieff, N.M., ed. *Environment and health.* Ann Arbor, Ann Arbor Science, 1980.
5. **Kates, R.W.** *Risk assessment of environmental hazard.* Chichester, John Wiley, 1978.
6. **Doll, R. & Peto, R.** *The causes of cancer.* Oxford, Oxford Medical Publications, 1981.
7. **International Agency for Research on Cancer.** *Monographs supplement 4.* 1982.
8. **Cohen, R.L. & Lee, Y-Sing.** A catalog of risks. *Health physics,* **36**: 707–722 (1979).
9. **Crouch, E.A.C. & Wilson, R.** *Risk/benefit analysis.* Cambridge, MA, Ballinger, 1982.
10. **Clark, D.** A view to the future of the air pollution control. *Environmental health,* (April): 96–97 (1983).

11. **Krzyzanowski, M. & Wojtyniak, B.** Ten-year mortality in a sample of an adult population in relation to air pollution. *Journal of epidemiology and community health,* **36**: 262–268 (1982).
12. *Estimating human exposure to air pollutants.* Geneva, World Health Organization, 1982 (Offset publication No. 69).
13. **Brochaus, A. et al.** Levels of cadmium and lead in blood in relation to smoking, sex, occupation, and other factors in an adult population of the FRG. *International archives of occupational and environmental health,* **52**: 167–175 (1983).
14. **Friberg, L. & Vahter, M.** Assessment of exposure to lead and cadmium through biological monitoring. Results of a UNEP/WHO Global Study. *Environmental research,* **30**: 95–128 (1983).
15. **Annest, J.L. et al.** Chronological trend in blood lead levels between 1976 and 1980. *New England journal of medicine,* **308**(23): 1373–1377 (1983).
16. **Spengler, J.D. & Sexton, K.** Indoor air pollution: a public health perspective. *Science,* **221**(4605): 9–17 (1983).
17. **Gyr, S. & Grandjean, E.** Industrial noise in residential areas: effects on residents. *International archives of occupational and environmental health,* **53**: 219–231 (1984).
18. **Pocock, S.J. et al.** Effects of tap water lead, water hardness, alcohol and cigarettes on blood lead concentration. *Journal of epidemiology and community health,* **37**: 1–7 (1983).
19. **Kmet, J. & Mahboubi, E.** Esophageal cancer in the Caspian littoral of Iran: initial studies. *Science,* **175**: 846–953 (1972).
20. Preliminary report: the epidemiology and etiology of esophageal cancer in north China. *Chinese medical journal,* **1**: 167–183 (1975).
21. **Tuyns, A.J. & Masse, L.M.F.** Mortality from cancer of the esophagus in Brittany. *International journal of epidemiology,* **2**: 241–245 (1973).
22. Report from the International Agency for Research on Cancer Intestinal Microecology Group. *Lancet,* **2**: 207–211 (1977).
23. **Terracini, B. et al.** High incidence of laryngeal cancer in the province of Torino (Italy). *Tumori,* **60**: 143–156 (1974).
24. **Beresford, S.A.A.** Cancer incidence and reuse of drinking water. *American journal of epidemiology,* **117**(3): 258–268 (1983).
25. **Knox, E.G.** Foods and diseases. *British journal of preventive and social medicine,* **31**: 71–80 (1977).
26. *Guidelines on studies in environmental epidemiology.* Geneva, World Health Organization, 1983 (Environmental Health Criteria, No. 27).

8.5 Appropriate provision and management of services[a] — *C. Montoya-Aguilar*

In measuring and evaluating the appropriate provision and management of services, four essential aspects of health care systems should be considered:

— the coverage of the system, that is, the proportion of people who actually avail themselves of specific health promotion or protection activities, out of those who would benefit from them;

— the effect of its activities, that is the changes in health status that can be attributed to health care or, in more general terms, the extent to which the broad objectives of the system are being attained;

— the efficiency of the system, or how economically the activities or the effects of the system are being produced or, in other words, the extent to which waste of resources is being avoided; and

— the structure and content of the system, in terms of the balance between different services (such as primary care and other services) and how the system meets relevant policy principles such as equity, intersectoral cooperation and community participation.

In this chapter issues relating to the measurement of these four aspects are considered. Many of the measurements discussed can be considered as equally relevant in other chapters in Part II, such as the chapters on personal protection (8.1) and the assessment of priority given to health promotion (8.6). Concepts of measurement related to community participation have also been discussed, although from a rather different perspective, in Chapter 8.3. Measurement of the effects of the activities of the health care system is dealt with in many other chapters; here they are briefly discussed in relation to evaluation.

Coverage of the System

Very succinctly, coverage is expressed as the ratio of the population served with an activity to the population in need of the activity. This definition, discussed and agreed upon by the participants in a WHO collaborative study *(1)* is essentially the same as that presented earlier by WHO *(2,3)*.

---

[a] This chapter has been largely drawn from a WHO document, *National assessments of health care coverage and of its effectiveness and efficiency.*

Coverage thus understood is the end result of a chain of circumstances:

— the existence of certain types and amounts of health care resources;

— the accessibility of these resources in physical, economic, socio-cultural and organizational terms;

— their acceptability to the population concerned; and

— the matching of health care activities to the actual needs of the population, or their relevance.

The extension of coverage depends on all these factors, as illustrated in Fig. 1.

Fig. 1. The concept of coverage and its determinants

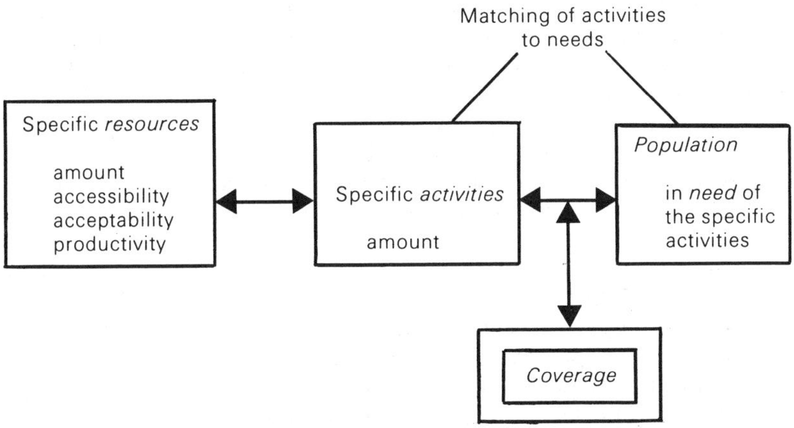

As indicated in a WHO-UNICEF joint report on primary health care *(4)* the concepts of coverage and its determinants have often been confused. National health reports frequently say that the coverage aimed at is to achieve a ratio of one primary health care worker per 1000 population, or that the aim is to have sufficient health care units so that nobody lives further than 5 km from such a unit. This can be misleading: coverage, as understood here, must refer to populations actually affected by the specific services or activities in question. Even the expression three consultations per caput does not indicate coverage. The numerator of the coverage ratio should indicate the number of population units (individuals, houses, villages) with which contact has been made within an area, and the denominator should refer to the population in the same area that needed the type of services indicated in the numerator.

Where true coverage is not being measured, it is understandable that an indicator of lesser specificity, such as the availability or accessibility of resources, be used instead. For political reasons it may be preferable to emphasize such achievements as the size and numbers of health care units, since these are the immediate, visible and durable results of decisions on financial allocations for health; these must not, however, be equated with coverage, the correct understanding of which is central to organizing, managing and evaluating health care systems.

Before leaving the subject of coverage, two important questions should be considered: coverage with what? and coverage for whom? For the first question, the general expression "coverage with health care" has no well defined meaning. Coverage indicates the proportion of population availing themselves of specific services that they need. Thus, if all children under five need regular health surveillance consultations, it makes sense to say that, for example, coverage for infant and preschool child consultations is, say, 50% or 100%. Here it is necessary to define what will be considered as appropriate coverage for a specific activity. Should there be at least one surveillance consultation per year for a preschool child? Are at least two consultations sufficient for antenatal control and three doses for poliomyelitis immunization in infants?

For many specific activities, coverage may be provided by the public and private health sectors, by other sectors, by the community, the family and the individual (self-care). Where there are many sources of care, coverage must be measured in a comprehensive way, or the source of the coverage reported must be specified.

The question of who is covered is basic for policy. The goal of health for all and the approach of primary health care imply a target of 100% coverage with all essential activities. In monitoring progress towards this goal, measurement should provide coverage figures for the different geographical subdivisions of the country or area under consideration. If possible, this should also be calculated separately for socioeconomic, age, sex, occupational and other significant population groups. This will help to assess the degree of equity being attained.

A particular example of the measurement of coverage is shown in Table 1. The data are taken from Egypt *(5)*. They show the variation among rural governorates in coverage for antenatal care provided by the maternal health services. In 1976, of an estimated 749 420 births, 280 432 (37%) occurred to mothers covered by clinic services during pregnancy. Three clinic consultations, as well as 1.8 home visits, were provided per woman covered. These were averages for the total rural population.

The figures in Table 1 were very useful for establishing a policy aimed at raising the coverage in all governorates to the level of those best covered. This policy would be on firmer ground if the differences found among provinces were explained. The first obvious possibility was that differences in coverage might be due to corresponding differences among governorates in availability and/or in physical accessibility of resources. The analysis of the pertinent indicators also shown in Table 1 suggested, however, that this was not the sole explanation. The health care resources of governorates were

Table 1. Coverage with antenatal care and average number of antenatal consultations per person covered, rural governorates of Egypt, 1976

Governorate	Percentage of mothers covered by antenatal care	Average number of antenatal consultations per person covered	Availability of resources		Physical accessibility (distance to health unit in km)	
			No. of persons per health care unit	No. of persons per nurse	Satellite villages	Hamlets
Kafr-el-Sheik	55	2.3	8 200	5 568	2.5	3.1
Fayoum	52	2.5	8 409	4 476	2.2	2.0
Kaliubia	49	2.9	8 636	3 435	2.0	2.0
Beni-Suef	45	2.3	6 851	2 392	2.1	2.8
Dakahlia	43	2.9	8 858	2 672	2.6	3.1
Menoufia	41	3.0	8 301	2 384	0.7	1.9
Behera	41	3.3	8 059	3 843	2.7	3.0
Damietta	40	2.6	8 394	2 570	1.2	2.2
Sharkia	39	3.9	8 650	4 781	2.4	2.9
Menya	38	2.6	7 939	2 876	2.3	2.2
Gharbia	34	2.8	11 791	1 704	2.0	2.7
Assiut	33	3.8	8 799	3 403	1.4	2.2
Guiza	32	2.5	9 211	3 953	0.8	2.0
Sohag	24	3.4	7 988	6 815	0.9	1.7
Aswan	15	2.6	4 976	3 818	1.4	2.2
Qena	10	3.1	8 245	6 862	2.2	1.8
All rural governorates	37	2.9	8 258	3 203	2.2	2.6

more similar than the coverage attained. A particularly clear example of this was provided by the three most southern governorates, Sohag, Aswan and Qena. Table 1 shows that the health units/population ratios in Sohag were similar to the general ratios for rural Egypt; in Aswan they were much better. Yet these governorates had the lowest antenatal coverage: 10–24%. In Sohag and Qena, but not in Aswan, the nurse/population ratios were the lowest in rural Egypt, but these ratios were almost equally low in Kafr-el-Sheik, where coverage was highest (55%). The settlements were smaller in the three governorates, as indicated by the finding that 41–66% of the people lived in hamlets, not in villages, as compared with 31% for all the rural population. Further enquiry revealed that most of the nurses posted in those three southern governorates came from northern Egypt, pointing to a possible cultural factor as an explanation for the findings and providing a guide for further investigation and interim action.

Effect of Health Care Activities

An effect of a health care intervention can be defined as the difference, in respect of some relevant health indicator, between populations with and without such care, which can be attributed to the intervention.

The concept of effect is most frequently applied to a positive change in respect of health, although the system has other broad goals also, such as the satisfaction of the social demand for health care or contributions to other aspects of economic and social development. With these qualifications, this definition is consistent with usage in WHO publications *(3,6)*.

A change in health status may result from various influences. For the evaluation of the appropriate provision and management of health services, changes attributable to interventions from the health care system matter most; only these can be considered to be the effects of that system. How can the fraction of an observed change attributable to health care be recognized? Certain types of positive circumstantial evidence can be sought, namely:

— the time trends of the assumed effect and of the intervention evolve in the expected directions;

— the assumed effect is observed in areas subject to the intervention and not in other areas;

— the size of the assumed effect is proportional to the magnitude of the health care effort, a dose–response relation;

— when the situation is replicated, the assumed effect appears again;

— the assumed effect persists even if other possible causes are eliminated either in the field or by means of statistical analysis;

— the nature of the association observed between the assumed effect and the intervention is congruent with what would be logically expected; and

— the intervention has been shown, under unbiased experimental conditions, to produce the effect in question.

Thus, although it is very difficult to have absolute proof in field conditions of the attributability of a change to a given health care activity, it is possible to reach a level of confidence that will be sufficient for decision-making. This is facilitated if natural experiments can be identified. One kind of natural experiment arises when a new resource or a new intervention is introduced in a phased manner to new places in successive years.

So far, three questions on effects have been implicitly referred to. These are:

— effects on what, health status or a non-health object?

— effects of what kind, positive or negative?

— effects from what, the health care system or another system?

Some additional considerations have to be taken into account when answering these questions for planning and evaluation. For example, a specific change attributable to the health care system may be the result of several interventions that may be complementary, may reinforce one another, or may be even necessary to one another. A single intervention may also be designed to affect several different areas (see the discussions about growth charts in Chapter 7.1 on child growth and development).

A fourth question is: effects for whom, or who benefits? The answer, of course, is closely related to the distribution of coverage. This is a key issue in the attainment of equity.

It is clearly important that the two categories of information, on health changes and on health activities, be collected and reported so that their mutual relationships can be analysed in regard to place, time and other possible related factors or causes of change.

Although the main purpose of health monitoring is not obtaining scientific evidence on effects, health managers must be regularly informed on whether health trends and differentials are behaving as expected to assess whether services are being provided appropriately. Many different measures appropriate to the task of monitoring are covered in the other chapters in Part II and will not be repeated here. For purposes of illustration, however, the question of what measures might be examined to assess the effects of clinic attendance presented in Table 1 can be considered. These measures could include the percentage of babies with low birth weight, the perinatal mortality rate, the maternal mortality rate, or gestational age at birth (for a fuller discussion, see Chapter 8.1).

The fifth and last question, which deserves clarification because of its fundamental importance in planning for health promotion and protection, is: what determines effect? Three immediate factors do so. One of these relates to the health problem addressed. It is the size of the problem in the population, such as the proportion of smokers for an antismoking campaign or the expected incidence of measles in the case of a measles immunization programme. The other two factors concern the health care system. They are the ability of the intervention to produce the intended effect under actual field conditions, which is called the effectiveness of the intervention (such as vaccination); and the degree of coverage with the intervention.

In other words, if for a health-related issue there exists an activity or intervention of a given level of effectiveness, this level will be fully realized if 100% coverage is attained. The absolute size of the effect in the total population will be proportional to the size of the problem. A very effective technology will produce only a small effect if used against a rare condition. On the other hand, high coverage with an ineffective intervention will be useless. Fig. 2 demonstrates the relationship between these factors and the health effect produced.

Fig. 2. Immediate determinants of a health effect

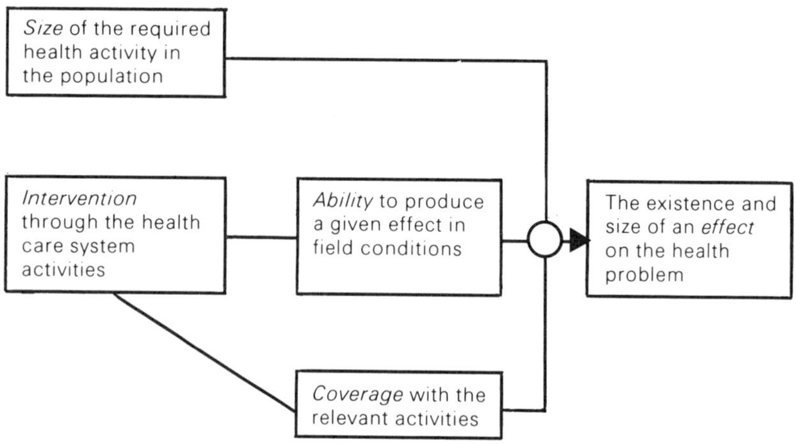

The last point is crucial. For the aims of health for all, what is needed is adequate coverage with promotive, preventive or curative activities that are highly effective under field conditions against the most prevalent and serious health problems.

How much of the potential effectiveness of an intervention, as determined under experimental conditions, is realized in practice depends upon the quality of the activities covering the population in need of them. This more qualitative aspect is sufficiently important to be mentioned here, even if the subject cannot be developed further in this chapter.

The examples of measurement of effectiveness shown here demonstrate clearly the relationship between effectiveness and the distribution of coverage mentioned above. The first of these is concerned with a rural primary health care programme, using paramedical personnel, implemented in Costa Rica *(7)*. A certain population is assigned to this programme in each area and the covered population is defined as the number of households that have received at least one home visit. Through the home visits a standard package of essential services is delivered. Thus defined, coverage by the rural programme had reached 83% of its assigned population in 1978, with an average density of three visits per household.

The Costa Rican Ministry of Health measured the health effect of the rural health programme, which began in 1973, by using life expectancy as the health indicator and comparing its levels and its modifications, before and after 1973, among districts with different levels of coverage. Some results are shown in Table 2 and Fig. 3.

From this comparison across both time and place, the Ministry concluded that the programme was associated with an increase in life expectancy at birth. There is a gradient in the gain in life expectancy that goes from 2.4 years in the districts with less than 25% coverage to 5.07 years in districts with 75% or higher coverage. Additional data would be needed to be sure that the observed differences, however suggestive of an effect of health care, are not due to other factors. For example, the people in areas with a greater increase in life expectancy might have had greater income increases or a higher educational coverage during the period in question.

The second example here is taken from the same source *(7)*, but relates to a more specific activity: a systematic programme of vaccination of each cohort of infants, begun in 1970.

Table 2. Increase in life expectancy according to coverage with the rural health programme, Costa Rica, 1970–1976

Groups of districts	Life expectancy at birth (years)		Increase in life expectancy at birth during the period	
	1970–1972	1974–1976	No. of years	Percentage increase
Without coverage (urban areas)	68.76	71.16	2.40	3.5
Less than 25% coverage	68.73	71.13	2.40	3.5
25–49% coverage	63.94	67.44	3.50	5.5
50–74% coverage	67.26	71.30	4.04	6.0
75% coverage and more	67.89	72.96	5.07	7.5

Fig. 3. Increase in life expectancy at birth according to rural health coverage, Costa Rica, between 1970–1972 and 1974–1976

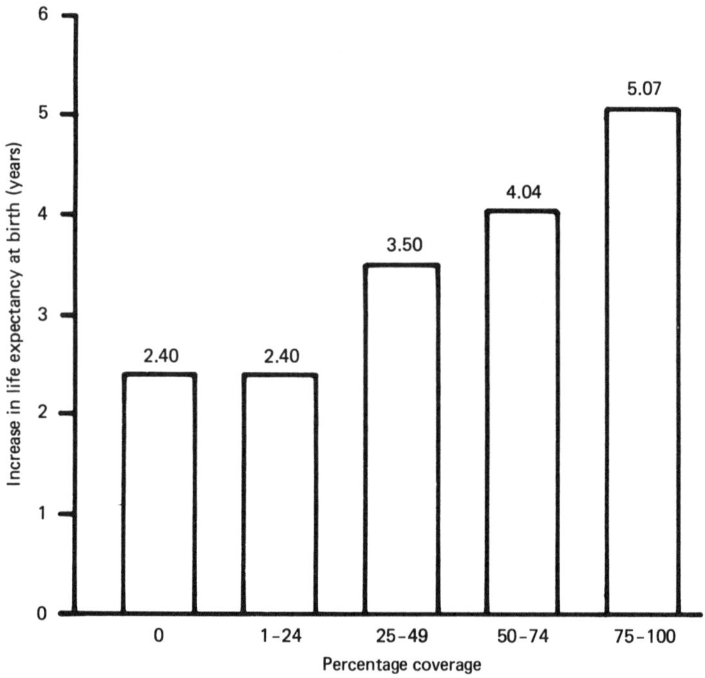

Coverage with immunizations was measured by means of a survey of a sample of children aged 12–14 months in 1979; the levels found were as follows:

Measles — rubella	68.9%
Poliomyelitis — third dose	73.5%
DPT — third dose	74.2%

Was the immunization programme effective? The recent trends of the corresponding diseases suggest that it was, as the following figures indicate.

	Incidence per 100 000 population		Mortality per 100 000 population	
	1970	1978	1970	1978
Measles	267.1	17.1	14.0	0.2
Pertussis	71.6	4.4	2.8	0.1
Diphtheria	3.3	0.0	0.9	0.0
Poliomyelitis	1.3	0.0	0.1	0.0

This evidence is supported by the more detailed analysis of trends made by the Ministry from year to year.

Efficiency of the System

The efficiency of the system is a comparative or relative concept, in the sense that a system or an activity is said to be more efficient than another one if its costs per unit of effect or per unit of activity are lower. Therefore, in measuring efficiency, ratios of costs to activities or to effects are compared among different systems that produce the same types of activity or effect.

Thus there are two categories of efficiency: one relating to the unit costs of the activities or outputs, which is purely economic and administrative; and the other relating to the unit costs of effects or outcomes, which includes consideration of the factors discussed in the previous section. Comparing ratios of cost to effect for various technologies is the method of choice for arriving at a decision, but this is unfortunately not always available.

It has been rightly stressed that high economic efficiency (minimization of the cost of activities) is useless if the resources are not being used in the most effective way to achieve the goals of the system. If a high percentage of patients admitted to hospital has diseases that should not occur given adequate preventive services, then the health system as a whole is both ineffective and inefficient, no matter what the cost per patient-day or the cure rate of the (avoidable) cases may be.

These two categories are obviously related. Fig. 4 is an attempt to show these relationships and to indicate the basic determinants of the two categories of unit costs.

As depicted, three factors determine the unit costs of the activities:

— the costs of the various resources (remunerations, cost of supplies and facilities) that are used to produce the activities;

— the proportion in which different resources, at different prices, are combined to produce the activities; for instance the unit cost will rise if highly qualified (and expensive) staff are used, inappropriately, to do simple activities; and

— the productivity of the combination of resources used, expressed as the number of activities produced by one unit of the resource combination (such as the number of houses sprayed per spray team per day).

The unit cost of the effects depends, in turn, on the unit cost of the activities and on the number of activity units required to produce one unit of effect. This number is a consequence of the effectiveness of the intervention selected. For example, the unit cost of avoiding one death from measles through an immunization campaign carried out in a given context is the result of multiplying two factors: the cost of vaccinating one child and the average number of children that must be vaccinated in order to avoid one death.

A second look at these factors will reveal that administration and programming underlie all the determinants of efficiency.

Fig. 4. Unit costs of activities and of effects: their connection and determinants

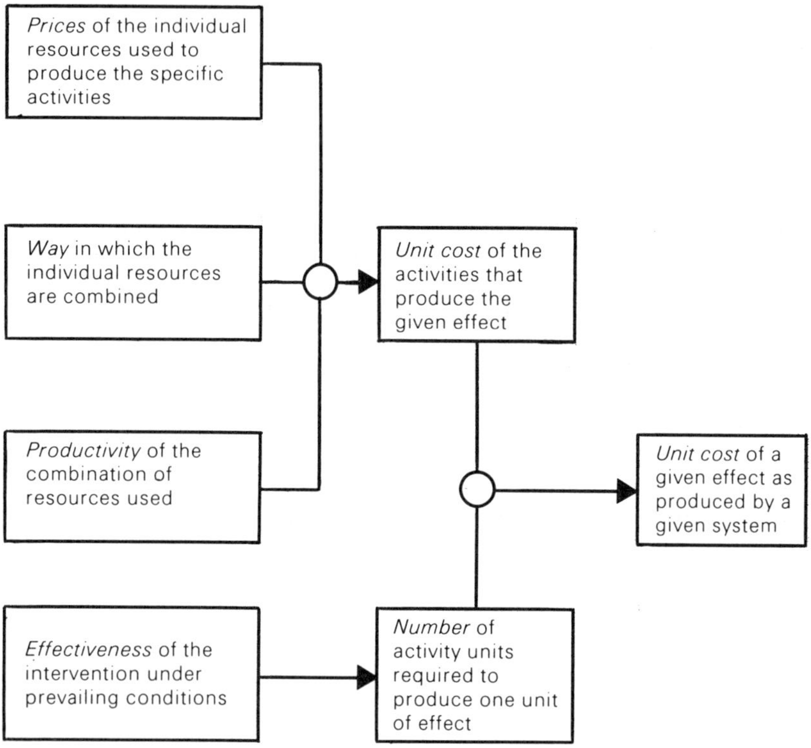

The concept of efficiency as presented here is an elaboration of the definitions offered by WHO *(2)*. It is easy to understand that there are very confusing variations in definitions and use of the term. Some authors use it only in the sense of cost/effect ratio; others use it only as cost/activities ratio; still others equate it with productivity or with skill in the use of resources, or with effectiveness. Knox *(8)* describes this confusion: "The concepts of cost-efficiency, cost-effectiveness, cost–benefit, borrowed from other contexts, are frequently used in ways which are mutually inconsistent . . .".

The concept of effect and the main questions related to it have already been considered. The other key concept, cost, deserves further examination before concluding this section on efficiency.

First the question should be posed: which costs? For the sake of simplicity, the above definitions took into account only organizational economic costs. In some circumstances, however, it may be necessary to extend the measurement of costs, for example, to include the economic costs for the users of health services, not only for fees, but for transport or for remuneration lost. There may be hidden costs in terms of subsidies provided to an activity from outside the health budget. Negative side effects on health of the interventions used should be taken into account. There may also be social costs, such as having to forgo the benefits that would arise from expenditure to boost industrialization, employment or housing. Political costs have obviously been taken into account in the past when deciding on health measures such as fluoridation or the use of traditional medicine.

The policy issue of equity crops up as a demand for information on the health care system. For whom are the costs incurred? Average per caput expenditures or costs give a general measure of the national effort, and even an idea of the national efficiency. Within a given country, however, it would also be useful to know whether the cost is borne in equal measure by all the population, or more by one group than another, and through which mechanisms *(9)*.

Structure and Content of the Health Care System

When problems are found in one or more of the three parameters analysed so far — coverage, effectiveness and efficiency — the first explanations may be looked for in the resources of the system and in the orientation of their organization and management. Is this orientation in line with the health policy stated by the country or region concerned? For example, is sufficient emphasis being placed on the application of primary health care principles such as equity, community participation, cooperation with other sectors for health promotion (cf. Chapter 8.6) and the assignment of priority to preventive activities?

In this regard, the way in which resources are allocated to the different levels and programmes of the system is of paramount importance. The indicators suggested by WHO at global *(10)* or regional *(11,12)* levels for measuring this aspect include the following:

- the percentage of national health expenditure devoted to local health care (first-level contact); and
- the proportion of different types of staff such as doctors and nurses working in primary health care.

Such measurements may also be calculated separately by population group or geographical area as appropriate, to assist in the assessment of equity and accessibility of services. When assessing these structural aspects of health care, particular attention should be addressed to the "district" or "area" units of territory and population in which most of the basic health and development needs should be met.

An essential prerequisite of appropriate provision of services is the development and availability of health care workers who are socially motivated and technically competent to carry out the tasks required to implement the policy. In this respect the simplest indicators are the ratios of personnel to population, but also the quality of the human resources and the support that they receive should be evaluated. The education of health workers may be assessed, as suggested by Katz *(13)*, in terms of the contents of the courses; their immediate results as regards knowledge, attitudes and skills; their long-term influence on the delivery of health care; and their ultimate effect on the health status of the population.

Measurement of the availability and accessibility of other essential resources, such as essential drugs, well maintained basic equipment and decent facilities, is also a necessary component of the evaluation of the structure of a health care system. This should be complemented by certain indicators of the adequacy of the organization and management of the system.

The explanation of the performance of the system should also go beyond the services themselves and take into account their environment. This includes the physical, demographic, social, economic, political and cultural contexts, all of which influence the health problems to be solved, the contents of the health policy, the availability of financial resources, the structure of the services, the morale of the staff, and the types of demands of the consumers. More specifically, two elements from the context should be carefully assessed with regard to current health policies: the involvement of countries and the close cooperation of all the main sectors dealing with the multiple causes and risk factors of priority health problems.

More and more people have realized that improved health status cannot be achieved without a great deal of involvement of the community to which services are directed. Taking health to the people, using the community's wants, and establishing health services that meet the community's cultural background are basic principles to which any positive indicator of community participation should refer *(14)*.

Community participation in health contributes both to health resources and to the effectiveness of health care. In addition, it is in itself the fulfilment of a policy principle, equity, that must be respected while striving for the most affordable and effective coverage. The extent and nature of community participation is thus a relevant measure in any consideration of the appropriate provision and management of services, it may be in any or all of the areas of policy determination, resource provision and health care delivery. Community participation does have a cost, although in budgetary terms this may be small. In health care delivery, for example, this would be mainly for training volunteers and for kits to enable them to function; such costs are usually accurately known.

Health education is closely related to the participation of the community. To a large extent it should be measured by its effects in terms of the number of people who have improved their health awareness and their behaviour in avoiding risks, caring for themselves and seeking help when appropriate. Coverage with health education activities may also be monitored and has been discussed earlier in this chapter.

The number of existing community groups such as health committees, neighbours' associations and Red Cross and other groups have been used as indicators of active community organization through which explicit health policy goals leading to improved health status may be implemented.

A study of the evaluation of a primary health and welfare programme in Cali, Colombia *(15)* provides an example of how some features of a given community might be used to predict the extent to which that community is likely to respond favourably to a health promotion effort. Characteristics such as internal organization, representativeness and democracy in the selection of the members of some community organizations condition the response of the whole community to attempts from health service staff to promote health. Those criteria were applied in the Cali programme to classify seven different community groups as strong, fair or poor as far as their organization was concerned. Since the aim of the programme was to mobilize the community for health improvement, those organizations classified as strong or fair were more likely to contribute to the programme, not only with physical resources, but also to the supplementary food programme and to the process of selection and training of community health workers *(15)*.

The collaboration of various sectors and institutes, with the aim of controlling the causes, risk factors and consequences of ill health, is best understood in the context of community participation and government support in local (district) areas, but it is also relevant at the national level and in international cooperation. The indicators for measuring progress in this important aspect may refer to the existence of health-related services provided by other sectors, to the establishment of mechanisms for co-ordination or, most important, to the processes and outcomes of multi-sectoral collaborative efforts aimed at the control of priority health problems *(11)*.

Conclusion

This discussion has centred around four important aspects of the health care system: coverage, effects, efficiency, and structure and content. Measurement of each of these four aspects is essential to any evaluation of the appropriate provision and management of services. However, if not all the required information is available, indicators for one parameter may be used as a partial proxy for another one: for example, the spatial distribution of coverage may to some extent be "represented" by the spatial distribution of facilities. Following a definition of the concepts used, various simple measures of each have been introduced and discussed, and, where possible, their use was illustrated with examples. In many places the discussion has been rather abstract, with guidelines on the desired properties of the measures required. Specific measurement instruments must be designed to fit the particular conditions in which they are used, and thus an exhaustive catalogue of possibilities is neither possible nor appropriate here.

References

1. *National assessments of health care coverage and of its effectiveness and efficiency: report and main lessons of a WHO collaborative study.* Geneva, World Health Organization, 1983 (SHS/83.7).

2. *Indicators for monitoring progress towards health for all.* Geneva, World Health Organization, 1981 ("Health for All" Series, No. 4).
3. **White, K.L. et al.** *Health services: concepts and information for national planning and management.* Geneva, World Health Organization, 1977 (Public Health Papers, No. 67).
4. *Alma Ata 1978 — Primary health care.* Geneva, World Health Organization, 1978 ("Health for All" Series, No. 1).
5. **Mobarak, A.B. et al.** *Study on coverage, effectiveness and efficiency of rural health delivery services in Egypt:* report on a WHO Collaborative Project, June 1979.
6. *Health programme evaluation.* Geneva, World Health Organization, 1981 ("Health for All" Series, No. 6).
7. **Ministerio de Salud, Unidad Sectorial de Planificación.** *Plan Nacional de Salud 1979-1982. Segunda Parte: AnSlisis de Cobertura, Eficacia y Eficiencia de los Servicios de Salud.* San José, 1979.
8. **Knox, E.G., ed.** *Epidemiology in health care planning.* Oxford, Oxford Medical Publications, 1979.
9. **Abel-Smith, B. & Leiserson, A.** *Poverty, development and health policy.* Geneva, World Health Organization, 1978 (Public Health Papers, No. 69).
10. *Development of indicators for monitoring progress towards health for all by the year 2000.* Geneva, World Health Organization, 1981.
11. *Targets for health for all.* Copenhagen, WHO Regional Office for Europe, 1985.
12. **Mya, D.Y.** Development and use of regional indicators for evaluation and monitoring progress towards health for all by the year 2000 in the WHO South-East Asia Region. *In:* Van Eimeren, W. et al., ed. *Proceedings of the Third International Conference on System Science in Health Care, Munich, July 16–20 1984.* Berlin, Springer Verlag, 1984.
13. **Katz, F.M.** *Guidelines for evaluating a training programme for health personnel.* Geneva, World Health Organization, 1978 (WHO Offset Publication No. 38).
14. **King, M.** *Medical care in developing countries.* London, Oxford University Press, 1966.
15. **Rojas, O.I.** *Evaluation of the Primary Health and Welfare Programme in Cali, Colombia.* Thesis. London School of Hygiene and Tropical Medicine, 1981.

8.6 Health promotion as an area of priority in health policy formulation — *C. Castillo-Salgado & V. Navarro*

In recent years considerable interest has been focused on the primary prevention of disease, in which the promotion of health is a major initiative. Important documents from international organizations *(1,2)* and governments of developed and less developed countries *(3–8)* have designated the promotion of health as a valuable alternative for coping with both present and emerging health problems in industrialized and economically dependent societies.

The acceptance of health promotion as an important health strategy carries with it the need for the conceptualization, recognition, identification and designation of indicators or observable conditions. This allows the quantification and measurement of different activities, outcomes and processes related to the primary prevention interventions of health promotion. Therefore, the conceptualization of health promotion and the use of its principal components are logical steps towards the application of this health intiative in concrete programmes.

Part of this concern is the analysis of the issues involved in the process of forming policies for health promotion. At present the health status of the people of the world is affected by many socioeconomic and political developments that need to be taken into account in health promotion. Unemployment, poverty, malnutrition, lack of public services and high military spending are some of the major threats to health and health promotion throughout the world.

Equally important are the limitations of the current over-emphasis on self-care, self-reliance and individual responsibility for health as basic strategies of health promotion without the implementation of social and environmental change in society.

Meaning and Scope of Promotion of Health

Although the promotion of health has become an increasingly accepted strategy, it still remains an undefined concept. Most of the major documents on the subject lack a conceptual or operative definition of the specific domain of health promotion (see Chapter 1 and references *9–11*).

In this chapter, health promotion can be seen as "a combination of environmental, social, political, educational, economic, recreational and other types of activities designed to provide a healthy condition and prevent the activation and/or emergence of any disease process in individuals and collectivities" *(9)*. This definition is basically similar to that given by Noack in Chapter 1.

In general terms, this suggests that health promotion is a broad concept in which the basic components are interventions intended to maintain the health of individuals and groups. In this sense, strategies are not necessarily related to particular diseases. Health promotion activities include those to provide healthy and safe working conditions, good nutrition and adequate housing, education and recreation. These health promotion activities can be carried out on the social and environmental level and on the individual level.

Moreover, individual decisions about health are not made in a vacuum but in a highly structured social situation in which pressures favouring or opposing specific behaviour strongly influence individuals and groups. Consequently, as the health of the population has mainly been influenced by social and environmental factors, measures for coping with these influences should include environmental and social intervention. Health promotion, in order to be postulated as a major health strategy, must therefore be analysed within the historical and social contexts that determine health.

Policy Formulations of Health Promotion

The process of assessing public policies on health promotion interventions requires, as a first component, the analysis of the political system within which they will be carried out. This in turn provides the framework for health policy assessment. Another basic part is the use of a theoretical framework of reference. Without a theoretical method of organizing empirical information, the incorporation of measures of ill health with indicators of socioeconomic conditions will result in a simple collection of information rather than in a unified articulation of the critical components of the health process in different social groups.

The concept of health promotion as a basic principle of any social policy requires the explicit recognition of the following ideas.

First, any health intervention should be targeted to eliminate existing inequalities among the different groups that constitute society. Consequently, the identification of health needs in specific social groups will assist the identification of health priorities.

In other words, rather than identifying groups of diseases, or negative outcomes, intervention should be directed towards the living and working conditions of specific social groups. The search for disease and illness is only a part of intervention. Instead of organizing action around the concept of disease, the target interventions are centred on the concept of social groups and their living conditions.

With this new idea, health promotion is a comprehensive strategy that recognizes the temporal and spatial distribution of social inequity, and its first task is the identification of the groups of people at higher risk and suffering a higher prevalence of disease.

Finally, the priority assignment of health and public resources is essentially a political act that should be defined in political terms. Technical and administrative considerations assist in the political decision-making process but they do not determine it *(12)*.

Health promotion interventions should use information provided not only by the health care sector but also by the socioeconomic sector. Societies are not homogeneous entities but totalities in which some groups have limited access to proper living conditions. Consequently, they are more exposed to diverse risk factors that determine a given disease distribution. Correlating information on health conditions with information on socioeconomic conditions is a required step in identifying social groups as target populations in the formulation of health promotion priorities and intervention. The variables that are required in health policy assessment are those dealing with living conditions such as work, income, housing and access to public services.

Under these conditions the concept and use of health promotion transcend their individual and biological connotations and presuppose the identification of a variety of socioeconomic, political and environmental conditions that determine the array of health problems in a given group.

The use of the comprehensive notion of health promotion is necessary for the assessment of social priorities that respond to specific health problems. The traditional biological and individual approach of the disease-oriented notion of strategy restricts the possibilities of any improvement in the health of some social groups. Information is not yet organized so that it can be used immediately to present the specific problems of these groups.

Shortcomings of the Modes of Analysis of Health and Health Promotion

The disease-oriented approach assumes that an adequate set of indicators of ill health (morbidity and mortality), linked to demographic characteristics, can provide the information needed for the characterization of the health status of the population and consequently support the process of forming health policy. This approach has dominated research on health policy analysis in recent decades.

By contrast, an approach based on historical and social contexts presents a more dynamic analysis. It holds that the study of health conditions must first identify the political system within which they are articulated. The analysis is not centred solely on the frequency and distribution of diseases in the general population. Rather, the core of the analysis consists of identifying specific socially deprived groups within their historical and social context. The study of the living and working conditions of these groups provides the critical knowledge essential for the recognition of their health status.

In other words, the strategy of health promotion should not be directed towards identifying single diseases in the general population but rather towards identifying social groups in relation to their own social conditions and, within these groups, the distribution of health conditions. Substantial differences in health status are constantly reported among different population groups. In the United States, for example, the infant mortality rates for non-white infants are much higher than those for white infants.

When all infant mortality rates from different social groups in the United States are pooled, the resulting figure is 16.1 deaths per 1000 live births in 1975 and 12.6 in 1980 *(13)*. When these rates are separated by race, the rate for white infants is consistently lower (14.4 in 1975 and 11.0 in 1980) than that for black infants (26.2 in 1975 and 21.4 in 1980) *(13)*. If the disaggregation is done according to social class, the difference in health status is even higher, as shown in Table 1, in which socioeconomic characteristics go farther than demographic variables to explain the poor health of the population.

This situation is worse in less developed countries. A series of socioeconomic and health indicators is included in the World Health Organization's global strategy for health for all *(14)* (see Fig. 1). These indicators illustrate the existing disparities in both socioeconomic conditions and health conditions between developed and less developed countries. The basic health indicator of infant mortality reflects some of the inherent inequities and disparities among countries. While infant mortality rates in developed countries have fallen to less than 20, or sometimes 10, per 1000 live births, in less developed countries this rate continues to be as high as 160 per 1000, or higher. Of 120 million children born in 1980, 12 million died before their first birthday. Fig. 2 illustrates the unequal worldwide distribution of infant deaths. In addition, there is a consistent pattern of disproportionate distribution of economic progress among and within countries, in favour of higher income groups that form a relatively small proportion of the world population. Some concrete figures on poverty provide a global framework of the world's socioeconomic conditions and account for the type of priorities and commitment to health and health promotion made by many nations.

Poverty

There is clearly a consensus about the overall negative impact of poverty on the health status of the population. Also of central concern are the extent, distribution and worldwide growth of poverty. By 1980 over 800 million people in the world were living in absolute poverty. Striking economic disparities among countries are reflected by current national income patterns. In 1979 the average gross national product (GNP) per capita in developed countries was US $7900 and US $740 in all developing countries *(15)*. According to the World Bank, by 1980 the GNP per capita in the world was distributed in the following categories:

— 19 developed countries with an average GNP per capita of US $6658 (at their 1975 value);

— 63 countries of middle income with an average GNP per capita of US $903;

— 33 countries of low income with an average GNP per capita of US $168.

In other words, the gap between the richest countries and the poorest countries in terms of the GNP per capita is equal to more than 40 times

Table 1. Percentages of those reported as in poor health in the 1975 health interview survey, USA

Demographic characteristic	Age				
	All ages	Under 15 years	15–44 years	45–64 years	65 years and over
Sex					
Male	2.8	0.5	1.3	6.4	9.5
Female	2.8	0.4	1.6	5.4	8.1
Colour					
White	2.6	0.4	0.1	5.3	7.9
Other	4.4	0.9	2.6	10.8	16.5
Family income					
Under US $5 000	7.9	1.1	4.1	17.8	12.3
US $5 000 to US $9 999	3.4	0.5	1.8	8.5	6.8
US $10 000 to US $14 999	1.5	0.4	0.9	3.9	5.1
US $15 000 and over	1.0	0.2	0.7	1.8	5.9

Source: Data from National Center for Health Statistics: Health United States 1975.

Fig. 1. Health and related socioeconomic indicators[a]

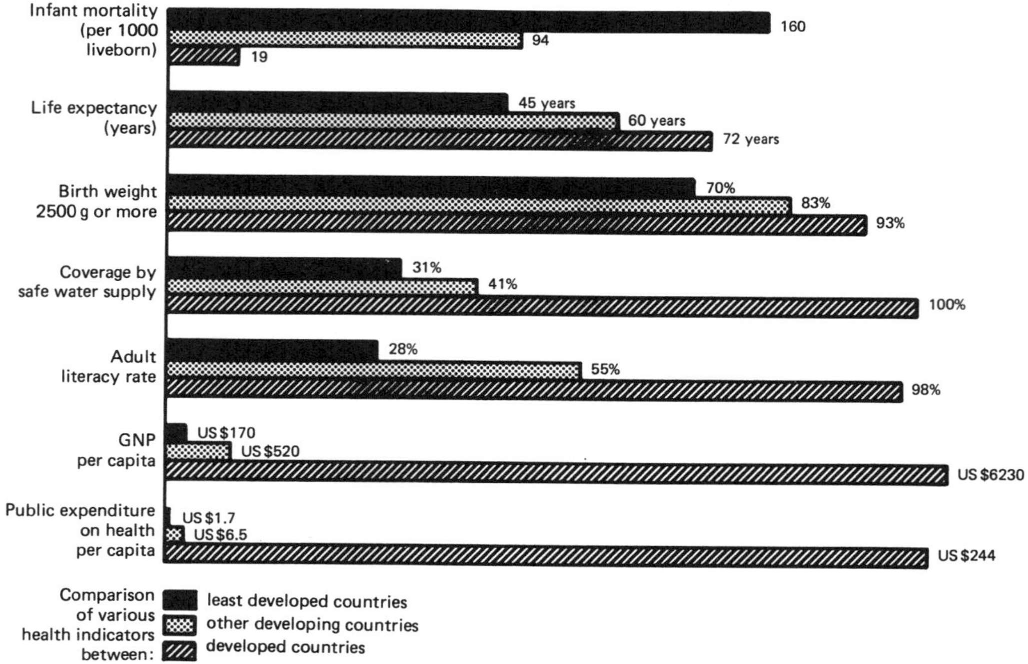

[a] Weighted average based on data for 1980 or latest available year.

Source: **World Health Organization** *(14)*.

Fig. 2. Infant deaths

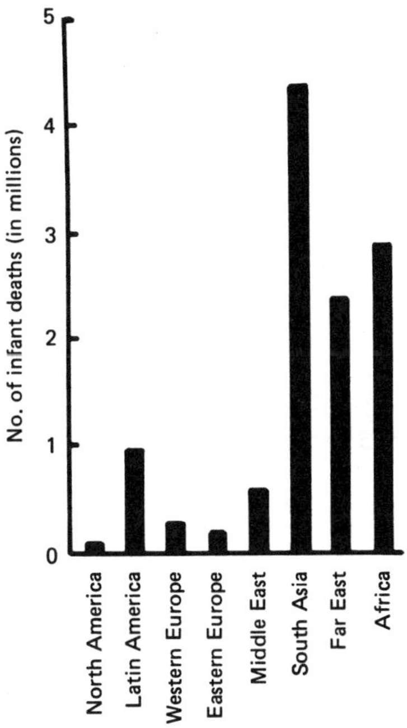

Note: Of 120 million babies born in 1981, 12 million died before their first birthday.

Source: **Sivard, R.L.** *(15).*

the GNP of the poorest countries. Table 2 illustrates these inequalities in terms of GNP and other measures.

The economic gap between countries can also be measured in terms of the number of years required by the less developed countries to reach the 1980 gross domestic product (GDP) per capita of the developed countries. For instance, if economic relations do not change, the less developed countries will not be able to reach the 1980 GDP per capita of the Federal Republic of Germany until the year 6508, or to reach the United States 1980 GDP per capita until 6007. These figures give grounds for genuine concern because, to eliminate the current economic gap, less developed countries would need several thousand years to reach the present level of GDP of the developed countries. This gap is the social cost of current worldwide economic relations as well as the economic structures within each country.

On the other hand, economic disparities within countries, particularly the poorest, seem even more extreme and inequitable. Such internal inequities and disparities also appear within developed countries. Recent figures estimate that 25 million people in the United States live below the

Table 2. The development gap, 1978

	Richest fifth of the world's population	Poorest fifth of the world's population
GNP per capita in US $	7718	163
Government education expenditure per capita in US $	429	4
Teachers per 1000 children	38	12
Percentage of literate adults	97	37
Government health expenditure per capita in US $	327	2
Physicians per 10 000 people	20	2
Life expectancy in years	72	50
Infant deaths per 100 births	2	14
Calories per capita as a percentage of requirements	120	86
Percentage of the population with safe water	95	31

Source: **Sivard, R.L.** *(15)*.

poverty line and, if the economic and health policies of the current administration continue, this figure will increase substantially. These economic disparities help to determine social differences, not only in deleterious living conditions but also in premature death. The richest fifth of the world's population lives 22 years longer, on average, than the poorest fifth *(15)*.

With this information in mind, any discussion on health promotion must take into consideration the socioeconomic conditions in these countries. The most important health promotion interventions are the political, economic and social activities aimed at changing these conditions.

Methodological Aspects of Measuring Health and Health Promotion

The emerging pattern of concern about promoting health in society has revitalized discussion about the idea of positive health and the new directions in the measurement of health and health promotion. The selection of suitable indicators of health and health promotion depends on the accepted definition of and basic postulates about these concepts. Accordingly, the individual lifestyle approach stresses the importance of individual-based indicators and promotes the establishment or implementation of health information systems that use indicators of changes in personal health habits as major components of health promotion interventions.

In the social and environmental approach, health promotion can be defined as a social and political strategy that provides a wide range of interventions (not only of a behavioural nature), conducive to the preservation and maintenance of the health status of the population, as well as to limiting the emergence of preventable diseases. Health promotion interventions emphasize the positive dimension of the health process. Because health and health promotion are complex categories that correlate with the quality of living and working conditions of the population, most of the indicators and measurable conditions of health promotion are linked to these components. Individual behaviour integrated in its social context is not, however, disregarded in this approach of health promotion. Behavioural components play a role in the development of ill health and in the maintenance of health status. They are not isolated elements in the social area but integrated in a complex network of economic, ecological and social conditions that mark the relationship between society and health.

In this approach, indicators of health promotion are measuring instruments that either describe or help to explain the particular process of a concrete social group in terms of the mediating structures (social, economic, political and ecological) that affect the ability of that group to maintain its health. The promotion of health in society is thus a preventive strategy that should be measured by accounting for the different social, economic and political mediating or determinant structures of health.

Regulation and Provision of Preventive and Curative Health Care Services

Among the important issues in the provision of health care services and health promotion activities is the notion that health and health care are the rights of all citizens. This concept involves the idea that care for the sick and the promotion of positive health are major public responsibilities. Issues in health and health care policies have long been of extraordinary importance and political concern. Major positive strategies such as health promotion have been influenced by both political and economic interests. As a consequence, the interpretation of health and health promotion has been affected by political forces involved not only in the health sector but also outside that sector. All national health policies are syntheses of power networks that define the boundaries and content of health promotion. Therefore, how health rights are being defined, by whom, and how they are implemented are important areas for describing and analysing health promotion. Legislation, constitutional provisions and health regulations are fundamental sources of information from which the political commitment of a government to the nation's health can be evaluated. Specific indicators of this commitment are:

(*a*) a declaration that health and health care are constitutional rights of citizens, that have a right to health and health care services regardless of the ability to pay;

(*b*) the adoption of universal, comprehensive and free national health services;

(*c*) the adoption of occupational health and safety legislation;

(*d*) the adoption of environmental and consumer protection laws;

(*e*) the adoption of right-to-know legislation;

(*f*) the adoption and enforcement of laws against the production and sale of health-threatening substances and products such as tobacco, asbestos, alcohol and vinyl chloride;

(*g*) the adoption of the prevention model of health and health care services; and

(*h*) the adoption of democratic procedures for popular participation in health promotion.

Indicators of Public Policy Priorities

Public expenditure provides one of the most obvious and important statements of the political goals and priorities of a nation. The comparison of the relative priorities, measured by public expenditure, assigned to defence, education and health is a useful measure of public policy for the promotion of health. The governmental budgetary allocation to health is a measure of social commitment to public health policy. A comparison between defence and health spending as proportions of GNP gives readable information about a government's commitment to health. It may also provide a way of classifying nations according to the commitment to health of the administration in power. Public health expenditure and proportionate spending on primary prevention interventions are another indicator of government commitment to the health of the nation. An important indicator of commitment to health promotion is the proportion of the health budget directed to preventive action and to research on prevention.

An exceptionally rapid increase in military expenditure in developing countries has been one of the most striking characteristics of public policy in recent years. Since 1960, military expenditure in the developing world has increased fourfold, while that in developed countries has gone up 44% *(16)*.

A review of the world's allocation of public funds raises serious concerns about the prospects for welfare and health in the world. Budget priorities show a persistent trend towards military expansion at the expense of social services such as health and education. Tables 3 and 4 and Fig. 3 provide summary information that illustrates the use of world resources for social and for military purposes. A critical difference between military expenses

Table 3. Military and social trends: world, developed and developing countries, 1961 and 1979

	1961	Value in 1978 US $	1979	Value in 1978 US $
Military expenditure (in millions of US $)				
World	102 000	262 000	360 000	400 000
Developed countries	92 000	237 000	280 000	310 000
Developing countries	10 000	25 000	80 000	90 000
Armaments exports (in millions of US $)				
World	2 400		19 000	
Developed countries	2 300		18 000	
Developing countries	100			
Armaments imports (in millions of US $)				
World	2 400		19 000	
Developed countries	1 300		5 000	
Developing countries	1 100		14 000	
GNP (in millions of US $)				
World	1 550 000	3 985 000	7 910 000	8 693 000
Developed countries	1 273 000	3 296 000	6 079 000	6 715 000
Developing countries	277 000	689 000	1 831 000	1 978 000
GNP per capita (in millions of US $)				
World	502 000	1 291 000	1 870 000	2 055 000
Developed countries	1 430 000	3 703 000	5 893 000	6 509
Developing countries	126 000	314 000	572 000	618 000
Population (in millions)				
World	3 093		4 240	
Developed countries	890		1 032	
Developing countries	2 203		3 208	
Armed forces (in thousands)				
World	18 960		23 181	
Developed countries	10 056		9 516	
Developing countries	8 904		13 665	
Physicians (in thousands)				
World	1 723		3 332	
Developed countries	1 265		2 228	
Developing countries	458		1 104	
Teachers (in thousands)				
World	15 149		27 446	
Developed countries	6 814		9 479	
Developing countries	8 355		17 967	

Source: **Sivard, R.L.** *(15).*

Table 4. Comparative resources, 1978

	Military (in millions of US $)	Education (in millions of US $)	Health (in millions of US $)	Armed forces (in thousands)
World	*418 209*	*474 450*	*326 282*	*23 817*
Developed countries	321 267	396 986	294 789	9 485
Developing countries	96 942	77 464	31 493	14 332
America				
North America	113 336	139 660	85 520	2 149
Latin America	7 431	18 139	7 068	1 139
Europe				
NATO Europe	76 644	112 654	112 811	2 678
Other Europe	11 119	24 792	21 959	801
Warsaw Pact	115 025	63 780	32 370	4 733
USSR	703 000	49 460	21 330	3 638
All NATO (including Canada and USA)	189 980	252 314	198 331	4 827
Asia				
Middle East	31 517	13 736	4 098	1 679
South Asia	4 713	4 056	1 584	1 792
Far East	46 424	77 470	52 916	7 789
Japan	9 211	56 130	44 730	240
China	26 000	15 000	5 900	4 325
Oceania	3 271	8 610	5 530	87
Africa	8 729	11 553	2 426	1 020

Source: **Sivard, R.L.** *(15).*

and budgets for health and education is that the social budget is directly related to the requirements of an increasing population and military expenses are not. According to data presented by Sivard *(15)*, the following statements reflect current public budget priorities.

- Military expenditure has now reached an estimated US $550 000 million annually. This is more than the annual income of the 2000 million people in the world's poorest countries.
- Between 1960 and 1980, the regular armed forces in developing countries rose from 8.7 to 15.1 million men. They now represent over 60% of the world total.

Top of page here.

Physicians (in thousands)	Teachers (in thousands)	GNP (in millions of US $)	
3 437.7	*28 477*	*9 279 213*	*World*
2 274.0	9 536	7 203 577	Developed countries
1 163.7	18 941	2 075 636	Developing countries
			Amcrica
943.2	2 703	2 333 378	North America
238.7	2 928	482 328	Latin America
			Europe
548.8	2 881	2 127 425	NATO Europe
156.4	710	483 867	Other Europe
1 107.5	3 018	1 394 939	Warsaw Pact
905.0	2 309	967 820	USSR
992.0	5 584	4 460 803	All NATO (including Canada and USA)
			Asia
80.4	862	254 803	Middle East
208.6	3 800	150 830	South Asia
584.5	9 760	1 670 463	Far East
139.0	850	1 028 231	Japan
258.5	6 300	424 620	China
26.6	210	135 705	*Oceania*
43.0	1 590	245 475	*Africa*

- Despite a per capita income that still averaged below US $670 in 1970, the non-OPEC developing countries spent US $64 000 million on foreign armaments between 1970 and 1979. The amount of money spent on importing armaments in these countries rose from US $3400 million in 1970 to US $10 900 million in 1979.
- On a global basis, society now invests US $16 000 a year on each soldier and US $260 a year on the education of each child.
- Worldwide, the support of national military forces costs US $92 a year per person; support of the United Nations, for all its programmes costs 57 cents a year and international peace-keeping operations, 5 cents a year.

Fig. 3. World military and other expenditures of governments, 1977

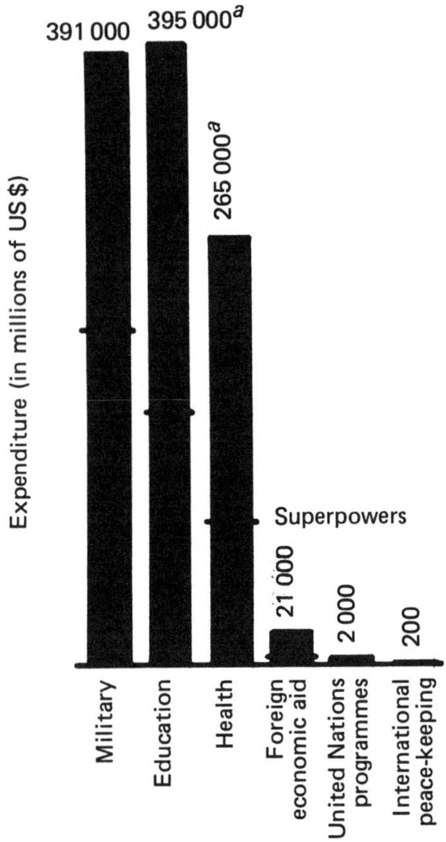

[a] Projected.

Source: **Sivard, R.L.** *(15)*.

- For the entire range of health needs, including preventive care, environmental health control and disease control, governments spent less than they did on space exploration.
- Finally, none of the top military powers stood as tall in social as in military ranking.

This global look into the current allocation policy in both industrialized and less developed countries shows that the two crucial components of government spending to be analysed are welfare and defence. The resulting problems of trade-offs between military spending and social and health investment is perhaps one of the most critical aspects of the current trend of public policies. For especially vulnerable groups, such as children, the elderly, pregnant women and people in the lower socioeconomic classes, the increase in military spending represents a real threat to both health and life, because military expenditure absorbs resources that are essential for improving their living conditions.

A recent report prepared for the United Nations Children's Fund *(17)* alludes to the major shifts in public policy and the current trends in expenditures per capita in the United States on defence and on programmes for low-income families and children (see Table 5).

This report includes a recent analysis from the US Congressional Budget Office *(18)* that shows how defence spending is increased at the expense of social programmes:

> Between 1982 and 1985 spending for national defense will increase from 25.7 per cent of the federal outlay. During the same years income security programs will decline from 11.1 to 9.4 per cent, federal expenditures for higher education will decline from 1.1 to 0.9 per cent, grants to state and local governments for education, employment and social services will decline from 2.3 to 1.9 per cent of the total federal outlay. The greatest cuts have been made in programs for poor people. *(17)*

Table 5. Per capita expenditure and projected expenditure on defence and on programmes for low-income families and children, United States, 1981–1988

Fiscal year	National defence (US $)	Programmes for low-income families and children (US $)
1981	695	416
1982	762	372
1983	825	379
1984	892	350
1985	983	342
1986	1054	334
1987	1097	327
1988	1133	325
Actual change, 1981-1988	+ US $438	- US $91
Percentage change, 1981-1988	+ 63.0%	- 21.9%

Source: **Miller, C. et al.** *(17)*.

A critical aspect of this change in public policy is the resulting problem of trade-offs. Obviously, the guns-versus-health problem goes beyond the mere identification of the trade-offs. However, it is crucial to identify the locus (who pays) and weight (degree of substitution) of the burden of military allocations on other sectors, such as the health sector. An interesting study of the costs of defence in the United States between 1938 and 1969 concludes that each dollar added to defence spending resulted in a reduction of:

> forty-two cents from personal consumption spending, twenty-nine cents from fixed capital formation, ten cents from exports, five cents from federal government civilian programs and thirteen cents from state and local governments' activities *(19)*.

This analysis is consistent with the present trend of budget allocations in the United States. The area losing substantially from the trade-offs is that of health and social services. This type of analysis requires diverse data on a variety of political and economic indicators. Indicators of health and health care, isolated from the indicators of direct government allocations, cannot provide evidence of the drastic effect that these trade-offs have on the health of the population, particularly vulnerable social groups.

In general, there is a tendency in the health sector to disregard the role of political factors in the analysis of public policy choices and government decision-making about health policy. Many studies rely on summary ill-health statistics, which in many instances obscure the impact of socioeconomic conditions on the health status of the population. In addition, studies frequently do not attempt to assess the political impact on policy decisions. They should also examine the political orientation of the allocation of public expenditure. Only through the consideration of information on the different social, economic and political areas can a policy analysis of the promotion of health interventions be made.

This discussion is of great importance because, as already mentioned, in both the industrialized countries and in less developed countries disease and health are distributed highly irregularly across different social groups. Health promotion as a suitable public health strategy must be understood in the political context and the socioeconomic structure of the different groups in countries. In this sense, the evaluation of measures of health or illness cannot be done by pooling all social groups together. A more valid approach is to identify those measures according to the degree to which a given group is separated from the opportunity for appropriate living and working conditions or, in other words, according to the level of socioeconomic deprivation.

Critical common deficiencies in the directions of health policy of both developed and less developed countries must also be considered. Among these deficiencies are the following:

(*a*) government expenditure tends to focus on curative, hospital-based, somatic and biological, and personal care services rather than preventive, community-based, occupational, environmental and social services;

(*b*) there are still large numbers of vulnerable groups: the disabled, the poor, the mortally ill, the elderly, the unemployed, rural populations, and others who do not receive appropriate health care services;

(*c*) present social and health policies are not only inefficient, but also inequitable;

(*d*) no active democratic involvement by users and potential users of services occurs in the decision-making process in the health services.

Living Conditions

A national health promotion programme cannot be effective unless fundamental human needs are met. Healthy living conditions should include full employment, adequate housing, adequate family income, education, good nutrition, access to better quality health care, improved public services (such as access to potable water and the elimination of wastes), and access to cultural and recreational activities. These provide the fundamental basis for positive health and for maintaining and promoting sound health in a nation.

To illustrate this point, a brief discussion of persisting disparities in nutritional status is included here.

Nutrition

The lack of sufficient and appropriate food, a major determinant of ill health, is a critical problem in a large part of the world. In contrast, developed countries are directing their attention to the overeating and inadequate diets of their people; these problems in turn contribute to the increased frequency of chronic disorders, a major health burden in industrialized societies. On the other hand, over 25 million people in the United States are malnourished *(16)*. Fig. 1 and Fig. 4 give the comparative figures for the distribution of low birth weight and hunger in the world. As a consequence of malnourishment and maternal disorders, 21 million children are born with low birth weights every year. In the least developed countries 30% of babies have a low birth weight, in contrast to 7% in the developed countries *(14)*. Many studies have revealed a wide range of adverse effects of malnutrition on human health. A WHO study reports that every year 250 000 children go blind; 100 000 of these do so owing to a lack of vitamin A *(16)*. As reported by the Food and Agriculture Organization of the United Nations, between 450 million and 750 million people in the world are seriously malnourished *(16)*. The malnourished tend to be concentrated among the poor, the unemployed and the elderly.

This brief account of nutritional conditions in the world highlights the importance of some of the most obvious social deficiencies and inequities. For fully effective health promotion, these deficiencies and inequities need to be addressed. Health promotion interventions not responding to the basic needs of the population, such as employment, adequate nutrition, clean water, sanitation and other social services, have limited value.

Fig. 4. Hunger in developing nations[a]

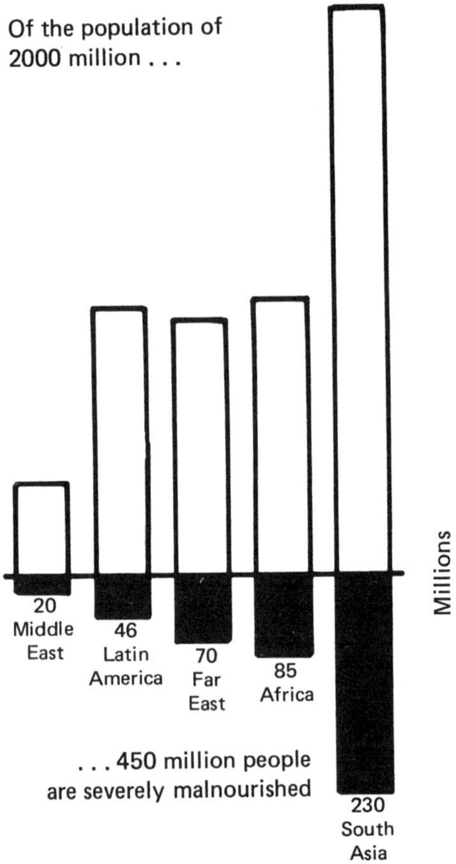

[a] Not including China and other centrally planned developing nations.

Source: **Sivard, R.L.** *(16).*

The following selected measures are examples of baseline information on the basic human needs linked to national health status.

1. The percentage of the population adequately nourished
2. The median income per family
3. The percentage of the population above subsistence level
4. The rate of employment

5. The percentage of households with drinking-water supply
6. The percentage of households with sanitation facilities
7. The ratio of people to rooms in a dwelling
8. The percentage of the population with a high-school education
9. The percentage of the elderly population with access to nursing homes or to facilities for the elderly
10. The enactment and enforcement of social security laws
11. The percentage of the population covered by medical care services
12. The percentage of families with access to social support networks
13. The percentage of families able to meet emergencies with existing funds

Use of Preventive Services as Indicators of Health Promotion

Primary prevention is the basic premise underlying health promotion. The use of preventive services is an important indication of the extent to which both the health system and the community are committed to the promotion of health. The following indicators are examples of measurements for primary prevention activities conducive to the promotion of health.

1. The percentage of children immunized against the major infectious diseases of childhood
2. The percentage of the population with access to dental health services
3. The percentage of the population using preventive services (number of prenatal visits by pregnant women, number of annual dental visits, annual check-ups in occupational settings, etc.)
4. The proportion of cities with fluoridation of the water supply
5. The proportion of television or radio programmes devoted to health promotion and health education

Health Insurance Coverage in Countries without a National Health Programme

The data gathered through such measurements as the percentage of people who can afford health insurance coverage and the percentage of people who have health insurance of any type provide insight into factors outside the health sector but with major impact in the health of the population. In the United States in the period from 1978 to 1980, 11.6% of the total population had no health insurance of any kind. If this percentage is disaggregated by ethnic groups, 8.7% of the white population, 17.8% of the black population and 25.7% of the Hispanic population have no coverage with health insurance *(20)*. Hispanics and black people are much more likely than white people to lack health insurance because of their limited ability to pay for it, and their high rates of unemployment. Consequently, the information provided by these two indicators permits the linkage of income, employment status and health insurance coverage — major determinants of the basic health status of the population.

Environmental Health Policy and Interventions as Basic Health Promotion Actions

The differences in the health status of a given population can also be attributed, in part, to risks in the living and working environment. The results of many epidemiological studies show the substantial responsibility for the rising morbidity and mortality from chronic diseases of the high levels of pollution, industrial wastes, industrial carcinogens, toxic substances and harmful physical agents present in the living and working environment *(21–25)*. A major initiative and health promotion intervention that logically emerges is the elimination and regulation of those substances, which threaten health and life.

The following indicators are some of the practices directed at providing the changes in the environment that are essential for promoting the health of individuals, groups and communities.

1. The existence and enforcement of environmental protection laws
2. The existence and enforcement of occupation and safety health laws
3. The proportion of occupational health standards that are stringent enough to fully protect the health of the worker
4. The existence of policies to eliminate hazardous conditions and toxic subtances in the work environment
5. The percentage of industries with environmental, equipment and engineering control and protection
6. The percentage of industries with more than 50 workers that have a health and safety committee with representatives of both workers and management
7. The percentage of industries that, in addition to engineering control equipment, provide personnel protection equipment to their workers
8. The percentage of industries that meet or surpass air quality standards
9. The percentage of industries that have adopted restrictive environmental monitoring for harmful substances
10. The percentage of industries that continuously provide information about the health conditions in the workplace
11. The percentage of industries in compliance with the threshold value limits for the substances that they use

12. The ratio of the total capital investment in industry and pollution control investments

13. The levels of major pollutants (carbon monoxide, hydrocarbons, nitrogen oxides) in the working and community environment

It is also worth considering indicators of enforcement of environmental or occupational health promotion activities, such as:

— the percentage of the working population with all occupational health rights, such as control over occupational health services, access to information, the option to stop work in risky conditions, and others;

— the number of occupational health and safety inspections per 100 000 workers; and

— the proportion of violations of occupational health and safety conditions that are the objects of sanctions.

The need to conceptualize the socioeconomic indicators and give them priorities does not preclude the need to consider the individual behaviour indicators. Both types of indicator should be examined together. In this area, Breslow *(26)*, using a more comprehensive approach, explains that health promotion:

> consists of all the measures that enhance the possibility of a full life, in both extent and quality. The activities of health promotion embrace steps to maintain and expand function generally and to build reserves against forces adverse to health.

Health promotion typically involves, in Breslow's interpretation, three approaches: prevention, environmental changes and behavioural modifications. Measures directed against economic and political forces adverse to health could be added, since the nature of the major threats to the health of the population is not limited to bacterial or microbial agents or personal conditions, but includes environmental, social and economic forces. These forces also account for the development of chronic diseases and the creation of barriers to health, and they should be regarded as the immediate focus of health promotion.

The greatest current opportunity to promote health is through preventive interventions that affect not only the behavioural features of living but strengthen the social and ecological environment in which they are articulated. Health promotion is a process with different components and areas of intervention. The crucial problem is the selection of the parts of that process that permit the most effective impact.

The overall picture of this process provides insight into the hierarchy of activities within health promotion. The greatest impact on the health status of a population naturally depends on the type and level of the health interventions.

Conclusions

Most of the current activities in health promotion follow a behavioural or individual model. This is insufficient to resolve many existing health problems. This behavioural model responds to a limited vision of health promotion. It ignores the socioeconomic and political context that is responsible for many of the health problems that exist today and for the types of individual behaviour that behaviourists want to change. A comprehensive health promotion programme should include different forms of intervention, not only in the individual but also in the socioeconomic and political spheres.

Health promotion as a social and public health strategy needs to be seen within the framework of public policy decisions. In this context, the analysis of health promotion interventions requires the articulation of the political components of the public decision-making process. Health promotion as a basic principle of social policy must be seen as political strategy for the assessment of social priorities that respond to the specific health needs of the population.

References

1. *Targets for health for all.* Copenhagen, WHO Regional Office for Europe, 1985.
2. *WHO regional programme in health education and lifestyles.* Copenhagen, WHO Regional Office for Europe, 1981 (unpublished document EUR/RC31/10).
3. **United States.** *The National Health Information and Health Promotion Act of 1976.*
4. **US Department of Health, Education and Welfare.** *Departmental Task Force on Disease Prevention and Health Promotion: Federal programs and prospects.* Washington, DC, US Government Printing Office, 1978.
5. **Office of Assistant Secretary for Health and Surgeon General.** *Healthy people: the Surgeon General's report on health promotion and disease prevention.* Washington, DC, US Government Printing Office, 1979 (DHEW Publication No. (PHS) 79-5007).
6. **Department of Health and Human Services.** *Public health services: promoting health/preventing disease. Objectives for the nation.* Washington, DC, US Government Printing Office, 1980.
7. **LaLonde, M.** *New perspective on the health of Canadians. A working document.* Ottawa, Government of Canada, 1974.
8. **Ministry of Health and Social Affairs.** *Health in Sweden. The Swedish health services in the 1990s.* Stockholm, National Board of Health and Welfare, 1982 (HS90).
9. **Castillo-Salgado, C.** Assessing recent developments and opportunities in the promotion of health in the American workplace. *Social science and medicine,* **19**(4): 349–358 (1984).
10. **Terris, M.** Epidemiology as a guide to health policy. *Annual review of public health,* **1**(7): 323–344 (1980).

11. **Wenzel, E.** Health promotion and lifestyles. *International journal of health education,* **1**(January): 57–60 (1983).
12. **Organizacion Panamericana de la Salud.** *OMS notas sobre las implicacions de la meta SPT/2000.* Programa de Desarrollo de Sistemas de Salud, 1983 (Documento Borrador HSS-1983).
13. **US Department of Health and Human Services.** *Health and prevention profile, United States, 1983.* Hyattsville, MD, Department of Health and Human Services, 1984 (DHSS Publication No. (PHS) 84-1232).
14. *Global strategy for health for all by the year 2000.* Geneva, World Health Organization, 1981 ("Health for All" Series, No. 3).
15. **Sivard, R.L.** World military and social expenditures. *In: World priorities.* Leesburg, VA, 1981.
16. **Sivard, R.L.** World military and social expenditures. *In: World priorities.* Leesburg, VA, 1979.
17. **Miller, C. et al.** The world economic crisis and the children: United States case study. *International journal of health services,* **15**: 95–134 (1985).
18. **Congressional Budget Office.** *Major legislative changes in human resources programs since January 1981.* Washington, DC, Congress of the United States, 1983.
19. **Russett, B.M.** *What price vigilance?* New Haven, Yale University Press, 1970.
20. *Health and prevention profile.* Hyattsville, MD, Department of Health and Human Services, 1983 (DHHS Publication No. (OHS) 84-1232).
21. **Tomatis, L. et al.** Evaluation of the carcinogenicity of chemicals: a review of the IARC monograph program. *Cancer research,* **38**: 877–885 (1978).
22. **Davis, D.L. et al.** Cancer prevention: assessing causes, exposures and recent trends in mortality for US males, 1968–1978. *International journal of health services,* **13**(3): 337–372 (1983).
23. **McKinlay, J.B. & McKinlay, S.M.** The questionable contribution of medical measures to the decline of mortality in the United States in the twentieth century. *Milbank Memorial Fund quarterly,* **55**(3): 405–428 (1977).
24. **Davis, D.L. & Rall, D.P.** Risk assessment for disease prevention. *In:* Ng Lky & Davis, D.L., ed. *Promoting health and preventing disease.* New York, Van Nostrand & Reinhold, 1981.
25. **Fraumeni, J.F.** Epidemiologic approaches to cancer etiology. *Annual review of public health,* **3**: 88–105 (1982).
26. **Breslow, L.** The potential of health promotion. *In:* Mechanic, D., ed. *Handbook of health, health care and the health professions.* New York, Free Press, 1983, pp. 50–55.

9. Information strategy as a basis for measuring health promotion and protection

V.D.L. Carstairs & M.A. Heasman

Categories of Information Relevant to Health Promotion and Protection

A wide variety of measures are described and illustrated in this book; among these particular categories of information may be identified:

(*a*) traditional (negative) measures of mortality and illness that may nevertheless be expressed in a positive format;

(*b*) service provision and the use of services aimed at health promotion and disease prevention;

(*c*) physiological (objective) measures of health status;

(*d*) self-reported (subjective) measures of health status;

(*e*) behaviour that has implications for health;

(*f*) physical, biological and social aspects of the environment that influence health;

(*g*) attitudes of the population towards management of health, including community participation; and

(*h*) decisions, action and legislation at governmental level that indicate priorities or determination to pursue the path of health promotion.

The variety of data that fall into this framework covers a much wider landscape than is normal for health information services. Their role has traditionally been restricted to a narrow view of health service resources, contacts and activity (and in some cases costs), rather than the extended panorama of health status, health behaviour and promotional activity that emerges in this volume. Any information service that seeks fully to support the measurement of health promotion and protection will need to adopt strategies that extend beyond documenting resources and the use of health services. Some of the traditional material may nevertheless be harnessed to this approach.

Traditional measures positively expressed

Data that report contacts with health services, as well as mortality, tend to present a picture of disease, disability and death. These are mainly interpreted as deficits in health. Falls in death rates over time nevertheless represent gains in health, as do increases in expectation of life, and the presentation of data in this manner is well established. Years of life lost is a measure more recently derived, and less familiar, but useful particularly to give additional weight to deaths occurring at younger ages. An indication of life expectancy free of disability is illustrated by Colvez (Chapter 11.8) and more sophisticated measures by Schach (Chapter 7.7). These measures may be calculated at a national level or for groups within the population. For flexibility in analysis, the development of easy retrieval systems is essential to meet the needs of users, as is the existence of complete and reliable vital statistics. These are by no means universally available and the determination of population size and numbers of births and of deaths must sometimes be obtained by indirect methods. Primary health care workers may be used to provide such information; van Lerberghe (Chapter 13.7) refers to the provision of population counts by a system of reporting based on visits by nurses to all families in a target area, which permits the derivation of population-based measures, while Blom (Chapter 13.1) illustrates the way in which a survival index may be calculated through a count of children still alive in relation to the numbers born to a mother.

The sentinel health events approach outlined by Rutstein (Chapter 7.6) also relies on routine recording of mortality or morbidity as a means of identifying unnecessary or avoidable events, and provides both a tool for inquiry that may lead to improvements in health and a measure to monitor whether such improvements are taking place. The application of this method in Britain, as illustrated by Charlton (Chapter 11.7) focuses on an analysis of deaths that might have been avoided by suitable and timely treatment; it shows comparative rates for subgroups of the population and provides an example of the selective use of the causes that Rutstein identified as avoidable. A further process of inquiry is necessary to search out the reasons for such deaths. While a few such inquiries, such as those conducted on maternal mortality in the United Kingdom *(1)*, have developed models in which the process of investigation is built into the data collection, it is unlikely that this approach can be used except when the number of events is relatively few.

Health service provision and use

Records of health service use generally relate to the sick members of society and do not, on the whole, lend themselves to measuring health promotion and protection. There are, nevertheless, exceptions to this general rule. Data may be available, for instance, on the use of services that prevent disease or promote health. Such data will identify the proportion of the population using the services (immunization, family planning and antenatal care, screening and early diagnosis) and thus provide a measure of the population's commitment to health promotion, as well as the success of campaigns to encourage their participation.

Considerations of equity also imply a need for information on the level of resources and the kinds of service available to monitor the provision of appropriate services to different subgroups in a population in relation to their needs. Such data will identify the balance between resources provided at primary care level compared to institutional services.

State of health

Routine systems

Changes in health status cannot usually be inferred from contacts that relate to treatment: hospital episode-based systems rarely provide information on individuals that may be used for epidemiological analysis, although systems that link the episodes for an individual may be able to identify first admissions. Disease registers overcome some of these problems by creating a record for an individual and may include patients seen at the primary care level as well as in hospital, but they are limited in giving information only about specific causes of ill health. Trend data from these sources, of which cancer registers are the most common, may be used to identify changes in the incidence of specific diseases, although the completeness of registration has always to be considered in interpreting these data. Where it is possible to link a subsequent death with the disease event, the system provides a basis for measuring changes in survival.

Few developed countries collect information on patient contacts at the primary care level on a routine basis, except where primary care practitioners are paid on a fee-for-service basis and where data collected via sample surveys mainly relate to patient-initiated contacts with the health services. In countries where primary care is the main resource for the delivery of health care, opportunities may exist to seek a more complete perspective of the health problems of a community. Data collection, however, is a luxury and systems to provide information should normally make use of the records required to support the delivery and functioning of a service. Van Lerberghe et al. (Chapter 13.7) report on an individual summary record completed at the health centre level in Kasongo, Zaïre; intended as an aid to individual patient management, aggregated data provide information on health problems and health care delivery. A sentinel information system based on volunteer health workers' reports of cases of specific diseases is described by Basu & Sokhey (Chapter 11.10). Cox *(2)* also describes some simple methods, such as mapping, to identify the location of specific problems; and the use of a tally sheet, with precise instructions for completion, to carry out small epidemiological inquiries. These low cost methods can rarely be used to estimate absolute levels of disease, but may be adequate to show trends in disease incidence and to provide an early warning of an increase in disease occurrence or to monitor a reduction. A number of the contributions thus describe methods that may be adopted or adapted for use in countries with few resources available for information collection.

Physiological measures
Measures of health status that refer to a total population require information from those not using services, as well as those who do, and normally imply a need for some kind of population survey. Although routine health services data rarely cover a total population, nevertheless there are exceptions. In particular, where there is a programme of surveillance of all children, the opportunity exists to observe change in successive cohorts. The records of primary care nurses can provide a source of information on the health status of preschool children and where systematic examination takes place, as on school entry, this provides data on physiological features such as height and weight, as well as on the prevalence of various defects. These data may be used to monitor changes over time. Charts on the distribution of height and weight by age are required in order to evaluate development and nutritional status in children and these are discussed by Falkner (Chapter 7.1) and Tremlett, Lovel & Morley (Chapter 12.2). Nabarro (Chapter 12.1) provides an example of an excellent simple chart for this purpose.

Data may also be collected at later ages about particular groups within the population that are subject to fairly universal screening procedures. More often, information on biological and physiological measures in adult populations will have to be gathered in health examination surveys. As reported in the contribution by Nissinen et al. (Chapter 11.3), information on blood pressure and serum cholesterol was obtained for test and control populations in this way, and the authors were able to report the beneficial effects of particular interventions.

Health examination surveys are much less common than interview surveys because of their greater cost, the enhanced skills required in the interviewer and the greater complexity of organizing the inquiry and obtaining a satisfactory response rate.

Self-reported measures
Population surveys have been shown to be reasonably reliable in obtaining fairly general indicators of health status, as well as more specific measures, as assessed by the respondent. They may cover both physical and emotional aspects of health experience, including the effects of ill health on social and work activities, as well as on functional capacity. Such surveys also commonly collect information on sickness experience in terms of days off work or in bed, and the prevalence of long-term and short-term illness. It should be recognized, however, that cultural differences in perceptions of illness that affect people's behaviour and attitudes, and changes in the social environment, such as the introduction of or a change in a welfare benefit, may influence people's assessment of their state of health. The comparison of data over time or between populations presents some problems on this account.

Such inquiries may serve to provide information on emotional reactions and pyschosocial functioning. John et al. (Chapter 7.3) describe some of the measures available, and McDowell (Chapter 13.3) discusses the scoring problems in providing an overall index and presents data showing gains in health for an experimental group.

Surveys are also used to elicit information on self-reported functional state or mobility and ability to carry out household tasks and personal care, although questions on these aspects of health status may be restricted to the elderly for whom functional incapacity is more common and the forms of questioning appear more relevant than they may to the general adult population. Measures particularly suitable for use for the elderly are reviewed by Fillenbaum (Chapter 7.4). Instruments developed primarily for the impaired and handicapped provide a basis for this approach. These may serve as simple tools for assessing changes in an individual's functional state and thus provide a measure of the outcome and effectiveness of health care on one particular dimension, although further work is required to improve their sensitivity at the individual level. Many models exist and the basic data set for long-term care developed in the United States *(3)* includes measures of this kind. The development of international standards to categorize impairment and disability is in train at WHO *(4)*; although somewhat elaborate at present for some purposes, parts of the classification provide a useful tool for general population studies, as well as in the clinical context for people with handicaps and impairments.

A simple measure from inquiries of this kind will normally reflect an easily identified aspect of health status such as days of disability or the percentage of the population reporting any health problems. A complex measure or index aims to summarize data on multiple aspects of health status to provide a single measure for individuals and to allocate individuals to a level on a scale of health that permits the derivation of data for a population. Complex measures of health are still in the process of development; terminology, schedule design, weighting and scaling, and validation are under examination. It is not yet possible to identify measures that are easily and cheaply available and applicable on a universal basis, and it may be some time before methods suitable for adoption as national standards become available. Goldberg & Dab (Chapter 7.5) describe some of these developments and Harnly & Williams (Chapter 12.3) cover some of the methodological problems. A fairly simple questionnaire, suitable for completion by individuals, which provides information on a number of dimensions of health status, is reported by McEwen et al. (Chapter 13.4).

Lifestyle characteristics and behavioural risk factors

Lifestyle characteristics and behavioural risk factors are also reported through population surveys and often incorporated in both specific and multi-purpose inquiries. The paper by Kar & Berkanovic (Chapter 8.2) develops a methodological framework and lists behaviour relevant to inquiries in this area, although instruments are not fully developed for all of these. Smoking and alcohol consumption are topics frequently covered and national standards for question design now exist in many countries. Comparison with data from other sources, such as import data, indicates that there may be some underreporting of absolute levels of consumption, especially for alcohol. Despite this, these data are believed to provide reasonably reliable evidence of trends. A number of examples of data on behavioural factors are included, demonstrating their use to monitor changes in lifestyle (see Chapters 11.1, 11.2, 11.3 and 13.3).

Public sensitivity to being questioned on what were once thought intrusive topics seems to be diminishing rapidly; contraceptive practice and sexual behaviour are now among the topics studied by this means. A decrease in sensitivity may, however, result in an increase in the reporting of some behaviour, which could affect trends. In addition to recording people's practices, changes in attitudes to behaviour and to public policies on drinking and smoking may also be monitored by these means. While interview methods are most commonly employed for population surveys, questionnaires completed by the respondents themselves have been successfully used in such inquiries and may both reduce costs and obtain more honest responses, especially from younger adults. Multi-purpose surveys are not generally considered suitable for collecting information on attitudes to health and health practices; this may require detailed questioning, and such information is more often obtained by periodic surveys on that topic alone.

Some aspects of lifestyle may not be readily obtained in a brief interview, and some topics require recall over a period. Subjects such as diet may require diary methods over a period, or even the weighing of foods consumed, for very accurate reporting. McDowell (Chapter 13.3) nevertheless reports on the use of a one-day recall approach to give an indication of dietary content including salt, sugar, fat and fibre content. He also describes instruments based on reported leisure activity for 7 days and the derivation of a physical activity index from the various activities that may form part of leisure and recreation. Methods of collecting information on diet, using community health workers and determining weights by volume, have also been reported *(5)*. Surveys on some practices, such as infant feeding and contraceptive practice, require some means of identifying these populations as a basis for drawing a sample, although it is possible, albeit expensive, to find subsets of the population through interviews or a postal sift to the general population.

Aspects of the environment which may influence health

Over the past century or more, interest in environmental influences on health has focused on the traditional public health concerns of the eradication of infectious agents from water, food and air, and improvements in waste disposal, to minimize the spread of infection from these sources. Such problems are still paramount as a focus for action in many countries. In others, environmental surveillance is increasingly directed towards monitoring and control of man-made pollutants in the air, water, soil and food supply. Many developed countries maintain inspectorates or bodies that monitor and control environmental pollution and working conditions; useful information is often reported as a result of these functions. Notification systems about the toxic effects of drugs, either on a patient or indirectly on a fetus, and about outbreaks of food poisoning also provide information on these specific aspects of the environment.

An unfavourable physical environment may directly affect health. The influence of social conditions, such as poor housing, overcrowding, low levels of literacy and education, unemployment and poverty, is less direct, but all of these have been shown to be associated with poorer states of health. Improvements in these social factors are generally associated with gains in health or health potential. Authorities responsible for social policy normally monitor these conditions, and data may not easily lend themselves to disaggregation into populations of interest to health services. Alternative potential sources are population censuses or sample surveys; these usually provide a range of information about these social indicators. Sample surveys are often of insufficient size to give more than a very broad area breakdown, but census data are often available for the smallest area for collection of data and these may serve as building bricks for aggregation into other areas. Coding systems that locate a health event or a death in a small area through a post-code open up possibilities for analysis of these events in relation to the characteristics of the area *(6)*. Such systems also permit the generation of population-based statistics that are not tied to the health facility used.

Population attitudes and participation in health management

Data on people's attitudes towards and participation in health management may be hard to find. Surveys are the main means of finding out about attitudes, but these may also be inferred to some extent from behaviour, such as participation in practices that promote health or willingness to make use of preventive services. Numerous self-help agencies exist, usually related to specific diseases; they may benefit people suffering from the diseases and campaign to influence policy and the allocation of resources in relation to needs. The number, membership and activities of these agencies may provide some "soft" information on participation.

Community participation belongs in the organizational framework and may be observed in the extent to which policy and management are subject to democratic procedures and in the influence of consumer representation in the determination of priorities (see Chapter 8.3 by Davies). Further work is required to develop measurement in this area.

Action at governmental level

The political will to promote health may be detected directly through legislation (on seat belts or measures designed to limit the exposure of individuals to noxious substances, for example) and its implementation. Less directly, action at this level may seek to reduce the appeal of substances such as alcohol or tobacco by controlling the nature or extent of advertising of these substances, or by the use of specific warnings about their harmful effects on health. Governments may also supply specific advice on healthy practices *(7)*. Willingness to use fiscal measures to influence health promotion may also form part of a central strategy. The amount of the health budget allocated to particular kinds of service or specifically to promotion is a useful indicator of this. The distribution of the health budget to supply resources in relation to population needs also provides an indication of the government's commitment to the equitable provision of health care.

Characteristics of the Information Base and Making Information Useful

Data are expensive to collect, but they provide essential information for determining policy, planning appropriate services and monitoring the effects of these decisions; without information, managers cannot evaluate the effects of their actions. Information requirements vary. At the lowest level they are met by the individual record. These include records kept as a result of a legal requirement to register an event such as a birth or a death; notifications of infectious diseases that serve an alerting function; notifications designed to monitor the operation of a particular policy, such as abortions; records with a purely statistical purpose, such as cancer registration; and the individual record that provides the basis for delivery of health care to a patient, or records the health status and the development of a child. These individual records, to fulfil various functions, may be standardized to provide a statistical abstract that enables them to be aggregated into data to serve the information needs of managers at the local level and to assist in the delivery of services. Henry & Rahaman (Chapter 11.5) provide an example of such use. At the regional or central level, information provides a basis for the development of policy, planning, and the allocation and deployment of resources to subregions or to groups within the population. Policy tasks should include setting targets, and for some countries the targets set by the WHO Regional Office for Europe *(8)* will be relevant. Whether it concerns service provision and use, or reductions in mortality, disease and disability, information is essential to monitor progress towards these targets.

Ways of collating and refining information can briefly be summarized as follows:

Records of:	*Statistics on:*	*+ Expert knowledge of:*	*Information leading to, and required for:*
registrations	health and disease	epidemiology	problem formulation
contacts	mortality	clinical care	setting priorities
events	environment	medical sociology	decision-making
notifications	manpower	pharmacology	implementation
questionnaires	facilities	health economics	evaluation
	finance	and other subjects	setting targets
	services		monitoring progress
	utilization		

To be of value, data should possess a number of qualities and some of the basic characteristics are described by Abelin & Noack (Chapter 5) and by Brzeziński (Chapter 6). To these may be added those required to make them informative, and to provide these qualities the individual record should contain such essential elements as personal data, and the date and place of the event. Provided that data recording is standardized, statistics can then:

— be related to a population in a given area

— provide trends over time

— have the potential for disaggregation

— be comparable between subgroups and over time.

Comparability is essential in making data informative and requires careful definition and classification of the various items in an information system. Minimum basic data sets identify the items for inclusion, and standardize the definitions and terms used and the conventions for completion. They are thus a necessary uniform framework for achieving many of the desired qualities in the data. Monitoring progress over time and towards targets requires that data are available and reported continuously or periodically and, for this purpose, measures must remain reasonably standard. This is not always easy, particularly where definitions are subject to change. Even apparently simple measures may pose problems in definition (as illustrated by the shifting basis for measuring a stillbirth), and complex measures are still evolving. Nevertheless, for many of the measures discussed in this book there is substantial agreement on definitions; a basis exists for monitoring improvements in health and progress towards targets that have been set.

Data should also be capable of being disaggregated to provide information for areas of health service provision and groups within the population; information on age, sex, area of residence, employment status, and social or ethnic group provides some of the key variables for analysis.

The appropriate presentation of statistical data has a big part in making it understandable and valuable to users of information who may not be familiar with statistical concepts. Basic numerical data should be converted into rates in relation to a population or into percentages to make them comparable. Data should be presented as clearly and simply as possible and the use of simple graphics may help to achieve this. It may be necessary to define any terms that are not in common use and to explain techniques such as standardization to allow for differences in the composition of a population that may be well known to statisticians but unfamiliar to many others. It should also be common practice to draw attention to problems and limitations inherent in the data which could affect interpretation. A WHO Regional Office report *(9)* provides a more comprehensive review of how to make statistics talk.

Fig. 1 provides an example that illustrates some of these concepts and conveys an immediate message. Definitions are constant and measurement over time identifies changes in the percentage of the population smoking cigarettes, broken down by sex and social group. Visual presentation enables the data to make an immediate impact.

Fig. 1. Prevalence of cigarette smoking, by sex and socioeconomic group, Great Britain, 1972–1982

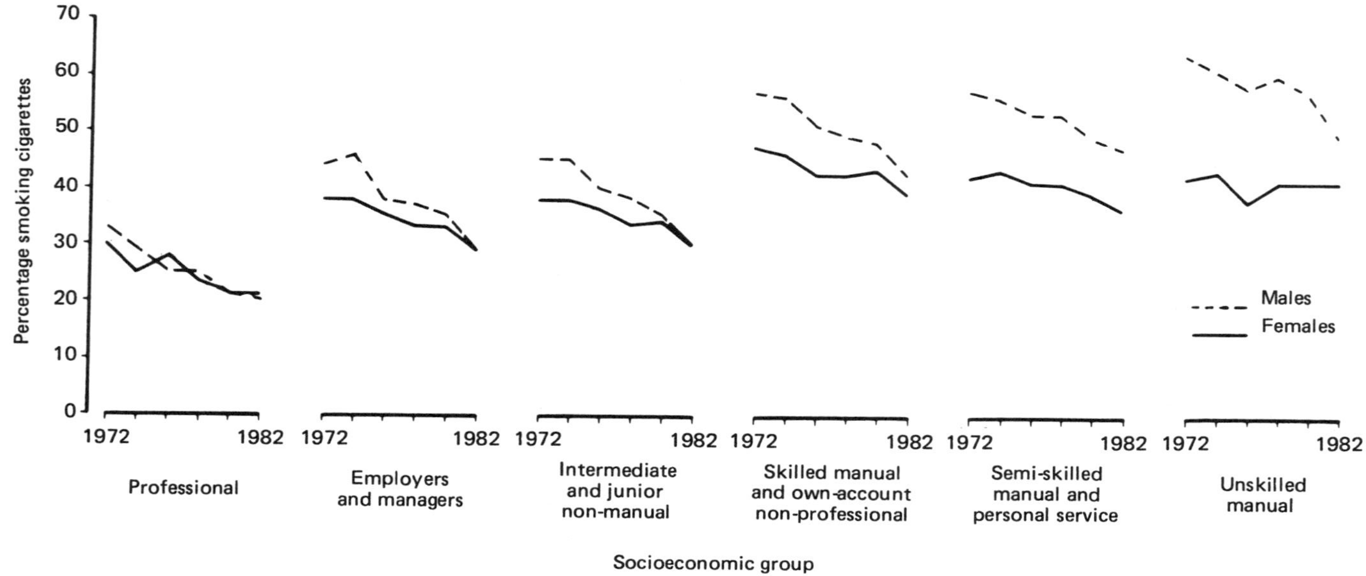

Source: **Office of Population Censuses and Surveys.** *OPCS population trends No. 37.* 1984, p. 15.

Developments in Methods of Data Acquisition and Information Technology: The Role of Information Services

It will be clear from this review that not all of the information that is relevant to the measurement of health promotion and protection lies within the territory of health information services; other areas of social policy or environmental control constitute useful and necessary sources. Where data acquisition lies primarily in the hands of another agency, the role of information services will be, at least, to assemble published data and interpret them for use in the health services. Too often, however, aggregate data from other areas of social policy provide information on indicators that are relevant to their policy interests and are convenient for administrative purposes but of lesser relevance to health service concerns. A more active role will therefore extend to influencing data acquisition in terms of content or data analysis to ensure that health policy is monitored.

Data relevant to health promotion will also often be required, covering a total population and not merely people making contact with the health services. Censuses or sample surveys of the population provide one of the main techniques of data acquisition. A national survey organization may control these population surveys and topics related to health may be only one of a number of interests in a multi-purpose survey. In some countries, on the other hand, the health services may themselves have resources to carry out or commission inquiries designed specifically to provide information for monitoring health and determining policy. Whatever the approach, it is essential that information from these sources should be compatible with that acquired directly by the health services.

Traditional data acquisition in the health service rests on continuous reporting of data on resources, use and activity, in which a considerable degree of stability can be established in the design and procedures. Population surveys require very different organizational structures and technical skills. The work is episodic and progresses through various stages. Management tasks include the training and supervision of interviewers, and methods of quality control differ from those commonly encountered in abstracting information from medical records. The technical tasks of question design, sample construction, treatment of non-response and statistical inference may overlap with those in normal health service statistical schemes, but they also demand additional skills. For these reasons it is normal to establish a survey team, to function as a separate resource, without responsibilities for routine data collection. There are, nevertheless, benefits in such a team's being part of the overall information function.

Both health interview and health examination surveys are expensive, particularly where specialized staff are required to carry out the field work. Many surveys have successfully contained the costs by employing primary care nurses as a local field force, and postal questionnaires and telephone interview methods have been used successfully in several inquiries. As most people are interested in their health, response is generally fairly good; high levels of response may, however, require fairly strenuous follow-up procedures and the elderly and the sick in particular may have difficulty in responding. Experiments have shown that people will complete fairly lengthy questionnaires by themselves when they are interested in the topic, but such questionnaires demand particularly clear, relevant and simple question design, a layout that is easy to follow, and a range of response options that assist people to complete the form.

In less developed countries the paucity of resources and trained staff will not usually permit very sophisticated, and hence expensive, population inquiries to be made. These countries may aim to build on systems of lay reporting that are developing on the initiative of WHO *(10, 11)*. In addition, WHO has published guidance on the training of primary health workers for information collection *(12)*. The people so trained (who may include village officers and headmen, community workers, teachers and sanitary workers, as well as primary care nurses) should provide a resource adaptable to the collection of other data. Conducting such inquiries is the topic of two publications that provide simple guidelines on sampling and on planning and organizing health surveys *(13, 14)* and various aspects of health surveys are also covered in a statistical report *(15)*. Some of the problems encountered in carrying out ad hoc inquiries are reviewed in a publication on maternal and child health *(16)*.

The National Household Survey Capability Programme of the United Nations Statistical Office *(17)* aims to collaborate with developing countries to establish a systematic programme of household surveys. Done on a continuing basis, these enable progress in health conditions to be monitored over time. Carlson reviews some surveys in developing countries *(18)*. One major benefit of these and other multi-purpose surveys is that they permit health conditions to be related to other social and environmental factors. They also ensure consistency and compatibility in measurement and establish a permanent infrastructure that overcomes many of the organizational problems encountered by ad hoc surveys, such as building a new organization and survey team, recruiting and training staff and interviewers, developing a field organization, sample design and selection, procedures of data collection, data transmission, and computer processing and tabulation. These are formidable tasks for most countries of the world. They are the reasons why many surveys run into difficulties and fail to meet objectives; even simple and limited inquiries require some trained staff for coordination and analysis. Using the organization set up to conduct population censuses (by means of follow-up surveys directed to a random sample or to households meeting certain characteristics) is one way of using an established survey capability to provide health information.

In some countries population surveys may be required to provide the basic information for planning health care, but their largest role is to provide additional information to that gathered by routine systems. One example of a survey that was designed to fill the gaps left by the traditional system is reported from Canada *(19)*. The findings from this inquiry were specifically intended to aid in the planning of health care, health promotion and disease prevention. Data collection was based on the model in Fig. 2.

Fig. 2. Model of health

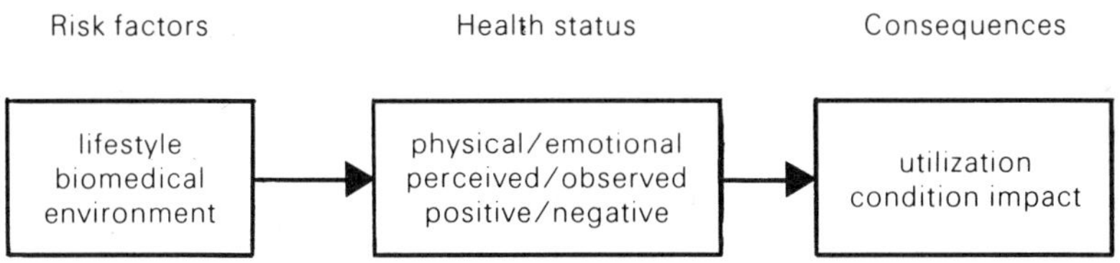

Source: *The health of Canadians (19).*

The survey was accomplished via the use of self-reports as well as interview techniques, and for a smaller sample a number of physical measurements were taken by public health nurses. The kinds of data collected are shown in Fig. 3.

This survey yielded a wealth of information which was intended to answer three main questions on:

— the people exposed to the risk of future illness

— the current health status of the population

— the impact of illness.

Table 1 reports on the proportion of the population with healthy lifestyles and an example of an instrument for data collection is given in Fig. 4. Further surveys, perhaps not on the same scale, will be required to monitor changes in lifestyle and health status, and to provide an assessment of whether policies are leading to improvements in these. Also from Canada, McDowell (Chapter 13.3) provides an example of the use of such data in evaluating the impact of health counselling in reducing harmful health practices in an experimental group.

Information services have a crucial role in pursuing and coordinating these developments, not least in selecting, amassing and presenting these data. In addition to continuing efforts to standardize, integrate and improve existing data bases, the provision of appropriate information in the terms described here will demand the adoption of a wider vision and expanded skills to shift the focus from monitoring the provision and use of services towards identifying achievements.

Innovations in technology are paralleling new methods of measurement. In developed countries investment in computer technology is accelerating sharply. Much of this investment is intended primarily for the administration of services, including patient administration, call-up for vaccination, immunization and screening, control of pharmacy and other supplies, laboratory and diagnostic services, manpower scheduling, payment of staff, and costs of services. These and other aspects of health care are all increasingly being managed by computer-based systems. In some countries

Fig. 3. A summary of data items

Lifestyle

Item	Source
alcohol use	LHQ
tobacco use	LHQ
physical activities	LHQ
use of seat belt	LHQ
female preventive behaviour	LHQ

Reported health

Item	Source
activity limitations	IAQ
short-term conditions	IAQ
accidents and injuries	IAQ
chronic conditions	IAQ
impairments	IAQ
hearing, vision, dental status	IAQ

Utilization

Item	Source
professional providing care	IAQ
location care received	IAQ
reasons care not sought	IAQ
drug use	IAQ
medical devices used	IAQ

Biomedical

Item	Source
immune status	BLOOD
cholesterol, glucose, uric acid	BLOOD
family disease history	LHQ

Physical health

Item	Source
cardiorespiratory fitness	PMQ
blood pressure	PMQ
percentage of body fat	PMQ
anaemia	BLOOD
liver function	BLOOD
kidney function	BLOOD

Condition impact

Item	Source
disability days	IAQ

Environment

Item	Source
lead, cadmium, copper, zinc	BLOOD

Emotional health

Item	Source
psychological wellbeing	LHQ
alcohol-related problems	LHQ

Household characteristics

Item	Source
area designation	HRC
household membership	HRC
dwelling characteristics	HRC

Demographic characteristics

Item	Source
social characteristics	IAQ & LHQ
economic characteristics	IAQ
mobility, immigration	IAQ
life events	LHQ

Note: HRC = Household record card
IAQ = Interviewer-administered questionnaire
LHQ = Lifestyle and your health questionnaire
(Interview component)

PMQ = Physical measures questionnaire
BLOOD = Blood sample
(Physical measures component)

Source: *The health of Canadians (19).*

Table 1. The health of Canadians, 1978–1979: population aged 15 years or more

Age group (years)	Sex	Percentage of the population: Not drinking more than 7 drinks weekly	Never smoked or stopped smoking	Moderately active or very active	With positive "Affect balance score"	Taking no drugs by medical advice
15+	Males	52.7	50.1	38.8	46.8	59.2[a]
	Females	75.5	56.5	33.9	44.2	45.2
15–19	Males	63.4	57.0	62.6	41.6	71.4
	Females	75.2	55.0	53.3	39.9	60.7
20–24	Males	44.0	44.0	45.6	47.0	71.4
	Females	76.3	47.7	34.3	45.8	49.7
25–44	Males	50.7	47.7	38.7	48.9	66.0
	Females	77.2	54.7	36.5	46.5	46.5
45–64	Males	51.4	49.8	29.1	48.9	51.4
	Females	72.6	57.5	29.8	44.4	32.9
65+	Males	58.7	58.1	22.2	40.6	33.6
	Females	75.2	70.0	15.0	40.1	23.0

[a] All ages.

Source: *The health of Canadians (19).*

Fig. 4. Sample instrument for data collection

ALCOHOL The following questions are about your experiences with alcohol.

1 In the last twelve months, about how often have you taken at least one drink of beer, wine, liquor or any other alcoholic beverage?

501 ☐ 1 Two or more times a day
☐ 2 Once a day
☐ 3 4 to 6 times a week
☐ 4 2 or 3 times a week
☐ 5 About once a week
☐ 6 2 or 3 times a month
☐ 7 About once a month

OR →

Answer the questions in Part "A" only

PART "A"

2 Not counting small sips, at what age did you start drinking alcoholic beverages?

At age 502 ⌊__⌋

3 Beginning with yesterday, how many drinks did you have on each of the last 7 days?

(a) Yesterday
503 ☐ 1 No drinks ☐ 2 1 ☐ 3 2 or 3 ☐ 4 4 to 7 ☐ 5 8 to 11 ☐ 6 12 or more

(b) 2 days ago
504 ☐ 1 No drinks ☐ 2 1 ☐ 3 2 or 3 ☐ 4 4 to 7 ☐ 5 8 to 11 ☐ 6 12 or more

(c) 3 days ago
505 ☐ 1 No drinks ☐ 2 1 ☐ 3 2 or 3 ☐ 4 4 to 7 ☐ 5 8 to 11 ☐ 6 12 or more

(d) 4 days ago
506 ☐ 1 No drinks ☐ 2 1 ☐ 3 2 or 3 ☐ 4 4 to 7 ☐ 5 8 to 11 ☐ 6 12 or more

(e) 5 days ago
507 ☐ 1 No drinks ☐ 2 1 ☐ 3 2 or 3 ☐ 4 4 to 7 ☐ 5 8 to 11 ☐ 6 12 or more

(f) 6 days ago
508 ☐ 1 No drinks ☐ 2 1 ☐ 3 2 or 3 ☐ 4 4 to 7 ☐ 5 8 to 11 ☐ 6 12 or more

(g) 7 days ago
509 ☐ 1 No drinks ☐ 2 1 ☐ 3 2 or 3 ☐ 4 4 to 7 ☐ 5 8 to 11 ☐ 6 12 or more

4 Has your drinking changed over the last 12 months?

510 ☐ 1 Drinking more now
☐ 2 Drinking less now
☐ 3 No change over last 12 months

5 What do you usually drink?

(Check one only)

511 ☐ 1 Beer
☐ 2 Wine
☐ 3 Liquor or mixed drinks
☐ 4 Other

OR → ☐ 5 It varies

6 Over the last 12 months, has your drinking played a part in any of the following problems?

512 ☐ Tension or disagreement with family or friends?
513 ☐ Trouble at work or school?
514 ☐ Problems with your health?
515 ☐ Difficulties with driving?
516 ☐ Trouble with the law?
517 ☐ Accidental injury to yourself or someone else?
518 ☐ Violent injury to yourself or someone else?

OR → 519 ☐ None of these

Source: The health of Canadians (19).

Fig. 4 (contd)

501 ☐ 8 Less often than once a month

☐ 9 Not at all in the last 12 months

Answer the questions in Part "B" only

The following table might help you answer some of these questions

One drink equals . . .

- One pint bottle of beer (12 ounces)
- One small glass of wine (4–5 ounces)
- One shot of liquor or spirits (1–1½ ounces) with or without mix

A shot with a beer chaser or a double should be counted as two drinks

PART "B"

2 What experience with alcohol have you had?

520 ☐ 1 Drink occasionally
☐ 2 Never drank
} Go to page 10

OR ☐ 3 Used to drink

3 *(a)* At what age did you start?

At age 521 ⌊_⌋_⌋

(b) At what age did you have your last drink?

At age 522 ⌊_⌋_⌋

4 About how often did you usually drink?

523 ☐ 1 Two or more times a day
☐ 2 Once a day
☐ 3 4 to 6 times a week
☐ 4 2 or 3 times a week
☐ 5 About once a week
☐ 6 2 or 3 times a month
☐ 7 About once a month
☐ 8 Less often than once a month

5 About how many drinks did you have at a time?

524 ☐ 1 One
☐ 2 Two or three
☐ 3 Four or five
☐ 4 Six or seven
☐ 5 More than that

6 What did you usually drink?

(Check one only)

525 ☐ 1 Beer
☐ 2 Wine
☐ 3 Liquor or mixed drinks
☐ 4 Other

OR ☐ 5 It varied

7 Were there any particular reasons why you stopped drinking?

(Please check all appropriate boxes)

526 ☐ Close friend or spouse did not drink
527 ☐ It was affecting my health
528 ☐ Joined the A.A.
529 ☐ Had a bad experience because of drinking
530 ☐ It was a source of conflict with family or friends
531 ☐ Didn't drink much and decided to quit
532 ☐ It was too expensive
533 ☐ Thought that I could use my time better
534 ☐ It was affecting my job, studying, or homemaking

OR 535 ☐ No particular reason

population registers kept in computers also contain information for all individuals on service use and health experience and these offer the prospect of allowing the health status of a population to be monitored automatically. In addition to the direct benefits to patient care, these systems provide a bonus of information on service use and patient care as a by-product.

While such systems provide a powerful resource for assisting the production of information, even greater benefits can be achieved if the potential for improved integration of the different data bases can be realized. This will happen only if developments are pursued with the objective of sharing data among the different systems as a part of the strategy. Information should be viewed as a corporate resource that demands the pursuit of compatible and integrated computer systems as strenuously as standardization in the information base. Developments in this direction are not easily achieved without a considerable degree of coordination and control.

The phenomenal and continuing fall in the costs of computer hardware also begins to bring microcomputers within reach of individual practitioners for the management of their caseloads and opens up yet further prospects for collecting data. It also makes the development and acceptance of standardization in data collection even more urgent. Solar-powered equipment is also on the horizon and may, before too long, enable even developing countries to employ small computers as an aid to management and in the information process *(20)*. Examples of the use of computer technology in a developing country are provided by Bernard & Sastrawinata (Chapter 11.6) and by Bertrand *(15)*. The marked decrease in hardware costs, however, has to be balanced against the increasing costs of software and the personnel required to maintain the systems and to assist and train the users. These are not negligible and underline the necessity for proper evaluation of the benefits and a carefully considered strategy for the introduction and continuing support of these tools.

Obviously, the relevant skills and resources for data collection, processing and analysis will facilitate the information process. A number of contributions show that data exist, often unrecognized, at the primary care level in many countries, and the improved use of available data, rather than investment in sophisticated health information systems, should be the first priority. Without major resources but with a little imagination and persistence, information can be identified and used to monitor progress in health. Although we may strive for excellence in the information base, this is not always possible or necessary. It is important not to let the best be the enemy of the good and arrest the progress that can be achieved.

References

1. **Department of Health and Social Security.** *Report on confidential enquiries into maternal deaths in England & Wales 1976–1978.* London, H.M. Stationery Office, 1982 (Report on Health and Social Subjects, No. 26).
2. **Cox, P.** Epidemiology and research at low cost. *British medical journal,* **288**: 1814–1816 (1984).

3. *Long-term health care: minimum data set.* Washington, DC, US Department of Health, Education and Welfare, 1979.
4. *International classification of impairments, disabilities and handicaps.* Geneva, World Health Organization, 1980.
5. **Pratinidhi, A.K. et al.** Diet surveys in rural areas. *World health forum,* **5**(2): 168–169 (1984).
6. **Carstairs, V.** Small area analysis and health service research. *Community medicine,* **3**: 131–139 (1981).
7. **Department of Health and Social Security.** *Prevention and health: everybody's business.* London, H.M. Stationery Office, 1976.
8. *Targets for health for all.* Copenhagen, WHO Regional Office for Europe, 1985.
9. *The use of health indicators — how to make statistics talk:* report on a WHO Workshop. Copenhagen, WHO Regional Office for Europe, 1980 (unpublished document ICP/SPM 043).
10. **Kupka, K.** Lay reporting of health information. *World health forum,* **2**: 211–217 (1981).
11. *Lay reporting of environmental health information.* Geneva, World Health Organization, 1981 (unpublished document ICD/LR/WP/81.3).
12. *Training trainers of primary health workers in the collection and use of health-related information:* report on a WHO Working Group. Geneva, World Health Organization, 1982 (unpublished document WHO/HS/NAT.COM/82.382).
13. **Lutz, W.** *Community health surveys: a practical guide for health workers. 1. Planning and organising.* Geneva, International Epidemiological Association, 1981.
14. **Lutz, W.** *Community health surveys: a practical guide for health workers. 2. Survey sampling.* Geneva, International Epidemiological Association, 1982.
15. *World health statistics quarterly,* **38**(1): 38–64 (1985).
16. *Meeting on maternal and child health indicators for health for all by 2000: evaluation of alternatives.* Geneva, World Health Organization, 1982 (unpublished document WHO/HS/NAT.COM/83.383).
17. *Handbook of household surveys.* New York, United Nations, 1981.
18. **Carlson, B.A.** National household surveys and their health components. *In: International conference on health statistics for the year 2000.* Budapest, Statistical Publishing House, 1984, pp. 121–136.
19. *The health of Canadians.* Ottawa, National Health and Welfare, 1981.
20. **Kholy, A.E. & Mandil, S.H.** Microcomputers and health improvement in developing countries. *WHO Chronicle,* **37**(5): 163–165 (1983).

Part III

Examples and applications of measurements

10. Introduction

M.C. Thuriaux & A.R. Taket

Part III, the largest section of this book, comprises illustrative examples of the types of measurement described in the chapters of Part II. They are presented in four separate sections, according to the level of application and degree of implementation of the measurements discussed.

Each of the contributions in this part is introduced by a paragraph highlighting points of interest in the material presented and relating the measurement tools and issues covered to the relevant chapters in Part II. In selecting material for Part III, a deliberate attempt has been made to include examples from both developed and developing countries to show that the measurement tools discussed in Part II are applicable in a wide variety of contexts. Differences in the subject matter presented in examples reflect the different health priorities of countries at various stages of development.

The primary aim of health promotion and protection activities is the improvement or maintenance of the health of a defined population. The first set of illustrations (Chapter 11) deals with examples illustrating the use of measurements for assessing health and monitoring progress in populations or communities. Examples include illustrations of the measurement issues discussed earlier in the chapters on personal protection (Chapter 8.1), behaviour conducive to good health (Chapter 8.2) and environmental protection (Chapter 8.4).

The contributions in this chapter include, *inter alia,* descriptions of the application of simple measurements to the evaluation of the effects of specific health campaigns (Catford & Nutbeam (11.1), Ramström (11.2) and Nissinen et al. (11.3)). Jedrychowski (11.4) reports on a study based on the measurement of physiological function and the extent to which this is maintained in a population exposed to a given risk. This is in contrast to the more traditional methods of measuring changes in incidence of dysfunction or disability. In the same chapter, Bernard & Sastrawinata (11.6) demonstrate, in the context of a developing country, how the use of modern computer technology can provide a suitable basis for an information system to monitor health services, in this case primary maternity care services. Henry & Mujibur Rahaman (11.5) apply measurements to environmental health.

The study and measurement of disability will constitute an increasingly important part of health status measurement as the importance of the problem increases, especially in developed countries, with the postponement of death to higher and higher ages. This is therefore an area where it will become increasingly necessary to develop appropriate measurement tools. Charlton (11.7), Greenwood & Wali (11.9) and Basu & Sokhey (11.10) all refer to the "sentinel events" mentioned by Rutstein (7.6). The contribution from Colvez et al. (11.8), on the use as a health indicator of life expectancy free from disability, provides an illustration of some of the possibilities in this area. Two papers in this chapter (Marti et al (11.11) and Dwyer et al. (11.12)) focus on the promotion of physical fitness and exercise, and demonstrate examples of measurement methods applicable in this field. The second of these looks specifically at the health benefits gained by schoolchildren from participating in a daily physical education programme.

Chapter 12 presents some examples of instruments primarily designed for use at the level of the individual. These can, however, be used at the level of the community and the potential for this is discussed. The examples given relate mainly to results used at the level of the individual rather than to evaluating the effects of health promotion and protection activities in communities or populations. The chapter contains two examples relating to the measurement of child growth and development (Nabarro (12.1) and Tremlett et al. (12.2)), both of which deal with charts used primarily in developing countries but which are (or should be) equally relevant in more developed societies. An example on the construction of various complex indices of health status and their use in the context of positive health counselling for individuals exemplifies the application of more sophisticated techniques of individual measurement. The final example in this chapter (Harnly & Williams (12.3)), which illustrates the participation of people in the maintenance or protection of their own health through the use of self-documentation of health status, is one which would be applicable in a large spectrum of development contexts.

Chapter 13 contains some applications in the research and development of methods. This chapter includes examples relating to programmes still in progress, for instance the paper by Srivastava & Verma (13.6) dealing with possible indicators for assessing the impact of safe water supplies on health, and also some measurement tools which, although they have not yet generally been used in the monitoring or evaluation of health promotion and protection activities, could easily be applied in such a way. Contributions in this category include that by Blom (13.1) on a child survival index that may be determined retrospectively, and that by McEwen et al. (13.4) on the Nottingham health profile, a measure of perceived health, by Krupinski (13.7) in a similar area, and by McDowell (13.2) and Rojas et al. (13.5) in relation to health promotion. In considering the evaluation or monitoring of any health promotion or protection activity, the information strategies in support of health promotion are of crucial importance. The contribution by van Lerberghe et al. illustrates many of the considerations involved in aligning the two.

Chapter 14 contains a paper by Uemura on the application of indicators for monitoring progress towards health for all by the year 2000. The indicators described deal with multiple aspects of health, though very few actually concentrate on the areas of health promotion and protection that form the focus of this book. The common framework and format discussed in this chapter, together with indicators selected by various WHO regions, provided a basis for the evaluation by Member States of their progress towards overall and regional targets for health for all.[a]

In 1984, the WHO Regional Office for Europe established a programme on health promotion, and a meeting was organized on "Concepts and principles in health promotion". Chapter 15, based on the report of this meeting, provides a further contribution to the discussion of the conceptual issues involved in health promotion and indicates recent developments in health promotion programmes within WHO as a basis for future efforts in this field.

[a] *Evaluation of the strategy for health for all by the year 2000: seventh report on the world health situation.* Geneva, World Health Organization, 1986, 7 volumes.

11. Assessing health and monitoring progress in populations

11.1 Use of positive measures: the Wessex experience — *J.C. Catford & D. Nutbeam*

This contribution illustrates the value of relatively simple, inexpensive and easily obtainable indicators in assessing the effects of various health measures. The examples given range across the subject matter of several of the chapters in Part II of this book, dealing with appropriate provision of family planning services, the effectiveness of a seat belt promotion campaign, and the level of smoking restrictions in health premises.

Over the last few years there has been increased interest and activity in health promotion and disease prevention in the Wessex health region of the United Kingdom, which lies in the central part of southern England and has a population of 3 million. An interdisciplinary approach has been adopted. Contributions have been made by the Regional and District Health Authorities, local government bodies and the Regional Sports Council. The Departments of Education, Community Medicine, Psychology and other departments at the University of Southampton have also been active.

Another important development has been the formation of the Wessex Positive Health Team, a regional health promotion group, one of the first of its kind in the United Kingdom. Membership includes representatives from across the region in a number of key disciplines. This was considered vital to the implementation of health promotion strategies. The team's objectives range from health status monitoring, research and evaluation, to policy formation, training and strategic support for local initiatives *(1)*.

A prominent part of the team's work has been to initiate the development of positive health measures and to use them to formulate policies and priorities, determine resource allocation, and evaluate the outcome of health promotion interventions. Three examples of areas where progress has been made in Wessex will be described, namely:

- measuring the effectiveness of a seat belt promotion campaign;
- assessing the level of smoking restrictions in health premises;
- determining the need for family planning education and services.

Other areas of work have concerned:

- surveying the level of preventive medicine practice among general practitioners *(2)*;
- measuring the level of breast self-examination in the community *(3)*;
- investigating the value of health workers as role models for health *(4)*;
- measuring the achievement of dental health promotion goals *(5)*;
- determining the need for exercise promotion in the community *(6)*;
- investigating ways of promoting increased participation in physical activity *(7)*;
- measuring the effectiveness of preventive child health services *(8)*;
- surveying dietary intakes in hospitals, schools and in the community *(9)*.

It should be pointed out that the United Kingdom as a whole lags behind many other developed countries in the implementation of health promotion programmes and particularly in the development of positive health indicators *(10)*. The comparative lack of progress in reducing rates of premature death from coronary heart disease is perhaps an indication of this inactivity.

Measuring the Effectiveness of a Seat Belt Promotion Campaign

In 1979 approximately one third of drivers and front-seat passengers in the United Kingdom wore seat belts. Despite the evidence that death and serious injury could be greatly reduced if seat belt wearing was raised to 85%, successive British governments had failed to introduce legislation to enforce the wearing of safety belts in the front seats of vehicles.

The Government's attitude at that time was that education could further raise the level of seat belt wearing, yet no controlled study had been performed to test this hypothesis. As a result of its concern to prevent death and injury from road accidents in the region, Wessex Regional Health Authority mounted a research project to evaluate the effectiveness of a substantial, coordinated programme of health education to promote the use of seat belts *(11)*.

Baseline measurements of seat belt wearing among front-seat occupants of vehicles were undertaken in two comparable city populations in

Wessex (Winchester and Salisbury). A pilot study had shown that it was not possible to measure seat belt wearing rates accurately among the occupants of moving vehicles as they passed a particular location on the roadside. However, it was found that the level of seat belt wearing could be assessed fairly easily by studying motorists entering public car-parks. Data was therefore collected from a sample of motorists entering two different types of car-park in the two cities; a central car-park for short-stay parking and a multi-storey car-park for long-stay parking.

Measurements covered six days of the week and the same sampling frame was used in both cities, so that motorists were selected from similar car-parks at the same time of the same day of the same week. Further details or methods have been described elsewhere *(12)*.

The study population in Winchester was the target of a large-scale, integrated campaign in the mass media over a six-month period. Health education was offered to the population generally as well as to the target group which comprised front-seat car occupants. The programme was divided into a main and a reinforcement activity and took a variety of forms. Twenty thousand leaflets/book marks were distributed personally to motorists and employees in the town. Posters were displayed in public buildings, health centres, clinics and doctors' surgeries during the study period. Television stations gave generous peak-time coverage to the case in favour of seat belt wearing, as did the local radio station throughout the campaign. Local newspapers also cooperated with marked enthusiasm, giving considerable space to press releases and the reporting of occasions when seat belts had saved lives. On virtually every publication day during the campaign, at least one local newspaper carried a major feature relating to the project.

Thus, over the six-month period, the study population received intensive and sustained information about the need to wear seat belts. The programme utilized the best skills and knowledge available and was generously supported by the media. Not surprisingly, it achieved a high level of penetration. Of a random sample of the electorate in the study population, asked to complete a postal questionnaire after the campaign, approximately one half replied that they were aware of the objectives of the project. The control population in Salisbury was subjected to no special intervention during the six-month period.

At the end of the campaign, seat belt wearing was again measured in the study and control populations. No major changes were observed; the level of seat belt wearing remained at around 35%, with some minor fluctuations. It was found that 39% of women wore seat belts compared to 33% of men, and 39% of front-seat passengers compared to 34% of drivers. The postal questionnaire survey of a random sample of the study population revealed that 66% of non-smokers wore seat belts as opposed to 38% of smokers. On direct questioning, only 10% of the respondents who did not wear seat belts thought that they were hazardous in some way.

The Regional Health Authority concluded that health education on its own was unlikely to raise the level of seat belt wearing further. It went on to examine the evidence in favour of compulsion, and subsequently agreed to support activities urging legislation. Accordingly, the Authority mounted a public relations exercise along with other national bodies. The Regional Health Authority's Chairman and officers lobbied politicians and other influential groups. The study was quoted in Parliament during several debates on seat belt legislation. In July 1981, in a free vote, legislation making the wearing of seat belts by drivers and front-seat passengers compulsory was finally approved and came into force in February 1983.

Three months after the introduction of legislation, a follow-up study on the use of seat belts among drivers was conducted in Wessex: 92% of the drivers questioned said that they now always wore a seat belt, whereas before the law was passed only 37% did; 61% of all drivers thought that the seat belt law was saving a lot of lives, and another 25% considered that a few deaths at least were being avoided; 75% of drivers indicated that they had no particular difficulties with wearing a seat belt, although an important minority (24%) reported having problems mainly related to discomfort and restriction of movement. Of the drivers questioned, 52% considered that seat belt legislation should be extended to include the compulsory fitting and wearing of seat belts in the rear of vehicles.

Twelve months after the law came into force, the Minister of Transport announced that during this period there had been 550 fewer deaths, 7000 fewer serious injuries and 16 000 fewer people slightly injured as a result of road traffic accidents. She attributed this welcome reduction to the 95% seat belt wearing rates that had been achieved.

Experience in Wessex has shown that the new seat belt law is widely viewed as being effective, necessary and fair. This is encouraging, given that there has been a vocal minority opposed to what it perceived as a "curb on the freedom of the individual". It appears, therefore, that sensible legislation for health promotion is acceptable to the public. However, there is still scope for further improvement; in particular, ways have to be found to overcome practical difficulties in the wearing of seat belts, and there is a need to promote the fitting and use of seat belts in the rear of vehicles.

Assessing the Level of Smoking Restrictions in Health Premises

Data on the prevalence of smoking at a national level are available for the United Kingdom. In 1982, 37% of the adult population smoked cigarettes. Over the last 10 years there has been a gradual reduction in smoking, most markedly among the male population and the higher socioeconomic groups. The restriction of smoking in public places, which aims to protect the non-smoker rather than to persecute the smoker, is of great relevance to this encouraging downward trend.

From a health promotion standpoint, smoking restrictions form an important part of an overall commitment to encourage non-smoking. In addition, they help to reduce the opportunities for smoking and may therefore have an impact on cigarette consumption. Restrictions can also act as a positive reinforcement to those who have already given up the habit. All of these points apply to health premises as "public places", but in addition to this, health services have an exemplary role to play in smoking prevention in that they are often viewed as "shop windows" for health.

The aim of non-smoking policies in health premises should not be an entirely prohibitive one, but rather that of promoting non smoking as the normal way of behaving. Visitors and patients attending outpatient clinics usually attend for such short periods of time that it is not necessary for them to smoke and facilities for them to do so need only be minimal. The situation of patients in hospital wards, and long-stay patients in particular, merits careful consideration. The aim in all cases is both to make a genuine effort to restrict smoking and to take account of the physical and mental capabilities of individual patients.

Using this rationale as the basis, the Wessex Regional Health Authority set goals and minimum acceptable levels of smoking restrictions for health premises as outlined in Table 1. The performance of individual hospitals and health centres could thus be monitored.

In 1982, a survey was conducted in Wessex to determine existing policies and practices relating to the promotion of non-smoking in health premises. Administrators of all 190 hospitals and health centres in the region were invited to complete a postal questionnaire. This enquired about (*a*) smoking restrictions in public areas of health premises (based on the percentage of floor space designated and clearly marked "no smoking"), (*b*) the identification and monitoring of restrictions, (*c*) the perceived level of cooperation of patients, visitors and staff, and (*d*) cigarette sales.

A 97% response was achieved and a sample validation based on more objective measurements indicated a high degree of accuracy in the answers received. For assessment purposes, individual health premises were categorized into five groups, i.e. acute, maternity, psychiatric and long-stay/geriatric hospitals, and health centres. Further details of the method and results are available *(13,14)*.

The results of the survey were encouraging but at the same time highlighted areas for further improvement. As shown in Table 1, 81% of all health premises achieved a total ban on smoking in outpatient clinical areas and consulting rooms, and the same percentage achieved the minimum acceptable level of "non-smoking" floor space (80%) in wards and public waiting areas. In addition, the vast majority of patients, visitors and staff were identified as cooperating with these restrictions.

However, there were two important exceptions to these encouraging results. The first was in hospital day-rooms, where only 25% of hospitals achieved the minimum level of 40% of floor space designated "no smoking" and less than 15% achieved the goal of 60% of floor space designated "no smoking". Such discrimination in favour of smokers is not necessary: not only are smokers in the minority, but there is evidence to suggest that smokers entering hospital either give up completely or cut down on their consumption *(15)*. The second exception concerned the sale of cigarettes in almost 25% of all acute hospitals. This was worrying, as the example set by the promotion of non-smoking in hospitals can be completely undermined by the sale of cigarettes there.

Table 1. Goals and minimum acceptable levels of floor space designated and marked "no smoking", and the percentage of health premises achieving these levels in Wessex

	Goal (percentage of floor space designated "no smoking")	Percentage of health premises achieving goal	Minimum acceptable level (percentage of floor space designated "no smoking")	Percentage of health premises achieving minimum level
Public areas				
Wards	100	63	80	81
Day-rooms	60	14	40	25
Waiting areas	100	68	80	83
Outpatient clinical areas and consulting rooms	100	81	100	81
Visitors' refreshment areas	80	48	50	73
Staff areas				
Canteen and restaurant	100	58	50	68
Coffee lounge and rest-room	60	15	40	20

When publishing the results, Wessex Regional Health Authority requested districts to achieve by 1984 the minimum levels of non-smoking provision set out in Table 1, and to impose a total ban on cigarette sales in acute and maternity hospitals. A flexible policy was suggested for patients in long-stay hospitals, but cigarettes should not be on sale to staff or visitors in any hospital.

Considerable interest and activity has resulted; many hospitals and districts have made or are making concerted attempts to reduce smoking in health premises. A follow-up study in 1985, using the original questionnaire, showed that real progress was being made in achieving the targets.

Determining the Need for Family Planning Education and Services

The Wessex Regional Health Authority has for some years been concerned about the level of unwanted pregnancy in the region. Together with the Southampton University Department of Human Reproduction, a number of studies have been undertaken to investigate the factors affecting the need for and outcome of fertility control services *(16)*. These included research into the attitudes and behaviour of general practitioners *(17)* and gynaecologists *(18)*. Importance was also placed on the need to determine women's knowledge, attitudes and behaviour regarding family planning *(19)*. It was hoped that this information would lead to improved educational and contraceptive services.

One hundred 18-year-olds randomly selected from the electoral roll (recently designated as new voters) and 100 mothers (with at least three children) randomly selected from the birth notification register were invited to be interviewed. The sample was drawn from two areas in Southampton Health District, which would give together a social class mix similar to that of the region. The two groups of women were chosen to reflect the ends of the fertility spectrum — i.e. those entering the reproductive period and those approaching the end of it. The experience of the mothers would be valuable in assessing the performance of services in hindsight and with maturity, while the teenagers, as potential customers, would be able to give their views on the current situation as they saw it. Both groups were also easy to identify.

A trained interviewer called by appointment to see the women in their homes. She administered a predominantly closed-answer questionnaire, which had been extensively tested. The response rate was 78% in the mothers and reasons for non-response included adverse attitudes of husbands and alleged invasion of privacy. Information was collected from 64% of the teenagers. The higher non-response rate was attributable partly to changes of address and partly to concern about anonymity, and to parental disapproval.

The attitudes and experiences of the women's introduction to family planning/sex education varied markedly between the two groups. Only 14% of mothers considered the school contribution to have been useful, compared to 55% of the teenagers. To assess which topics had been covered in the school curricula, the women were handed a list of ten topics and asked to indicate those about which they had received or would have liked to receive information.

The results are presented in Table 2, categorized into four topic areas: biological (e.g. animal reproduction), physiological (e.g. human birth, menstruation, breastfeeding), technical (e.g. methods of contraception, advantages, disadvantages), and personal relationships (e.g. sexual feelings and their control, responsibility for self and others). The percentages of women (*a*) receiving information, (*b*) wanting but not receiving information, and (*c*) not wanting and not receiving information are given.

The table shows clearly that there had been some dramatic improvements in the type and availability of sex education in schools during the time-span of a generation. For example, 61% and 72% of teenagers had received information about the physiological and technical aspects respectively, compared to 36% and 16% of the mothers. Yet there remained considerable scope for improvement. Whereas 9% of mothers and 34% of teenagers had had instruction on personal relationships, 69% and 33% respectively had not, but specifically wanted it. Many of the women considered this a major omission in their education.

One half of the teenagers reported that they were sexually active and, of these, 64% were using the pill and the remainder mostly the sheath. However, two girls (6%) reported relying solely on the withdrawal method. Among the mothers it was found that there was a high degree of dissatisfaction with contraceptive measures. This had led 14% of them to seek irreversible methods of contraception either for themselves or their husbands while still aged below 30 years. The wariness of teenagers towards professional advisers was also very evident; 28% said they would prefer to have an independent pregnancy test before seeking professional advice, if they thought they were pregnant.

The majority (61%) of teenagers and mothers would not normally consider abortion as an option if they found themselves pregnant. However, given a hypothetical situation, 82% of mothers and 62% of teenagers said they would prefer to have a termination carried out within the National Health Service and in their own health district. This was in sharp contrast to the availability of abortion services within the National Health Service in Wessex, which varied considerably from district to district; 50% of women seeking an abortion resorted to the private sector in the region and, because of the relatively high costs of treatment, an unmet need for abortion among some women was suspected.

A number of important recommendations were made following these studies and accepted by the Regional Health Authority. They included improved training of doctors in family planning and the setting up of multidisciplinary youth advisory centres. More appropriate health education courses in schools and improved availability of pregnancy test facilities were also recommended. Relevant activities have already begun in some districts. Educational seminars for health professionals and teachers have been organized. In one area with a particularly high teenage pregnancy rate, a walk-in counselling service has started. Perhaps of greatest importance has

Table 2. Experience and attitude of women to family planning/sex education in school

Type of information	Percentage receiving information		Percentage wanting, but not receiving, information		Percentage not wanting, and not receiving, information	
	Teenagers	Mothers	Teenagers	Mothers	Teenagers	Mothers
Biological	44	49	6	24	50	26
Physiological	61	36	10	47	29	17
Technical	72	16	16	62	13	22
Personal relationships	34	9	33	69	34	22

been the setting up of contractual arrangements with a charitable organization so that more teenagers can receive pregnancy testing and counselling and abortion services free of charge in the region.

Conclusions

The experience in Wessex has in part led to renewed interest in the United Kingdom in the development of data bases at local level for health promotion and disease prevention. Ad hoc approaches such as those described above are time-consuming, often complex and hence expensive. There is a need for routine, low-cost and valid information systems to provide useful data on health-related behaviour and its determinants. At present most of the United Kingdom has insufficient information to identify local priorities for health promotion initiatives and to monitor local trends and progress. Perhaps this is one reason why the United Kingdom lags behind many other European countries in health status.

In Wessex higher priority is being given to the development of improved and continuing information systems for health promotion. Emphasis is being placed on the importance of finding cheap, simple and reliable data-collecting procedures. To this end, the potential of the self-administered questionnaire sent by post to a random sample of the population (drawn from computerized primary health care registrations), and supplemented by household interviews is particularly attractive. Once the methodological obstacles are overcome, there will be an opportunity to publish regular district health profiles. These should greatly help both the planning and monitoring of health promotion activities at a local level, and should provide an essential lead to the community and to health professionals in their efforts to achieve health for all by the year 2000.

References

1. **Wessex Positive Health Team.** *Terms of reference and membership.* Wessex Regional Health Authority, 1981.
2. **Catford, J.C. & Nutbeam, D.** Prevention in practice: what Wessex general practitioners are doing. *British medical journal,* **288**: 832–834 (1984).
3. **Nicholls, S. & Waters, W.E.** The practice and teaching of breast self examination in Southampton. *Public health,* **97**: 1, 8–17 (1983).
4. **McCullough, W.** A taste of their own medicine. *Health and social service journal,* **90**: 4185, 1138–1139 (1982).
5. **Wessex Positive Health Team.** *Filling gaps: dental health in Wessex.* Wessex Regional Health Authority, 1982 (Lifeline report No. 3).
6. **Wessex Positive Health Team.** *Exercise and health in Wessex: what should the NHS be doing?* Wessex Regional Health Authority, 1983 (Lifeline report No. 7).
7. **Nutbeam, D.** *The Dorset get fit campaign: feasibility study of a community fitness testing programme.* Wessex Regional Health Authority, 1984 (Wessex Positive Health Team Technical Report No. 4).

8. **Catford, J. & Weeks, D.** *Preventive child health services in Wessex — a review of current policies, programmes and resources.* Wessex Regional Health Authority, 1984 (Wessex Positive Health Team Technical Report No. 3).
9. **Wessex Positive Health Team.** *Towards a healthier diet in Wessex.* Wessex Regional Health Authority, 1984 (Lifeline report No. 8).
10. **Catford, J.C.** Positive health indicators: towards a new information base for health promotion. *Community medicine,* **5**: 125–132 (1983).
11. **Wessex Positive Health Team.** Promoting the use of seat belts. *British medical journal,* **281**: 1477–1478 (1980).
12. **Wessex Positive Health Team.** *Promoting the use of seat belts — an evaluation of integrated health education.* Full report. Wessex Regional Health Authority, 1980.
13. **Catford, J.C. & Nutbeam, D.** Smoking in hospitals. *Lancet,* **2**: 93–96 (1983).
14. **Wessex Positive Health Team.** *Smoking prevention in Wessex health premises.* Wessex Regional Health Authority, 1982 (Lifeline report No. 4).
15. **Seymour, H.** Health education and smoking related disease. *In: Smoking and smoking related diseases: proceedings of a seminar, December 3–5, 1980.* University of Manchester, 1981.
16. **Ashton, J.R. et al.** The Wessex Abortion Studies: I, Interdistrict variation in provision of abortion services. *Lancet,* **1**: 82–85 (1980).
17. **Edwards, C.A. et al.** *General practitioners' attitudes to abortion services.* University of Southampton, 1981.
18. **Chamberlain, A. et al.** *Consultant gynaecologists' attitudes to induced abortion in Wessex.* University of Southampton, 1979.
19. **Edwards, C.A. et al.** *Women's attitudes to induced abortion and related services.* University of Southampton, 1981.

11.2 Monitoring the decline of smoking in Sweden — *L.M. Ramström*

In presenting an analytical framework for the construction of indicators of behaviour conducive to good health, Kar & Berkanovic (Chapter 8.2) discuss the need for measures relating to different stages of health behaviour, their health outcome, and the social structural and environmental factors which can affect them. The example presented next, dealing with smoking behaviour in Sweden, illustrates some of the possible relevant measures in each of these categories.

It is a well established fact that tobacco smoking impairs health in several ways. Smoking is a major or contributory factor in the causation of several serious diseases, as well as aggravating the course of some common diseases caused by other factors. It has also been shown that the cessation of smoking has beneficial health effects. Consequently, smoking control, both in terms of prevention of the onset of smoking and in terms of cessation-oriented intervention among smokers, can be an important means of disease prevention. In this connection it is appropriate to note an observation by a Swedish group of scientists who were studying the potential of disease prevention as a means of improving public health *(1)*. They pointed out that large health benefits could only be obtained by measures that were broad enough to influence several of the most important categories of diseases, for example cancer and cardiovascular diseases, at the same time. Smoking control is one of the few types of disease prevention activity that can actually have such a broad impact.

It could further be noted that smoking control is not to be regarded as merely a disease prevention activity. Both prevention of the onset of smoking and smoking cessation are among the "healthy lifestyle" factors that strengthen health in a general sense. To summarize, smoking control can in several ways be an important, positive factor in health promotion.

In this paper, Swedish efforts in the field of smoking control will be outlined, general aspects of measurements of smoking and health-related parameters will be discussed, measurements carried out in Sweden will be described and some concluding remarks will be made.

Smoking Control Action in Sweden

Establishing a programme

The modern history of smoking control in Sweden began in 1963, when a group of 25 prominent scientists sent a petition to the Government urging regular government funding of information and education on smoking and health. The petitioners were successful, in that from the fiscal year 1963/1964 the Swedish governmental budget has included a grant for funding such action. These funds have been used partly for activities carried out by the National Board of Health and Welfare, and partly as a contribution to the National Smoking and Health Association (NTS). This organization was thus able as early as 1964 to establish a secretariat of full-time staff. This meant that Sweden was perhaps the first country in the world to acquire a specialized agency for smoking and health, serving as a focal point for all kinds of questions regarding smoking and health. It should also be mentioned that in September 1978 the World Health Organization designated the NTS a WHO collaborating centre for reference on smoking and health.

It is a general principle of the Swedish programme for smoking control that the programme as a whole should be of a long-term, multicomponent nature. No single activity should be expected to generate an overall effect, while at the same time every single activity should be contributing to the strength of the programme as a whole. All activities should as far as possible be mutually supporting parts of the programme.

Education and information

Programmes intended to reach millions of people cannot function without the involvement of numerous collaborators at the local level. Therefore the basic implementation technique adopted in Sweden has been to involve professionals, e.g. health workers, teachers and leaders of civic organizations, who have day-to-day contact with people and can thus incorporate smoking control efforts in their ordinary work. However, such a system cannot work unless these key people are given assistance by the central leadership of the national programme. The following tasks have therefore been important for the central agencies, i.e. the National Board of Health and Welfare and NTS: the development of methodologies for local work according to various categories; the organization of training courses for the persons in question; and the provision of teaching aids and similar material. This enables these key people to perform smoking control tasks as an integral part of their daily work. Specific manuals have been produced and distributed to a number of groups, e.g. teachers in the comprehensive school system, and medical personnel at maternity health centres and primary health care units. This kind of work is continuously going on to cover an increasing number of categories.

While many major tasks require personal efforts of the kind described above, a good deal of information can be given by the mass media, at both local and national levels. Therefore, mass media activities have also been an important part of the programme as a whole.

Special efforts have been made to ensure that the educational activities forming part of the programme are really comprehensive. As far as the message content is concerned, this means that traditional, medically-oriented information is amply supplemented by material relating to everyday psychology, environmental protection, the economy, etc. New ways of presenting the message have also been sought. An important feature here are the efforts to adopt as far as possible a "positive" approach, i.e. first of all emphasizing the favourable aspects of non-smoking rather than creating a sense of fear about the ill effects of smoking.

Special treatment for smoking cessation

Large-scale cessation-oriented action predominantly consists of educational and counselling activities incorporated in the daily work of health professionals. In some cases, however, specific treatment procedures can be added. Some such procedures may be used at any doctor's surgery, for example the use of certain medications such as nicotine chewing-gum. Other more complex procedures can only be used at particular smoking cessation clinics. In Sweden such clinics exist at eight hospitals.

Legislation

The mandatory nature of smoking and health education in schools is established by law. Another important piece of legislation is the Tobacco Labelling Act, which became effective at the beginning of 1977. According to this Act, all tobacco packages have to carry health warnings. In addition, cigarette packages have to bear a declaration of contents. Such declarations indicate the yield of carbon monoxide, tar and nicotine and, as a comparison, the averages for all brands on the Swedish market. Health warnings on cigarette packages are varied, so that 16 warnings appear in rotation at any given time.

From 1979 onwards there has been a specific Act regulating tobacco advertising. Under this Act there is a total prohibition of outdoor advertising and of advertising in certain publications directed at young people. In ordinary newspapers, advertisements for tobacco products are restricted in size, and there can be no picture other than that of a single package shown against a neutral background. The text of the advertisements has to be confined to factual information on the product, and each advertisement must include a health warning and, in the case of cigarettes, a declaration of contents.

Possible Methods of Measuring Smoking-related Parameters

Monitoring a country's development with regard to smoking and health requires the measurement of certain parameters. One basic parameter is tobacco consumption. There are two major ways in which tobacco consumption can be measured: (*a*) by reviewing sales data, and (*b*) by analysing survey data. As pointed out by a WHO Working Group *(2)*, sales data may often deviate from consumption data in several respects, so that the former do not always truly reflect consumption. Further, sales data can never reflect differences in consumption between sexes or population groups. Survey data can also be subject to uncertainties, but generally they provide better estimates of consumption than do sales data.

For many reasons it is necessary to have information about people's smoking behaviour, both in terms of the prevalence of various forms of tobacco use and in terms of the intensity of its use, e.g. the number of cigarettes smoked per day. It is also important to have this kind of information for each of various subgroups according to sex, age, educational level, place of residence, etc. This can be achieved only by appropriately designed surveys.

The long-term public health aspects of smoking depend not only on the actual smoking pattern at a given time but also on its future development. This makes it important to map out the various determinants of future behaviour as far as possible. One way of measuring this kind of parameter is to include in smoking surveys questions regarding attitudes and beliefs.

From a health promotion point of view, smoking behaviour is in some respects an intermediate variable that is of interest only because of its known relation to health conditions. When evaluating the success of smoking control, the "final" output indicator would have to deal with morbidity and mortality. The relation between changes in smoking behaviour and changes in disease-related variables is complicated by time lag and other factors, but, first of all, good records of the incidence and prevalence of smoking-related diseases are necessary when it comes to assessing the impact of smoking control.

In a wider health policy perspective, it would also be desirable to estimate the costs of smoking-related diseases to the national economy. This would, for example, enable governments to see the size of the smoking problem in comparison with other problems and to set priorities accordingly when allocating funds for smoking control and other purposes.

Measuring Developments in Sweden with regard to Smoking and Health

As pointed out above, the monitoring of a country's smoking and health situation has to include measurements at several levels. In Sweden a number of such measurements have been carried out, some of them covering longer, some shorter, periods of time. The more important measurements are described below.

Sales of tobacco

Certain sales data have been available since the middle of the nineteenth century. Per capita sales of all types of tobacco product taken together have remained surprisingly constant at about 2 kg per person aged 15 years and above from the 1890s up to now. Before the First World War, tobacco was sold almost entirely in the form of snuff. Then cigarettes were introduced and gradually took the lead. Cigars and pipe-tobacco have had a fairly constant, but rather modest, share of total tobacco sales. Snuff sales were steadily falling until 1967, when the sale of snuff accounted for some 18% of total tobacco sales by weight. Since then, the sale of snuff has increased and now represents about 29% of total tobacco sales by weight.

Table 1 gives some selected data on cigarette sales at three different periods during the time when there has been smoking control action of any kind. It is worth noticing that since 1967–1969 sales of cigarettes have gone up in number but down in weight. This reflects a changes in the proportions of heavy and light cigarettes sold, with a consequent decrease in the average weight of cigarettes. It would be reasonable to infer that weight is a better measure of tobacco consumption than the more commonly published figures for the number of cigarettes sold.

Table 1. Annual average cigarette sales in Sweden

Period	Total		Per adult	
	Number per year (millions)	Weight per year (tonnes)	Number per year	Weight per year (kg)
1962-1964	7 720	7 890	1 290	1.3
1967-1969	9 580	8 740	1 540	1.4
1981-1983	11 710	8 040	1 730	1.2

The statistics for 1982 illustrate another weakness of sales figures as a measure of consumption. The sale of cigarettes in 1982 was actually 5% above that in 1981, but according to the calculations of the Swedish Tobacco Company, consumption increased by only 1%. The sales increase was largely due to the increased purchase of stock before the end of the year, in anticipation of a scheduled increase in the duty on tobacco. Some of the sales increase was also attributable to a sharp growth in trade along the Norwegian border.

Prevalence and intensity of tobacco use

From 1976 onwards, NTS has made annual surveys of the adult population's smoking habits *(3)*. Each year the study comprises around 2000 individuals randomly selected in such a way as to constitute a representative sample of the total Swedish population. In 1963 a comparable study was made by the national Bureau of Statistics. The period 1963–1976 is not covered in detail. However, some data from unpublished studies by the Swedish Tobacco Company make it possible to trace the main lines of development in the prevalence of tobacco use.

In the above-mentioned annual surveys the respondents' sex, age, educational level, occupation, residence area and a few more background variables are recorded. With regard to smoking behaviour, respondents are identified as daily smokers, occasional smokers or non-smokers. Among daily smokers, certain subgroups are identified, namely: daily smokers of cigarettes only, daily smokers of cigarettes and other tobacco products ("mixed smokers"), and daily smokers of other tobacco products only. All cigarette smokers are asked to indicate in figures the average number of cigarettes smoked per day. Answers to this question are presented both as averages of the numbers indicated and as percentage distributions over five levels: 1–7, 8–12, 13–17, 18–22, 23 or more cigarettes per day. It should be noted that these classifications and procedures for the processing and presentation of data are exactly those recently recommended in the WHO guidelines for smoking surveys *(2)*.

Prevalence data for daily smoking are shown in Fig. 1. Throughout the 1960s there was an increase among both males and females. Around 1970 the trend among males became a downward one. Among females the increase was arrested around 1970; prevalence remained level for some years and began to show signs of a downward trend just a few years ago.

Virtually all female smokers are cigarette smokers. Among males there are a small number of daily smokers of pipes and cigars only, but this group is decreasing in size. In 1976, 43% of the males were daily smokers, 36% smoked cigarettes and 7% smoked pipes or cigars. In 1981, 30% of the males were daily smokers, 27% smoked cigarettes and 3% smoked pipes or cigars. In both years some of the cigarette smokers were using a pipe or cigars as well.

During the period 1976–1981, when the number of cigarette smokers decreased by around 15%, cigarette consumption decreased in numbers by only about 5%. This discrepancy is due to an increase in the average daily consumption level of the remaining smokers. Survey data show that this increase in smoking intensity has taken place almost entirely among females, especially the younger ones. For example, in the female group aged 18–24 years the average daily consumption level was 11.3 cigarettes in 1976 and 13.1 cigarettes in 1981, i.e. an increase of 16%.

Fig. 1. Prevalence of daily smoking in the Swedish adult population (aged 18–70 years), as percentages

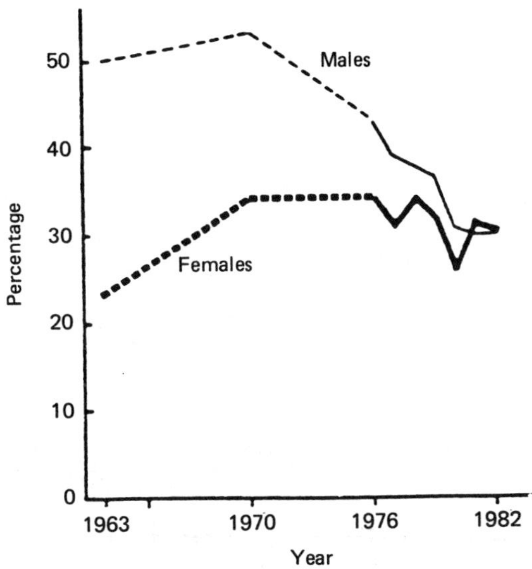

Source: **Nordgren, P., ed.** *(4)*.

Throughout the period since 1976 smoking has been more common in the less educated than in the highly educated groups. However, a decrease in smoking rates among males during that period has occurred in all groups.

The use of snuff is exclusively a male habit. In 1981, 13% of males were using snuff daily, 8% being non-smokers and 5% being smokers as well. The proportion of non-smoking snuff-users has been increasing during the same period as a great many smokers have become non-smokers. It appears that some of those who stop smoking may continue to use tobacco in the form of snuff.

As far as adolescents are concerned, annual nationwide smoking surveys have been carried out by the National Board of Education since 1971. The results are shown in Fig. 2. The positive trend demonstrated in this figure is most probably due to the combined effect of specifically youth-oriented efforts and favourable interaction with the development that has taken place simultaneously in the adult population.

Determinants of future behaviour

For most smokers, the decision to abandon the habit is not taken suddenly; the individual who stops smoking has usually built up a readiness to do so over a period of time. One of the effects of the various smoking control

Fig. 2. Prevalence of teenage smoking in Sweden

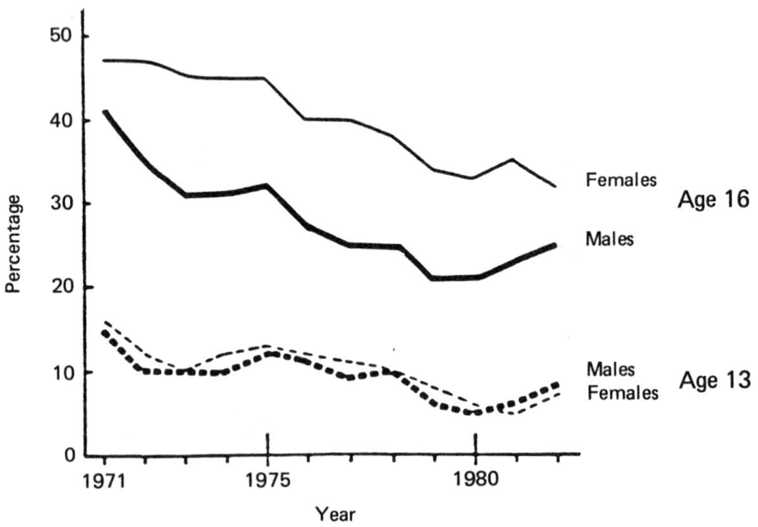

Source: **Nordgren, P., ed.** *(4).*

measures may well be to increase receptiveness to the idea of cessation, while an actual change in behaviour may not appear until later.

The NTS surveys have for some years included a question to smokers about whether they wish to continue smoking or whether they would like to stop. Those who reply that they want to continue smoking have decreased in number. In 1980 just 20% of male and 16% of female daily smokers belonged to this group, while in 1976 the corresponding figures were 27% and 29%.

Lung cancer rates

Epidemiological studies have shown that individual smokers who stop smoking will reduce their lung cancer risk gradually over the following 10–15 years. Where smoking prevalence begins to go down in a population one would therefore expect a decrease in lung cancer rates after a number of years.

In Sweden, smoking rates among men reached a peak and began to fall around 1969 or 1970. According to the Swedish Cancer Registry, the age-standardized lung cancer rate for males reached a peak of 46.2 per 100 000 person-years in 1976 and has since then shown an annual decrease. Among females there has been no such definite turning-point in the smoking rate and the lung cancer rate is constant or rising slightly, the 1979 incidence rate being 11.1 per 100 000 person-years. The annual development from 1971 to 1979 is shown in Table 2 *(5)*.

Table 2. Age-standardized incidence rates of lung cancer in Sweden per 100 000 person-years

Year	Males	Females
1971	40.2	8.4
1972	41.9	9.2
1973	42.4	9.7
1974	43.9	10.6
1975	43.4	10.5
1976	46.2	10.1
1977	44.3	10.2
1978	43.8	10.7
1979	42.2	11.1

Source: Sweden, National Board of Health and Welfare.

The above patterns of development of smoking and lung cancer rates are consistent with the hypothesis that the decline in the lung cancer rate among males is a result of the reduced proportion of male smokers. This idea is further supported by data from the Stockholm area. Here the turning-point in the smoking rate for males came earlier, around 1963, and the turning-point in the lung cancer rate also came earlier, namely in 1970. The situation as it developed in the Stockholm area has been analysed separately for different histological tumour types. Analysis indicates that the tumours most closely related to smoking (squamous cell carcinoma) are those that show a development consistent with the trend in smoking rates, while incidence rates for tumours that are less clearly related to smoking (e.g. adenocarcinoma) continue to rise slowly. Further details are given in Fig. 3 and 4 *(6)*.

Fig. 3. Age-standardized incidence of lung cancer (squamous cell carcinoma) in Stockholm county

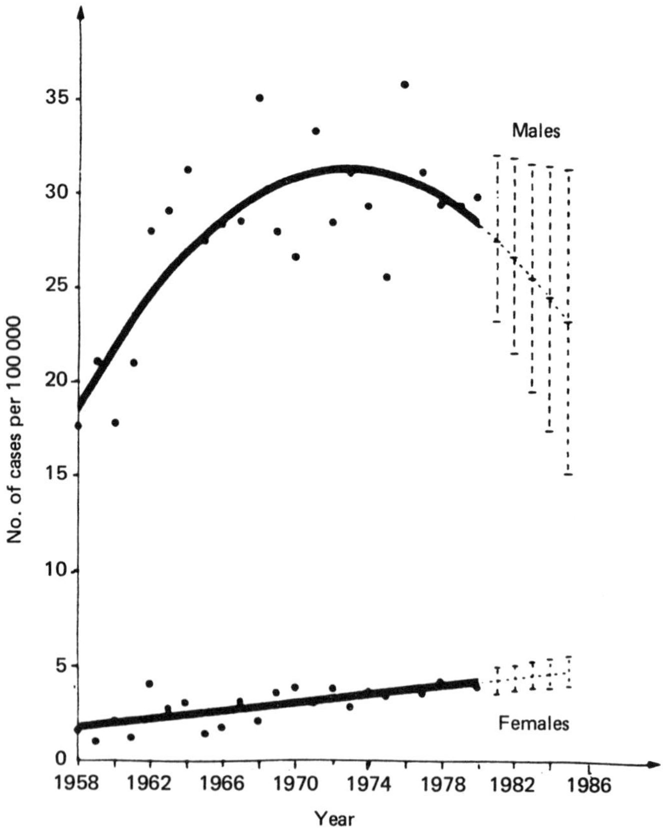

Source: **Wiman, L.-G. et al.** *(6)*.

Fig. 4. Age-standardized incidence of lung cancer (adenocarcinoma) in Stockholm county

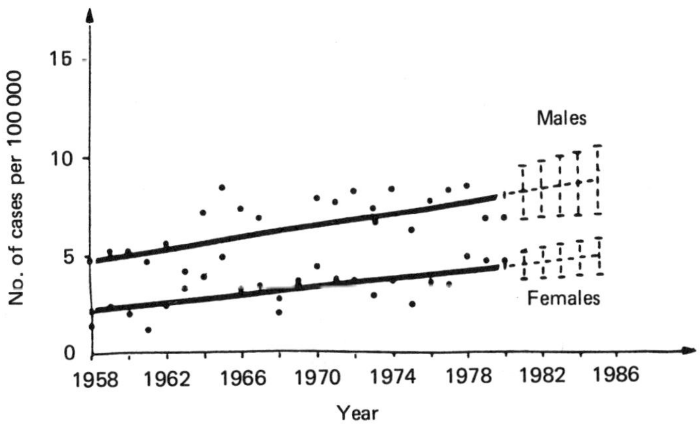

Source: **Wiman, L.-G. et al.** *(6).*

Costs to the national economy

Smoking gives rise to deaths before retiring age, chronic disablement, and excess morbidity causing absenteeism from work. All three of these effects will result in a fall in the number of days worked, this in turn leading to a reduction in the Gross National Product (GNP). Since the size of the GNP is often taken as a measure of a country's wealth, it is obvious that smoking control is justified not only on health grounds but for economic reasons as well.

In Sweden it has been calculated that the GNP around 1980 was reduced by about 2000 million Swedish kroner by the above smoking-related factors; one half of that amount relates to premature deaths and one quarter each to the other two categories. The corresponding burden to society resulting from road traffic accidents has, likewise, been calculated to be of the same magnitude. In view of this, it seems quite astonishing that governmental expenditure on smoking control is only about $^1/_{40}$ of the well justified expenditure on the prevention of road traffic accidents.

Evaluation of some Specific Programmes

The various kinds of measurement dealt with above can all contribute to the task of monitoring the situation with regard to smoking and health and can also provide the basis for some evaluation of the smoking control action as a whole. However, when it comes to evaluating individual activities within the comprehensive smoking control programme there are certain specific difficulties. For example, most measurable parameters come under the combined influence of several programme activities and it is very difficult to attribute the effects to specific influences. However, some evaluations of single activities have been performed in Sweden; a number of these are described below.

Introduction of health warnings on cigarette packages

In order to evaluate the impact of health warnings on cigarette packages, a number of items were added to the regular NTS smoking survey at the end of 1976, immediately before the introduction of the labelling system, and also one year later, at the end of 1977, when the labelling system had been in operation for almost a year. Knowledge, attitudes and behavioural variables were measured by identical questions in both years, and in the second year a number of specific questions were added concerning explicit reactions to the labelling system.

As a result of publicity in the mass media and activities of a similar nature, the warning labels as such are generally known to most Swedish people. However, there is a striking difference between smokers and non-smokers, in that the former have a much better and more detailed knowledge of the system. This should most probably be seen as indicating that smokers in general have really studied the labels, noticing them rather than neglecting them. About one half of the population believes that the warning notices have a favourable effect. The two major ways in which these effects are believed to occur are: (*a*) making people better aware of the health hazards related to smoking, and (*b*) encouraging people to stop smoking or encouraging young people to remain non-smokers. The belief that the warnings might encourage smokers to stop is held equally by smokers and non-smokers, which strengthens the credibility of these answers. The majority of respondents also think that a rotation system, whereby a number of different messages are publicized, is better than having a single text. The main reason is stated to be that the rotation system evokes curiosity, so that the notice is actually read and not neglected. Again, this is an opinion held equally by smokers and non-smokers.

In both 1976 and 1977 those questioned were asked to what degree they approved or disapproved of statements like "Smokers are more susceptible than non-smokers to general air pollution". (This statement is similar in content to one of the 16 warning notices.) Among those exposed to the warning notice, i.e. smokers, there is a definite change towards increased acceptance of the statement, while there is a less significant change among non-smokers, who serve as a "control group". This could be interpreted as evidence that the change in people's knowledge is directly linked to the degree of their exposure to the warning labels. This means not only that the warnings have been noticed and understood, but also that they have made an impact.

The campaign: "A Non-Smoking Generation"

A short specific campaign has been concentrated on influencing the way teenagers look upon smokers and non-smokers, i.e. by advertising non-smoking as the popular, modern, smart, attractive lifestyle. The focus of the campaign could be described as an effort to improve the "image" of non-smokers. This has served as a guideline for the evaluation procedure that has been adopted. In interviews with teenagers, the subjects were shown a picture of two young people who appeared to be identical: one was identified as a smoker, the other as a non-smoker. The respondents were then asked to indicate "Which one of these do you think your pals would prefer to have in your group?".

Among non-smokers of both sexes in the age group 12–24 years the smoker was preferred by only 3–7%. Comparing non-smokers of different age groups, it is found that, with increasing age, the preference for the smoker remains very low and the preference for the non-smoker remains high, although there is an increasing "tolerance" in older age groups in terms of a greater proportion indicating "Doesn't matter". Even among smokers, the preference for the non-smoker is higher than for the smoker, although "Doesn't matter" is the dominating answer here.

Unfortunately these measurements have not been going on long enough for any real trends to be established, but the results do yield an unexpectedly strong image of the non-smoker's attractiveness, a view that was probably less widely held some years ago.

The "Smoke-free Pregnancy" programme

A programme to promote "Smoke-free Pregnancy" was launched in 1976, starting with one-day training courses for all midwives serving at maternity health stations in the province of Stockholm. A special manual about smoking and health-related activities at maternity health stations was given to the midwives. A year later, material was produced to help midwives when counselling and giving instructions. A poster entitled "Please ask us about smoking" is now to be found in waiting-rooms, while in examination rooms midwives have a teaching poster headed "Important facts to remember when pregnant". A special folder, to be handed to the mother, is entitled "Smoking when pregnant?" and mainly reiterates the points made on the teaching poster and by the midwife. A fourth aid is a diary for a person giving up smoking.

One evaluation activity consisted of informal interviews with a sample of pregnant women who had been visiting maternity health stations. Very few reported any negative reactions to the midwife's initiatives with regard to smoking. There was, rather, a common view that the information on smoking should have been more comprehensive. A considerable number of the women said that they had already known most of the facts provided.

Another evaluation activity consisted of a special monitoring system established at selected stations. There the midwives had to make notes about actual smoking behaviour at every visit made by the pregnant women to the station. These records indicate that a surprisingly large number stopped smoking immediately upon learning that they were pregnant. Among the rest, quite a few stopped completely, while others decreased their consumption.

A third evaluation activity was linked to a larger study carried out in 1983 with regard to several smoking-related variables in various groups of health professionals. Here the midwives enrolled in the "Smoke-free Pregnancy" programme could be compared to similar groups without any smoking-specific training. It was found that the trained midwives came out favourably in several respects. Compared to similar groups, they smoked less, had a better knowledge of smoking and health and intervened more actively in their patients' smoking habits. At the same time, it was noted that several midwives limited themselves just to educating patients and failed to give them active assistance to stop smoking. This clearly indicates a need for continued and expanded training.

Concluding Remarks

The feasibility of smoking control

Health policy planners have to establish priorities among several courses of possible action. When considering smoking control, there are three basic questions that have to be answered:

1. Can large-scale changes in smoking behaviour be achieved by health promotion activities?

2. Can a change in smoking patterns be expected to have a major impact on public health?

3. Can favourable results of smoking control be achieved at a reasonable cost?

The first of these questions can be answered "Yes", as the experience of several countries, including Sweden, demonstrates.

An affirmative answer to the second question is supported by earlier findings from studies among specific groups, such as British doctors. The findings described here regarding smoking and lung cancer in Sweden may be one of the first pieces of evidence to apply to the total male population of a country.

The Swedish calculations of economic factors suggest that the economic benefits to be gained from smoking control are very large compared with the costs of operating a smoking control programme. There are some other Swedish calculations which demonstrate further that smoking control could be economically advantageous *(7)*.

Standardization of measurements — international collaboration

In connection with the planning, design, conduct and evaluation of smoking control programmes, it is necessary to carry out measurements of relevant parameters. As shown above, there is a need to make measurements at several levels. It is therefore desirable to have some standards about the kinds of measurement to be made as well as the methods of conducting them. Such standards should preferably be international, since this would also facilitate intercountry comparisons. Many of these requirements are already met by WHO guidelines. With regard to measurement questions not covered in these guidelines, WHO should be able to assist Member States either directly or in liaison with other bodies.

References

1. **Carlsson, G. et al.** *Liv och hälsa. En kartläggning av hälsoutvecklingen i Sverige* [Life and health. A study of the development of health in Sweden]. Stockholm, Liber, 1979, p. 167.
2. *Guidelines for the conduct of tobacco smoking surveys of the general population.* Geneva, World Health Organization, 1983 (document WHO/SMO/83.4).
3. **Nationalföreningen för upplysning om tobakens skadeverkningar (NTS)** [National Smoking and Health Association (NTS)]. *Tobaks vanor i Sverige — en kort historik* [Smoking habits in Sweden — a short history]. Stockholm, NTS, 1983.
4. **Nordgren, P., ed.** *Smoking control in Sweden.* Stockholm, National Smoking and Health Association (NTS), 1983.
5. **National Board of Health and Welfare. The Cancer Registry.** *Cancer incidence in Sweden 1971 resp. 1972 . . . 1984.* Stockholm, 1975 resp. 1976 . . . 1986.
6. **Wiman, L.-G. et al.** Lungcancer i Stockholmsregionen — aarlig incidens 1958–80, prognos 1981–85 [Lung cancer in the Stockholm region — annual incidence 1958–80 and projections 1981–85]. *Läkartidningen,* **80**: 3290–3293 (1983).
7. **Ramström, L.M.** Public health effects of smoking control. *In:* Arvidsson, O., ed. *Health and society IV.* Stockholm, Committee for Future Oriented Research, 1979, pp. 1–22.

11.3 Experiences from the North Karelia Project — *A. Nissinen, P. Puska & J. Tuomilehto*

This contribution presents an overview of some of the experiences from the North Karelia Project, which are relevant to the subject matter of many of the chapters in Part II. In particular, they discuss the measurement of behavioural change associated with the North Karelia programme, and provide examples of the methods discussed in Chapter 8.2.

During the past hundred years the impact of infectious diseases has been dramatically reduced as a result of improved levels of hygiene, general social measures and specific preventive and therapeutic activities in the industrialized countries. Chronic diseases, especially cardiovascular diseases, have now emerged as the main public health problem. Analysis of data from several industrialized countries shows that the control and prevention of cardiovascular diseases has the greatest potential impact on longevity among the adult population *(1)*. Thus, further advances in public health are dependent on the success achieved in controlling cardiovascular and related noncommunicable diseases. Considerable differences in both the cardiovascular disease and coronary heart disease rates, even between industrialized countries, have been shown repeatedly in mortality statistics *(2,3)*. A WHO-coordinated acute myocardial infarction registration study *(4)* found the rates highest in Finland. The data showed also that, within Finland, the cardiovascular disease rates were higher in the east than in the west of the country.

These findings aroused the awareness and concern of the Finnish public. The people of North Karelia county in eastern Finland, where the study had started in the 1950s, were particularly concerned. The statistics showing high disease rates matched people's own observations. At the beginning of the 1970s, among the county's total population of 180 000 (1972 figure), some 1000 myocardial infarctions took place annually, about one half of these being among men below 65 years of age. Some 40% of these cases were fatal. In 1972, among people aged 45–59 years in North Karelia, 27% were pensioned owing to disability, about one third of them as a result of cardiovascular diseases *(5)*. The North Karelia Project was then formulated, and this major community-based preventive cardiovascular study was started in spring 1972.

North Karelia is the most eastern of the 11 Finnish counties. It has an area of 18 000 km^2, with great forests, lakes, hills, small farms, small towns and numerous small villages. The area has a relatively low socioeconomic status, a high level of unemployment, an income based on farming and forestry, and sparse medical and other services.

The programme was aimed at the total population of the area, with special reference to middle-aged men, among whom the disease rates were especially alarming. Evaluations were designed to assess the feasibility, effects, process of change, costs, and other consequences related to this programme. The original project was set up for the programme to be carried out and evaluated for a five-year period (1972–1977). Since the experience gained was encouraging, it was decided to continue the programme. In spring 1982 a major ten-year survey was completed *(6)*.

General principles

The historical background of the North Karelia Project led to the adoption of a community approach. Also, since cardiovascular diseases are a widespread health problem and their precursors are present in a major proportion of the population, a community-wide scale was necessary. The community approach included the integration of the programme with the existing social and health service structure. When the North Karelia Project was set up, much was already known about the precursors of and risk factors for coronary heart disease. Numerous studies indicated that a few factors, notably smoking, elevated serum cholesterol and elevated blood pressure, predict a major part of subsequent coronary heart disease risk, independent of other potential factors studied *(7,8)*. Results from basic biochemical studies, as well as results from a few experimental and quasi-experimental studies on the different risk factors, have also long been available with regard to smoking cessation *(9)*, cholesterol-lowering diets *(10)* and treatment of blood pressure *(11)*.

In the light of existing information, the choice of the main risk factors calling for intervention was relatively easy in the North Karelia Project. The international work had highlighted the obviously important roles of smoking, serum cholesterol (related to dietary habits) and blood pressure. At the same time, it was already well known that the levels of these risk factors were high in the Finnish and, more specifically, in the North Karelian population. Furthermore, some other possible risk factors, such as physical inactivity, obesity or type-A behaviour, were not common in the area.

The theoretical frameworks on which the North Karelia Project is based are summarized as follows.

(*a*) *The behaviour change approach,* which relates to social psychology and deals with the determinants of individuals' behavioural changes *(12–15)*; the modified model used in the project *(16)* emphasizes that programme planning and evaluation should relate to the following key steps, so as to help the individual modify his or her behaviour:

— improved preventive services, to help people identify their risk factors and to provide appropriate facilities and advice;

— information, to educate people about the relationship between types of behaviour and health;

— persuasion, to motivate people and to encourage them to adopt healthy lifestyles;

— training, to increase the skills required for self-management and environmental control;

— social support, to help people maintain the initial action;

— environmental change, to create the opportunities for health-promoting action and to improve unfavourable conditions;

— organization, to mobilize the community to implement wide-ranging changes (through increased social support and environment modification), and to support the adoption of new lifestyles in the community.

(*b*) *The communication–behaviour change approach,* based on Bandura's social learning theory *(12)*, the classical communication–persuasion model of McGuire *(17)*, its modification by Flay et al. *(18)* and the belief–attitude–intention model of Ajzen & Fishbein *(19)*; this approach has been developed in the North Karelia Project, especially in connection with health education programmes about the project on national television *(20)*.

(*c*) *The innovation-diffusion approach,* which emphasizes that the new lifestyles are innovations that diffuse with time through the natural networks of the community to the members of a given social system *(21)*.

(*d*) *The community organization approach,* which emphasizes the efforts of the project to influence the various organizations and to structure them in accordance with needs; the concept of community organization refers both to community self-development (the community initially detecting a problem and organizing itself to cope with it) and to the various degrees of outside influence needed to effect the necessary reorganizations.

The previous approaches have been unified in Fig. 1, which shows the behavioural/social model of community intervention most relevant to the North Karelia Project. The external project input works both in the form of communication via the mass media to the population (where its effect is further mediated through interpersonal contact) and even more so as an agent of change (formal and informal leaders of opinion influencing various aspects of community organization). The overall aim is to increase knowledge, to motivate, to teach practical skills and to provide the social and environmental support necessary for the population to exercise and maintain its health skills. These activities and the ensuing new lifestyles will, it maintained, ultimately lead to a more favourable risk factor profile, reduced disease rates, and improved health for the population.

Although the main project features and the evaluation design were clearly established during the initial planning phase, many theoretical aspects relating to community intervention became understood and were developed only in the course of the project's implementation.

Fig. 1. Model of community intervention as used in the North Karelia Project

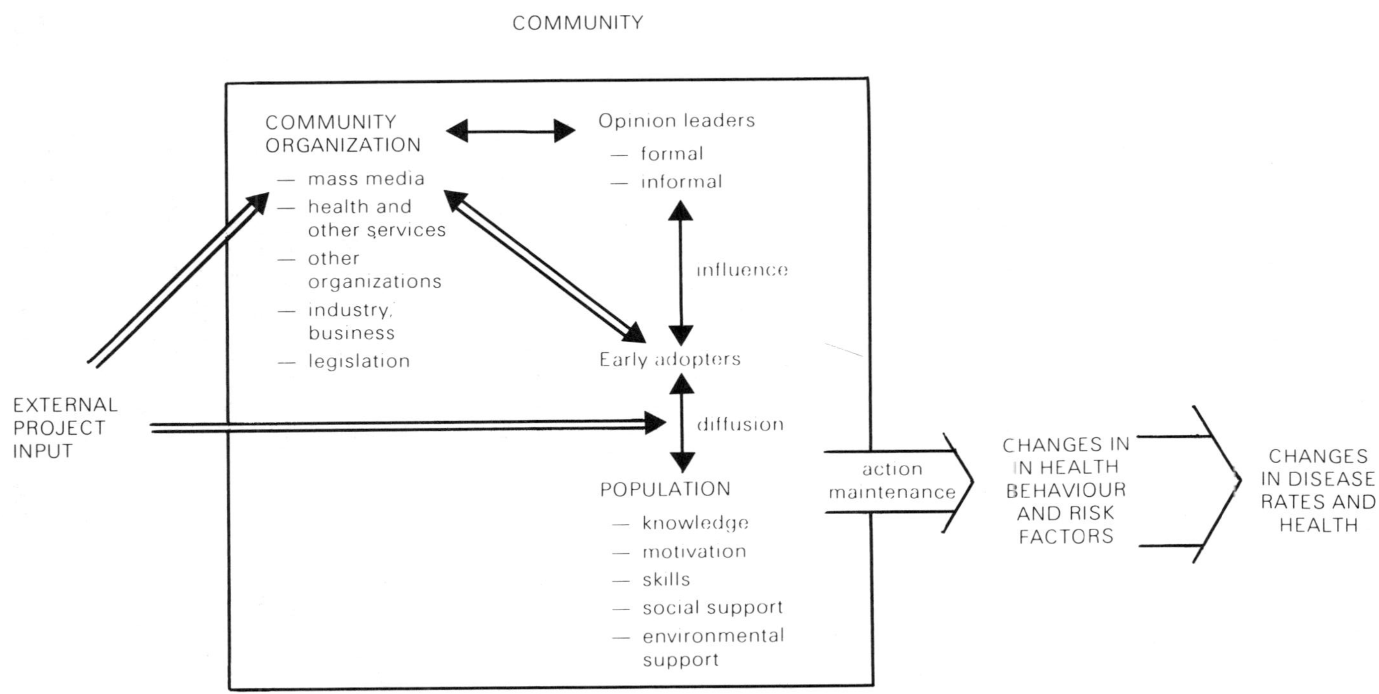

The Main Project Components

The practical framework of the North Karelia Project consists of three components: (*a*) planning, (*b*) intervention programme implementation, and (*c*) evaluation (see Fig. 2). Although this is also the main chronological sequence, in many cases these measures take place simultaneously as the project proceeds.

Within the overall aims and framework, the actual implementation of the project in North Karelia was flexible, so that it could be adjusted in response to opportunities in the community. Integrating the programme into the community social organization was a necessity, because it ensured the community's participation and made its resources available. Thus, the project set the objectives and developed the general framework, while the activities were carried out mainly by the community. The project catalysed this work by providing materials, training, necessary official support, mass media support and follow-up.

The programme activities were simple and practical, so as to facilitate their implementation in the community at large. They may be divided into the following groups:

- media-related and general educational activities;
- training of local personnel and other active groups;
- organization of health services (primary health care, other);
- other community organization activities; and
- activities for monitoring developments for management and feedback purposes.

A detailed description of the intervention activities has been published in a monograph on the North Karelia Project in 1972–1977 *(5)*.

Evaluation

Evaluation in the North Karelia Project covers the following five aspects of the programme: (*a*) feasibility, (*b*) effects (behaviour, risk factors, disease rates), (*c*) process, (*d*) costs, and (*e*) other consequences (see Fig. 2).

The evaluation of *feasibility* assessed the extent to which it was possible to implement the planned activities in the community. This concerned the amount of resources available to the project, how they were used in the community, and how effectively the activities reached the target populations. The results of the feasibility assessment were based on survey and other data (project statistics) collected during and after certain programme periods.

Evaluation of the programme's *effect* was carried out, using a quasi-experimental study design, to assess whether and to what extent the main and intermediate objectives were achieved.

Fig. 2. Model of elements in the community-based project as used in the North Karelia Project

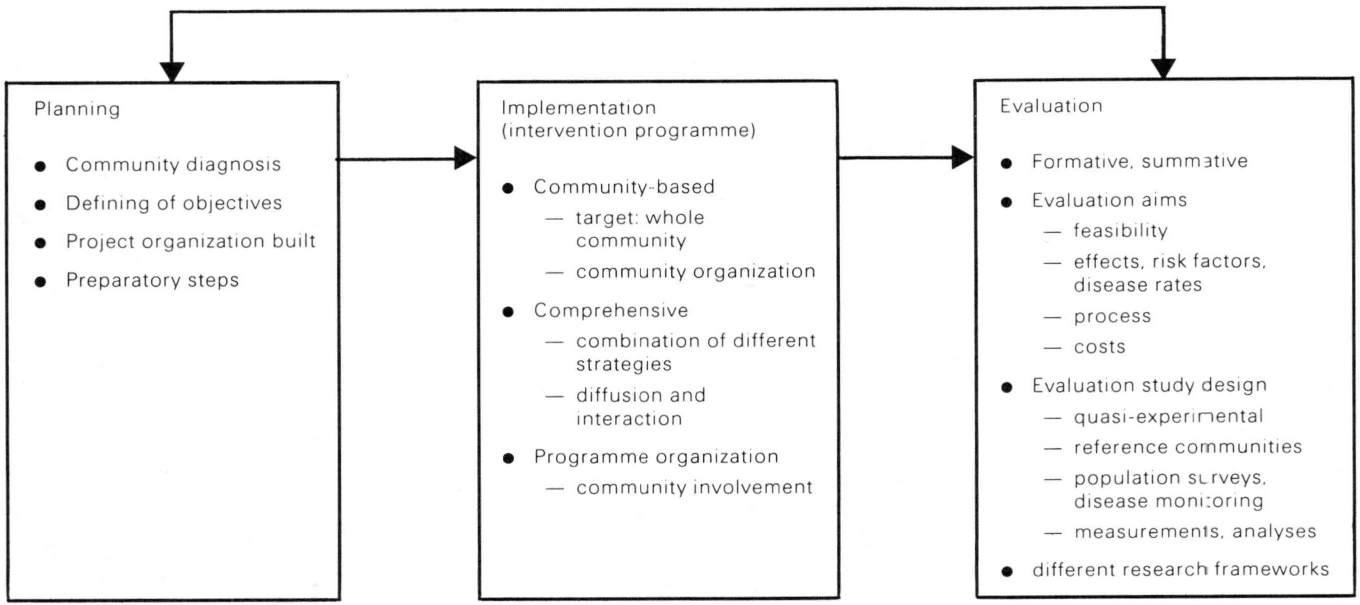

Since the programme target was the whole community, information was collected from representative independent population samples at the outset (the baseline survey in 1972) and at the main evaluation points: after five years (in 1977) and after ten years (in 1982). The sample sizes were large in order to detect changes in risk factors that would be small for individuals but significant for the population as a whole. The large sample sizes also enabled some interesting subgroup analyses to be made. In each survey nearly 10 000 subjects were examined, participation ranging between 80% and 94%. To assess changes occurring during the period for reasons other than the activities of the intervention programme, a reference area was used.

The baseline and follow-up surveys were carried out simultaneously in the reference area and in North Karelia with strict adherence to identical methodology and sampling procedures. Survey results concerning changes in the reference area represent changes occurring independently of the programme ("national changes, "secular trends", "spontaneous changes"). The programme effect was regarded as the observed change in the programme area (North Karelia) minus the observed change in the reference area (the so-called "net change").

Mortality rates were collected by disease category and analysed for North Karelia and the reference area (and also all other counties of the country). Additional information concerning related hospital discharges was available from a national register, and data from the national cancer register were also used. Special acute myocardial infarction and stroke registers were established in North Karelia in accordance with WHO criteria to monitor the respective incidence rates. Since these registers were themselves thought to be powerful intervention tools and part of the comprehensive programme to be evaluated, no permanent new registers were established in the reference area. Thus the registers served the process evaluation and also served for validation of the other mortality and morbidity data.

Process evaluation was twofold, i.e. it concerned both the change in trends over time during the programme and changes in the intervening variables. Thus, it examined when the changes actually took place during the period, and also covered the behavioural/social framework adopted and the definition of the intended intervening (independent) variables. Measurement of these factors gave a picture of how the process of change in the community led (or did not lead) to the desired behavioural and risk factor changes.

Cost evaluation assessed the total project resources and how they were allocated (especially for intervention and evaluation purposes). In addition, efforts were made to assess the cost to the community. This information was collected using statistical data sources, project surveys and other data *(5)*.

Other consequences of the programme apart from those intended were also assessed. Fig. 3 gives a summary of the main evaluation study design in the North Karelia Project. A more detailed discussion on the various evaluation principles and issues can be found in other publications *(12,22–24)*.

Fig. 3. Main evaluation study design in the North Karelia Project

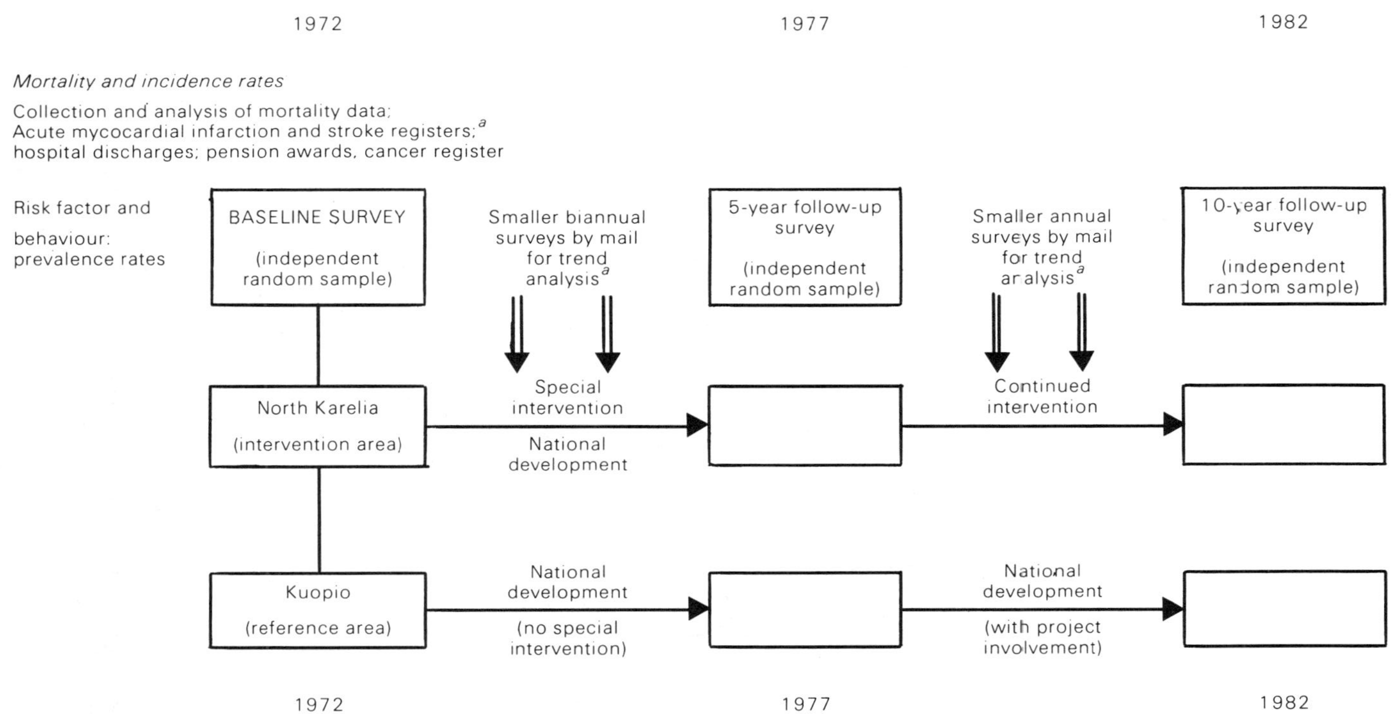

[a] Refers to North Karelia only (acute mycocardial infarction register in the reference area in 1977 and since 1982).

Results

The results of the first five-year period (1972–1977) of the project have been published in a number of scientific publications and in a WHO monograph *(5)*. They showed that:

- the feasibility of the programme was good;
- the programme had distinct effects on lifestyles and risk factors;
- cardiovascular morbidity and mortality rates decreased during the period in the region, but no significant difference between the study and reference area was observed with regard to mortality trends;
- the costs of the programme were modest and were considerably less than the sums saved as a result of reduced expenditure on disability payments;
- the inhabitants participated actively in the programme and were very satisfied with it — no major adverse emotional effects were observed in the population.

The results of the programme indicated that smoking and serum cholesterol levels among the North Karelian population continued to decline during the second five-year period (1977–1982). Table 1 shows the net reduction (adjusted for changes in the reference area) in the risk factor levels during the 10-year period 1972–1982 for both men and women. On the whole, the net reductions achieved in 1972–1977 were maintained during the follow-up period *(6)*.

Analysis of the latest available mortality data for the period 1969–1979 *(25)* has shown that age-standardized coronary heart disease mortality among the middle-aged male population in North Karelia decreased by 24% (12% nationally, $P < 0.05$). Most of this decrease in North Karelia took place after 1973. During the period 1974–1979, when the impact of the risk factor changes became clear, the reduction in coronary heart disease mortality was 22% in North Karelia, 12% in the reference area and 11% in Finland as a whole (excluding North Karelia) ($P < 0.05$). Coronary heart disease mortality also decreased among women, with a decline of 51% among the middle-aged female population in 1969–1979. This decline among women in North Karelia was also significantly greater than that in the rest of the country ($P < 0.001$). Because the mortality rates from coronary heart disease are much smaller among women than among men, the number of male deaths avoided was much greater (see Table 2).

Process aspects

As part of the process analysis, time trends and changes in subgroups and intervening variables were examined. A sharp reduction in smoking took place among men during the first year. Dietary changes took place gradually throughout the project period. Major changes in government price policy were reflected in these trends. The frequency of blood-pressure measurements increased in the area during the first two years of the intervention. The

Table 1. Relative net reductions (±SD) in risk factor means, males and females aged 30–59 years, North Karelia, 1972–1977 and 1972–1982 (values expressed as percentages of the baseline value in North Karelia)

	Percentage change over the period:			
	1972–1977		1972–1982	
	Males	Females	Males	Females
Daily smoking	-15 (±10)**	-12 (±27)	-28 (±11)***	-14 (±38)
Serum cholesterol	- 4 (± 1)***	- 1 (± 2)	- 3 (± 2)***	- 1 (± 2)
Systolic blood pressure	- 3 (± 1)***	- 5 (± 1)***	- 3 (± 1)***	- 5 (± 1)***
Diastolic blood pressure	- 3 (± 1)***	- 4 (± 1)***	- 1 (± 1)*	- 2 (± 1)*

* $P<0.05$; ** $P<0.01$; *** $P<0.001$

proportion of men receiving antihypertensive treatment increased from 3% in 1972 to 10% in 1975 and that of women from 9% to 14%. These new levels remained constant throughout the rest of the period.

Changes in risk factors were generally greater among men than among women; this was in accordance with the aims of the project. The population's knowledge of risk factors increased somewhat during this period, but the increase was only slightly greater in North Karelia than in the reference area. Various measures to influence health attitudes showed no major changes during the period and there was little difference between the areas in this respect.

Physicians and public health nurses had generally been more active in North Karelia than in the reference area in their contacts with various community organizations concerning health promotion activities. Local decision-makers had received advice from health personnel about cessation of smoking and changes in dietary habits twice as often in North Karelia as in the reference area.

Other consequences and cost aspects

From 1972 onwards, both the surveys and the statistics of the National Social Security Institution showed a favourable trend in the number of disability pensions awarded in North Karelia compared with the reference area. According to the surveys, between 1972 and 1977 the proportion of all disability pension awards increased by 16% in North Karelia and by 25% in the reference area.

Table 2. Average annual regression-based change in age-standardized mortality from coronary heart disease in North Karelia, the reference area and Finland (excluding North Karelia), 1974–1979 (± 95% confidence intervals)

Area	Annual percentage change in the period 1974–1979	
	Males	Females
North Karelia	- 3.7 ± 1.5	- 2.2 ± 3.4
Reference area	- 1.9 ± 2.3	- 1.8 ± 1.4
Finland (excluding North Karelia)	- 1.7 ± 2.2[a]	- 1.2 ± 2.4

[a] Difference from North Karelia in relation to random variation $P < 0.05$.

The project budget was used for the extra input to intensify cardiovascular prevention in North Karelia. The direct project budget was US $1.75 million for the period 1971–1977 (with evaluation up to 1979). Out of this budget, US $0.73 million was for intervention expenditures and US $1.02 million for evaluation costs. It was possible to keep the budget so modest because many of the actual costs involved were covered by the university or other institutions.

The direct project costs were only 1% of the total general health service operation costs and 4% of similar cardiovascular disease-related costs in North Karelia during the period 1972–1977. During the same period, the reduced numbers of acute myocardial infarction and stroke cases represented a saving of US $2 million. A substantial relative reduction in cardiovascular disease disability pension awards, specific to North Karelia, took place from 1972 onwards. The savings in these pension awards amounted to US $4 million during the period 1972–1977.

The survey questionnaires included standard precoded questions that were used to assess the psychosocial consequences of the programme. After ten years, in 1982, people tended to report their health status as "very good" or "good" more often than was the case in 1972. This improvement in subjective health status was significantly greater for North Karelia than for the reference area ($P < 0.005$). A similar pattern was found in the perceived risk of heart disease; the decline in North Karelia was again greater than in the reference area ($P < 0.01$).

In addition to covering these two variables, the questions dealt with measures of psychosocial stress, social interaction, psychosomatic symptoms, somatic symptoms, subjective fitness, days of illness, etc. The total score of these complaints (altogether 20 variables and 56 questions) showed a decrease in both areas. This was greater in North Karelia, resulting in a net decrease of 6% for men ($P < 0.05$) and 10% for women ($P < 0.001$).

These findings exclude the possibility of the preventive programme having any general unwanted emotional consequences; rather, they suggest a general positive effect of the intervention in terms of subjective health and quality of life.

In the 1977 survey of local physicians, public health nurses and local decision-makers, these groups were asked how they felt about various cardiovascular disease prevention- and control-related activities in their own communities. The degree of satisfaction with all these activities among the groups surveyed was markedly greater in North Karelia than in the reference area. With regard to other types of activity, the responses differed little between the areas (see Table 3).

These results, together with the personal experiences of the project team, clearly indicate that there was broad general satisfaction among the population of North Karelia with the preventive programme initiated and coordinated by the project team. People participated well in the activities, cooperation with various community organizations and opinion leaders was good and, in terms of subjective feelings, reaction to the project activities was generally positive.

Conclusions

The results achieved so far support the initial hypothesis that a well conceived comprehensive community-based programme can have a beneficial impact on the lifestyles and cardiovascular risk factors of an entire population and that such a development is associated with reduced cardiovascular mortality rates. These results thus give further support to the now widely accepted risk factor theory. Furthermore, they demonstrate the potential of a community-based approach in changing risk factors, as well as affording practical experience in organizing such activities within health services and other community settings.

For some considerable time there has been little question about the role played by smoking and elevated blood pressure in the development of cardiovascular diseases. After the results of the Lipid Research Clinics study were published *(26)*, the importance of elevated serum cholesterol as a coronary heart disease risk factor has also been firmly established. The question now is whether such changes should concern only people at high risk or the entire population and, in the latter case, how such changes can be promoted.

Even if some of the evidence may be questioned, there are good reasons to strive for a reduction in the general risk factor in whole populations. Many health benefits result from ceasing to smoke; reduced obesity and an increase in vegetable and fibre consumption are likely to be beneficial; and treatment of hypertension is warranted. People should be helped to make changes which a large proportion of them desire and which reduce the risk of several chronic diseases and premature death and promote health. These factors are common in the community and are closely linked with lifestyles. Any intervention limited to a small group of people at high risk cannot by itself have much of a long-term impact on the community. In community-based interventions people themselves ultimately take the decisions about

Table 3. Opinions of health personnel and local decision-makers about local cardiovascular disease control activities in North Karelia and the reference county

Cardiovascular disease control activity	Percentage considering the activity at the local health centre to be sufficient					
	Physicians		Public health nurses		Local decision-makers	
	North Karelia	Reference county	North Karelia	Reference county	North Karelia	Reference county
Cardiovascular disease control in general	52	18	49	7	20	7
Anti-smoking	45	30	34	19	28	18
Nutritional education	35	13	31	18	24	10
Hypertension control	79	42	90	47	45	31
Heart disease patients' rehabilitation	52	13	44	9	21	8
Health examinations	59	35	49	23	28	22

their health practices and lifestyles. The changes recommended, for example, by a recent WHO Expert Committee on the prevention of coronary heart disease *(27)*, are moderate and safe, can be enjoyable, and are likely to reduce the risk of several major noncommunicable diseases and to promote health in general. People have a right to this information and to be helped to make such changes.

The greater potential of the community strategy compared with the high-risk strategy in reducing coronary heart disease rates in the community has been demonstrated by modelling the different approaches and using the data from the North Karelia Project *(28)*. The differences are shown in Fig. 4. The same effect has also been well described by Rose using the Framingham data *(29)*. The North Karelia Project results also show that in the community lifestyle changes are not predicted by people's initial risk factor levels but rather are related to a general community-wide process of change *(30)*.

The results achieved by the programme in North Karelia continue to underline the favourable development observed so far. This is considered important for national and international demonstration and training purposes. At the same time, it is important to continue to monitor the risk

Fig. 4. Projected effects of different prevention strategies on reduction of acute myocardial infarction rates in the community: North Karelia Project data

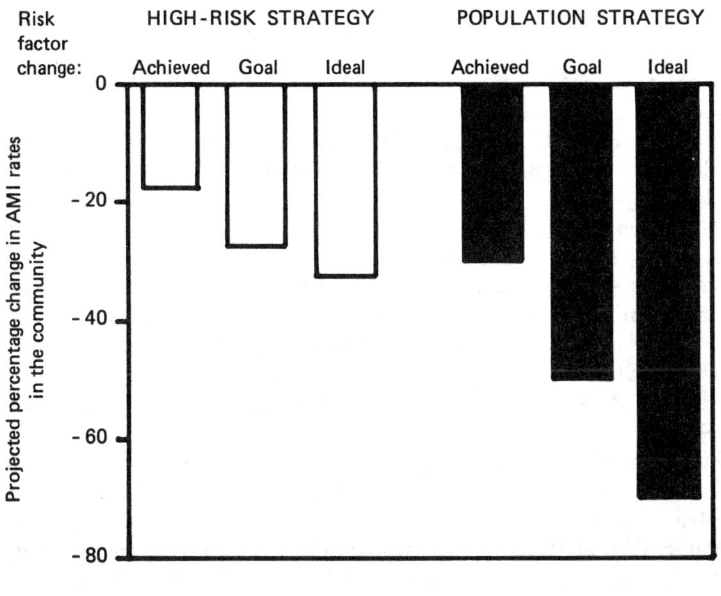

Note. "Achieved" and "goal" refer to experiences in recent studies (see Kottke, T.E. et al. *(28)*).

factor and disease trends and to assess fully the long-term impact of the activities. Furthermore, the scope of the programme is being enlarged to consider related major noncommunicable diseases in an integrated way and to emphasize also the promotion of "positive" health. With careful evaluation on a nationwide basis, the experience gained during the project continues to be applied through the national health service system, through several mass-media channels and by means of health education and other material.

References

1. **Fejfar, Z.** Prevention of cardiovascular diseases. *In: Chronic diseases.* Copenhagen, WHO Regional Office for Europe, 1973 (Public Health in Europe, No. 2).
2. *World health statistics quarterly,* **31**: 208–346 (1978).
3. *World health statistics quarterly,* **35**: 11–17 (1982).
4. *Myocardial infarction community registers.* Copenhagen, WHO Regional Office for Europe, 1976 (Public Health in Europe, No. 5).
5. **Puska, P. et al.** *The North Karelia Project: evaluation of a comprehensive community programme for control of cardiovascular diseases in North Karelia, Finland, 1972–1977.* Copenhagen, WHO Regional Office for Europe, 1981.
6. **Puska, P. et al.** Change in risk factors for coronary heart disease during 10 years of a community intervention programme (North Karelia Project). *British medical journal,* **287**: 1840–1844 (1983).
7. **Dawber, T.R. et al.** Epidemiological approaches to heart disease: the Framingham Study. *American journal of public health,* **41**: 279–286 (1951).
8. **Tibblin, G.** Risk factors in coronary heart disease. *Advances in cardiology,* **4**: 123–130 (1969).
9. **Doll, R. & Hill, A.B.** Mortality in relation to smoking: ten years' observations of British doctors. *British medical journal,* **1**: 1399–1410 (1964).
10. **Turpeinen, O.** Effect of cholesterol-lowering diet on mortality from coronary heart disease and other causes. *Circulation,* **59**: 1–7 (1979).
11. **Veterans Administration Cooperative Study Group.** Effects of treatment on morbidity in hypertension. Results in patients with diastolic blood pressure averaging 90 through 114 mmHg. *Journal of the American Medical Association,* **213**: 1143–1152 (1970).
12. **Bandura, A.** *Social learning theory.* Englewood Cliffs, NJ, Prentice Hall, 1977.
13. **Fishbein, M. & Ajzen, J.** *Belief, attitude, intention, and behavior: an introduction to theory and research.* Reading, MA, Addison-Wesley, 1975.
14. **Kar, S.B. et al.** Psychosocial model of health behavior: implications for nutrition education, research and policy. *Health values,* **7**: 29–37 (1983).
15. **Lewin, K.** *In:* Cartwright, D., ed. *Field theory in social science, selected theoretical papers.* New York, Harper & Row, 1951.

16. **McAlister, A. et al.** Theory and action for health promotion: illustrations from the North Karelia Project. *American journal of public health,* **72**(1): 43–50 (1982).
17. **McGuire, W.J.** The nature of attitudes and attitude change. *In:* Lindsay, G. & Aronson, E., ed. *Handbook of social psychology.* Reading, MA, Addison-Wesley, 1969, Vol. III.
18. **Flay, B.R. et al.** Mass media in health promotion. *Health education quarterly,* **7**: 127–143 (1980).
19. **Ajzen, J. & Fishbein, M.** *Understanding attitudes and predicting social behavior.* Englewood Cliffs, NJ, Prentice Hall, 1980.
20. **Puska, P. et al.** Television in health promotion: evaluation of a national program in Finland. *International journal of health education,* **24**: 238–250 (1981).
21. **Rogers, E.** *Diffusion of innovations.* New York, The Free Press, 1983.
22. **Farquhar, J.W.** The community-based model of lifestyle intervention trials. *American journal of epidemiology,* **108**: 103–111 (1978).
23. *Proposal for the multinational monitoring of trends and determinants in cardiovascular disease and protocol (MONICA project).* Geneva, World Health Organization, 1983 (WHO/MNC/82.1).
24. **Williams, P.T. et al.** A comparison of statistical methods for evaluating risk factor changes in community-based studies: an example from the Stanford Three Community Study. *Journal of chronic diseases,* **34**: 565–571 (1981).
25. **Salonen, J.T. et al.** Decline in mortality from coronary heart disease in Finland from 1969 to 1979. *British medical journal,* **286**: 1857–1860 (1983).
26. **Lipid Research Clinics Program.** The lipid research clinics coronary primary prevention trial results. I. Reduction in incidence of coronary heart disease. *Journal of the American Medical Association,* **251**: 351–364 (1984).
27. WHO Technical Report Series, No. 678, 1982 (*Prevention of coronary heart disease:* report of a WHO Expert Committee).
28. **Kottke, E.T. et al.** Projected effects of high risk versus population-based prevention strategies in coronary heart disease. *American journal of epidemiology,* **121**: 697–704 (1985).
29. **Rose, G.** Incubation period of coronary heart disease. *British medical journal,* **284**: 1600–1601 (1982).
30. **Salonen, J.T. et al.** Change in health behavior in relation to estimated coronary heart disease risk during a community-based cardiovascular disease prevention programme. *International journal of epidemiology,* **10**: 343–354 (1981).

11.4 Measuring the biological impact of air quality at population level — *W.A. Jedrychowski*

The study in occupational health that follows is based on an elaboration of the tool developed in the mid-1960s by the Medical Research Council in the United Kingdom. This has led to an approach based on the use of measurements of active physiological function rather than the traditional approach based on the presence or absence of symptoms or the number of days lost through occupational disease.

Epidemiological surveys performed in various countries in the past 20 years have provided much evidence about the impact of atmospheric air pollution on chronic obstructive lung disease, but the results are so far rather controversial. At present the prevailing opinion is that atmospheric air pollution, although harmful to the respiratory tract, does not play a substantial role in the etiology of these diseases.

Since Ramazzini's investigations in the eighteenth century, it has been thought that dust and chemical pollution in the industrial environment is an important factor in the spread of pulmonary diseases among workers. In industry, a large number of chemical substances are strong irritants of the respiratory tract. However, as with atmospheric air pollution, there is often a lack of consistent research results concerning industrial air contamination that would convincingly indicate to what extent various substances used in industry can be regarded as damaging the health status of workers; most studies rely on the presence of such negative indicators as the development of disease.

The purpose of this study was to assess the biological effect of air polluted with styrene and methyl methacrylate in an occupational environment, using a positive approach based on measurements of function. The health status of the workers was determined at two levels:

— respiratory symptoms (chronic bronchitis and asthma);

— lung function testing.

In the analysis performed, workers were diagnosed as healthy when they had no chronic respiratory symptoms and when their lung function, measured by FEV_1 (forced expiratory volume), was equal to or greater than 91% of the expected values. This working example is based on a previous publication *(1)*.

Materials and Methods

A total of 454 males at a styrene and methyl methacrylate plant (exposed, group A) and 683 males at a carbon derivatives plant (controls, group B), were examined. The workers in group B had been chosen as controls because they had never been exposed to styrene and methyl methacrylate and because low concentrations of other substances not harmful to the respiratory tract, such as methanol, phenol and carbon monoxide, were present in their occupational environment. The workers from both plants performed the same kinds of task, i.e. operation and maintenance of industrial installations. Some important characteristics of the population under study are presented in Table 1.

The health status of the workers was evaluated by means of standardized interviews on chest symptoms, using a questionnaire based on that developed in the United Kingdom by the Medical Research Council *(2)*. Further information included anthropometrical measurement (height) and lung function testing with the Zimmermann water spirometer. A diagnosis of chronic bronchitis was made when the respondent had a persistent cough and phlegm on most days in three consecutive months in the previous 2 years or longer *(3)*. Asthmatic syndrome was diagnosed when attacks of breathlessness with wheezing in the chest occurred independently of colds or fever.

For lung function assessment, five tests of one-second forced expiratory volume (FEV_1) were carried out on each person. For the final analysis, the highest value of FEV_1 from a series of five tests of a given person was chosen and corrected to body temperature, pressure saturated coefficient (BTPS). The lung ventilatory function was evaluated comparing the observed FEV_1 with the expected normal value, which had been calculated for a representative sample of non-smoking inhabitants of Cracow who in the previous 5 years had had no chest diseases *(4)*.

Table 1. Characteristics of the population under study — mean values (standard deviations in brackets)

	Plant A (n = 454)	Plant B (n = 683)
Age	35.8 years (9.8)	41.1 years (9.6)
Height	170.6 cm (6.1)	170.3 cm (6.4)
Weight	69.8 kg (9.9)	73.6 kg (9.9)
Duration of employment	12.9 years	18.5 years
Employment in the plant under study	7.4 years	12.4 years
Current smokers (%)	68.3	60.0
Average number of cigarettes smoked daily by current smokers	18	18

The workers examined were divided into three subgroups according to their smoking habits:

- non-smokers, i.e. those who had never smoked regularly;
- ex-smokers, i.e. those who had smoked regularly in the past but had stopped smoking at least 3 months before the survey;
- current smokers, i.e. those who confirmed that they regularly smoked at least one cigarette daily for a period longer than 6 months before the survey.

The measurements of styrene and methyl methacrylate in the environment were carried out at 18 workplaces in plant A, and those of phenol, methanol and carbon monoxide at 17 workplaces in plant B. The instruments measuring the air pollution were constructed in such a way that the dust was collected on filter and chemical substances in the bubbler after passage of the sampled air. The instruments were mounted about 1.5 m above floor-level on a special framework. Air samples were taken at each site every working hour during the three daily shifts in the week chosen (Monday to Sunday). Although the air was sampled throuthout the 24 hours of each day, the filter discs and bubblers were changed at the end of each shift. Styrene concentrations in the sampled air were determined, using the method recommended by the Polish Committee for Normalization (PN-71, Z-04035). The principle of the method is the reaction of styrene with dinitrogen trioxide in the presence of acetic acid with formation of alfa-nitroso-beta-nitroethylobenzene, measured by polarography. Methyl methacrylate sampled from the air was measured by the colorimetric method after reacting with chromotropic acid.

The results may be summarized as follows.

Plant A (378 measurements):

- styrene: range 0.06 to 31.81 mg $\times$ m^{-3} (mean: 2.66; median: 0.81)
- methyl methacrylate: range 0.20 to 382.2 mg $\times$ m^{-3} (mean: 11.06; median: 17.6)

Plant B (357 measurements):

- phenol: range 0.013 to 0.89 mg $\times$ m^{-3} (mean: 0.41; median: 0.17)
- methanol: range 0.00 to 0.72 mg $\times$ m^{-3} (mean: 0.009; median: 0.01)
- carbon monoxide: range 0.00 to 20.0 mg $\times$ m^{-3} (mean: 4.67; median: 5.9)

Results and Discussion (see Tables 2–4)

The proportion of symptom-negative persons in the non-exposed group (80.8%) does not differ significantly from that in the exposed workers' group (82.4%). The same pattern was found in non-smokers (87.5%

Table 2. Positive health status in exposed and non-exposed workers in relation to the smoking habit

	Exposed (Plant A)		Controls (Plant B)	
	Non-smokers[a] (n = 143)	Smokers (n = 311)	Non-smokers[a] (n = 272)	Smokers (n = 411)
Without chronic chest symptoms	130 90.0%	244 78.5%	238 87.5%	314 76.4%
FEV_1% not less than 91%	28 19.6%	45 14.5%	180 66.2%	239 58.2%
Without chronic chest symptoms and FEV_1% not less than 91%	25 17.5%	40 12.9%	166 61.0%	190 46.2%

[a] Including ex-smokers.

Table 3. Comparison of mean values of FEV_1 observed and FEV_1 expected (in litres) in relation to the smoking habit among symptom-negative workers

		n	FEV_1 'observed	FEV_1 expected	Difference
Exposed subjects (Plant A)	Non-smokers[a]	130	3.4	4.2	-0.8
	Current smokers	244	3.4	4.2	-0.8
Controls (Plant B)	Non-smokers[a]	238	3.8	3.9	-0.1
	Current smokers	314	3.7	4.0	-0.3

[a] Including ex-smokers.

Table 4. Relative risk of non-healthy versus healthy status in relation to smoking and occupational exposure

	Total	Healthy[a]	Non-healthy	Odds[b] ratio	95% confidence interval
Non-exposed[c] non-smokers	272	166	106	1.0	—
Non-exposed smokers	411	190	221	1.822	1.801– 1.842
Exposed non-smokers[c]	143	25	118	7.392	7.123– 7.670
Exposed smokers	311	40	271	10.610	10.157–11.084

[a] No chest symptoms, FEV_1% at least equal to 91%.

[b] Odds ratio calculated to non-smokers in the non-exposed group *(12)*.

[c] Including ex-smokers.

and 90.1% respectively) and in smokers (76.4% and 78.5% respectively). However, the proportion of "healthy" workers (symptom-free, with FEV_1 91%) was nearly four times higher (61.0% and 16.0%) among the non-exposed workers (plant B) than among the exposed workers (plant A); this difference is significant at $P < 0.01$. In the control group, the proportion of healthy workers is significantly different in non-smokers and in smokers (61.0% and 46.2%). The corresponding difference among exposed workers is not significant (17.5% and 12.9%).

The comparison of lung function indices in the exposed subjects and the controls also showed an excess of lower values among all the exposed workers (see Fig. 1 and Table 5). The distributions of spirometric values FEV_1, observed as a percentage of FEV_1, expected in both groups were significantly different ($\chi^2 = 236.198$, df = 4, $P < 0.05$). The symptom-free workers in the exposed group had very poor lung function indices (see Table 3).

To measure the effects of smoking and occupational exposure to styrene and methyl methacrylate, the relative risks (odds ratio) were calculated (Table 4). The effects of both factors proved to be statistically significant, but the effect of smoking was less (odds ratio = 1.822) than that of occupational exposure (odds ratio = 7.392). The results of the analysis showed no interaction between the factors under study.

Fig. 1. Distribution of lung function indices among exposed subjects and controls

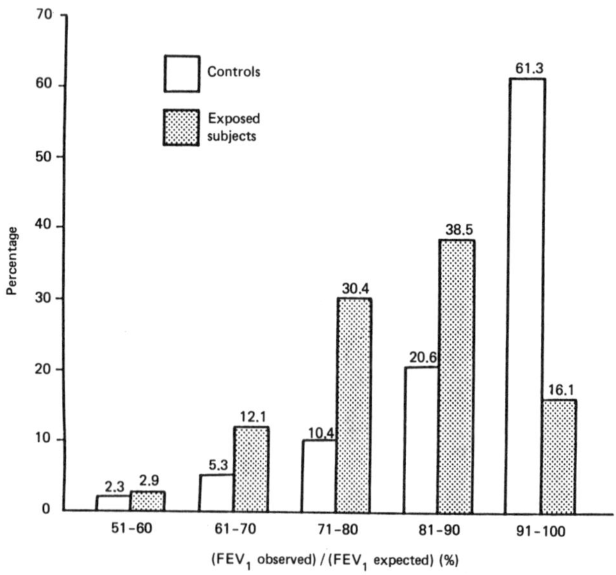

Table 5. Distribution of lung function indices among exposed subjects and controls

FEV_1 observed/FEV_1 expected	Exposed subjects	Controls
51- 60%	13	16
61- 70%	55	36
71- 80%	138	71
81- 90%	175	141
91-100%	73	419
Total	454	683

The clinical picture of the styrene effects has been dealt with in the literature. Symptoms of styrene exposure have been listed as skin, eye, nose and throat irritation, tiredness, loss of appetite, difficulties in concentration and, at higher exposure, dizziness *(5)*. Studies on respiratory symptoms and lung function have until now been rather scarce. Results of the study performed by Chmielewski et al. *(6)* suggest that long-term exposure to styrene can cause obstructive changes. In another survey, Lorimer et al. *(7)* confirm styrene to be an important factor responsible for airway obstruction.

The results of the study described here also showed that the harmful effect of styrene and methyl methacrylate on lung function was unexpectedly strong despite the rather low prevalence of chronic chest symptoms, which was similar to that observed in the general population *(8)*. In this respect the findings were consistent with the results of the study by Lorimer et al. However, contrary to the suggestions in their paper and other reports *(7,9,10)*, no significant interaction was found here between smoking and industrial exposure. It thus appears that this particular environmental factor has developed a much stronger effect on lung function than smoking and that one effect is independent of the other.

It is very difficult to explain the low prevalence of chronic chest symptoms in contrast to the high risk of lung function damage. One can assume that it may be the result of a developed tolerance in industrial populations. However, when the environmental factor does not cause a defence reaction in the upper respiratory tract in terms of coughing or phlegm production, this factor is nevertheless harmful to the small bronchioles, although the association between symptoms and lung function deterioration may not be observed. Usually, chemical substances present in the inhaled air, if soluble in the bronchial mucus, cause an irritant reaction in the upper respiratory tract *(11)*. Styrene and methyl methacrylate, being insoluble in water, are not absorbed in the mucus of the upper respiratory tract and may reach the smallest bronchioles, which are very sensitive to external factors, in high concentrations.

Taking into account the fact that the presence of chronic bronchitis or asthmatic symptoms was not a valid predictor of environmental hazards, spirometric monitoring of workers employed in the chemical industry is necessary, as there are many substances which have not been fully evaluated in relation to health risks. The present study, in addition to providing preliminary data on the harmful effect of low concentrations of styrene and methyl methacrylate in the industrial environment, shows the importance of using measurements related to effective physiological function (i.e. "positive aspects of health") rather than the absence of symptoms.

It is hoped that the use of such indicators in comparative studies of the occupational environment may lead to improved monitoring of environmental hazards and to more sensitive assessment of interventions designed to reduce the risks of environmental pollution.

References

1. **Jedrychowski, W.** Styrene and methyl methacrylate in the industrial environment as a risk factor of chronic obstructive lung disease. *International archives of occupational and environmental health,* **51**: 151–157 (1982).
2. *Questionnaire on respiratory symptoms and instructions for its use.* London, Medical Research Council, 1966.
3. **Medical Research Council.** Definitions and classification of chronic bronchitis for clinical and epidemiological purposes. *Lancet,* **1**: 775–777 (1965).
4. **Jedrychowski, W. & Flak, E.** [Standard normal spirometric values of FVC, FEV_1, $FEF_{25-75\%}$, $FEF_{50-75\%}$ and $FEF_{200-1200}$ in a random sample of healthy non-smokers]. *Przeglad lekarski,* **37**: 643–646 (1980) (in Polish).
5. **Härkönen, H.** Styrene, its experimental and clinical toxicology. A review. *Scandinavian journal of work, environment and health,* **4**(Suppl. 2): 194–214 (1978).
6. **Chmielewski, J. et al.** Clinical and experimental studies on the pathogenesis of toxic effects of styrene. II. The effect of styrene on the respiratory system. *Bulletin of the Institute of Marine Tropical Medicine (Gdynia),* **26**: 299–302 (1975).
7. **Lorimer, W.V. et al.** Clinical studies of styrene workers: initial findings. *Environmental health perspectives,* **17**: 171–181 (1976).
8. **Sawicki, F. et al.** [*Chronic nonspecific respiratory disease in the City of Cracow*]. Warsaw, PZH, 1977 (in Polish).
9. **Elmes, P.C.** Relative importance of cigarette smoking in occupational lung disease. *British journal of industrial medicine,* **38**: 1–13 (1981).
10. *Smoking and health. A report of the Surgeon General.* Washington, DC, 1979 (Department of Health, Education and Welfare publication 79-50066).
11. **Gross, P. et al.** The pulmonary reaction to toxic gases. *American Industrial Hygiene Association journal,* **28**: 315–321 (1967).
12. **Fleiss, J.L.** *Statistical methods for rates and proportions.* New York, John Wiley, 1973.

11.5 Measuring the health impact of water and sanitation investments in less developed countries — *F.J. Henry & M. Mujibur Rahaman*

Measurements of the impact of water and sanitation programmes have tended to focus on reduction in mortality and morbidity from water-related diseases and on the reduction in the amount of work required to obtain sufficient water for personal and household purposes. This is, in the main, the approach adopted here. The importance of taking into account the sociocultural setting in the determination and standardization of relevant measurements is stressed. Also demonstrated is how the results of the measurements can be applied by health planners in formulating appropriate local policies, and in planning the management and deployment of resources.

This chapter examines the use of measurements which relate to water, sanitation and health, and tries to show how measurements can influence the decision-making process regarding investments in these fields. It also points out the opportunities and limitations of using various measurements in different sociocultural settings.

The lack of financial resources for intervention programmes in less developed countries often forces decision-makers to rank competing development projects, and cost-effectiveness analyses devised for other purposes are now increasingly applied in the field of health to achieve the most efficient allocation of resources. However, measuring and forecasting the benefits of such projects is difficult owing to the many political, social, educational and environmental variables which affect health. The best way of minimizing the effects of these interrelated factors is to conduct large-scale longitudinal studies, but this approach is costly. In most developing countries the available health data are an inadequate basis for determining relative priorities for communities. Field studies are therefore necessary, but these are often difficult to undertake in rural areas.

The ideal design in intervention studies is to compare disease incidence in communities with and without sanitary facilities and also to monitor disease patterns before and after the installation of such facilities. Admittedly, this ideal design will not be available in many projects, but the possible benefits must be expressed in a form that would be appropriate for decision-making, whether in medical or financial terms. In some circumstances, rapid assessment might be required, using a few key health indices, while in others sophisticated research techniques might be necessary.

No set number or type of measurements will be effective in all situations, but factors of particular importance include the quantity of water used for personal and domestic hygiene, water source and quality, distance from source, and level of sanitation. The outcome measures that can be examined also have differing strengths and weaknesses. The decision to measure mortality, diarrhoea morbidity, bacteria, viruses, parasites, clinical cases, nutritional status or behavioural changes will depend on the resources available and on the reason for the particular study.

Because of the influence of various socio-environmental factors, the impact of water and latrine improvement is often difficult to assess. Consideration of intermediate effects is therefore a justified approach, particularly in less developed countries where only partial improvements can be afforded. These intermediate variables might include: method of food preparation; collection of water; disposal of waste; level of personal and domestic hygiene; reliability, convenience and maintenance of the supply system; and habits and cultural customs associated with the use of water. The importance of a variable will change according to the particular setting, and in some situations the additional measurements of socioeconomic or educational level can be crucial.

The studies discussed below illustrate how measurements of the impact of water and sanitation investments have produced critically important information that can be used by public health administrators.

The Studies

The two studies considered here were undertaken in differing cultural environments. One was performed in St Lucia, a Caribbean island *(1)*, and the other in Teknaf, Bangladesh *(2)*. Table 1 contrasts the settings of the two studies.

The designs of the two studies are different. In St Lucia three similar rural valleys were compared. One valley, comprising three settlements, had both improved water and latrines. The second valley, where there were three settlements, had improved water only, and the third, comprising five settlements with no sanitation improvement, served as a control. In this way the impact of water and latrines could be determined individually and collectively. In Bangladesh only two areas were considered: one for the intervention and the other as a control. In the study area, improvements were made step by step. Water was supplied first, then latrines, then health education. In this way, time-series evaluations would be able to separate the effects of each additional facility.

Cohorts of children were surveyed regularly in both studies for 2–3 years. In both locations the study teams had the advantage of established field research institutions to support their activities. In St Lucia, a Research and Control Department has been in existence since 1965. In Bangladesh, the International Centre for Diarrhoeal Disease Research (formerly the Cholera Research Laboratory) started work in 1960 and moved to Teknaf in 1974. Several years of pre-installation data were, therefore, available from routine surveillance carried out for other related projects. Hence, analyses and comparisons were made of independently collected data in which high quality control was achieved and maintained.

Table 1. Comparative data for St Lucia and Bangladesh

	St Lucia	Bangladesh
Total population	130 000	90 000 000
GNP per capita (US $)	600	100
Literacy (%)	70	20
Size (sq. miles)	239	55 000
Infant mortality rate (per 1000)	20	140
Religion	(Catholic) Christian	Muslim
Ethnicity	African (Caribbean)	Indian (subcontinent)
Improvement (water)	From public to private pipe	From surface to tube-well water
Improvement (latrine)	From pit to pour-flush	From defaecation in the fields and around houses to pour-flush

Water use

It is customary to measure the impact of water and sanitation interventions by comparing the incidence of related diseases in communities with and without a particular facility. However, confounding factors usually prevent the valid interpretation of such studies. Because the valleys in St Lucia did not differ in other respects such as income, education, population density and feeding pattern, it was justifiable to ascribe differences in morbidity to the different levels of sanitation. Monthly diarrhoea surveys using a calendar card system *(1)* were carried out on the same children for two years after the intervention. In the upgraded areas the quantity of water used was doubled, hence it can be concluded that this level of improvement lowered diarrhoea[a] prevalence by 33% (see Table 2). After latrines were improved with a pour-flush facility, diarrhoea was further reduced by 31%. However, the level of morbidity which is considered acceptable for a community will be a major influence on the extent of an intervention programme.

Doubling the quantity of water used will only cause a reduction of morbidity within a specific range. In St Lucia that crucial range was found to be between 10 and 40 litres per head per day. Above this, infections were not significantly reduced, hence 40 litres/head/day might be a minimum target to aim for here. It should be stressed that the relation between the costs of improvements and the health benefits is not linear. Moreover, it is a mistake to assume that *any* improvement will create benefits. In fact, minimal

[a] Diarrhoea is defined here as "three or more abnormally loose stools in 24 hours". Both mild and serious cases reported in the home are included.

Table 2. Percentage distribution of children with diarrhoea by valley and age, St Lucia

Age (months)	Control		Water		Water plus latrine	
	No.	%	No.	%	No.	%
<6	89	30.3	112	28.6	72	19.4
7-9	121	23.1	149	26.8	106	18.9
10-12	178	30.3	188	26.2	135	18.5
13-15	191	23.0	194	16.0	175	13.1
16-18	197	26.9	191	14.1	173	10.4
19-21	204	21.1	176	11.9	167	3.0
22-24	165	18.2	126	8.7	133	8.3
25-27	113	18.6	68	5.9	65	4.6
28-30	68	17.6	19	0.0	42	0.0
Total[a]	1326	23.5	1223	15.7	1068	10.8

[a] Percentages are corrected for age, the control being used as a standard.

interventions can even be detrimental and should be avoided. This is why these types of measurement are crucial to engineers and public health administrators who wish to implement effective projects when only limited budgets are available. If it is accepted that the study areas in St Lucia are typical of rural Caribbean communities, then findings such as these can assist planning on a regional basis.

Age

Table 2 also shows the value of grouping the data according to the subjects' ages. In this way it may be seen that the highest prevalence of diarrhoea occurs during the first year of life and the decline is faster in the upgraded valleys. In contrast, the diarrhoea peak in Bangladesh occurs during the second year, so it is important to identify the age groups that are more likely to benefit from improved water supply and sanitation.

Water source

In St Lucia no one returned to the traditional sources for water after the household pipes were provided. The standard of general education was high and health education in particular was given through the school system, at health centres, and by community health aides at home. There was no problem in gaining acceptance of the new facilities, and the water supplied was reliable, convenient and palatable. In Bangladesh, on the other hand, nearly everyone used tube-well water for drinking, but it was not exclusively used for all domestic purposes. The failure of these wells to control or significantly reduce cholera and other diarrhoeas is well documented *(3)*. The iron content of the water was relatively high and rendered it less readily acceptable. Furthermore, the level of health and general education was poor and parents were not commonly aware of the dangers of using traditional supplies. In such circumstances, careful consideration has to be given to the most suitable approach for measuring improvement in health status.

Because some households used the tube-wells exclusively, the possible benefits of this practice were assessed in a quantitative way. Households in the upgraded area were grouped according to their exclusive or non-exclusive use of tube-well water. As Table 3 shows, diarrhoea incidence was consistently lower in the "exclusive use" group. It seems appropriate to advocate sustained and specific health education messages that encourage the exclusive use of tube-well water, but the reasons for the continued use of traditional water sources should also be identified so that the health education package can be suitably formulated.

Seasonality

In Bangladesh, where there are large seasonal fluctuations in the incidence of diarrhoeal diseases, it is important to monitor the rates over several seasons and in various villages so that sporadic and local epidemics do not lead to spurious quantitative estimates of impact. Table 3 also demonstrates the usefulness of this approach.

Table 3. Incidence of diarrhoea per 100 children aged 0–4 years according to source of water used

Three-month period	Tube-well and other water sources used	Tube-well water used exclusively
July - September 1980	95.8	51.3
October - December 1980	98.1	71.9
January - March 1981	77.0	73.7
April - June 1981	108.9	107.2
July - September 1981	94.9	67.2
October - December 1981	107.5	83.5
January - March 1982	79.5	77.6
April - June 1982	97.2	73.3
July - September 1982	62.6	54.7
October - December 1982	52.5	54.7
January - March 1983	50.3	34.6
April - June 1983	56.3	43.7

Distance

Residents of rural communities are willing to walk varying distances to obtain clean and safe water, depending usually on the terrain to be traversed, the aesthetic quality of the water, and the proximity and attractiveness of alternative sources. Ultimately, the decision rests with individual households, so for planning purposes it is difficult to judge the critical distance for an entire community. In Teknaf, children living in households more than 150 yards from a tube-well experienced significantly more diarrhoea than those living nearer. Where distances of less than 150 yards are concerned there is no difference in incidence (see Table 4).

Table 3 shows that the exclusive use of tube-well water leads to lower infection rates. Almost all the residents concerned use tube-well water for drinking. These observations thus point to three hypotheses.

1. Residents are not willing to walk more than 150 yards to obtain tube-well water for non-drinking purposes.

2. Tube-well water becomes critically more contaminated when carried for distances over 150 yards.

3. Much less tube-well water is carried and used when distances from the pipe are greater than 150 yards.

Although these hypotheses have not yet been tested, the findings remain important for planning purposes. For example, (*a*) the minimum number of tube-wells for a community can be calculated and possible locations planned with some confidence of reducing diarrhoeal diseases; (*b*) installing an excessive number of tube-wells (i.e. reducing distance) will not further reduce diarrhoea unless concomitant inputs such as health education are added. It is noteworthy that this distance is not relevant to St Lucia, because few people there walk more than 150 yards to a pipe.

Table 4. Relationship between distance from tube-well and incidence of diarrhoea per child per year, July 1980 - June 1983

Distance (yards)	Control area		Study area	
	No.	Incidence	No.	Incidence
<25	299	2.94	620	2.72
26- 75	512	3.35	468	2.67
76-150	347	3.13	186	2.65
151+	188	4.10	50	4.24

Nutritional status

The synergistic interaction between infection and malnutrition points to nutritional status as a necessary indicator of impact in water and sanitation projects. Improvements in environmental sanitation can improve the growth of children by reducing the load of infection and preventing anorexia and loss of appetite. In addition, a better water supply can reduce the time spent collecting water, and this time can be used to improve child care and enhance growth. As to the measurements and cut-off points that should be used, the choice of an indicator of nutritional status will depend largely on the type and level of nutritional disorders locally.

Sanitation and behaviour

It is not easy to measure behaviour patterns. In Bangladesh, households were grouped according to their hygienic practices and level of sanitation. An appropriate score was then assigned to each household (see Fig. 1). The relationship between the scores and the incidence of dysentery is presented in Table 5.

Fig. 1. Scoring scale for standards of sanitation

Behaviour	Points scored		
	3	2	1
1. Water: drinking washing bathing	Tube-well (hand pump) Tube-well Tube-well	Tube-well Ring-well/ditch Ring-well/ditch	Ring-well[a] Ditch Ditch
2. Defaecation (children < 5)	Takes place outside courtyard, or faeces thrown away soon after defaecation	Takes place within yard; faeces left in the open	Takes place anywhere; old faeces seen in yard
3. Hand-washing by mother before handling or eating food	Hands washed in water	Fingers only washed	Hands not washed
4. Hand-washing by mother after defaecation	Hands washed with soap or ash	Hands rubbed with earth or some other material and water	Hands washed with water only
5. Appearance of mother's hands and clothes	Both clean	Only one clean	Both unclean
6. Water storage for drinking	None; direct tube-well use	Clean covered container inside house	Unclean, un-covered container inside house
7. Water storage for washing	None; direct tube-well use	Clean covered container inside house	Unclean, un-covered container inside house

[a] Only a few use ring-well water for drinking.

Categories (based on total score): good = 18–21; fair = 13–17; poor = 7–12.

Table 5. Distribution of dysentery episodes (per child aged 0–4 years per year), by sanitation score

	Sanitation score		
	Poor	Fair	Good
Year 1	2.3	1.8	1.6
Year 2	1.8	1.8	1.4
Year 3	1.4	1.1	0.8
Years 1-3	2.2	1.6	1.2

A clear reduction in incidence is noted for each sanitation score, but the effect of sanitation on the incidence of nondysenteric diarrhoeas was not as consistent, perhaps because the different etiological agents are not similarly influenced by water and sanitation. This observation can prove important, even within Bangladesh, because the main disease in Teknaf is dysentery, whereas in Matlab Thana it is watery diarrhoea, including cholera. For intervention, the emphasis (on quality or on quantity) might have to be varied according to the primary cause of diarrhoea in a given location *(4,5)*.

Most water and sanitation studies fall short of providing the crucially important quantitative information often desired. Moreover, there are not many instances where cost-effectiveness analyses have led directly to public decisions. Value judgements invariable contribute to the process. Ultimately, the decision is a political one; hence, measurements can only serve as an aid to informed decision-making.

References

1. **Henry, E.J.** Environmental sanitation, infection and nutritional status of infants in rural St Lucia, West Indies. *Transactions of the Royal Society of Tropical Medicine and Hygiene,* **75**(4): 507–513 (1981).
2. **Rahaman, M.M. & Azez, K.M.** *Interim report of the Water and Sanitation Intervention Project – Teknaf.* Bangladesh, International Centre for Diarrhoeal Disease Research, 1983 (unpublished document, Centre file 3-p-77-0095).
3. **Briscoe, J.** The role of water supply in improving health in poor countries (with special reference to Bangladesh). *American journal of clinical nutrition,* **31**: 2100–2113 (1978).
4. **Feachem, R.G.** Is cholera primarily water borne? *Lancet,* **2**: 957 (1976).
5. **Levine, R.J. & Nalin, D.R.** Cholera is primarily waterborne in Bangladesh. *Lancet,* **2**: 1305 (1976).

11.6 Hospital-based maternity care monitoring as a tool for improvement of primary maternity care services — *R.P. Bernard & S. Sastrawinata*

This paper, which describes a maternity care monitoring system in use in Indonesia, provides an excellent illustration of how a system for the collection and analysis of data can support decisions as to the appropriate provision and management of services. The use of visual display methods to present complex information and relationships in this example demonstrates an innovative aid for use in discussions with health planners.

Although most deliveries in Indonesia occur in rural homes and are assisted by traditional birth attendants, the teaching and planning of antenatal and obstetric care depends mainly on the large university obstetric departments. Helping the university departments to understand relationships between socioeconomic factors, family planning behaviour and the use of antenatal care, on the one hand, and the outcome of deliveries on the other, was therefore considered to be a high priority in a long-term programme to improve nationwide obstetric care in particular and reproductive health care in general. Candidate obstetricians for peripheral centres would thus learn the whys and hows of ubiquitously needed reproductive health care provision. Their practical example would then form a strong input to the education of those responsible for delivery and supervision of peripheral services.

However, the records of health services in developing countries kept for service statistics or clinical management leave much to be desired. Little interest is shown in these records by service providers, primarily because no arrangement has been made for recording quality and for systematic feedback to them in such a way as to provide a learning experience. In spite of this neglect of such clinical records at all levels, they are of value for epidemiological research, policy decisions and continuous training. The clinical conditions to be observed are unique to developing countries and information on them is a resource that could be utilized everywhere for health promotion and prevention.

What is needed is a system that can tap this potential by utilizing the information revolution for the benefit of the service providers. One such new information system has been developed for the reproductive health care services after successful pretests *(1,2)* with maternity care monitoring (MCM).

MCM was developed jointly by the International Fertility Research Program and the International Federation of Gynaecology and Obstetrics *(3,4)* for major maternity centres and adapted to peripheral maternity services by the International Federation for Family Health *(5)*. This paper illustrates the diagnostic process, utilizing data from a standard MCM record at 11 maternity centres in Indonesia *(6)*.

Materials and Methods

The analytical framework pertains to 36 802 singleton births recorded on a single-sheet MCM record from September 1978 to June 1980 at the following university departments of obstetrics and gynaecology: Jakarta, Bandung, Semarang, Yogyakarta, Surabaya, Malang, Medan, Padang, Palembang, Ujung Pandang and Manado. The MCM form was published in many journals and publications (e.g. *1,3,4,5,6*) and addresses the following themes: (*a*) reproductive history and some socioeconomic characteristics, (*b*) reproductive health and its care, (*c*) management of the current delivery and its outcome, and (*d*) reproductive planning. The form is shown in Fig. 1.

The forms are filled in by the attending physician or midwife, with clear-cut delegation to the social worker for specific sections. A data collection coordinator keeps a close check on the completeness and quality of recording. For this first multicentre monitoring scheme, the records were reviewed in Bandung and monthly batches forwarded to the International Fertility Research Program, USA, for processing and the running of a specially designed, richly labelled, standard computer output. These centre-specific standard computer outputs were returned to Indonesia for study and for review sessions and reports, both national and regional. The transfer of software and the acquisition of microcomputers led to technical independence. After careful study of centre variation for some 25 variables, the 11-centre pool was created for many detailed analyses. The current report uses this pool.

The strategy of analysis for this report is sketched in Fig. 2. Module 1 gives perinatal death as a function of education, breastfeeding and antenatal visits. Module 2 shows the lack of antenatal visits as a function of education, breastfeeding and family planning shortly before the current conception. Module 3 gives the mean latest birth interval by breastfeeding of latest live birth and family planning before current conception. Finally, Module 4 gives the additional children desired and family planning intentions/acceptance by number of living children postpartum. Experience has taught that tables of incidence and prevalence do not really convey the information to the doctors and midwives. There was an information gap, and hence a felt need to experiment with a graphical presentation that would convey the basic messages to the service providers, while keeping the entire information for statistical documentation. Fig. 3 illustrates this process. Two-way tables are turned around and the information drawn to scale on isometric, open-angle paper with the totals fitting a "roof" over the three-dimensional display. In this way, "dry" statistical tables are being "brought to life", since the "dual control" indices are sculptured onto paper. Appropriate connection of block edges gives easy optical access to relative risks and prevalence ratios.

Fig. 1. Maternity care monitoring form

INTERNATIONAL FERTILITY RESEARCH PROGRAM

MATERNITY RECORD

Please circle appropriate numbers and fill in appropriate boxes and blanks. All boxes and appropriate blanks should be filled.

Example: 11. Patient's status: 1) private (2) not private 8) other [2] 20

PATIENT IDENTIFICATION: 1. Hospital or clinic no. ____ 2. Admission date ____ *day month year*

3. Patient's name ____ Husband's name ____

4. Address ____

STUDY IDENTIFICATION

5. Center name ____ and number: [ ] 1-3
6. Study number: [9 0 3] 4-6
7. Patient order number: [ ] 7-11
8. Delivery date: [ ] *day month year* 12-17
9. Registration status: 0) not booked 1) booked, patient's choice 2) referred by physician 3) referred by midwife 4) emergency 8) other ____ [ ] 18

PATIENT CHARACTERISTICS

10. Residence: 1) urban 2) rural 3) urban slum 4) rural slum [ ] 19
11. Patient's status: 1) private 2) not private 8) other [ ] 20
12. Patient's age: *(completed years)* [ ] 21-22
13. Patient's education: *(school year completed)* 0) 0 1) 1-2 2) 3-4 3) 5-6 4) 7-8 5) 9-10 6) 11-12 7) 13-14 8) 15+ [ ] 23
14. Marital status: 1) never married 2) currently married 3) divorced 4) separated 5) widowed 6) consensual union 8) other [ ] 24
15. Age at first marriage/union: *(completed years)* [ ] 25-26

OBSTETRIC HISTORY (Not Including This Pregnancy)

16. Total live births: [ ] 27-28
17. Children now living: number of males *(8 or more = 8)* [ ] 29; number of females [ ] 30
18. Duration of breast feeding of last live birth: 0) did not breast feed 1) < 3 months 2) < 6 3) < 9 4) < 12 5) < 15 6) < 18 7) < 21 8) 21+ months [ ] 31
19. Number of stillbirths: *(8 or more = 8)* [ ] 32
20. Number of infant deaths: *(less than 12 completed months) (8 or more = 8)* [ ] 33
21. Number of spontaneous abortions: *(8 or more = 8)* [ ] 34
22. Number of induced abortions: *(8 or more = 8)* [ ] 35
23. Outcome of last pregnancy: 0) not previously pregnant 1) live birth, full term, still living 2) live birth, full term, deceased 3) live birth, premature, still living 4) live birth, premature, deceased 5) stillbirth 6) induced abortion 7) spontaneous abortion 8) other [ ] 36
24. Number of months since last pregnancy ended: *(98 or more = 98)* [ ] 37-38
25. Contraceptive method mainly used before conception: 0) none 1) IUD 2) orals/injectables 3) female sterilization 4) male sterilization 5) condom 6) withdrawal/rhythm 7) foam/diaphragm/jelly 8) other ____ [ ] 39

MEDICAL DATA

26. Number of antenatal visits: *(8 or more = 8)* [ ] 40
27. Primary antenatal condition: *(see code list)* [ ] 41-42
28. Hospitalization required during this pregnancy: 0) no 1) yes, for condition indicated in Item 27 2) yes, for condition other than the one indicated in Item 27, specify condition ____ [ ] 43
29. Tobacco smoking during pregnancy: 0) none **During part of pregnancy** (cigarettes/day): 1) 1–10 2) 11–20 3) 21 or more **Throughout pregnancy** (cigarettes/day): 4) 1–10 5) 11–20 6) 21 or more 8) cigars, pipes, etc. [ ] 44
30. Number of previous cesarean sections: [ ] 45
31. Estimated duration of pregnancy: *(menstrual age in completed weeks)* [ ] 46-47
32. Hemoglobin at admission for delivery (to nearest gm): 1) 5 gm or less 2) 6 gm 3) 7 gm 4) 8 gm 5) 9 gm 6) 10 gm 7) 11 gm 8) 12 gm or more 9) not done [ ] 48
33. Rupture of membranes: **Spontaneous:** 1) < 24 hrs. before delivery 2) ≥ 24 hrs. before delivery **Artificial:** 3) < 24 hrs. before delivery 4) ≥ 24 hrs. before delivery 5) during cesarean section [ ] 49
34. Type of labor: 0) no labor 1) spontaneous 2) spontaneous, augmented with artificial rupture of membranes (ARM) 3) spontaneous, augmented with drugs 4) spontaneous, augmented with ARM and drugs 5) induced, with ARM 6) induced, with drugs 7) induced, with ARM and drugs 8) other ____ [ ] 50
35. Type of presentation during labor (for Item 38 delivery): 0) vertex, occiput anterior 1) vertex, occiput transverse or posterior 2) breech, frank 3) breech, footling 4) complete breech 5) brow/face 6) transverse lie 7) compound 8) other ____ [ ] 51
36. Anesthetic administered: 0) none or psychoprophylaxis only 1) analgesic, systemic or inhalation 2) local 3) paracervical/pudendal 4) spinal/epidural 5) general 6) 1 and 2 or 1 and 3 7) other combination 8) other ____ [ ] 52
37. Episiotomy: 0) none 1) midline 2) midline, with extension 3) midline, with hematoma 4) mediolateral 5) mediolateral, with extension 6) mediolateral, with hematoma 8) other [ ] 53
38. Type of delivery (if multiple birth, code most difficult): 0) spontaneous 1) outlet forceps 2) vacuum extractor 3) mid- or high forceps 4) manual rotation 5) breech extraction 6) cesarean section 7) destructive procedure 8) other ____ [ ] 54
39. Primary injury during labor and/or delivery: 0) none 1) vulva 2) vagina 3) perineum 4) cervix 5) uterus 6) rectum 7) bladder 8) other ____ [ ] 55
40. Primary complication of labor and/or delivery: 0) none 1) prolonged/obstructed labor 2) placenta previa 3) placenta abruptio 4) hypotonic uterine contractions 5) hypertonic uterine contractions 6) hemorrhage 7) retained products 8) other ____ [ ] 56
41. Secondary complication of labor and/or delivery: *(use Item 40 codes except code 2)* **cord prolapse = 2** [ ] 57
42. Duration of labor: *(in completed hours)* 0) none 1) < 2 2) 2-6 3) 7-12 4) 13-18 5) 19-24 6) 25-48 7) over 48 [ ] 58
43. Attendant at delivery: 0) none 1) nurse 2) qualified midwife 3) student nurse/midwife 4) paramedic 5) medical student 6) general physician 7) OB/GYN physician 8) other ____ [ ] 59
44. Birthweight: *(grams; for multiple births, refer to Item 38 delivery) (9988 or more = 9988)* [ ] 60-62
45. Sex of infant(s) born at this delivery: *(write number of each)* number of males [ ] 63; number of females [ ] 64

Items 46 and 47 refer to Item 38 delivery

46. Apgar score: 9) not done *(8 or more = 8)* at 1 minute [ ] 65; at 5 minutes [ ] 66
47. Primary fetal/neonatal condition: 0) normal 1) fetal distress during labor 2) minor malformation 3) major malformation 4) respiratory distress syndrome 5) isoimmunization 6) neonatal sepsis 7) trauma 8) other *For codes 2), 3), 7), 8), specify* ____ [ ] 67
48. Associated or secondary fetal/neonatal condition: *(use Item 47 codes) Specify* ____ [ ] 68
49. Death of fetus/newborn: 0) none 1) antepartum, one 2) antepartum, two or more 3) intrapartum, one 4) intrapartum, two or more 5) postpartum, one 6) postpartum, two or more 7) combination 8) other ____ *For each death, complete Perinatal Mortality Record* [ ] 69
50. Primary puerperal condition: 0) normal 1) fever requiring treatment 2) bleeding requiring treatment 3) urinary tract infection 4) mastitis 5) phlebitis 6) dehiscence 7) death *(complete Death Report)* 8) other ____ [ ] 70
51. Maternal blood transfusion during hospitalization: 0) none 1) yes, before delivery 2) yes, during delivery 3) yes, after delivery 4) 1 and 2 5) 1 and 3 6) 2 and 3 7) 1, 2 and 3 [ ] 71
52. Number of nights hospitalized this admission before delivery: *(8 or more = 8)* [ ] 72

SPECIAL STUDIES

53. ____ [ ] 73
54. ____ [ ] 74
55. ____ [ ] 75

COMPLETE THESE ITEMS AT TIME OF DISCHARGE

56. Number of nights hospitalized this admission after delivery: *(8 or more = 8)* [ ] 76
57. Female sterilization: 0) none 1) before this delivery 2) at cesarean section 3) immediately after delivery 4) same day 5) 1-2 days later 6) 3-4 days later 7) 5-9 days later 8) 10 or more days later [ ] 77
58. Number of additional children wanted: *(8 or more = 8)* [ ] 78
59. Contraceptive method planned or provided: 0) none 1) IUD 2) orals/injectables 3) female sterilization 4) male sterilization 5) condom 6) withdrawal/rhythm 7) foam/diaphragm/jelly 8) other ____ [ ] 79

Recorder's name ____ [1] 80

 MAT 5/77

PLEASE AIRMAIL TO: International Fertility Research Program, Research Triangle Park, North Carolina 27709 USA

Fig. 2. Strategy of analysis: four analytical modules leading to four figures

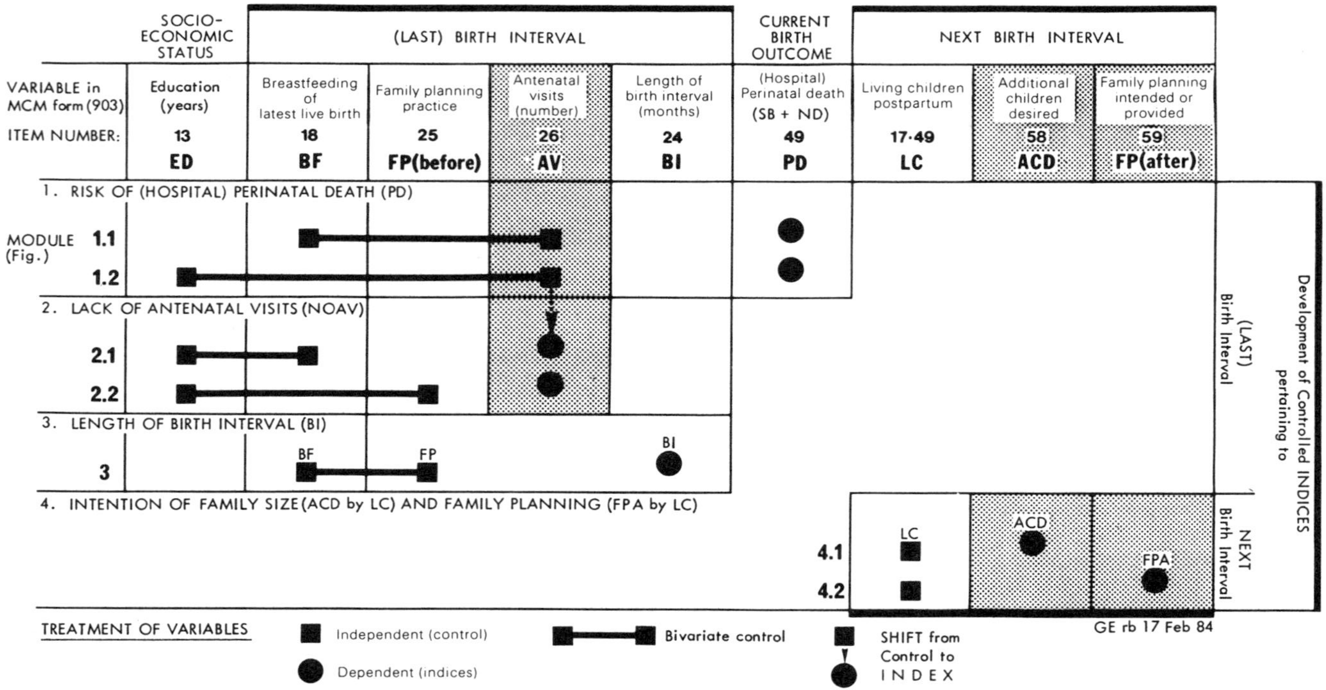

Fig. 3. From two-way control tables to three-dimensional display of indices: a standardized feedback system

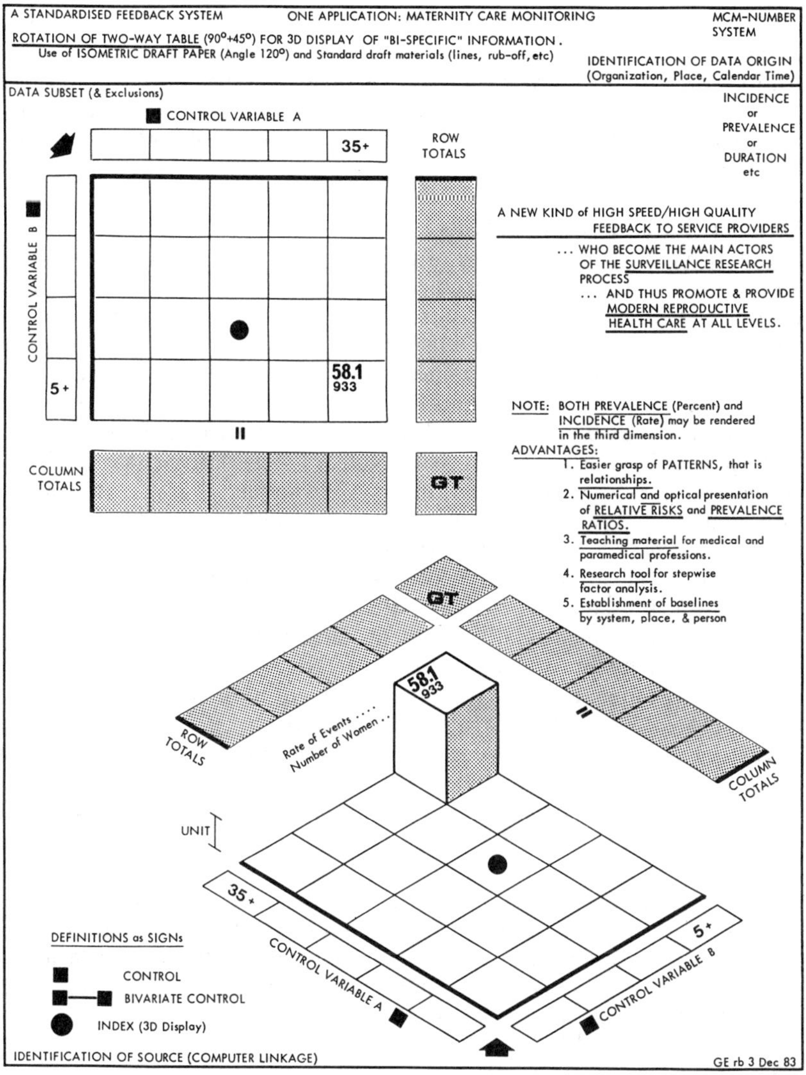

Results

Selected findings are given in four figures pertaining to (*a*) the risk of hospital perinatal death by antenatal visits, (*b*) lack of antenatal visits by education, (*c*) length of latest birth interval by breastfeeding of latest live birth and contraceptive use during the latest birth interval, and (*d*) additional children desired and family planning intentions/acceptance by living children postpartum. The figures are self-contained graphical illustrations of statistical tables that may serve as reference in time and place. Background information is programmed into the figures (data set, place, time, source, unit, etc.). Succinct technical reading is provided (suggested reading and epinotes).

Perinatal death by antenatal visits

Fig. 4 displays the hospital risk of perinatal death by antenatal visits with additional control for breastfeeding of previous live birth (4.1) and education (4.2). Within the latter control categories, the risk of perinatal death decreases multifold with increasing number of antenatal visits (8 dotted lines flowing towards the left). For women who breastfed their previous live birth for between 1 and 5 months and had 7+ antenatal visits for the current pregnancy, the rate of perinatal death is 11.3 per 1000 as compared with 112.1 per 1000 for no antenatal visits (NOAV) — a relative risk of 9.92. For women with 3–6 years' education and 7+ antenatal visits, the rate of perinatal death is 16.6 per 1000 as compared with 140.3 per 1000 NOAV — a relative risk of 8.45. Equally important, antenatal visits appear to "erase the education effect on perinatal death", since the pattern of perinatal death (PD) assumes a stepwise decline with increasing antenatal visits, quite independent of educational attainment. One may confront the two competing effects by putting to ratio the relative risks of perinatal death (*RR*(PD)) by antenatal visits ((AV)*RR*(PD)) within the four education categories (15.76, 8.45, 6.89, 4.34) against the relative risks of perinatal death by education ((ED)*RR*(PD)) among women with no antenatal visits (3.74, 2.31, 1.40, 1). For the four education levels, the AV effect carries over the education (ED) effect by a factor of around 4 (4.21, 3.66, 4.92, 4.34), as summarized in Fig. 4.2. This documented preponderance of the AV effect over the ED effect has implications for pregnancy care programmes in general and social obstetrics in particular. One cannot imagine a greater preventive impact on the risk of perinatal death than making available pregnancy care services to the uneducated segments of the population across an entire nation. Universities should thus promote antenatal care clinics throughout their catchment areas.

Lack of antenatal visits by education

The previous finding emerged unaltered when controlling for parity, haemoglobin level, type of labour, type of presentation, type of delivery, type of complication of labour and/or delivery, and attendant at delivery. For high perinatal survival, antenatal visits appear to be more important than formal education *(7)*, so it is reasonable to accept that antenatal visits stand for a

Fig. 4. Perinatal death, by antenatal visits and (4.1) breastfeeding of previous live birth and (4.2) education

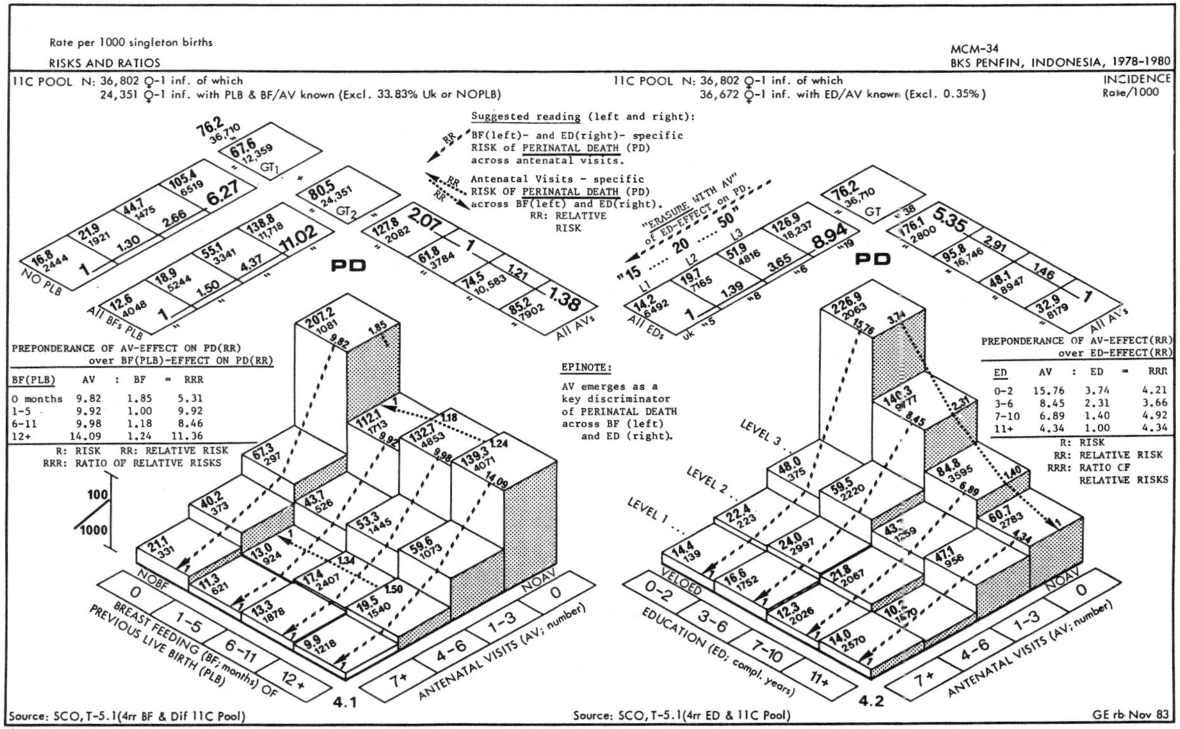

reduction in the risk of perinatal death. It is thus desirable to quantify the extent of lack of antenatal care (NOAV), since it stands for unmet need during the pregnancy. Fig. 5 displays the proportion of women with no antenatal care during the current pregnancy by education and with additional controls for breastfeeding of previous live birth (5.1) and family planning shortly before the current conception (5.2). Within these co-control categories, the lack of antenatal visits strongly decreases with education (dotted lines flowing towards the right). For women who breastfed their previous live birth for 6–11 months, there were only 32.1% without antenatal visits (NOAV) for 11 + years' education, against 71.5% NOAV for 0–2 years' education — a ratio of 2.23. For women who used oral contraception shortly before the current conception, there were only 17.8% with NOAV for 11 + years' education, against 60.4% with NOAV for 0–2 years' education — a ratio of 2.17. Just as important, within the four education categories the extent of NOAV is lower for women with contraceptive use than for women with no contraceptive use (4 dotted lines showing to the left). For instance, among women with 3–6 years' education, the occurrence of NOAV is 43.2% for women with oral contraception before the current conception, against 60.2% for women with no family planning before the current conception (NOFP) — a ratio of 1.39. One may confront the two competing effects on antenatal visits by putting to ratio the relative rates of NOAV (PR(NOAV)) as suggested in Fig. 5.2. Among women with low education (0–6 years), the ED effect carries over the family planning (FP) effect (RPRs of 1.70 and 1.22), whereas among women with 7 + years' education it is the FP effect that carries over the ED effect (RPRs of 0.74 and 0.78). The patterns suggest that recourse to antenatal visits is governed not only by education but also by contraceptive behaviour before the index pregnancy. The programme implication is that among segments of the population with no or low education the combined availability of information and services for both family planning and antenatal care may substantially increase the use of such services, and thus contribute significantly to a reduction in the risk of perinatal death of the index pregnancy. Combination of family planning programmes with pregnancy care programmes may thus emerge as a feasible option.

Birth interval by breastfeeding and family planning

The two previous co-controls — breastfeeding of previous live birth (BF) and family planning shortly before current pregnancy (FP) — govern the duration of the latest birth interval and may be monitored *(8)*. Fig. 6 gives the mean duration in months of the latest (closed) birth interval by both BF and FP. Three-dimensional display of the index allows the interaction of the two factors to be studied by the service personnel. Overall, the mean duration was 31.8 months (top cell), as compared with 23.5 months for women with short breastfeeding (1–5 months) and no contraception (NOFP), compared with 46.3 months for women with 12 + months' breastfeeding and use of the intrauterine device — a difference of 22.8 months.

Among non-contraceptors, prolonged breastfeeding (12 + months) associates with an interval of 34.8 months — an increase by 11.3 months over

Fig. 5. Lack of antenatal visits, by education and (5.1) breastfeeding of previous live birth and (5.2) family planning before current conception

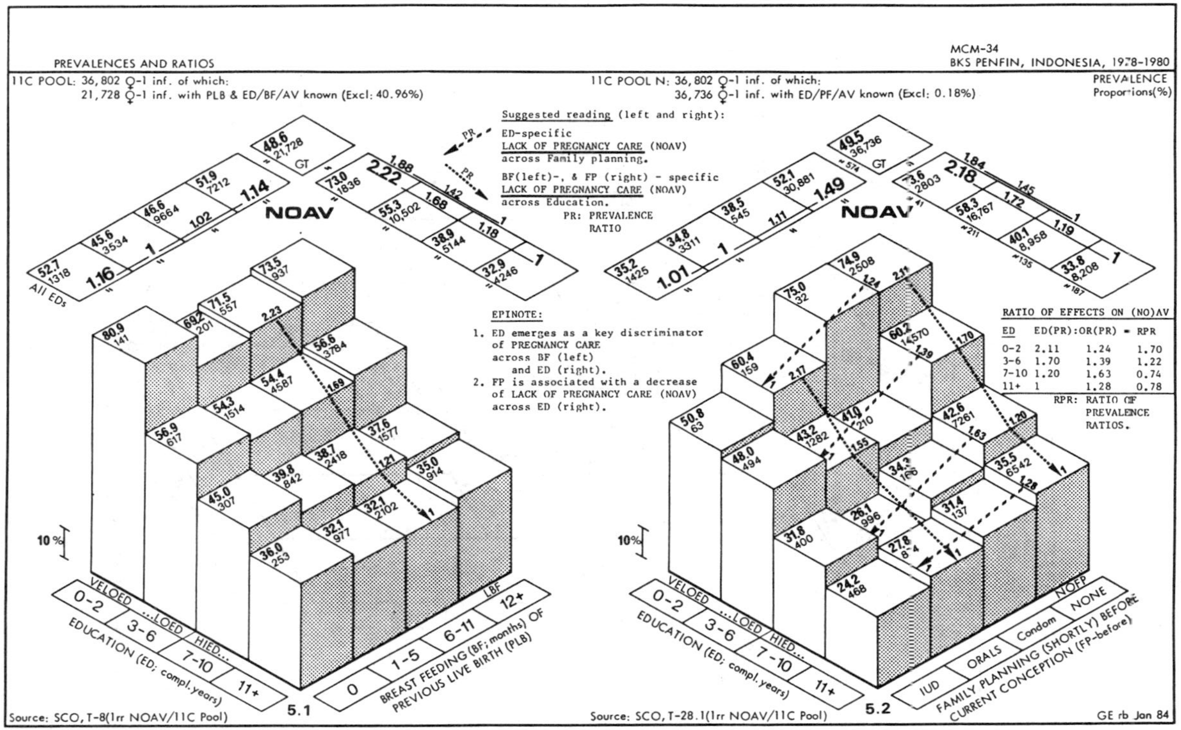

Fig. 6. Length in months of latest birth interval, by both breastfeeding of previous live birth, and family planning before current conception

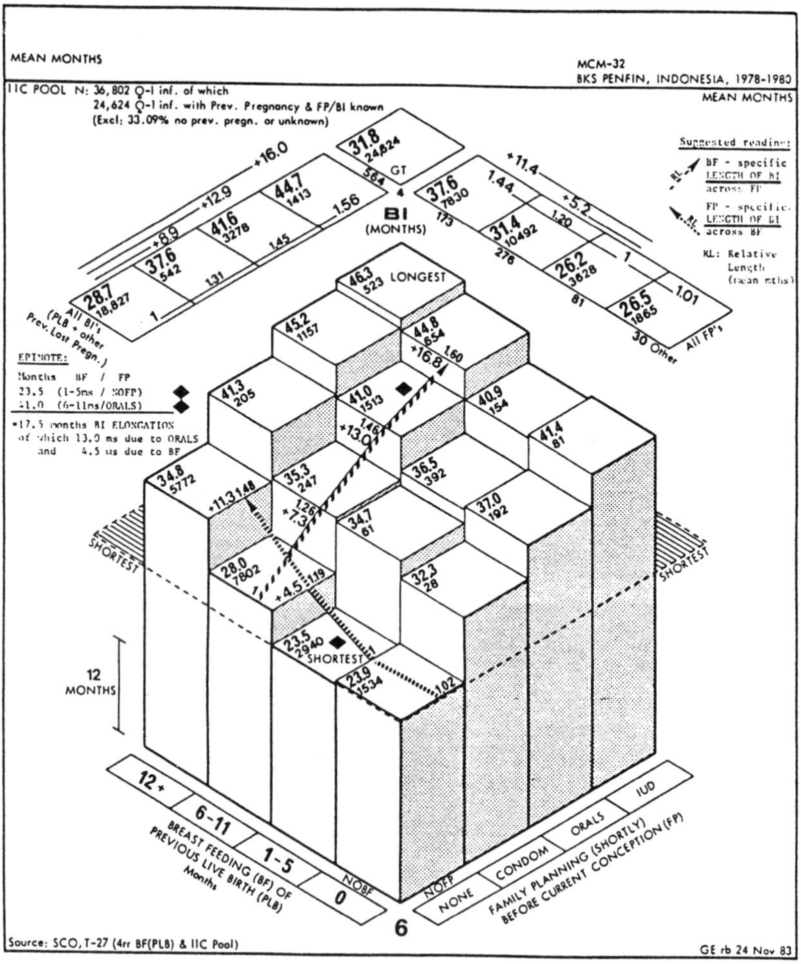

the duration for women with short breastfeeding (1–5 months; 23.5 months). By contrast, among women with 6–11 months' BF and NOFP, the increase in months of the birth interval is 4.5 months over that of short breastfeeding, but it rises by 7.3 months with condom use, by 13.0 months with pill use, and by 16.8 months with IUD use. This instructive "live statistical sequence" demonstrates to the service providers, both medical and paramedical, the relative effects of birth interval elongation by the two factors they are to promote as specific birth interval input, not only at the university clinics but above all in the primary reproductive care services across the nation. As tallied in Fig. 6 (epinote), and following the dotted lines, three quarters of the birth interval elongation among women with less than 1 year of breastfeeding is to be ascribed to pill use (13.0/17.5 = 0.74), compared with the remaining quarter ascribed to breastfeeding proper (4.5/17.5 = 0.26). Finally, the absolute elongation of the birth interval as a consequence of pill use is 13.0 months among women with either 6–11 or only 1–5 months' BF, suggesting an independent contraceptive effect on birth interval elongation for this range of duration of breastfeeding.

To social obstetrics — the promotion of "preventive input" by way of the "protective triad": breastfeeding, family planning, antenatal visits *(8)* — the findings of Fig. 6 are encouraging, since the use of contraceptives did lead to marked pregnancy/birth spacing within controlled breastfeeding durations. The active promotion of family planning is thus a critically significant "spacing support" to breastfeeding, whose primary impact remains infant nutrition and selective immunological protection *(9)*. It is, then, important to monitor the reproductive plans in the routine service situation of these women. The crucial consideration is to control for number of living children postpartum and — for each attained "family build-up level" — to look both at the number of additional children desired and at the intention/acceptance of family planning postpartum.

Additional children desired (ACD) and family planning intention/acceptance (FPA), both by living children postpartum (LC)

The new family size postpartum is the new base upon which indices of family size attitudes and family planning attitudes are to be developed. Fig. 7 gives, by number of living children postpartum (LC), the proportion of women wanting additional children (Fig. 7.1) and the proportion of women selecting a given method of family planning (Fig. 7.2). The current analytical round gives concepts developed nationally in a preliminary analysis with half the current data base *(6)*.

As shown in Fig. 7.1, the likelihood of wanting additional children assumes, with increasing family size postpartum, a somewhat reversed S-shaped curve, with marked variation among centres regarding the 50% intercept. For the two extremes, the interpolated number of living children postpartum (LC) at which 50% of the women want, and 50% do not want, additional children (ACD50) is 4.84 LC for the Medan centre and 2.35 for the Manado centre, with the 11-centre pool's value of 3.53 LC falling in between. Furthermore, at controlled family size level of three living children postpartum, the corresponding proportions of women wanting additional

Fig. 7. (7.1) Additional children desired, by number of living children postpartum, and (7.2) family planning intentions/acceptance, by number of living children postpartum

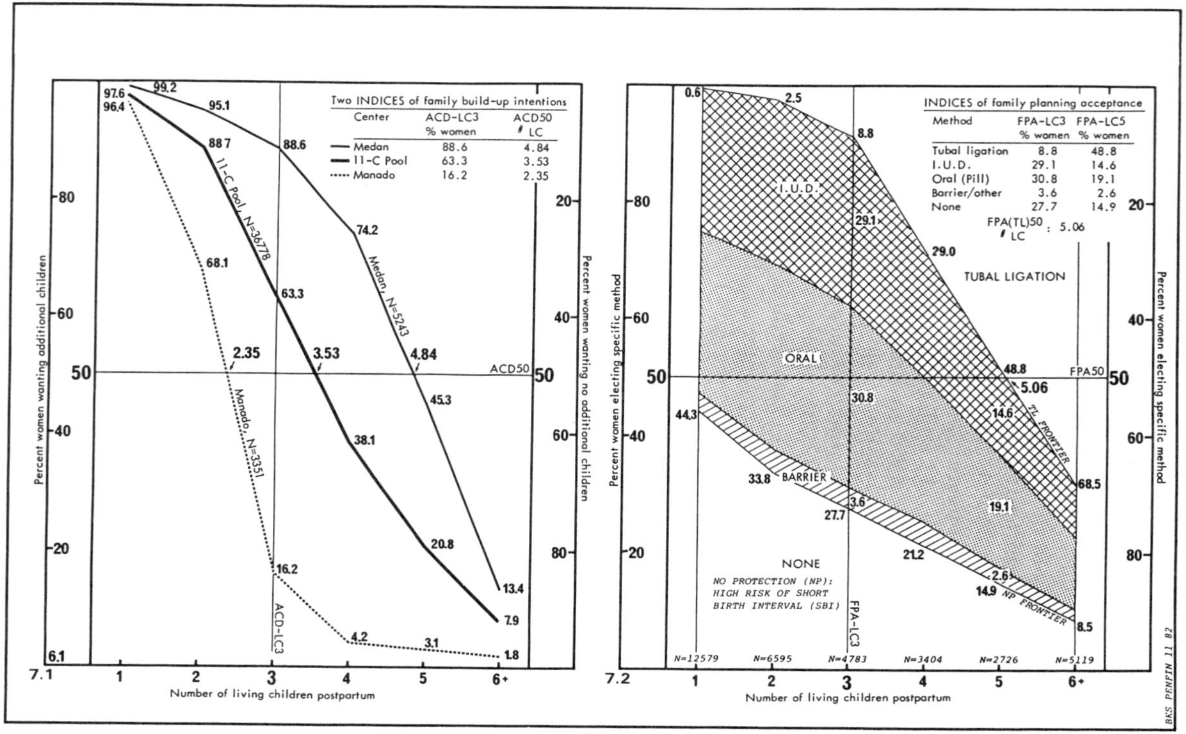

children are still 88.6% for Medan against only 16.2% for Manado, with 63.3% for the 11-centre pool in between (ACD-LC3). These two indices of family build-up intentions, as given in Fig. 7.1, may be followed by place and over time. Viewed together, they quantify the transition in family size desired within defined population groups.

As shown in Fig. 7.2, the likelihood of selecting a specific contraceptive shifts, with increasing family size postpartum, towards tubal ligation (TL). At LC order 3, only 8.8% opted for tubal ligation, at LC4 29.0%, at LC5 48.8% and at LC6 + 68.5%. This "tubal ligation frontier" (TL-frontier) also has its 50% intercept. FPA(TL)50 is the interpolated number of living children postpartum at which 50% of the women select tubal ligation: 5.06 LC for the 11-centre pool (5.48 and 4.20 for Medan and Manado, respectively). Furthermore, at controlled family size level of three living children postpartum, the "contraceptive mix" selected is instructive. This index series (FPA-LC3) for the 11-centre pool series is as follows: 27.7% NOFP, 3.6 barrier methods, 30.8% orals, 29.1% IUD, and 8.8% tubal ligation. The comparison of the contraceptive mix at three and five living children postpartum, as shown in Fig. 7.2, should be part of the routine evaluation and monitoring of PHC programmes pertaining to reproductive health care provision. The information is of constant interest to programme planners and directors. One may also study the "no protection frontier" (NP-frontier) by giving the proportion of women intending no family planning protection. The intentional non-protection against a likely short birth interval by number of living children is an important diagnostic index of the relative ignorance of various risks associated with short birth interval. This diagnostic index may thus be used for assessing the relative need for developing means to promote longer birth intervals for family health reasons. Finally, the two frontiers of NP and TL move "diagonally" from the right top to the left bottom: hence the dynamics of the contraceptive mix may be monitored by place and over time *(6)*.

In summary, routine MCM at the institutional level gives insights into prevailing relationships between socioeconomic factors, family planning behaviour and use of antenatal care, on the one hand, and the outcome of deliveries on the other. In addition, since antenatal visits emerge as a key determinant of pregnancy outcome quite independent of education, the measurement of the extent of uptake of pregnancy care becomes essential for monitoring progess in the provision of this vital service. The unmet need (percentage of women with NOAV) measured at the hospital is to a great extent "originating" in the hospital's catchment area and thus implies that the promotion of this service is required throughout the systems providing primary health care services. The interactive impact of breastfeeding and family planning on the duration of the birth interval extends also into the community. The findings at the hospital may thus be used in promoting these inputs in slum and rural areas. Finally, monitoring of the intentions pertaining to family size and family planning after the current birth provides insights into two kinds of transitions: family size desired and contraceptive intentions. Local, regional and national programmes of reproductive health care provision need this information for optimal steering and management of social change. In general, tubal ligation services lag systematically behind the people's level of readiness, due to the lack of specialized services apart from a very few centres at the university level.

While the long-term goal of the nation must be education — with its documented associated pregnancy care, family planning and increased survivals — the shorter-term goal is the active promotion of pregnancy care together with family planning, particularly among segments of the population with lower education in the slum and rural areas. In general, the improvement of family planning programmes would mean their linkage with maternal and child health services. MCM may serve as a routine evaluation tool of maternal and child health and family planning services by using the index delivery as the entry point *(10)*. However, focal endpoints for evaluation of maternity care provision are not only perinatal death and its components, but also low birth weight, fetal distress during labour, suboptimal Apgar score, and maternal death. Parallel analysis of both maternal death and perinatal death, and their relationships with some 10 variables, provided additional insights with this data set *(11)*.

Discussion

Potential biases. The data collection method of MCM is both retrospective and prospective. The population studied here is the obstetrical universe of Indonesian university centres, with the most professional care in attendance, both for cases with an unfavourable delivery outcome and for cases with a favourable delivery outcome. A prominent aim of the analysis of such institutional data is to identify factors related to improved infant survival. Education and prenatal visits emerged as the most salient factors related to improved infant survival around birth, and were therefore included in this presentation aiming at the positive promotion of both reproductive health and reproductive health care. The clinicians and paramedical personnel in a country with a population of 160 million have no other choice than to try to learn from their professional universe, while being fully aware that the latter is not representative of the prevailing situation of unattended deliveries. They know that this approach will have to be taken — preferably in successive programmed steps — at all levels of reproductive health care provision, including modest rural maternity homes and the services of traditional birth attendants. The top referral system can develop a model of monitoring that must then be adapted in methodology and focus on different attributes at the other, more peripheral levels *(5)*.

In retrospective studies, risk factor data are collected after the disease or mortality status is known and are thus subject to potential bias. By contrast, the MCM system records the risk factor data before the index delivery in professional attendance. The potential measurement bias is thus minimized. In general, the MCM system provides *a priori* for the identical collection mechanism of risk factors among women with perinatal death (cases) or with infant survival (non-cases). The information is recorded by one category of professionals. Delegation of certain sections of the form from the physician to the midwife or social workers is worked out in advance.

As long as the MCM system is restricted to top referral hospitals, a possible source of bias may lie within the selection mechanisms, leading some women to give birth in the top-level obstetric hospital, whereas others give birth in less specialized institutions or in their homes. In particular, the association between the use of antenatal visits and low perinatal mortality might be a spurious one, if women having used antenatal care regularly are more likely to deliver in obstetric hospitals regardless of their risk status, whereas women not having had regular antenatal care would be brought to the hospital only when difficulties with the delivery have started to appear. Analyses, including the type of admission (booked cases, emergencies, etc.), showed, however, that the frequency of antenatal visits remains a strong determinant of birth outcome even within these categories *(15)*.

Before hospital discharge, with or without a living infant, the woman is asked about intentions for the next birth interval with respect to both the number of additional children desired and intended family planning. The woman bases her answer on her "updated family size", hence the control for this variable as proposed in Fig. 7. This postpartum information cannot be obtained in any other way and is critically needed for programmatic plans of reproductive health promotion. In pool analyses at defined levels of health care provision, potential biases are small, due to a cancelling-out effect. The dual retrospective and prospective outlook of MCM provides this new information system with a unique advantage: linkage of reproductive past, present and future.

Visualization of patterns. So far, computer-generated feedback in the form of standard computer outputs has not aroused major interest among the service providers: the "ciphered messages" do not pass. The current report describes some of the types of graphical illustration developed for standard feedback of statistical messages that pass. Fig. 4–7 show incidences of unfavourable infant outcome around birth (Fig. 4), the extent of lack of pregnancy care (Fig. 5), mean durations of the latest birth interval (Fig. 6), and family size-dependent proportions of women wanting additional children and the intended contraceptive mix (Fig. 7). One important feature of the illustrations is that they retain all the statistical information for additional calculations. They become a document of continuous reference value and hence, over time, provide accurate trend studies within defined health care systems. Prevalence ratios and relative risks are marked and inscribed for immediate comprehension of the strength of studied associations. Indices are inscribed for specific groups and controls. An overall inventory of associations studied is given in Fig. 2. This transparency in strategy of analysis and feedback leads the service providers to grapple with epidemiological perceptions — a rewarding pay-off in terms of continuous medical education. Above all, this factual approach leads to further questions by the service providers. In practical terms, they would develop their own "Fig. 2" and request data display according to their perceptions. This new curiosity leads to new inquiries and a sense of commitment to the service of patients they now better understand, medically and socially, as far as their preventive needs are concerned. Since future directors of more peripheral centres are trained at university level, the spirit can travel peripherally, and monitoring at that health care level with adapted data collection instruments *(5)* will lead to feedback for that level, in turn preparing the ground for the most peripheral level of health care provision.

Monitoring versus studies. In obstetrics, there is a particular need to introduce a standardized recording system that may be applied to each attended birth. MCM is such an advanced experimental information system that aims at professionalization of the service providers. Any first pooled analysis may be viewed as a baseline. Reactive curative, preventive and promotive intervention necessarily follows in the light of intelligible feedback. For instance, the level of consciousness of the need for ubiquitous pregnancy care availability was raised in Indonesia through university level MCM. Regional and national workshops at regular intervals discussed the MCM findings in much detail and depth, with the pay-off that peripheral and rural management of reproductive health care provision would be reviewed. In one province, all 22 hospitals adopted a simplified MCM system. The monitoring revealed a high prevalence of grand multiparity and a persisting great family size norm. Prenatal care emerged as the most important method of intervention to decrease perinatal mortality *(12)*. The hospital incidence of maternal death was found to be three times as large as that observed in the top referral centre, which in turn pointed to the need to review the referral system. This need was corroborated by independent findings at the university level: 10% of all university admissions were prolonged/obstructed labour with an associated risk of stillbirth of 144.8 per 1000 — a 5.28-fold risk when measured against that for women with no complications (27.4 per 1000) *(13)*. But booked cases (implying antenatal visits) of prolonged/obstructed labour were associated with a very low risk of stillbirth (14.7 per 1000), suggesting once more the vital importance of antenatal visits *(14)*. A detailed analysis of the pool of monitored data at the university level showed the antenatal visits to be an important preventive determinant of late fetal death if co-controlling for registration status, maternal morbidity at admission, complications of labour and/or delivery or infant birth weight *(15)*. The last three references point to a model-like inquiry with monitoring data, whereby members of the obstetrical profession of Indonesia become aware of the notion of risk of stillbirth as a function of all binary combinations of five important variables.

In summary, monitoring is very different from studies, since epidemiological analysis and interpretation are applied to all cases receiving a certain health care service, in this case attendance at delivery. The strength of this approach, if data are collected completely and correctly, lies with the possibility of controlling for variables at the stage of analysis. A valid study presumes a carefully thought out and enforced protocol, whereas the monitoring system shifts the main design work to the stage of analysis. Analytical guidance thus becomes very important. Since the MCM data are technically comparable in regard to collection (form, manual), processing and tabular display (standard printout), the clinics refer to "their findings" as measured with other clinics' findings, or, for instance, with the latest "national baseline". This diagnostic process, involving all professionals, spells progress, since informed decisions and recommendations can be formulated for the improvement of reproductive health.

Health information. MCM emerges thus as an "on-the-job" approach to reproductive health promotion that is to affect the entire nation. In Indonesia, an *esprit de corps* among professionals, spanning the sectors of reproductive health provision (MCH/obstetrics/family planning), was noted. In order to maximize the use of the monitoring feedback initiated by Indonesian obstetricians, the wealth of information now available should be linked with the kind of national health information centre envisaged in a conceptual paper on national health planning *(16)*. Such a centre could also provide guidance, in particular, on additional "pathways of analysis" and on technical support for the obstetricians' laudable efforts. Also, issues of national interest could be re-examined by submitting the data to multivariate and regression-type analyses and feeding back the most important findings in the form of graphical illustrations to the professional corps who generated the data in the first place. This kind of closure of the information loop would elevate the service providers' monitoring efforts to a genuine health systems research component *(17)*. The comparison of "different-level" (horizontal) pool information, the extremes being finally TBA-monitoring (TBA = traditional birth attendant) and top referral monitoring, would thus generate the true profile of the nation's reproductive health status, the major effort resting with the specialized service providers. In essence, motivation for improvement would have come to the rescue of service statistics.

Conclusion

The diagnostic process illustrated with feedback from MCM is useful for many policy decisions. Fig. 4 shows, for instance, the importance of some antenatal care for women of low educational level, if perinatal mortality is to be lowered. Fig. 7 illustrates the marked differences in desired family size that can occur between maternity centres and the changing pattern of contraceptive choice with increasing family size. The relative influence of contraception and breastfeeding on the length of the birth interval, as shown in Fig. 6, is of interest to countries which have or are still without a policy of reproductive health and/or population. The current unmet need regarding the provision of pregnancy care is shown to be dependent on both education and family planning, as illustrated in Fig. 5. One major goal is to supply this information to committees on perinatal mortality, since MCM provides the necessary information to reduce all three components (i.e. antepartum, intrapartum, and postpartum deaths) of mortality around birth *(18–20)*.

The most important uses of this diagnostic process relate to training and what may be called the process of professionalization. Experience has shown that important indices show wide variation between centres *(1,2,4,6,8,10,11)*. When such variation is graphically presented to a group of peers, an interesting discussion ensues that leads to a consensus regarding standards of maternity care and a sense of responsibility for that care. This peer review of epidemiologically developed indices is applicable at any level of the referral chain and is even generic, with potential for use in other areas of primary health care. What is needed is interesting information of educational value shown in ranked order *(10)* to peers who provide a service and who have actually collected the necessary data. The result is a process of professionalization that is probably more cost-effective than the present emphasis on improved supervision, while at the same time more consistent with the philosophy of primary health care *(5)*.

Transferring responsibility for health care policy and services to peripheral centres and communities is an important part of primary health care provision. In the process, however, higher health authorities must design information systems that enable health workers in peripheral centres and community leaders to obtain the information needed for intelligent decisions, as well as providing a continuous learning process and a mechanism for consensus formation regarding standards of care *(16)*. MCM is one successful illustration of such an information system.

This presentation has shown how delivery and pregnancy outcome in university hospitals — despite the obstetric technology and know-how available there — depends very largely on social factors and the use of services integrated in the primary health care system. The observed relationships, based on data collected in university hospitals, are being used for teaching university hospital staff and candidate heads of peripheral maternity centres about the important priorities in improving health in general and reproductive health in particular.

The three-dimensional form of presentation was chosen in order to make the message more graphic, because the goal here is health promotion rather than research *per se,* for which multivariate and regression-type analyses should be considered. Ideally, the two approaches should converge, since the key findings from sophisticated statistical analyses may also be presented by three-dimensional display, in order to achieve greater understanding of the subject among members of the service profession and for health promotion purposes.

References

1. **Bernard, R.P.** Maternity care monitoring: a new opportunity in service statistics. *Population reports.* Baltimore, Johns Hopkins University, 1977 (J-17).
2. **Bernard, R.P. et al.** International maternity care monitoring: results of a pretest. *International journal of gynaecology and obstetrics,* **17**: 24–39 (1979).
3. FIGO news. *International journal of gynaecology and obstetrics,* **18**: 476–478 (1980).
4. **Bernard, R.P. et al.** International maternity care monitoring: a beginning. *In:* Aladjem, S. et al., ed. *Clinical perinatology.* St Louis, C.V. Mosby, 1980, pp. 521–559.

5. **Kessel, E.** Maternity care monitoring: a new information system. *In:* Mundo, F. et al., ed. *Primary maternal and neonatal health care: a global concern. Proceedings, First International Congress for Maternal and Neonatal Health* of IAMANEH, Manila, 2–7 November 1981. New York, Plenum Press, 1983, pp. 253–264.
6. **Bernard, R.P. et al.** Maternity care monitoring in Indonesia: early findings and implications for the 1980s. *Indonesian journal of obstetrics and gynecology,* **6**: 191–290 (1980).
7. **Bernard, R.P. & Sastrawinata, S.** Maternity care and perinatal mortality in Indonesia. *In:* Mundo, F. et al., ed. *Primary maternal and neonatal health care: a global concern. Proceedings, First International Congress for Maternal and Neonatal Health* of IAMANEH, Manila, 2–7 November 1981. New York, Plenum Press, 1983, pp. 265–305.
8. **Bernard, R.P. & Sastrawinata, S.** Breast-feeding, birth spacing and pregnancy care: prevalence and outcome. *Journal of tropical pediatrics,* **30**: 279–285 (1984).
9. **World Health Organization.** Breast feeding and fertility regulation: current knowledge and programme policy implications. *Bulletin of the World Health Organization,* **61**(3): 371–382 (1983).
10. **Bernard, R.P. et al.** *Maternity care monitoring (MCM): where next?* Report presented at the IGCC/IFRP East and South East Asia Seminar on Regional Fertility Research, Bangkok, Thailand, July 18–20, 1979. Kuala Lumpur, Malaysia, IGCC Secretariat, Inter-Governmental Coordinating Committee.
11. **Bernard, R.P. & Sastrawinata, S.** Maternal and perinatal death in Indonesian university obstetrics: risk display for selected social and biological determinants. *In:* Laaser, U. et al. *Primary health care in the making.* Berlin/Heidelberg, Springer-Verlag, 1985.
12. **Sastrawinata, S.** Maternity care monitoring in twenty-two hospitals in West Jawa. *In:* Mundo, F. et al., ed. *Primary maternal and neonatal health care: a global concern. Proceedings, First International Congress for Maternal and Neonatal Health* of IAMANEH, Manila, 2–7 November 1981. New York, Plenum Press, 1983, pp. 323–345.
13. **Bernard, R.P. & Sastrawinata, S.** 3D display of stillbirth in Indonesian obstetrics. Part 1: Birth weight, complications, and morbidity. *Sozial- und Präventivmedizin,* **28**: 208–209 (1983).
14. **Sastrawinata, S. & Bernard, R.P.** 3D display of stillbirth in Indonesian obstetrics. Part 2: Booking, referrals and emergency arrivals. *Sozial- und Präventivmedizin,* **28**: 210–211 (1983).
15. **Bernard, R.P. & Sastrawinata, S.** 3D display of stillbirth in Indonesian obstetrics. Part 3: Antenatal visits as preventive determinant. *Sozial- und Präventivmedizin,* **29**: 94–97 (1984).
16. **White, K.L.** Health planning: a new look at health information. *World health forum,* **4**: 368–373 (1983).
17. **Taylor, C.E.** Health systems research: how can it be used? *World health forum,* **4**: 328–335 (1983).

18. FIGO report. *FIGO Workshop on Monitoring and Reporting Perinatal Mortality and Morbidity,* Heidelberg, March 19–21, 1982. London, FIGO, 1982.
19. **Bernard, R.P. & Sastrawinata, S.** 3D display of stillbirth in Indonesian obstetrics. Part 7: Expansion to neonatal death. *Sozial- und Präventivmedizin,* **31**: 225–227 (1986).
20. **Sastrawinata, S. & Bernard, R.P.** 3D displays of stillbirth in Indonesian obstetrics. Part 8: Component analysis (intra-/antepartum). *Sozial- und Präventivmedizin,* **31**: 227–229 (1986).

11.7 Avoidable deaths and diseases as monitors of health promotion — *J.R.H. Charlton*

The "sentinel events" approach described by Rutstein (Chapter 7.6) can be used for comparing different geographical regions. The application of this approach to "avoidable deaths", whilst not immediately linked to health-enhancing measures, has important potential implications for the provision of health services and the allocation of health resources.

Assessing the success of health promotion activities in influencing the health of the target population is difficult because of the complexity of the concept being measured and the variability of disease itself. The WHO Constitution's definition of health as a "state of complete physical, mental and social well-being, and not merely the absence of disease or infirmity" does not easily translate into practical terms. Health promotion activities include actions aimed at prevention (e.g. immunization, water purification, health education and public hygiene legislation), cure (e.g. treatment of tuberculosis), and the care of individuals with incurable conditions, particularly in old age. One approach to health promotion is to identify avoidable events; this may then lead to specific interventions in terms of changing behaviour, modifying hazards, improving clinical practice and other similar activities. It is possible to count the number of events which should be wholly or largely avoidable in a perfect health care system, and which may thus reflect progress and failures.

A working group in the United States, led by Rutstein, drew up lists of causes of disease, disability and death which are preventable or manageable by appropriate medical and government intervention, and could thus be used to monitor the outcome of medical care defined in its broadest sense *(1,2)*. The method is described in the earlier chapter on sentinel health events (Chapter 7.6).

The incidence of disease, disability and mortality in a particular place and at a particular time may depend upon social, environmental and genetic factors as well as on the nature of the disease itself, which may vary geographically and over time. For certain conditions the progress of disease, the disability caused and the likelihood that it will lead to death may be modified by the preventive and remedial activities of health services and the legislative policies of governments, although the sequence of events leading up to avoidable disease, disability or death can be complex. Regional and time-series comparison of these "sentinel events" may pinpoint regions with particular problems in health service delivery and the effect over time of intervention in these areas. Diseases may be chosen whose occurrence or consequences are influenced predominantly by health education, immunization practices, continuity of care, surgical care, or other aspects of the health care system.

Although ideally the thorough evaluation of a specific intervention calls for a carefully designed randomized controlled trial, large-scale trials can be prohibitively expensive to conduct, or even impractical for ethical or logistic reasons, especially when the effect on a whole population rather than a selected subgroup is to be measured. Observational studies such as those utilizing sentinel events are generally much less expensive to conduct and can provide hypotheses for testing by more thorough investigation. However, improvements in quality of life and reduction of level of disability will not necessarily be measured adequately by such counts, and these aspects of care may require a more detailed approach. Such information may be gathered in household surveys, although achieving geographical coverage that will provide estimates for small areas may be expensive.

Using "Avoidable Deaths" to Compare Geographical Regions

In developed countries, data on mortality by cause are almost universally available, often for small geographical areas, with nearly complete recording, while this is rarely the case for data concerning disease prevalence or disability. Thus, counting avoidable deaths provides an inexpensive solution to monitoring a number of aspects of health promotion. However, for disease and disability, mortality data are subject to inaccuracies in diagnosis, which may vary from site to site and over time. Variations in mortality rates from a particular disease will depend on variations in the incidence of that disease, in disease severity, and in case fatality rates. It is also important to have reasonably accurate estimates of the population. The inaccuracies which limit the usefulness of mortality data are difficult, if not impossible, to quantify. Also, differences in diagnostic habit and precision may affect the observed pattern of variation. Studies based on routine autopsy findings provide information on diagnostic accuracy but are not representative of the community as a whole, since post-mortem examinations are more frequently conducted on cases where there is some doubt regarding the diagnosis *(3)*. There may also be variations in coding practice. Diagnostic and coding inaccuracies are generally greater in the older age groups, and so the problem is reduced by concentrating attention on younger people (e.g. those under 65 years).

Observation of sentinel events is not intended, however, to produce definitive verdicts, but to raise questions which may be answered by a series of further investigations, and as such may prove to be a valuable tool in spite of possible inaccuracies. The monitoring of avoidable deaths may yield information for a broad range of health services or for other areas of public policy, although some aspects of health care (e.g. relief of symptoms) may still remain outside the scope of this approach. Once areas with relatively high avoidable mortality have been identified from routine data, it may then be necessary to mount further investigations to try to identify the reasons.

Analysis and Interpretation

The absolute numbers of avoidable deaths in different geographical regions are of importance in themselves, but it is impossible to compare geographical regions without taking into account differences in population size. Data should be collected in, say, five-year age groups for males and females, giving the size of population and the number of deaths in each group. It may be necessary to aggregate data for several years in order to obtain sufficient numbers of deaths to enable statistically valid comparisons to be made. These data can then be conveniently summarized for each region and disease group into a standardized mortality ratio (SMR), which is the observed number of deaths divided by the number of deaths the geographical region would be expected to have if each age/sex group experienced the same death rates as that of a "standard" population. This standard population is usually taken to be the aggregate of all the regions being studied. Of the various approaches to standardization, the SMR has theoretically the smallest standard error, and is described in most standard textbooks on medical statistics. Some assumptions are implicit in the use of SMRs, and these can be tested *(4)*. If a region has an SMR which is high relative to others, this provides a warning signal that that region might experience greater shortcomings in health promotion than others, although there may well be other reasons which would account for the observed differences.

The investigator should examine, with the data at his or her disposal, the possible reasons for these differences, and more detailed studies should be performed if they are considered justified. Variations in mortality may result from both variations in disease incidence and variations in case fatality. If variations in disease incidence are to be ruled out as the reason for the mortality differences, and reasonable incidence data exist, these could be incorporated into the analysis and used to adjust the mortality data. One method by which it is possible to "adjust for incidence" if incidence data are available is to use multiple regression, suitably weighted to take account of the different population sizes of the regions *(5)* and thus form a predictive equation for mortality. The difference between the observed SMR and the SMR predicted on the basis of incidence provides a mortality index standardized for incidence. Reliable incidence data seldom exist, although some hospital admission data (which identify first admissions) or disease registration data may be used for some causes. Otherwise, proxies for incidence (e.g. factors known to be strongly related to incidence) might be considered and a similar statistical approach used. Regression analyses based on data describing aggregate characteristics of geographical areas are subject to a number of potential sources of bias, for example the "ecological fallacy", and these limitations should be considered when interpreting findings. The results of such analyses cannot be definitive, and warning signals provided by both the unadjusted and the adjusted indices will have to be considered when deciding whether further detailed examinations are justified.

Any explanation of variations in mortality from the selected avoidable causes will have to take into account all potential influences. Further investigations into the reasons for high avoidable mortality in a particular area might begin with an audit of the medical and other records of the patients concerned. This would commence with examination of the accuracy of the recorded deaths, and the associated causes of death. For those cases where death is considered avoidable, patient records could be examined to determine whether correct treatment was given, and, if so, whether there were delays in giving treatment. If there were unacceptable delays, then reasons should be sought, e.g. lack of facilities and inadequate access to medical care. These investigations should also provide information on quality of care and on patient characteristics such as attitude, education, environment, use made of medical facilities, and compliance. Where justified, intervention studies could be designed to attempt to alter the pattern of mortality. Available routinely collected resource data may also shed light on the reasons for shortcomings in health service delivery in certain areas, but more sophisticated information may well be required to establish the reasons for variations in mortality rates.

Deaths may be avoidable by prevention or by timely and appropriate treatment. The example given below is of geographical variation in mortality from conditions amenable to medical intervention in England & Wales.

In the first stage of a study of medical intervention and the avoidability of death in England & Wales *(6)* the main concern was the development of a set of outcome indicators sensitive to the curative aspects of care provided through the National Health Service. The lists drawn up by Rutstein et al. *(1,2)* were for international use, covering the avoidability and treatability of unnecessary disease, disability and untimely death, and can be used as a framework for selection by countries in relation to specific problems or policies. Some of the conditions listed are rare in developed countries, and some relate mainly to the curative aspects of health services. In selecting causes of mortality appropriate for the study objectives, diseases whose control depends mainly on prevention (e.g. lung cancer) were excluded, although some of the diseases chosen are dependent to a certain extent on secondary prevention.

It was decided to examine mortality data because they are readily available and more reliable than data on disability or on the occurrence of disease. Surveys of morbidity tend to be infrequent in the United Kingdom and not geographically representative, while other routine systems such as hospital activity analysis are episode-dependent, suffer greatly from inaccuracy and incompleteness *(7)*, and the level of admission depends on the availability of health care resources. Although the limitations of mortality data have been noted by a number of authors, no other routine system of data collection rivals it in terms of availability, economy and completeness.

Causes were chosen to cover a broad range of health service activities within the curative services. Perinatal, maternal and "all causes" mortality were also studied for comparative purposes. Age limits were set for each cause to increase the proportion of potentially avoidable mortality. A further requirement of the data was that in England & Wales the number of deaths in the period studied (1974–1978) should exceed 200 in order to ensure sufficient numbers for statistically valid comparisons. The mortality causes selected were not intended to provide a definitive evaluation, but rather to indicate where problems may exist and thus stimulate further investigation. The chosen disease groups, in order of mortality incidence in England & Wales, were the following.

Hypertensive disease *(ICD8 400–404, ages 5–64 years)*
Intervention has been shown to decrease morbidity and mortality *(8–10)* and thus variations in mortality may reflect differences in medical care.

Cervical cancer *(ICD8 180, ages 5–64 years)*
Although the efficiency of cervical screening programmes is still debated, the early detection and treatment of cervical cancer appears to be effective in reducing mortality from this disease *(11–13)*.

Pneumonia and unqualified bronchitis *(ICD8 480–486, 490, ages 5–49 years)*
The vast majority of pneumonias should respond adequately to antibiotics *(14)*. Where timely antibiotic therapy with supportive medical care is provided, the survival rate should be high in the more resilient age groups chosen. Some deaths will occur in immunologically compromised individuals with cancer or other debilitating conditions, but observance of the correct coding procedure will ensure that these deaths are certified as due to the underlying cause and not to pneumonia or bronchitis. "Unqualified" bronchitis excludes chronic bronchitis and emphysema.

Tuberculosis *(ICD8 011–019, ages 5–64 years)*
Many factors are associated with morbidity and mortality due to tuberculosis, including nutrition and housing. However, effective antituberculosis chemotherapy is available, and has been associated with a reduction in mortality rates *(15)*.

Asthma *(ICD8 493, ages 5–49 years)*
In the United States the introduction of steroid therapy in the early 1950s coincided with a progressive decrease in the mortality rate *(16)*, but the mortality rate in the United Kingdom for people aged 5–34 years has hardly changed since 1867 *(17, 18)*. Although the effectiveness of medical treatment in preventing asthma deaths is somewhat contentious, studies in the United Kingdom of asthma fatalities, both in and out of hospital, have shown that improved availability of appropriate services, and greater doctor and patient awareness, should prevent a substantial number of deaths *(19–24)*.

Chronic rheumatic heart disease *(ICD8 393–398, ages 5–44 years)*
The progressive fall in the occurrence of acute rheumatic fever over the last 40 years has been followed by a reduction in the incidence of chronic rheumatic heart disease. Although environmental factors, and possibly an unexplained change in the pathogenicity of beta-haemolytic streptococcus, explain most of the change, current medical therapy has been shown to be effective in reducing the incidence of rheumatic fever *(25)*. In addition, many patients with rheumatic valvular disease will benefit from surgical and medical therapy.

Acute respiratory infections and influenza *(ICD8 460–466, 470–474, ages 5–49 years)*
Included here are influenzas and other acute infections of the respiratory tract, mostly viral, with death usually occurring after secondary bacterial invasion. Good medical care, with immunization of high-risk individuals and antibiotic therapy of secondary infections, should reduce mortality in this age group.

Bacterial infections *(ICD8 381–383, 390–393, 680–686, 710, 720, ages 5–64 years)*
These comprise bacillary dysentery, streptococcal sore throat and scarlet fever, meningitis, otitis media, mastoiditis, rheumatic fever, chorea, infections of the skin and subcutaneous tissue, acute arthritis due to pyogenic organisms and osteomyelitis and periostitis. For the age group chosen, the majority of these should respond adequately to antibiotics if treated promptly and correctly.

Hodgkin's disease *(ICD8 201, ages 5–34 years)*
Early recognition with accurate identification of the stage and appropriate therapy can lead to recovery in most cases *(26)*. Many centres are reporting 5-year survival rates of more than 90% for stage IA and IIA, and over 85% for all groups under 35 years *(27)*. By restricting attention to the age groups under 35 years, the proportion of cases of this cancer with favourable histologies was increased.

Abdominal hernias, cholecystitis and cholelithiasis, appendicitis *(ICD8 550–553, 574–575, 540–543, ages 5–64 years)*
Medical/surgical intervention would be expected to result in decreased mortality from the complications of these conditions. Increased surgical activity may have a paradoxical effect on observed mortality, in that surgical mortality may be attributed to the condition itself *(28)*. In general, however, it is accepted that surgery is of positive value in reducing mortality from these disorders.

Deficiency anaemias *(ICD8 280–281, ages 5–64 years)*
Most of the deaths from this condition should be preventable in western countries. Deaths due to other causes but featuring anaemia should be coded to the primary disease and not to the anaemia itself.

As a first step the variation in mortality from these selected causes among the 98 area health authorities comprising England & Wales *(29)* was analysed. Socioeconomic conditions are associated with geographical variation in mortality, and they also influence disease incidence and the uptake of medical services. Indicators of socioeconomic conditions were therefore used in an attempt to control for disease incidence, although they may also be associated with case fatality, which was of particular interest in this study. The residual variation after controlling for socioeconomic factors was thus examined. This was done by regressing mortality on socioeconomic indicators for each disease, using iteratively reweighted least squares *(5)* to take account of differences in population size. The differences between observed SMR and SMR predicted on the basis of socioeconomic factors provided a mortality index standardized for socioeconomic factors. The socioeconomic indicators used were social class, housing tenure and car ownership (the last two being measures of wealth). The source was an 8% national sample survey, since this provided contemporary data, although such data are also collected in decennial censuses. There was wide variation among the area health authorities for a number of causes. Socioeconomic factors explained a large part of the variation for some causes, e.g. tuberculosis and cervical cancer. However, considerable variation among area health authorities remained even after standardizing for these factors, and the relative rankings of authorities remained little altered.

As an example, Fig. 1 shows the variation in mortality from pneumonia and bronchitis in people aged 5–49 years in areas of England & Wales, before and after standardization for socioeconomic factors. In both cases there was wide variation among area health authorities. Although standardizing for socioeconomic factors narrowed the range, the variation remained significantly greater than could be expected by chance. It is not possible to establish on the basis of this particular analysis that this degree of variation is due to differences in the quality of medical care. However, if a relationship is confirmed, it may have important implications for the provision and delivery of health services.

The relationships between these indicators, other measures of disease incidence, and measures of health service resources were also examined *(30)*. Although mortality levels were generally found to be related to indicators of morbidity, significant heterogeneity persisted after these and socioeconomic factors were taken into account. These findings suggest that morbidity and socioeconomic factors were not the only determinants of mortality variation among areas for these particular diseases. Measures of health care input were also examined, the hypothesis being that fewer deaths would be expected where there were more resources, although a strong relationship could not be expected owing to the crudity of the resource data readily available. There was wide variation in provision of resources in different parts of the country, such as hospital revenue spent per head of resident population and general practitioners per 1000 population. Resource availability was weakly but significantly ($P < 0.01$) related to mortality as hypothesized, consistent with fewer deaths occurring where there were more resources, but the results need to be treated with caution. For example, areas that were socially deprived also tended to have significantly fewer resources per head of population. Although the analyses are not conclusive, they do suggest possible reasons for variation in mortality that can be examined further. Furthermore, several of the areas identified by the study as having high mortality have mounted clinical audits of the individual patients dying from selected causes, to identify at what points in the chain of events leading up to death the health services may have failed *(31)*. The first of these to be published has identified potentially avoidable factors that contributed to death from the two causes studied, hypertension and cervical cancer *(32,33)*.

Fig. 1. England & Wales: mortality from pneumonia and bronchitis in persons aged 5–49 years, before and after standardization for socioeconomic factors

Original data
(standardized mortality ratio (SMR))

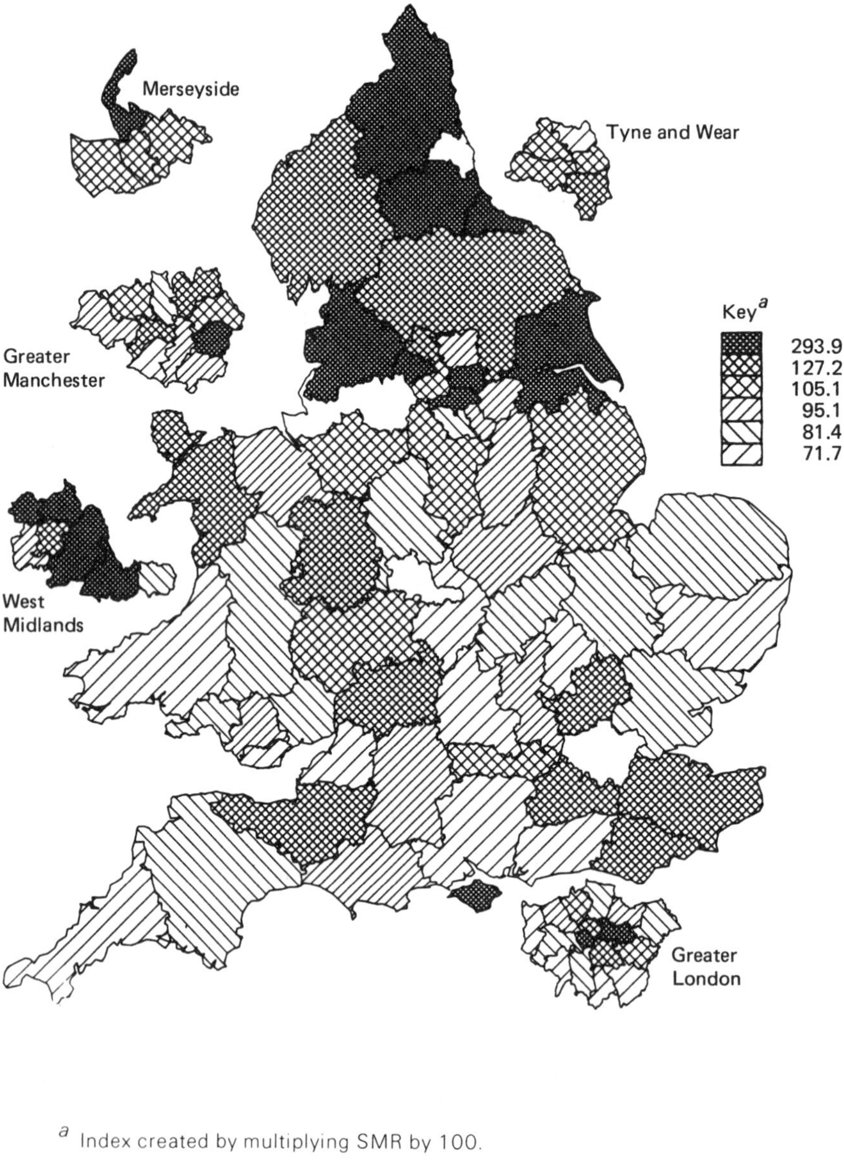

[a] Index created by multiplying SMR by 100.

Fig. 1 (contd)

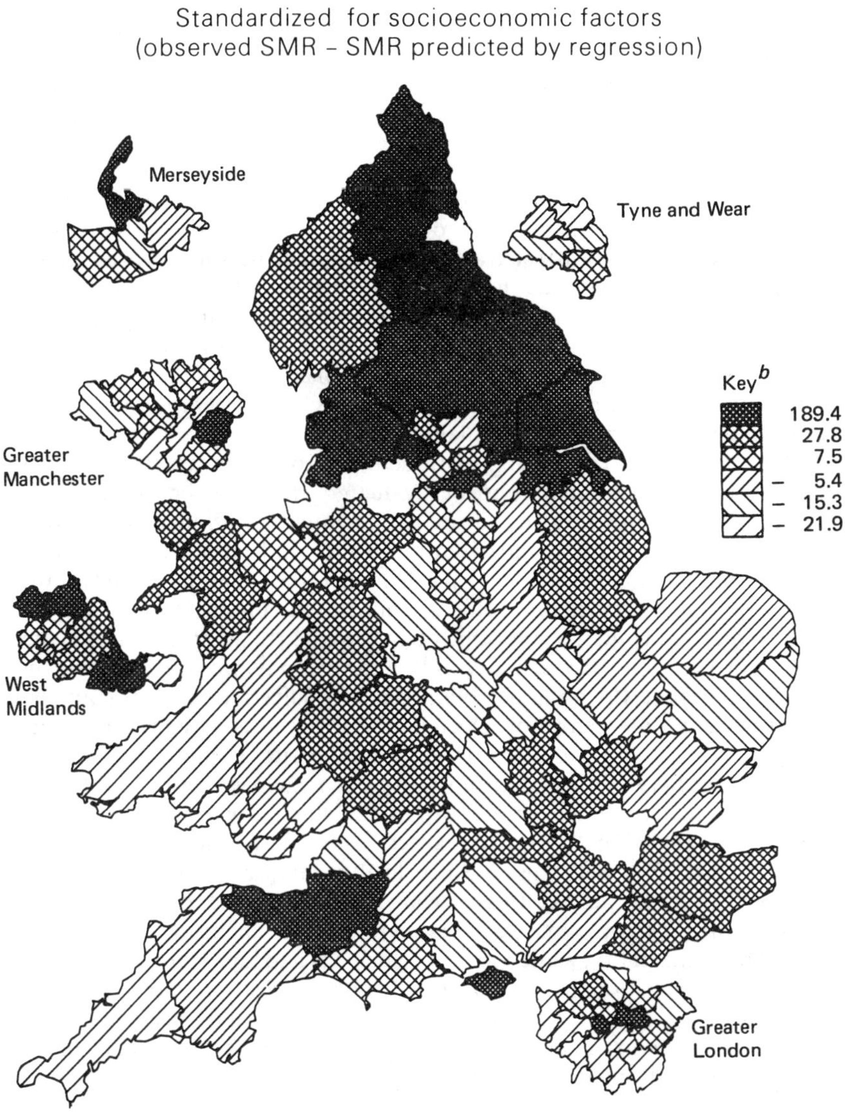

[b] 100 × (observed SMR – SMR predicted by regression).

These detailed investigations will have to be based on individual patients, since the sequence of events leading up to an avoidable death may be complex. For example, the likelihood of contracting a disease will depend upon characteristics of the individual, including attitude and education, and his or her environment, which may also influence when and whether the illness is recognized and treatment is sought. Where timely contact is made, the individual's willingness to comply with treatment may affect outcome, particularly where long-term medication (e.g. antihypertensive treatment) is prescribed. Once a diagnosis has been made, death from an avoidable cause may result from inaccurate diagnosis, human error or shortage of resources. Insensitivity of diagnostic tests might lead to a certain proportion of cases ending in death instead of recovery. The availability of health service resources may affect the outcome of treatable illness at several points in the chain from illness to recovery or death. The level of primary care and screening services will affect travelling and queueing time and hours of opening, and may influence the individual's decision to make timely first contact with the health service. Pressure on staff time and facilities may reduce the degree of detail or accuracy of initial investigations and thus delay treatment. Where a correct diagnosis has been made, the lack of availability of specific treatment resources (e.g. radiotherapy) may delay timely intervention or lower its quality.

The usefulness or otherwise of these indicators as measures of health service performance remains to be evaluated. This will be achieved by probing more deeply into the causes of mortality variations between different parts of the country, and over time. If these indicators are established as valid measures of health care performance they may have important applications in achieving more effective allocation of health care resources. These indices and others are currently being applied to other countries in the European Economic Community *(34)*, and this may provide information additional to that which can be obtained from analysis for a single country.

At present, time trends for selected mortality causes amenable to treatment are being compared in six developed countries. Preliminary data for the years 1951–1974 show that mortality from each of these "avoidable" causes has fallen to a much greater extent than mortality from other causes. Fig. 2 shows the fall in "avoidable causes" as previously defined compared with that for all other causes. Since health care, and access to it, has improved over the period, this is what was expected. Japan, which has changed most in terms of medical treatment, has also changed most in terms of avoidable mortality, while Sweden, which has had high standards of care throughout the period, has consistently had the lowest avoidable mortality rates. However, over-interpretation of such results should be resisted, since comparisons are not made between similar populations with similar diets, social habits and genetic characteristics.

References

1. **Rutstein, D.D. et al.** Measuring the quality of medical care. *New England journal of medicine,* **11**: 582–588 (1976).

Fig. 2. Comparison of fall in mortality from "avoidable[a] causes" with that from all other causes

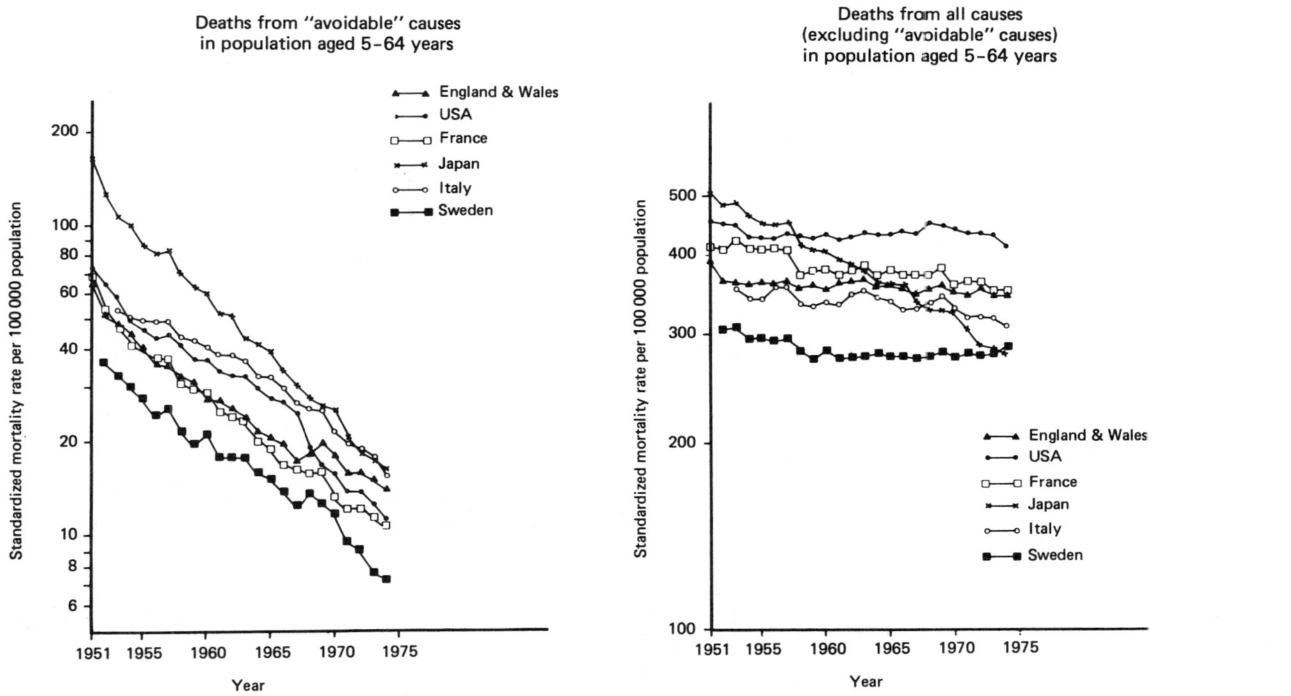

[a] Includes maternal mortality, tuberculosis, malignant neoplasm of cervix uteri, hypertensive disease, acute appendicitis, chronic cholecystitis, chronic rheumatic heart disease, acute respiratory infection.

2. **Rutstein, D.D. et al.** Measuring the quality of medical care: second revision of tables of indexes. *New England journal of medicine,* **302**: 1146 (1980).
3. **Armitage, P.** *Statistical methods in medical research.* Oxford, Blackwell Scientific Publications, 1971.
4. **Gail, M.** The analysis of heterogeneity for indirect standardisation mortality ratios. *Journal of the Royal Statistical Society, Series A,* **141**: 224–234 (1978).
5. **Pocock, S.J. et al.** Regression of area mortality rates on explanatory variables: what weighting is appropriate? *Applied statistics,* **30**: 286–295 (1981).
6. **Charlton, J.R.H. et al.** Geographical variation in mortality from conditions amenable to medical intervention in England and Wales. *Lancet,* **1**: 691–696 (1983).
7. **Whates, P.D. et al.** Accuracy of hospital activity analysis operation codes. *British medical journal,* **1**: 1857–1858 (1982).
8. **Hypertension Detection and Follow-up Program Co-operative Group.** Five-year findings of the hypertension detection and follow-up program. 1. Reduction in mortality of persons with high blood pressure, including mild hypertension. *Journal of the American Medical Association,* **242**: 2562–2571 (1979).
9. The Australian therapeutic trial in mild hypertension. Report by the Management Committee. *Lancet,* **1**: 1261–1267 (1980).
10. **Veterans' Administration Co-operative Study Group on Antihypertensive Agents.** Effects of treatment on morbidity in hypertension. II. Results in patients with diastolic blood pressure averaging 90 through 114 mmHg. *Journal of the American Medical Association,* **7**: 1143–1152 (1970).
11. Canadian Medical Association screening for carcinoma of the cervix. *Canadian Medical Association journal,* **114**: 1031–1026 (1976).
12. **MacGregor, J.E. & Teper, S.** Mortality from carcinoma of cervix uteri in Britain. *Lancet,* **2**: 774–776 (1978).
13. **Clark, B.A. & Anderson, T.W.** Does screening by "PAP" smears help prevent cervical cancer? *Lancet,* **2**: 1–4 (1979).
14. **Hook, E.W.** Pneumococcal pneumonia. *In:* Beeson, P.E. et al., ed. *Cecil textbook of medicine,* 15th ed. Philadelphia, W.B. Saunders, 1979.
15. **Johnston, R.F. & Wildnick, K.H.** State of the art. Review of the impact of chemotherapy on the care of patients with tuberculosis. *American review of respiratory disease,* **109**: 636–664 (1974).
16. **Karetzky, M.E.** Asthma mortality: an analysis of one year's experience; review of the literature and assessment of current modes of therapy. *Medicine,* **54**(6): 471–484 (1975).
17. **Clark, I.J.H. & Godrey, S.** *Asthma.* London, Chapman & Hill, 1971, pp. 303–388.
18. **Office of Population Censuses and Surveys.** *Mortality statistics, Series DH2 1–7.* London, H.M. Stationery Office, 1974–1980.
19. **MacDonald, J.B. et al.** Asthma deaths in Cardiff, 1963–74: 53 deaths in hospitals. *British medical journal,* **1**: 1493–1495 (1976).

20. **MacDonald, J.B. et al.** Asthma deaths in Cardiff, 1965–74: 90 deaths outside hospital. *British medical journal,* **2**: 721–723 (1976).
21. **Hetzel, M.R. et al.** Asthma: analysis of sudden deaths and ventilatory arrests in hospital. *British medical journal,* **1**: 808–811 (1977).
22. **Osmerod, D.P. & Stableforth, D.E.** Asthma mortality in Birmingham, 1975–77: 53 deaths. *British medical journal,* **1**: 687–690 (1980).
23. **British Thoracic Association.** Death from asthma in two regions of England. *British medical journal,* **2**: 1252–1255 (1982).
24. **Compton, G.K. et al.** Edinburgh emergency asthma admission service: report on 10 years' experience. *British medical journal,* **2**: 1199–1201 (1979).
25. **Gordis, L.** Effectiveness of comprehensive programs in preventing rheumatic fever. *New England journal of medicine,* **289**: 331–335 (1973).
26. **Aisenberg, A.C.** The staging and treatment of Hodgkin's disease. *New England journal of medicine,* **299**: 1232 (1978).
27. **Kaplan, H.S.** *Hodgkin's disease,* 2nd ed. Cambridge, MA, Harvard University Press, 1980, pp. 548–597.
28. **Lichtner, S. & Pflanz, M.** Appendectomy in the Federal Republic of Germany: epidemiology and medical care patterns. *Medical care,* **9**: 311–330 (1971).
29. **Charlton, J.R.H. et al.** Geographical variation in mortality from conditions amenable to medical intervention in England and Wales. *Lancet,* **1**: 691–696 (1983).
30. **Bauer, R.L. & Charlton, J.R.H.** Area variation in mortality from diseases amenable to medical intervention: the contribution of differences in morbidity. *International journal of epidemiology,* **15**: 408–412 (1986).
31. **Charlton, J.R.H. et al.** Outcome measures for district and regional health care planners. *Community medicine,* **6**: 306–315 (1984).
32. **Charlton, J.R.H. et al.** How have "avoidable death" indices for England and Wales changed? 1974–78 compared with 1979–83. *Community medicine,* **8**: 304–314 (1986).
33. **Single, G.M. et al.** *A confidential enquiry into premature preventable deaths. Pilot study.* Report to Walsall Health Authority. Walsall, 1985.
34. **EC Working Group on "Avoidable Mortality".** An analysis of some causes of mortality possibly affected by health care delivery and national policies for prevention. *In: EC atlas of avoidable mortality (1974–78).* Oxford, Oxford University Press, 1987.

11.8 Quebec planners' choice of health promotion indicators — *A. Colvez, M. Blanchet & P. Lamarche*

Many measurements of health status rely on mortality or morbidity-related concepts, such as that of years of life lost. The increasing importance of disability, linked mainly to the ever-increasing proportion of elderly people in many communities, emphasizes the importance of "potential years of wellbeing". This concept of "life expectancy free from disability" is presented here as a planning and evaluation tool in the health programmes of Quebec.

In 1979, the Directorate of Health Care Planning and Evaluation of the Ministry of Social Affairs of Quebec (Canada) gave its Department of Epidemiological Studies the task of developing new health indicators, with a view to facilitating the definition of priorities and evaluation of programmes.

At that time, health planning in Quebec was based on three criteria: *(a)* the geographical distribution of facilities and personnel (number of beds, doctors and dentists per 1000 inhabitants); *(b)* mortality and hospital morbidity statistics; and *(c)* morbidity diagnoses in outpatient care. Why, then, was it necessary to develop further indicators? The obvious answer is that the limitations of those indicators were increasingly apparent.

It was becoming more and more difficult to accept without qualification the view that the development of medical facilities invariably brings about an improvement in health status, and this meant that the quantity of services provided could no longer be used to assess the level of health of the population. Mortality is a more relevant criterion for that purpose, and this was the factor used in orienting the planning of a number of programmes (e.g. those covering the perinatal period, cancer of the uterus, nutrition and accidents). However, mortality is not a sufficient criterion either, since it fails to take account of other problems that are equally important but which do not involve a life-threatening prognosis (physical disabilities, sequelae of accidents, sensory impairments, rheumatic complaints, mental disorders).

The use of diagnosed morbidity (in hospitals and outpatient care) was an initial attempt to go beyond mortality, but even this information is not enough, especially so far as chronic diseases are concerned, since the same diagnosis (e.g. diabetes) can cover a whole range of functional states (from coma to the mere constraint on a stabilized diabetic of a daily drug regimen).

New criteria therefore had to be considered and integrated with "traditional" indicators in a wider view of health that would take account not only of patent morbid states but also of the whole range of health situations, the aim being not merely to prolong life but to foster the quality of life or, in other words, to extend healthy life.

The present paper reports on this experiment and gives some examples to illustrate the results obtained.

The Base Options

Conceptual framework

Health — a multidimensional phenomenon, the result of an adaptational process

In the view *(1)* subscribed to in this paper, health is regarded as a complex phenomenon with physical, mental and social components, the attainment of which depends on the organism successfully making a continuous effort to adapt to its environment *(2)*. Disease is thus the result of an imbalance caused by either a deficiency in the organism or an unfavourable environment. These two factors in turn give rise to the concept of risk, which may be defined as a state of deficiency in the organism or a particular factor in the (physical, biological or social) environment linked to an unacceptably high probability of causing disease, loss of function or death. According to this definition, neither the deficiency nor the environmental factor itself implies a state of disease, but a disease may result from the relationship between them when the organism fails to adapt to its environment.

Distinction between measuring the intensity of morbid phenomena and analysing underlying causes

The individual's failure to adapt to his environment, which constitutes the diseased state, cannot therefore be described in terms of either a risk or a diagnosis; it must be seen as the deviant behaviour adopted by the individual compared with that of the members of his reference group. Health indicators will accordingly be based on the behaviour patterns observed during a disease or pathological state. In this approach, the operation of measuring health status is considered separately from the assessment of causes and mechanisms. However, these two aspects are not mutually exclusive but complement each other. The overall measurement of a level of health based on outcome gives a clearer definition of the objective to be attained, but offers no information on the interventions required. These are described in diagnostic terms or derived directly from the diagnosis. Thus, a diabetic stabilized by insulin treatment need not necessarily be classified as "ill", as he would be in conventional morbidity statistics; on the other hand, only the diagnosis of diabetes gives information on the intervention required, namely, insulin treatment.

Measuring health status is based on certain concepts contained in the International Classification of Impairments, Disabilities and Handicaps

There is an unbroken spectrum between health and death, but only the most serious states are easily registrable. The intensity of mortality is easily measured by the classic indices (rates and quotients). In order to assess the intensity of morbid states, four of the dimensions proposed by WHO for measuring the consequences of diseases were adopted *(3)*:

— *physical mobility* related to the movement of individuals in their living space;

— *physical independence,* which concerns carrying out the elementary tasks of daily life unaided;

— *customary occupations* or activities which a subject regularly carries out and which depend on his sex, age and occupation;

— *social integration:* although by nature fundamentally different from the previous dimensions, this was adopted because of its important links with mental health.

Analysis of causes
It was envisaged that the causes of the following states would be analysed in conjunction with indicators of functional disability, but only at a secondary level: mortality, hospitalization and restriction of activity. Analysis is primarily based on the conventional diagnoses as arranged in the various categories and subcategories of the International Classification of Diseases.

Choice of an aggregate indicator of health status

Choice of life expectancy free from disability as the overall indicator of health status
For the limited and well defined purposes of geographical planning of services and overall evaluation of health policies, it is of interest to replace the indicator of mortality alone with an aggregate indicator of health status that takes account of both mortality and functional disability. Mortality was indeed formerly used in Quebec as an overall index to measure the results of the health care system.

The Department chose life expectancy free from disability as described by Sullivan *(4)*. This indicator, which combines mortality and disability, expresses the health status of a population in the form of the average number of years of life without disability. The principle of the calculation is a simple one: it consists in taking a current mortality table, subtracting the number of years lived in a certain state of disability or poor health, and recalculating a new life expectancy, namely life expectancy free from disability.

There are several advantages in using an index of this kind.

- From the methodological point of view, life expectancy free from disability is calculated using normal demographic methods, since it is merely an extension of the concept of life expectancy.

- Both health professionals and other users can easily understand this index. To the extent that life expectancy is widely used, life expectancy free from disability may be said to have its own frame of reference, since by comparing life expectancy free from disability and life expectancy an immediate picture is easily obtained of the extent of disability within a population.

- Life expectancy free from disability enables the objectives of a health care system to be more precisely defined; these are to increase not merely life expectancy but also the average number of years lived free from disability. An upward trend in the index accurately reflects rising aspirations concerning the quality of life, and it is a good expression of the latter in the health field.

Development of a statistical instrument for measuring the effect of pathological causes on life expectancy free from disability: potential gains in life expectancy free from disability

Using life expectancy free from disability, it is possible to rank different populations by health status, but not to classify the various pathological problems according to their repercussions on health. In order to assess these repercussions, a simple method has been developed to measure the effect of pathological causes on life expectancy free from disability *(5)*. This method consists in taking as the "weight" of each cause the sum of the theoretical gains in life expectancy free from disability that would be obtained if the deaths and restrictions of activity due to that cause were removed.

This method means that conventional statistics on mortality and morbidity by pathological cause can be linked to measurement of life expectancy free from disability. From the weights of these causes on life expectancy free from disability, a hierarchy of priorities can be drawn up in each pathological field, taking full account of mortality and disability.

Application

These options were applied under operational conditions. This called for rapid collection of the data required for initial estimates, together with identification of data that were not available and which should be obtained in future.

Sources of data

For *mortality,* data were taken from Canadian national statistics on mortality by province (Statistics Canada). Mortality tables were drawn up from the mortality rates using conventional demographic methods.

Three kinds of *disability* were distinguished: institutionalization, temporary limitation of activity and permanent limitation of activity.

- Data on *institutionalization* were derived from the Ministry of Social Affairs' hospital statistics, giving the total numbers of inpatients *(6)*.

- Data on *temporary limitation of activity* were derived from the Canada Health Survey *(7)*. They are expressed as the number of days in the two weeks preceding the interview during which the subject was unable to carry out his customary activities for health reasons (confined to bed, principal activity given up or limited).

- Data on *permanent limitation of activity,* derived from the Canada Health Survey *(7)*, are measured by the number of subjects stating that their activities were limited for health reasons during the past 12 months. This indicator was subdivided into four categories: no limitation; slight limitation, not in main activity but in other activities; limitation of main activity; and unable to carry out main activity.

These various types of disability are expressed in the same units. Each day of temporary limitation of activity is counted as 1/365th of a "man-year" of limited activity, and each person with permanent limitation corresponds to one "man-year" (i.e. 365 days) of limited activity.

An example of calculation of life expectancy free from disability for women is given in Table 1.

Findings

Life expectancy free from disability in Quebec

The findings published below have been taken from Dillard *(8)*. Life expectancy free from disability was calculated by breaking down life expectancy at a given age into the following categories: life expectancy in institutional care, life expectancy with temporary limitation of activity, and life expectancy with permanent limitation of activity.

In Quebec in 1980, "ordinary" life expectancy at birth was 70.31 years for men and 78.23 years for women (Fig. 1). The total number of years of disability amounted to 11 years in men and 18 years in women, i.e. 16% and 23% of life expectancy respectively (Table 2).

Life expectancy free from disability in Quebec in 1980 was accordingly 59 years in men and 60 years in women. It should be noted that the difference in disability between the sexes means that men and women have almost the same life expectancy free from disability, whereas life expectancy at birth is 8 years lower in men. Permanent limitation of activity accounts for some two thirds of all limitations. Whereas women had more limitations, men were far more affected by severe permanent limitations (3.0 compared with 0.8 years, i.e. nearly four times more). On the other hand, institutionalization was markedly higher in women (1.8 compared with 0.8 years).

Comparison between Quebec and the other provinces of Canada

Using the health survey of the whole of Canada, Wilkins et al. *(9)* have compared life expectancy free from disability in the various provinces (Fig. 2). With regard to mortality, British Columbia was best placed for both women and men, while Quebec had the lowest life expectancies at birth.

The way in which limitations of activity are perceived would appear to differ from one province to another: despite having the lowest life expectancy, Quebec had the highest life expectancy free from disability, because of the low rate of limitation of activity in this province.

Table 1. Example of calculation of life expectancy free of disability for women

Age (years)	Survivors	Total person-years lived	*Ordinary life expectancy*	Rate of institution-alization	Total person-years lived in institutions	*Life expectancy in institutions*	Total person-years lived outside institutions	Rate of (permanent and temporary) limitation of activity	Person-years lived with limitation of activity	*Life expectancy with limitation of activity*	*Life expectancy free of disability*
	(1)	(2)	(3)	(4) (in %)	(5) = (2) × (4)	(6)[a]	(7) = (2) - (5)	(8) (in %)	(9) = (7) × (8)	(10)[b]	(11) = (3) - [(6) + (10)]
0	100 000	1 483 184	78.23	—	—	1.76	1 483 184	3.721	55 192	16.24	60.23
15	98 653	983 964	64.26	0.0834	821	1.78	983 143	8.333	81 925	15.90	46.58
25	98 121	1 946 723	54.58	0.1743	3 393	1.78	1 943 330	14.506	281 899	15.15	37.65
45	96 124	1 838 726	35.46	0.5598	10 293	1.79	1 828 433	28.296	517 373	12.53	2.1.14
65	85 037	1 570 321	18.47	10.2728	161 316	1.90	1 409 005	48.754	686 946	8.08	8.49

[a] (6) is calculated as the total number of years lived in institutions by the initial population in a given age group, divided by this initial population.

[b] (10) is calculated as the total number of years lived with limitation of activity by the initial population in a given age group, divided by this initial population.

Source: **Dillard, S.** *(8)*.

Fig. 1. Total life expectancy and life expectancy free from disability at birth, by sex, Quebec, 1980

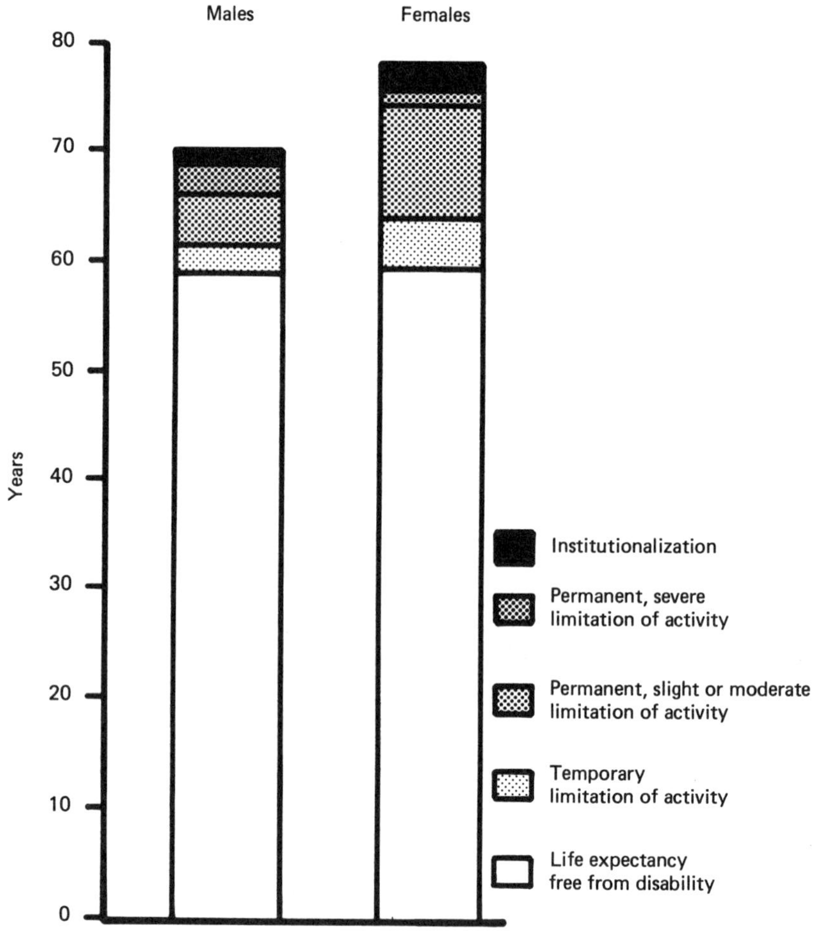

Source: **Dillard, S.** *(8).*

Table 2. Total life expectancy and life expectancy free from disability at birth, by sex, Quebec, 1980

Type of indicator	Males		Females	
	No. of years	%	No. of years	%
Total life expectancy	70.31	100	78.23	100
Long-term institutionalization	0.80	1.1	1.76	2.2
Permanent limitation of activity	7.70	11.0	11.71	15.0
of which: severe	3.01	4.3	0.83	1.1
Temporary limitation of activity	2.77	3.9	4.53	5.8
Total years lived with limitation of activity	*11.27*	*16.0*	*18.00*	*23.0*
Life expectancy free from disability	59.04	84.0	60.23	77.0

Source: **Dillard, S.** *(8).*

Ontario and the Prairies may be regarded as best placed, since they combine high life expectancy with high life expectancy free from disability, and the rates of limitation of activity are lower than the average for all age groups in Canada. The Atlantic regions (Maritime provinces), on the other hand, would appear to be in the worst position: life expectancy is low, and limitation of activity compounds this disadvantage. Quebec and British Columbia are in an intermediate position, albeit with differences between them. Quebec combines the lowest life expectancy with rates of limitation of activity slightly below the average, while British Columbia holds the double record of the longest life expectancy and the highest rates of limitation of activity *(8)*.

Wilkins & Adams *(9)* have studied life expectancy free from disability trends in Canada on the basis of a previous survey carried out in Canada in 1950/1951. They found that the improvement in life expectancy free from disability over the past 30 years has been far less than that of overall life expectancy (Table 3).

Fig. 2. Life expectancy at birth, with and without limitation of activity, Quebec and other regions of Canada, 1978/1979

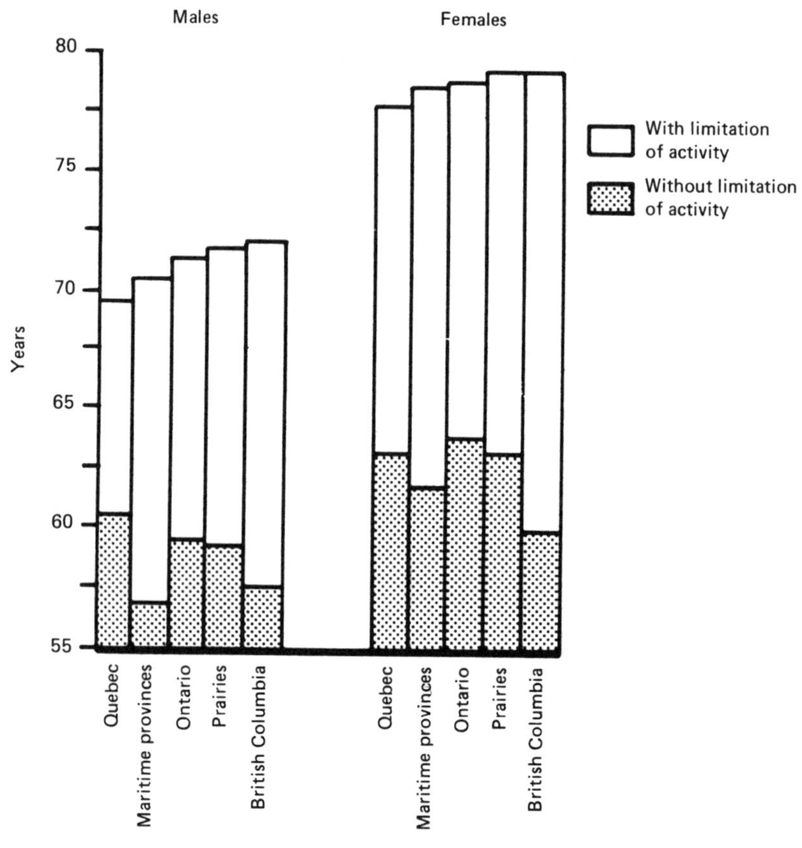

Source: **Wilkins, R. & Adams, O.B.** *(9).*

Table 3. Life expectancy at birth, by sex, Canada, 1951 and 1978

	Males			Females		
	1951	1978	Change in the period 1951–1978	1951	1978	Change in the period 1951–1978
Total life expectancy	66.3	70.8	+ 4.5	70.8	78.3	+ 7.5
Life expectancy with limitation of activity[a]	6.6	9.7	+ 3.2	6.1	12.2	+ 6.1
Life expectancy free from disability	59.8	61.1	+ 1.3	64.7	66.1	+ 1.4

[a] Permanent only.

Source: **Wilkins, R. & Adams, O.B.** *(9).*

The impact of various pathological problems on life expectancy free from disability

The impact of a given cause is measured by the sum of two components: the potential gain in life expectancy that would be obtained by removing deaths due to that cause, and limitations of activity (institutional, permanent or temporary) caused by it. Of course, this calculation requires identical classification of the causes of mortality and limitation of activity.

The calculations of Dillard *(8)* make it possible to rank the main disease categories in terms of their repercussions on life expectancy free from disability in Quebec (Fig. 3 and 4).

The position of cardiovascular diseases as a top priority for life expectancy free from disability is strengthened by the fact that these diseases are also major causes of disability; however, musculoskeletal disorders and impairments are also a high priority. They occupy second position in women and fourth position in men, relegating tumours to third place. In men, accidents and injuries are the second most important cause of disability.

By this method, the consequences of each field of pathology can be ranked in terms of mortality and disability, thereby giving a markedly different view of priorities from that obtained from mortality alone.

Prospects for Development of Indicators in Quebec

As a result of the work described above, planners in Quebec now have an assessment of the health status of the population in 1980, taking into account not only the duration and quality of life but also a ranking of the various health problems according to these criteria. This has been the foundation for continuing work on measuring health status.

Development of mental health indicators

All public health planning departments have to take account of mental health problems. However, few satisfactory instruments have yet been developed to tackle this problem in large populations. Quantifying mental diseases does not necessarily require a totally different approach from that used for physical diseases, since the two are often interlinked. General indicators such as limitation of activity may be applied to certain consequences of mental disorder, but they are probably inadequate. The Quebec Ministry of Social Affairs is therefore now developing suitable indicators *(10)*.

Introduction of new dimensions of disability

Limitation of activity continues to be the basis on which disability is measured. Although this is a sensitive indicator, it must be advantageous to take account of other dimensions of functional capacity. Two further dimensions have been selected, namely limitation of mobility and deterioration of physical independence; these have been proposed by WHO for measuring the consequences of diseases. These concepts will be introduced in future health surveys carried out in Canada.

Fig. 3. Potential gains in life expectancy free from disability (at birth) that would be obtained by eliminating certain disorders in women, Quebec, 1980

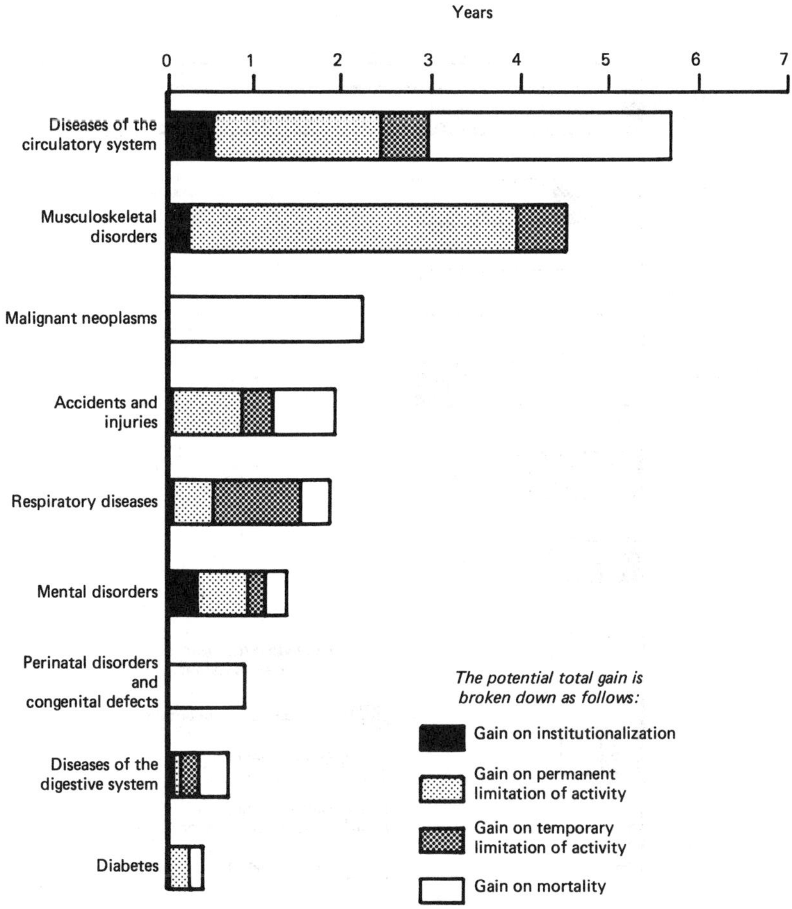

Source: **Dillard, S.** *(8).*

Fig. 4. Potential gains in life expectancy free from disability (at birth) that would be obtained by eliminating certain disorders in men, Quebec, 1980

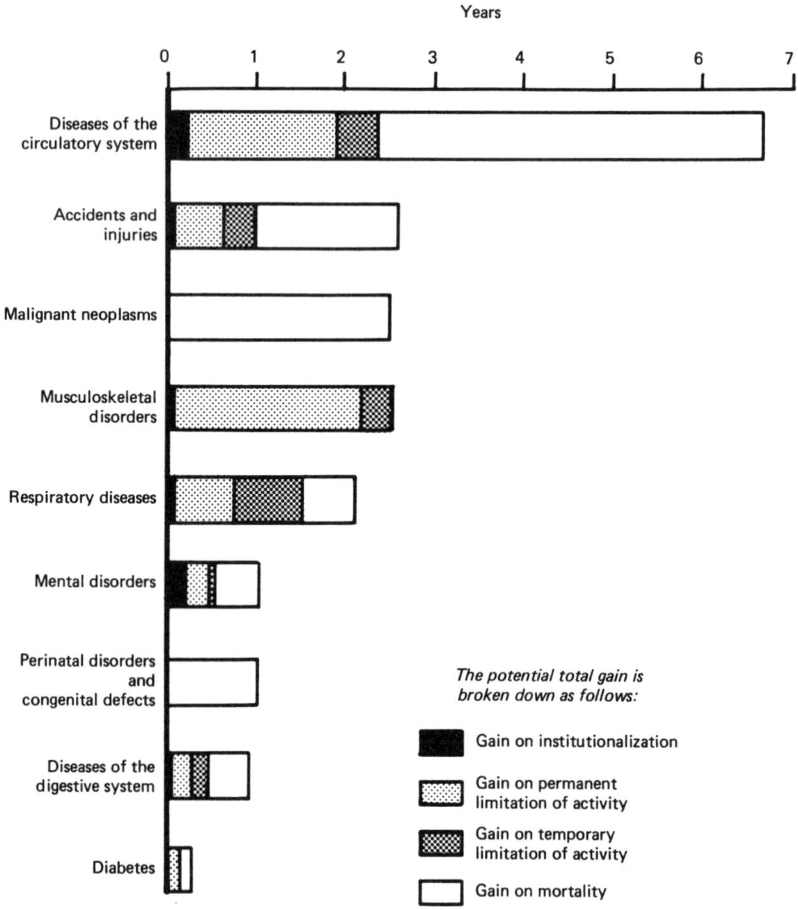

Source: **Dillard, S.** *(8).*

Towards the concept of social disadvantage by taking account of environmental conditions

Any health action, whether individual (medical) or collective (health policy), has always been aimed at removing or reducing the social disadvantage (or handicap) that results from a state of disease. Statistics must therefore be developed to show not only functional capacity but also the concept of disadvantage; the latter is directly linked to the collective recognition of a need in the population. Determining a degree of social disadvantage involves making a judgement on the extent to which the behaviour patterns considered above are disturbed. This judgement, in turn, depends on the state of the individual and the values attributed by the social group to the various states of health.

This is an extremely difficult undertaking, except for the most serious states where survival is at stake. In these cases, the social handicap may be seen as the result both of a certain level of functional performance and of the environmental conditions that may aggravate or compensate for a certain degree of limitation of activity. A third development project in this field would consist in developing suitable indicators for taking account of environmental conditions *(11)*.

Development of economic indicators

Planning objectives cannot be redefined unless economic aspects are also taken into consideration. The development of relevant indicators that can be applied to these new criteria of health status is also an important objective which is being pursued by planners in Quebec, in particular those working at the Conseil des affaires sociales et de la famille *(12)*.

Conclusion

The development of new health indicators is justified by the political will to adopt a new health strategy. Planning objectives must be redefined in the light of new criteria; the mere reduction of mortality is no longer an adequate planning objective. The optimism commonly felt after consideration of mortality statistics alone is sharply moderated when one turns to those concerning limitation of activity. The rise in life expectancy in the United States between 1966 and 1976 would appear to have been accompanied by a notable increase in the number of years lived with limitation of activity *(13)*, while in the same period, the proportion of GNP spent on health increased from 5.3% to 9% *(14)*. Under these circumstances, health action must be reconsidered. Quebec's initiative in developing new health indicators represents the first step towards new strategies for health promotion *(15)*.

References

1. **Colvez, A.** *Quatre documents sur l'introduction de nouveaux indicateurs de santé pour la planification.* Québec, Service des etudes épidémiologiques, Ministère des affaires sociales, 1979 (unpublished report).

2. **Dubos, R.** *L'homme et l'adaptation au milieu.* Paris, Payot, 1973.
3. *International classification of impairments, disabilities and handicaps.* Geneva, World Health Organization, 1980.
4. **Sullivan, D.F.** A single index of mortality and morbidity. *HSMHA health reports,* **86**: 347–354 (1971).
5. **Colvez, A. & Blanchet, M.** Potential gains in life expectancy free of disability: a tool for health planning. *International journal of epidemiology,* **12**(2): 224–229 (1983).
6. *Evaluation des bénéficiaires en centres d'accueil d'hébergement et en centres hospitaliers de soins prolongés.* Québec, Service de l'évaluation des programmes de santé, Ministère des affaires sociales, 1982.
7. **Statistics Canada and Ministry of Health and Social Welfare.** *Canadians' health: report of the Canada Health Survey.* Ottawa, Ministry of Supplies and Services, 1981.
8. **Dillard, S.** *Durée ou qualité de la vie.* Québec, Editeur officiel du Québec, Direction générale des publications gouvernmentales du ministère des communications, 1983 (report of the Conseil des affaires sociales et de la famille).
9. **Wilkins, R. & Adams, O.B.** *Healthfulness of life: a unified view of mortality, institutionalization and non-institutionalized disability in Canada.* Research on public policy, 1982.
10. **Kovess, V. et al.** *Les indicateurs de santé mentale.* Québec, Unité de recherche psychosociale, Centre hospitalier Douglas, 1982 (unpublished report prepared under contract for the Ministère des affaires sociales).
11. **Pampalon, R.** *Environnement et santé. Eléments d'une problématique québecoise.* Québec, Ministère des affaires sociales, 1980.
12. **Camirand, F.** *Les coûts de la maladie au Québec en 1980/1981.* Québec, Conseil des affaires sociales et de la famille, 1983 (unpublished report).
13. **Colvez A. & Blanchet, M.** Disability trends in the United States population 1966–1976. Analysis of reported causes. *American journal of public health,* **71**(5): 464–471 (1981).
14. **National Center for Health Services Research.** *Health United States 1980.* Washington, US Department of Health and Human Services, 1980.
15. **Blanchet, M. et al.** La santé des québecois. Priorité d'hier et d'aujourd'hui. *Carrefour des affaires sociales,* **5**: 19–24 (1983).

11.9 Control of meningococcal infection by selective vaccination linked to a surveillance system[a] — *B.M. Greenwood & S.S. Wali*

The following is a report on a study demonstrating the effectiveness of a strategy of selective vaccination on the control of meningococcal infection. The contribution illustrates many of the points raised in the discussion of vaccination in Chapter 8.1 on personal protection. Rutstein (Chapter 7.6) has described a set of untoward "sentinel events", the occurrence of which constitutes a sign that health programmes are not preventing disease or disability. The vaccination strategy suggested here can be regarded as a widening of the concept of sentinel events to health protection measures such as vaccination programmes, and not only to disease occurrence and notification.

There have been major epidemics of meningococcal disease in the savannah region of sub-Saharan Africa every 5–10 years throughout this century *(1)*. These epidemics have affected hundreds of thousands of people, many of whom have died. Most of the epidemics have been caused by group A meningococci, but recently there have been outbreaks of group C meningococcal disease in Nigeria, Niger and Upper Volta. Effective group A and group C meningococcal polysaccharide vaccines provide a means of controlling these devastating epidemics. However, it is still not certain how meningococcal vaccines should be used in the African meningitis belt *(2)*. If protection conferred by vaccination is only short-lasting, mass vaccination betweeen epidemics would be of little value. Vaccination of those with an enhanced risk of contracting the infection is an alternative, and much more economical, approach. Household contacts of patients with meningococcal disease (subjects at high risk of contracting the infection) can be protected by vaccination *(3)*. This approach has been developed to see whether an outbreak of meningococcal disease could be controlled by selective vaccination of affected villages.

[a] Meningococcal polysaccharide vaccines are now much cheaper than they were at the time that this study was done, so that the financial savings of selective vaccination as opposed to mass campaigns are less. The authors would now recommend vaccination of all members of a population, such as the one described here, who are at risk. Nevertheless, there remains the need for an effective surveillance system to ensure that large vaccination campaigns are not started too late.

Materials and Methods

Epidemic

During the 1979 dry season the Zaria area of northern Nigeria was affected by an epidemic of group A meningococcal disease for the third consecutive year. It was soon apparent that most cases were in a restricted area north of the town and a study population was therefore defined in that region. The population of this area (estimated from the number of villages and their approximate size) was between 100 000 and 150 000. During the epidemic in February – April 1979, 208 of the 360 cases of meningococcal disease (58%) admitted to Ahmadu Bello University Teaching Hospital, Zaria, came from this area.

Vaccination study

Owing to the limited amount of vaccine available, immunization was restricted to villages in which there had been two cases of meningococcal disease, since a more widespread outbreak was likely in such villages. These villages were identified by interviewing all patients with meningitis admitted to Ahmadu Bello University teaching hospital throughout the epidemic, or their relatives. Villages with two cases were allocated by random numbers to vaccination or control groups. Vaccination was performed within a week of presentation at the hospital of a second case from the same village (mean, 3 days). Vaccination was offered to all members of the village over the age of one year. Questioning of village elders at the end of each vaccination session suggested that at least 80% of the population in each village accepted.

Cards were issued in all vaccinated and control villages to ensure that any member of the village presenting at hospital with suspected meningitis was referred to the study team. Study villages were visited regularly throughout the epidemic. In addition, a record was kept of the home village of all patients with suspected meningococcal disease admitted to hospital in Zaria or admitted to a rural treatment centre which had been set up on the edge of the study area towards the end of the epidemic. Thus, most cases of meningococcal disease in the study area were identified.

Results

There were cases of meningococcal disease in 23 of the 44 villages in the study area and in 3 towns on its margin. Affected and unaffected villages were intermingled. In 20 of the 23 affected villages there was more than one case of meningococcal disease. Fig. 1 shows the number of cases recorded throughout the epidemic in 14 villages in which vaccination was not performed.

About 8600 members of 9 villages in which there had been 2 cases of meningococcal disease were vaccinated. The estimated population of these villages was 10 600, the size of individual villages ranging from 600 to 2300. Of the 10 cases of meningococcal disease identified in these 9 villages after vaccination, only 2 were in vaccinated people. In contrast, during the same period there were 38 cases of meningococcal disease in 7 control villages with an estimated population of 11 000 ($P = 0.001$) (Fig. 2). All patients in vaccinated and control villages had group A meningococcal disease.

Fig. 1. Incidence of meningococcal disease in 14 non-vaccinated villages during a 3-month epidemic (populations ranged from 600 to 4000 with a mean of 1300)

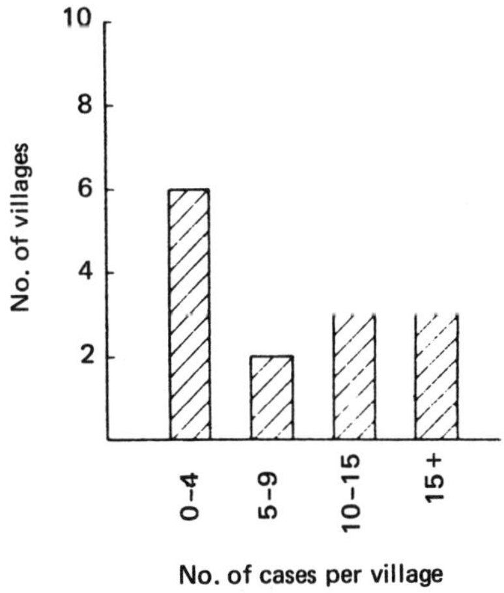

Fig. 2. Effect of vaccination on the incidence of meningococcal disease in villages where two cases of infection had been recorded

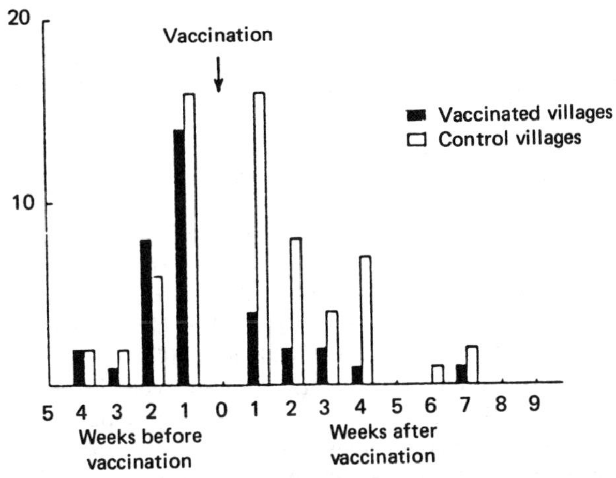

Note. Only two of the ten cases recorded in vaccinated villages had been immunized.

Discussion

Within the African meningitis belt, once a case of meningococcal disease has occurred in a village with a population of about 1000 or more, further cases of meningococcal disease are very likely. There was more than one case in all but 3 of 23 affected villages, and in 8 of 14 non-vaccinated villages there were 5 or more cases.

In view of the limited supply of vaccine available, vaccination was restricted to villages in which two cases of meningococcal disease had been identified. Analysis of the data in Fig. 2 indicates that this policy was too restrictive and resulted in vaccination being given at least one week too late. Since, during an epidemic, a single case of meningococcal disease in an average-size village will almost certainly be followed by more cases, the authors would now empirically recommend that, in villages with a population of 500 or more, vaccination should be performed as soon as possible after the first case of meningococcal disease has been identified. Defining criteria for selected vaccination of large villages and towns is more difficult. If a figure of one case per 5000 population per week had been applied to the three towns on the edge of the study area, vaccination would have been undertaken during the first two weeks of the epidemic and might have prevented the 86 cases of meningococcal disease which subsequently occurred in two of these three towns.

The spread of meningococcal disease in affected villages was rapidly controlled by vaccination. Of ten cases of meningococcal disease recorded in villages where vaccination had been performed, only two had been vaccinated, and in both these patients symptoms began on the day of vaccination (see Table 1). Five of the other eight patients came from households in which most of the members had been vaccinated.

Because only a limited amount of vaccine was available to the study team, the team's intervention had only a small effect on the overall outcome of the epidemic. However, the authors believe that with meningococcal polysaccharide vaccines selective vaccination is cost-effective. In their study, vaccination prevented about one case of meningococcal disease per 300 doses of vaccine per year. This figure contrasts with that of about one case per 5000 doses of vaccine per year obtained by pooling the data of the four controlled trials previously undertaken in Africa which involved nonselective vaccination *(4–7)*. On the basis of the study data, the 1979 epidemic of meningococcal disease in the Zaria district (which has a population of at least one million) could probably have been controlled by selective vaccination with between 100 000 and 200 000 doses of vaccine.

Within the African meningitis belt, meningococcal disease is most common in those aged 5–15 years *(1)*. Thus, in affected populations, vaccination of children in this age group only would probably considerably reduce the incidence of meningococcal disease and save a great deal of vaccine. This approach has been used successfully in Rwanda, where an outbreak of group A meningococcal disease was controlled by vaccination of those aged 2–20 years *(8)*. A policy of age-restricted vaccination would not, however, be popular with those threatened by a serious epidemic. Because of the poor

Table 1. Features of ten cases of meningococcal disease recorded in villages where vaccination had been performed

Patient	Age (years)	Sex	Vaccinated (V) or not vaccinated (NV)	Comments
1	8	F	V	Symptoms started on day of vaccination
2	10	M	V	Symptoms started on day of vaccination
3	<1	M	NV	Not vaccinated because aged 8 months — 4 out of 5 members of household vaccinated
4	4	M	NV	Away on the day the village was vaccinated — 6 out of 8 members of household vaccinated
5	2	M	NV	Away on the day the village was vaccinated — 5 out of 9 members of household vaccinated
6	6	M	NV	Away on the day the village was vaccinated — 5 out of 9 members of household vaccinated; sibling of patient 5
7	15	M	NV	Away on the day the village was vaccinated — 7 out of 10 members of household vaccinated
8	4	M	NV	From outlying non-vaccinated hamlet
9	8	F	NV	From outlying non-vaccinated hamlet
10	15	F	NV	No family details available

response of young infants to meningococcal polysaccharide vaccines, the study team restricted vaccination to those over the age of one year. There was much local criticism after meningococcal meningitis developed in an eight-month-old infant who had been refused vaccination.

A selective vaccination scheme can only be effective when there is a good surveillance system for detecting cases of meningococcal disease and when vaccine is available as soon as it is required. In the Zaria area of northern Nigeria, where there is an adequate number of hospitals and dispensaries, outbreaks of meningococcal disease are usually detected rapidly. In other, more sparsely populated areas of the Sahel a mobile surveillance system may be needed *(9)*. Simple assays for bacterial antigens can be of considerable value in establishing the cause of an outbreak of meningitis in areas where conventional bacteriology is not possible. Once the decision to vaccinate a village has been made, vaccination must be performed as soon as possible. Adequate supplies of vaccine must therefore be available locally; there is rarely time for it to be ordered from the manufacturers. At first, storage of meningococcal vaccines in the tropics was difficult, since early preparations were very heat-labile. Heat-stable preparations, based on lactose rather than mannitol *(10)*, are now available and these can be safely stored for several years in the tropics near to where they are likely to be needed.

Acknowledgement

This chapter is based on material drawn from a paper originally published in the *Lancet* (**Greenwood, B.M. & Wali, S.S.** Control of meningococcal infection in the African meningitis belt by selective vaccination. *Lancet,* **1**: 729–732 (1980)). The authors are grateful to the publishers for permission to use this material.

References

1. **Lapeyssonnie, L.** La méningite cérébrospinale en Afrique. *Bulletin of the World Health Organization,* Suppl. 28: 3–114 (1963).
2. Who should be given meningococcal vaccine? (Editorial). *Lancet,* **2**: 1185–1186 (1978).
3. **Greenwood, B.M. et al.** Prevention of secondary cases of meningococcal disease in household contacts by vaccination. *British medical journal,* **1**: 1317–1319 (1978).
4. **Ettori, D. et al.** Le vaccin antiméningococcique du type A : premiers essais contrôlés en Afrique de l' Ouest. *Médicine tropicale,* **37**: 225–230 (1977).
5. **Wahdan, M.H. et al.** A controlled field trial of a serogroup A meningococcal polysaccharide vaccine. *Bulletin of the World Health Organization,* **48**: 667–673 (1973).
6. **Wahdan, M.H. et al.** A second controlled field trial of a serogroup A meningococcal polysaccharide vaccine in Alexandria. *Bulletin of the World Health Organization,* **55**: 645–651 (1977).
7. **Erwa, H.H. et al.** A serogroup A meningococcal polysaccharide vaccine. Studies in the Sudan to combat cerebrospinal meningitis caused by *Neisseria meningitidis* group A. *Bulletin of the World Health Organization,* **49**: 301–305 (1973).
8. **Bosman, E.** Field trials with Mencevax in an epidemic situation in Rwanda. *In:* André, F.E., ed. *New developments in vaccines.* Rixensart, Smith-Kline RIT, 1979, pp. 113–130.
9. **Sanborn, W.R. et al.** *A system for epidemic meningitis control in West Africa.* Paper presented at the WHO Third International Conference on Immunity and Immunization in Cerebrospinal Meningitis, Marburg, October 1979.
10. **Tiesjema, R.H. et al.** Enhanced stability of meningococcal polysaccharide vaccines by using lactose as a menstruum for lyophilization. *Bulletin of the World Health Organization,* **55**: 43–48 (1977).

11.10 Sentinel surveillance of health events: application to the Expanded Programme on Immunization in India — *R.N. Basu & J. Sokhey*

Rutstein (Chapter 7.6) initially described and developed sets of untoward "sentinel events", the occurrence of which constitutes a sign that health programmes are not preventing disease or disability. After considering some of the possible strategies for collecting evaluative information on epidemiology, Basu & Sokhey discuss here how this concept of sentinel events could be expanded to apply to health-enhancing measures such as immunization programmes, and not only to disease occurrence and notification. The chapter discusses several possible data collection systems, describes how a model sentinel surveillance system could be established, and illustrates how this might be used by considering examples based on a single institution's records.

A major goal of health for all by the year 2000 is the reduction of morbidity and mortality by meeting the minimum health needs of people at their doorstep. Many programmes have been launched for the training of primary health care workers, the control of communicable diseases, the extension of maternal and child health services (including the immunization programme), the provision of safe drinking-water, and the treatment of minor ailments in the community. All these services must be supported by a regular and reliable flow of information, in order to identify problems and to monitor and evaluate programmes. While the need for reliable information is clearly understood, the collection, compilation and analysis of the necessary data pose enormous problems, especially in large developing countries with diverse geographical and socioeconomic characteristics and a limited health infrastructure.

Methods commonly used in the health information system include routine reporting of cases and deaths recorded at treatment centres, active surveillance, the investigation of outbreaks, special studies, sample surveys and the use of sentinel centres. Each has its advantages and limitations and can be used either separately or in combination. All the methods have been applied with varying results in the Expanded Programme on Immunization (EPI) in India and the present discussion is based on this experience.

Some Traditional Methods of Data Collection

Routine reporting

The routine reporting of cases and deaths or other health events is the most widely practised way of collecting information. The major disadvantage of the system lies in the difficulty of ensuring the quality or regularity of the reports. The information asked for is kept to the bare minimum, as most of the peripheral units have limited facilities for recording and reporting. Diagnostic criteria may vary, since a large number of health centres are involved. Most centres are heavily burdened with the treatment of the daily influx of patients and have little time for or interest in submitting reports. Experience has shown that even those centres that do send in reports are not always regular. Moreover, subjects with mild or moderately severe forms of disease who do not seek treatment at the centre are not recorded under the system. Sample surveys conducted in India confirm a gross underreporting of cases *(1,2)*.

The organization of the EPI at the national level in 1978 was justified by the large number of cases of vaccine-preventable diseases recorded by the routine reporting system. The data compiled at the Central Bureau of Health Intelligence of the Directorate-General of Health Services were based mainly on monthly returns from some of the health institutions in the country. On average, 45 000 cases of tetanus were reported to the Central Bureau of Health Intelligence annually over the last decade (with extremes of 27 000 and 76 000), to take one example. There were, however, no reliable data on incidence or other relevant epidemiological information for planning and monitoring the services. Neonatal tetanus, for example, was not recorded separately from other cases of tetanus. Moreover, most cases of neonatal tetanus, especially in the rural areas, result in death before the patient can be taken to a health centre for medical care and may therefore not be officially recorded as such.

Similarly, very little information was available regarding poliomyelitis. The recorded data led one to believe that poliomyelitis was indeed an urban problem. There was practically no information on age-specific incidence rates. The data could not be analysed to show seasonal patterns of the disease because the reports were not received regularly from month to month.

Surveys

Sample surveys were organized to collect reliable baseline epidemiological information; neonatal tetaus and poliomyelitis were taken up initially for the following reasons.

- Both diseases were considered to be far more serious public health problems than indicated by the routine reporting system.
- Effective and safe vaccines were available for their control.
- It was possible to organize surveys without the support of sophisticated laboratory methods.

These surveys yielded extremely useful information. From the mortality rates for neonatal tetanus in 12 states, it was estimated that between 91 000 and 116 000 neonatal deaths due to tetanus occurred annually in the areas covered by the surveys. Up to 67 deaths per 1000 live births could be attributed to neonatal tetanus in one state, in which 72% of neonatal deaths were caused by tetanus *(3)*. By extrapolation, it would appear that each year over 300 000 children die from tetanus within the first month of life in the country, nearly two thirds of them in one state alone in northern India.

Poliomyelitis, far from being an urban problem, is widespread in the rural areas. Less than one case in ten is recorded under the routine reporting system *(4,5)*. Since the majority of the children develop the disease before their second birthday, efforts have been concentrated on vaccination coverage of infants as early as possible. Resources have also been mobilized to extend the services to the rural areas.

Surveys are, however, difficult to conduct, relatively expensive, and call for technical qualifications and organizational abilities. The sample size, questionnaires and forms must be well designed to avoid bias and misinterpretation of data. Some diseases require laboratory back-up for accurate diagnosis; this makes surveys even more expensive and difficult.

Investigation of outbreaks

This provides useful information, but is dependent mainly on the communication system for reporting the outbreaks in time, and on adequate provision for their investigation at short notice. The attack rate and the case fatality rate during an epidemic differ from the rates for endemic disease.

Active surveillance

This has as its main purpose the detection of changes in trend or distribution in order to initiate investigative or control measures, and is useful in that it can involve the active participation of health personnel as well as that of the community, keeping both groups alert about priority problems and control measures undertaken. The degree of reporting is more complete than for any other method, especially for the clinically distinct and easily recognizable diseases. Active surveillance played a very important role in the eradication of smallpox, the global eradication of which was possible only because of the highly efficient surveillance system.

A search for fever cases suspected of being due to malaria is carried out in the country so that blood slides can be taken and presumptive treatment started. Active surveillance for suspected poliomyelitis (cases of paralysis following fever in children) is being introduced in selected areas where poliomyelitis vaccination coverage is high. The reported number of lame children is expected to be small enough for a medical officer to examine each child individually.

Sentinel Centres

Definition

A sentinel information system can be developed to obtain more reliable and extensive disease incidence data than would be available through the routine information system. Sentinel information services have been used for several years in various countries, including Belgium, the Netherlands and the United

Kingdom, to obtain information on the occurrence of a limited set of diseases. A sentinel service can be defined as one which, on a voluntary basis, records and forwards systematic information on a limited number of health problems or events in a standardized form; this reporting is usually undertaken on a monthly or, preferably, a weekly basis *(6)*. As regards the EPI, the following criteria are suggested.

> A sentinel centre for a particular disease is specially selected for its representativeness, willingness and capability to report regularly, completely and accurately on diseases covered by the EPI and on the related indicators. These centres can collect and report additional data on the morbidity and mortality in the population served by these institutions.

Any hospital, health centre, laboratory, or rehabilitation centre which attends to a large number of cases can be considered a sentinel centre. Sentinel centres have several advantages and the data supplied by them can complement information gathered from other sources. The quality of the information is usually dependable and the regularity of the reports can be maintained. Since the centres are already in existence, very little additional input is required. Many of the centres, such as teaching hospitals and national institutes, may already be collecting the information desired; others may be motivated to do so if basic facilities are made available. The additional available data help to identify specific population groups at risk and facilitate monitoring of the services provided.

Organization

The organization of sentinel centres involves at least three levels of functioning: the sentinel centre itself, the local health office, and a central cell. The major responsibilities of each are broadly as follows.

Sentinel centre	to collect and forward information
Local health office	to undertake immediate action on reports when and where necessary (elementary analysis)
Central cell	to monitor and analyse reports in depth
	to coordinate the work of different centres
	to provide periodical feedback and encouragement/control for the sentinel centres and local health offices
	to determine data needed
	to devise forms
	to identify sentinel centres
	to use data for policy decisions and future plans

Selection of sentinel centres

When selecting a sentinel centre, the following should be considered

- What is the information needed? In the case of the EPI, this is usually the number of cases of a specific disease or specific diseases occurring (incidence), together with one or more patient characteristics (e.g. age, sex, race, occupation, locality) and information on changes in vaccination coverage.

- What is this information needed for? What is the status of the control programme in the area and how fruitfully would the information be applied in the field? The information collected must be limited to what is needed for planning and monitoring the programme. Questions of academic interest must not be included. The minimum information for an immunization programme is the number of cases by:

  — geographical area or administrative unit, age at onset of disease, and vaccination status;

  — *desirable:* address of patient and agency of vaccination in cases where the disease developed after the full course of the vaccine; type of disease (e.g. for tuberculosis);

  — *optional* (in areas where the programme is well developed and where numbers of patients are expected to be small): address of all patients.

- Can the centre supply the information required? This usually implies:

  — large attendance of patients with the particular disease;

  — diagnosis reasonably accurate;

  — good recording and reporting facilities available;

  — willingness to submit regular reports.

In some cases, even schools can act as sentinels, e.g. for screening lameness, vision, or the health status of children starting school. Understandably, data obtained through schools reflect the quality of the services provided some years earlier.

- Can the patients coming to the centre be considered representative of the area? This involves such subquestions as accessibility, both physical (Is the centre too remote and not easily accessible? What is the percentage of the rural population using the services if the clinic is situated in an urban area?) and cultural (Is the centre too expensive or specialized, so that certain groups of people are prevented from attending the clinic?), and catchment population (Are people from neighbouring administrative units also using the treatment facilities and can they be identified from the records?).

- Do the staff understand the importance of the work and are they motivated to send the reports regularly?

- Could the same information be obtained from other centres in the area?

- What are the possiblities of analysing the data?

- How well can health centres and central units provide operational answers to the situations uncovered by the sentinel centre? This is critically important.

In summary, the type of information collected would be determined by three factors:

(*a*) the needs of the programme,

(*b*) the ability of the centres to provide the information, and

(*c*) the facilities available for compilation, analysis and response.

Response

Use of data

The data collected by the sentinel centres can be effectively used both for immediate implementation in the field and for future plans and policy decisions.

1. The report of a larger number of cases than in the corresponding period of the previous year(s) serves as an early warning of a potential epidemic. An unusual increase in the number of cases calls for an immediate investigation and the initiation of preventive measures by the local health officer.

2. The seasonal pattern of the childhood diseases is clearly established from reports of the sentinel centres and plans for preventive programmes must be made with this in mind.

3. The sentinel centres serve as indicators of the impact of the services provided. At the same time, they can be efficient watch-dogs of the quality of services, for example, as to whether the children are getting the diseases after completing the recommended vaccination course.

4. Data provided by sentinel centres can be used to check on the quality of routinely reported data in areas not covered by such centres.

5. An indication of the changing patterns of disease may be obtained from the data, and plans can be modified accordingly. The information may indicate the shifting of a disease to higher age groups or the clustering of cases in selected localities.

6. In areas where vaccination coverage is high and no EPI disease has been reported for some time, sentinel centres provide an early warning if new cases appear.

As an indirect advantage, it often happens that institutions which were clinically oriented become involved in community medicine because of close and regular liaison with the health officers responsible for the disease control programmes.

Limitations

Sentinel centres can at best show the trend of disease incidence in the area. The information cannot always be generalized to give accurate incidence rates because the degree of underreporting is usually not known and the geographical/administrative areas of residence at the onset of disease are often not clearly defined. Furthermore, since attendance at a clinic may fluctuate, depending on various factors, an absolute rise in the number of cases need not be taken as an indication that the situation is worsening or that the programme has proved ineffective. As the facilities for diagnosis and treatment improve, and knowledge about health services spreads, the number of recorded cases often increases, even without an increase in true incidence. If most of the centres are located in cities and towns and not easily accessible to the rural population, the data may be slanted, giving an impression that the problem is predominantly urban.

A general problem of sentinel centres is how to maintain a high level of interest and reporting. Two approaches have been used with regard to sentinel physicians in disease surveillance, singly or in combination:

(*a*) positive motivation of reporters through appropriate feedback or through financial reward;

(*b*) regular modifications in emphasis over time, the reporting being limited to a small number of disease groups, parts of which are modified at intervals.

The second approach is unlikely to be easily applicable in EPI activities, which have to be undertaken on a long-term basis. Most areas where these activities are being undertaken could not bear the burden of rewarding sentinel centres financially, even if this procedure were considered acceptable in principle. It is therefore necessary to emphasize the need for regular feedback to the reporting centre, in order that the use to which information is being put is properly appreciated. It is just as important that the number of topics to be covered should be kept to the essential minimum so as to avoid straining local resources and to ensure consistent quality of reporting.

Findings

The data collected from some of the sentinel centres and analysed at the national level have influenced the formulation of strategies for the immunization delivery system in India. Some findings are given below as examples.

Data from the Institute of Child Health, Madras, showed that 91% of the children examined in 1980 who were affected by poliomyelitis were below 3 years of age. This has been confirmed by reports from other centres. The poliomyelitis vaccination programme in India is now specifically aimed at children aged under 2 years.

Information on the vaccination status of patients is necessary for monitoring the services. In 1981, out of 2140 children admitted with poliomyelitis to one Calcutta clinic, 24 had a history of 3 doses of oral polio vaccine. A high failure rate, while not necessarily indicative of poor vaccine efficacy, would call for an investigation of the conditions of storage and transportation of the vaccines, and also of methods of administration. In places with low vaccination coverage, the number of children with a history of completed vaccination would also understandably be low. Vaccination coverage assessment surveys carried out in urban slums in Calcutta in 1981 showed that 34.8% of children aged 12–23 months had received 3 doses of oral polio vaccine. The coverage of children in other parts of Calcutta is expected to be higher. The number of polio cases from outside Calcutta who were included in the 2140 cases investigated in 1981 is not known.

Admissions of new polio cases to the Kalawati Saran Children's Hospital, Delhi, have shown a peak incidence of the disease in the month of August. A similar rise in the number of cases between July and September has been noted in other parts of the country.

Conclusions

Sentinel centres have many advantages and could be a major source of information not only for the assessment of health problems, but also for the monitoring of health services. The quality of the information provided by sentinel services is dependable, unlike that of the routine reporting system. Why? Surveys give useful data, but these are valid only for the period and the area in which the surveys were conducted. In addition, surveys are expensive to organize. Sentinel centres are a continuous source of epidemiological information and their format and scope of reporting can be adapted to reflect the changing patterns of diseases, depending on environmental and social factors and on the control programmes initiated.

Since a major thrust of primary health care is in the rural and urban slum areas, sentinel centres must be chosen with care so that the status of the health programmes in these areas can be reflected. Centres in rural areas or those catering for the rural population should be encouraged to participate.

It is essential that information from the sentinel centres should flow in two directions: to the local health officer in charge of the programme for action in the field and to the state or central officer, so that the information can be used in policy matters and adequate feedback from these authorities to the sentinel centres can be organized. This close liaison between sentinel centres and the agencies responsible for the disease control programmes is an indispensable feature of good reporting.

The sentinel information system can be developed even in countries with a relatively poor health infrastructure. During the initial phase of the programme, when information may be required for preparing rational plans, data from the past few years could be collected and a retrospective study made of patterns of morbidity and mortality. Such information is doubtless available at many centres in each country, but it has to be collected, collated and analysed at a central place in order to achieve more meaningful use of the data. Such centres could continue at regular (usually monthly) intervals to provide information required for the monitoring and evaluation of programmes.

References

1. **Basu, R.N. & Sokhey, J.** A baseline study on neonatal tetanus in India. *Pakistan paediatric journal,* **6**: 184–196 (1982).
2. **Basu, R.N. & Sokhey, J.** *Methodology of disease surveys and their use in supplementing surveillance systems:* report on the National Programme Managers Consultative Meeting, Bangkok. New Delhi, WHO Regional Office for South-East Asia, 1983 (document EPI/SEAR/6.2/1983).
3. Expanded Programme on Immunization. Prevention of neonatal tetanus. *Weekly epidemiological record,* **57**: 137–142 (1982).
4. **Basu, R.N.** Magnitude of problem of poliomyelitis in India. *Indian pediatrics,* **18**: 507–511 (1981).
5. **Prabakar, N. et al.** The epidemiology and prevention of poliomyelitis in a rural community in South India. *Indian pediatrics,* **18**: 527–537 (1981).
6. **Thiers, G. & Stroobant, A.** Enregistrement de données de morbidité par un réseau de médecins généralistes «vigies». *Archives belges de médecine sociale,* **42**(1–2): 38–49 (1984).

11.11 Promotion and measurement of physical fitness in Switzerland — *B. Marti, T. Abelin, H. Howald & B. Bissegger*

Lange Andersen & Rutenfranz discussed the measurement of physical functioning in Chapter 7.2. This chapter illustrates some of the possible measurements in this field and their application to measuring levels of physical fitness in the Swiss population. Simple measures of participation in various forms of physical exercise promotion activities are also considered.

In Switzerland, as in many other countries, efforts are being made to improve the fitness of the population by promoting physical exercise. The purpose of this chapter is to show how progress in this respect is being monitored and how the need for further efforts is being determined.

Promoting Physical Fitness

There are many reasons for promoting physical fitness in a country. These range from long-term health considerations to the need for a strong and fit army, from the desire to offer young people meaningful leisure activities to hopes of developing first-class performers for international sports competitions. In many cases, when efforts are made to promote physical activities, the reasons are not explicitly stated, but from the health point of view there is reason to ensure that the right parameters of fitness are being considered and that all age groups are being appropriately reached.

In the past 10–15 years, several initiatives have been taken to encourage the Swiss population to participate in sports activities. Some were at governmental level, while others were sponsored by private bodies. Some of the most important efforts are described below.

Legislation on compulsory physical education at vocational school level

During the period of compulsory school education (8–9 years, with regional differences), Swiss law provides for three physical activity lessons per week. In order to counteract the usual decrease in physical trainig after pupils have left school *(1)*, legislation was introduced in 1972 making sports lessons of at least one hour's duration per week compulsory for all young people in vocational training. The law formerly provided for federal financial support for the construction of sports facilities, and it still makes federal funding available for sports teachers in this context.

The purpose of the law was to ensure that each apprentice in the country would participate in at least one weekly period of sport. Evaluation of progress in this field was carried out by means of a questionnaire survey in connection with the procedures by which 19-year-old men are recruited to the army *(2,3)*.

The proportion of participants rose from 29.4% in 1977 to 36.5% in 1982. A supplementary survey conducted in 1982 indicated a large variation between regions, ranging from 0% (4 of the 26 cantons) to 100% (also 4 cantons), and from 19.4% in one linguistic region to 44.8% in another.

Fitness tracks

In May 1968, the first of a large number of standardized fitness tracks was opened in Switzerland. These tracks are sponsored by a commercial insurance company, and their construction and maintenance is usually the responsibility of the communes. They include a 2–3 km running-track in a forest, interrupted by 20 posts at which exercises have to be carried out. These are specified in written and pictorial form, and in turn emphasize muscle strength, flexibility and muscle relaxation. They are equipped with the necessary horizontal bars, balancing-poles, etc.

Between 1968 and 1983, 490 such tracks were open in the proximity of towns, or at highway rest areas. According to a survey conducted for the sponsoring company (methodological details are not available, however), 90% of adults in Switzerland seem to be aware of these tracks, and hundreds of people — often families with children — can be seen using them on sunny summer evenings. According to this survey, 45% of respondents say they use the tracks at least from time to time.

A similar concept underlies a new type of "meeting-point for joggers", established by the Swiss Sports Council near larger towns and comprising three marked runs of 3–12 km in length. Thirty-six of these points are available free of charge at present and 100 more are planned for the next 5 years.

Mass running events

In the last 15 years, jogging has become a mass phenomenon. The number of joggers in Switzerland is not known, but participation in mass running events has grown sharply. The oldest event of this type is the 17 km Murten-Fribourg run, a competition started in 1933 with 18 participants. On its fiftieth anniversary in 1983, 13 970 runners participated, and its popularity is still growing. In 1984, there were 10 other running competitions in Switzerland, with more than 3000 participants each. Special events worth mentioning are the 100 km Biel/Bienne competition with 4248 participants in 1983, and the Engadine ski marathon, with over 10 000 participants each year. These events are given wide publicity in the mass media, aimed at encouraging more persons of all ages to take up jogging and competitive running.

A community-oriented health promotion programme

From 1977 to 1980 a community intervention study concerning the major risk factors for coronary heart disease was conducted in two Swiss towns, with two other towns serving as controls. Although the explicit purpose of the project was a scientific one, it served as a model for testing the practical implementation of health promotion programmes which emphasized physical fitness. Public events in the framework of the project received wide media coverage, and in many towns efforts are now under way to establish similar programmes on an ongoing basis.

Table 1 summarizes some of the activities related to physical exercise and sports. One of the features of the programme is that it offers events that are organized, but open to everybody and not tied to membership of any organization. A good example is the popular "around the world" community running event, in which 3800 people (out of 15 000 inhabitants) participated, contributing larger or smaller distances to an overall total of more than 43 300 km.

Measurement of Fitness

Together with the promotion of physical exercise, an attempt was made to measure fitness and thus to monitor progress of the population's fitness level and to document the need for further efforts.

Self-evaluation instruments for individual use

As a tool for stimulating individual training activities, several brochures were prepared, giving training instructions and demonstrating how different dimensions of fitness can be individually tested. The biggest effort in this respect was when, in 1973, 14 000 visitors to the largest Swiss trade fair performed a test which included the following three components of fitness.

- *Flexibility* of spine and hip was measured by the distance between fingertips and shoe soles at maximum trunk bending with legs outstretched ("sit and reach" test).

- *Strength* of arm and shoulder girdle muscles was measured by the length of time that the chin could be kept at the height of a horizontal bar, while hanging on this bar with bent arms (bent-arm hang).

- *Endurance* was measured among 199 participating visitors by an ergometric test using a treadmill and (at a later date) a 12-minute run according to Cooper (see also Chapter 7.2). Performance capacity in the two tests was highly correlated ($r = 0.79$).

The results of these measurements *(5)* were used as age- and sex-specific standard values in a widely publicized three-part fitness test described in a brochure (more than 500 000 copies distributed). In order to obtain an overall fitness score, scores from the three tests are added, giving double weight to the endurance score.

Measuring endurance capacity in adult populations

Along with the community health promotion project described above, a bicycle ergometer test was performed among 952 men and 1064 women

Table 1. Physical exercise promotion activities, Aarau (Switzerland), 1978/1979

Activity	Description	Media	Number of participants
"Around the world" run	Community action, the aim being jointly to run a distance corresponding to the earth's circumference in 6 days	Newspaper advertisements, editorial text; invitation to enterprises, clubs; posters, mass mailing campaign	3800
Sports festival	Community event with 17 clubs, information booths, performances, competition	Newspaper advertisements, editorial text; monthly bulletin, mass mailing campaign, progamme booklet	700
Jogging track	Marked 5 km circuit, creation of jogging groups	Newspaper advertisements, reports, mass mailing, monthly bulletin	— in groups: 110 — other: ?
Bicycle track	Circuit with marked distances	Advertisements, posters, official opening ceremony, maps	?
Ice hockey tournament for adults	Tournament preceded by training	Invitation to enterprises, clubs; posters; sale of special sweaters	480
"Crossing the sea"	Invitation to those not away on holiday to swim a distance corresponding to the width of the Strait of Gibraltar	Mass mailing, posters, editorial text in newspaper, distribution of bags to successful entrants	— successful: 528 — unsuccessful attempt: 420

Source: Examples taken from **Autorengruppe Nationales Forschungsprogramm 1A** *(4)*.

between the ages of 16 and 80 years. The 6-minute test was done in a sitting position with constant workload at 50 pedal revolutions per minute. Submaximal workload level was chosen between 50 and 200 watts so as to obtain a steady-state heart rate of 140–160 for persons aged under 35 years and 130–150 for those above that age *(1)*. Maximum aerobic capacity (VO_2max.) was estimated according to Astrand *(6)* by extrapolation of the measured heart rate to the age-specific maximum heart rate.

Fig. 1 presents the results. It shows that, in an average population in which one half of the men and two thirds of the women report little physical exercise either during their work or in their spare time, maximum aerobic capacity decreases clearly with advancing age, the decline starting around the age of 20 years.

This decline in endurance performance in adult age is often regarded as an expected phenomenon following biological rules. However, examination of the performance capacity of well trained persons demonstrates that, under conditions of vigorous physical training, performance capacity can be maintained at maximum levels up to an age of about 35 years, and that the fitness of a well trained person even of advanced age is much higher than that of an untrained young person.

To study this question more fully, the 6800 contestants who finished the so-called "Grand-Prix of Berne", a 10-mile run, conducted for the third time in the spring of 1984, were investigated. The age range of participants was 8–75 years, with an average of 33 years. In relation to the general population, the age group 33–44 years was rather overrepresented. Those over 60 years were strongly underrepresented. Only 9% of the participants were women. The proportion of female runners was highest at ages 10–12 years (21%) and decreased with increasing age. About one third of the participants lived in the city or suburbs of Berne (about 250 000 inhabitants), one third in the Berne region (1 million inhabitants) and one third in the rest of Switzerland (5–6 million inhabitants).

Ten-mile running times were transformed into equivalent values for maximal oxygen consumption, using regression equations that had been obtained several times in the past *(6–8)*. A small comparative study of 20 athletes performing both in an ergometric test two weeks before the race and in the race itself resulted in an almost identical equation *(9)*. Fig. 2 compares the means and 90-percentile equivalent values of VO_2max. of the male participants older than 16 years in the 10-mile race (n = 5703) with the mean values obtained in a sample of the adult male population in connection with the community health project described above. It is clear from the figure that physical performance capacity is much higher among the runners than in the general population, and that even elderly trained men perform much better than untrained younger men. Performance capacity remains at about the same high level for well trained runners up to the age of 35 years, whereas there is a steady decrease beginning at the age of 20 in the general population. It thus appears that health potential, in terms of endurance capacity, can be maintained at top levels well into middle age by regular intensive physical training.

Fig. 1. Maximum aerobic capacity (VO_2max.) in relation to age

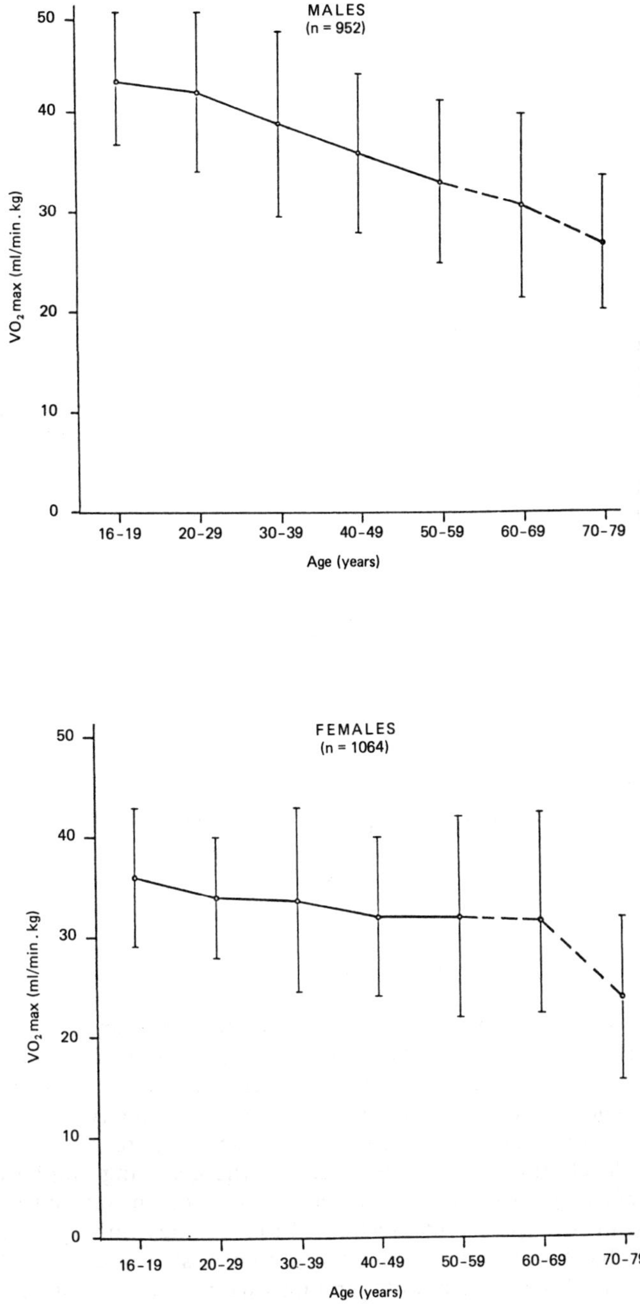

Fig. 2. Endurance performance capacity (VO_2max. equivalents) in relation to age — male participants in a 10-mile running competition and male population sample (see also Fig. 1)

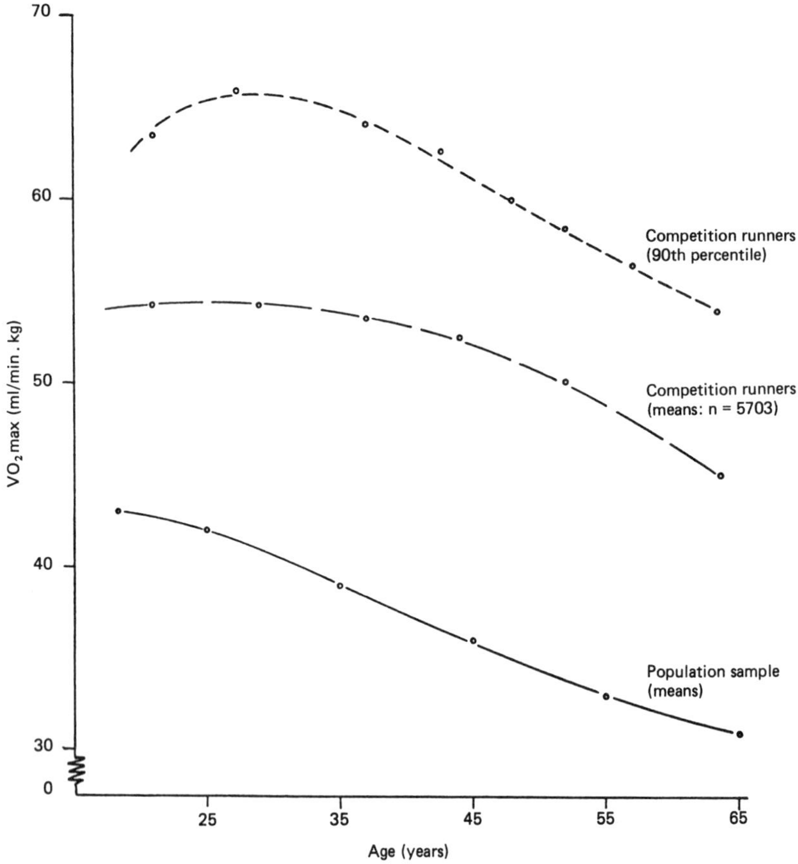

Measuring the sports performance of Swiss army conscripts

The sports test of all 19-year-old male citizens at the time of recruitment into the army is the only measurement of fitness regularly conducted in Switzerland. The sports test, which takes place yearly, is linked every 5 years with a questionnaire survey of habitual physical activity, lifestyle, etc. *(2,3)*.

The development of the test reflects the changing emphasis in the assessment of physical fitness. When the test was introduced in 1905, it included an 80 m sprint and long jump. In 1943, pole climbing and throwing a 500 g object were added, and the present test was completed by the addition, in 1974, of a 12-minute running test (see also Chapter 7.2). The test is conducted on 300 m or 400 m tracks. Up to about 30 participants start together. In 1977, a 20% sample of those tested (8917 conscripts) completed a questionnaire on lifestyles. An analysis of the results of performance in the 12-minute running test shows that endurance capacity depends on several factors, of which training intensity is the strongest.

Table 2 shows this relationship. Whereas those reporting daily training reached a mean distance of 2811 m in 12 minutes, the distance achieved by those training less than once a week was well below 2400 m.

Table 2. Performance in 12-minute running test in relation to frequency of physical training: Swiss army conscripts, 1977

Frequency of physical training	No.	%	Mean running distance in 12 minutes
Daily	299	3.4	2811 m
More than twice a week	3088	34.7	2696 m
Once a week	2295	25.7	2488 m
Once to three times a month	1124	12.6	2412 m
Less than once a month	1957	22.0	2318 m
Never	154	1.6	2238 m
Total	8917	100.0	2527 m

Source: *Statistische Quellenwerke der Schweiz,* 1980 *(2).*

Within a certain range, the type of sports activity is of less importance. Track and field, fitness training and cross-country skiing were related to higher running distances (>2650 m), whereas bowling and table tennis were related to shorter distances (<2500 m).

A very clear association could be shown with smoking habits *(10)*. Non-smokers reached a distance of 2623 m, whereas the distance decreased steadily among smokers according to the increasing amounts of cigarettes or tobacco smoked (Table 3).

A similar pattern emerges when drinking habits are compared with endurance performance. Multivariate analysis shows that training frequency remains the principal predictor of endurance performance among Swiss conscripts and that smoking is also an important factor. Alcohol consumption, on the other hand, seems to be related more to reduced motivation to perform than to performance capacity itself.

Table 3. Performance in 12-minute running test in relation to smoking habits: Swiss army conscripts, 1977

Smoking habit	No.	%	Mean running distance in 12 minutes
Non-smokers	4097	45.9	2623 m
Occasional smokers	849	9.5	2564 m
Smokers of 1–10 cigarettes/day	1030	11.6	2538 m
Smokers of 11 + cigarettes/day	2867	32.2	2365 m
No information	74	0.8	2665 m
Total	8917	100.0	2527 m

Source: Statistische Quellenwerke der Schweiz, 1980 *(2).*

In 1982, 45 977 young men (89% of the entire 19-year-old male population of the country) were tested and completed a comparable questionnaire. The remaining 11% were excused for health reasons and were not included in the analysis. The average distance reached in the 12-minute running test was 2588 m, which is 61 m more than in 1977. This improvement of 2.4% is highly significant ($P < 0.001$).

It was of interest to know what factors could have led to an increase in the endurance capacity of 19-year-old men in the space of 5 years. In Table 4 the training frequencies are compared for the two years. There was an increase among those reporting training more than once a week, but also among those reporting no sports activities at all. Overall, changes in training frequency are unlikely to explain the improvement in the running test.

On the other hand, as Tables 5 and 6 show, smoking and drinking habits changed rather remarkably during the same 5-year period. Whereas the proportion of smokers of more than 20 cigarettes per day decreased from 12.6% in 1977 to 7.0% in 1982, the proportion of non-smokers increased from 46.8% to 56.0%. Similarly, the proportion of those drinking more than 60 g of alcohol per week (as calculated from the number of glasses of wine, beer and distilled drinks reported) decreased from 38.5% in 1977 to 30.6% in 1982.

Detailed analyses are being conducted in an attempt to understand better the factors related to the improvement of endurance capacity among young men in Switzerland, but it is already clear that several elements of the health promotion campaign seem to be involved.

Conclusions

In Switzerland centralized government action in matters such as the promotion of health and physical fitness are not very popular. As a consequence,

Table 4. Frequency of physical activity among Swiss army conscripts, 1977 and 1982

	Year	
	1977	1982
Number of respondents	8917	44598[a]
	%	%
Frequency of physical activity:		
Daily	3.4	4.6
More than twice a week	34.6	37.1
Once a week	25.8	23.8
Once to 3 times a month	12.6	11.3
Less than once a month	21.9	16.0
Never	1.7	7.2
Total	100.0	100.0

[a] 3% with "no information" excluded from analysis.

Source: *Statistische Quellenwerke der Schweiz*, 1984 *(3)*

Table 5. Smoking habits of Swiss army conscripts, 1977 and 1982

	Year	
	1977	1982
Number of respondents	8917	44000[a]
	%	%
Grams of tobacco smoked per day:		
Non-smokers	46.8	56.0
1–10 g/day	21.4	21.0
11–20 g/day	19.2	16.0
21–40 g/day	11.1	6.2
41 + g/day	1.5	0.8
Total	100.0	100.0

[a] 4.3% with "no information" excluded from analysis.

Source: *Statistische Quellenwerke der Schweiz*, 1984 *(3)*

Table 6. Alcohol consumption habits among Swiss army conscripts, 1977 and 1982

	Year	
	1977	1982
Number of respondents	8 917	43 954[a]
	%	%
Grams of pure alcohol drunk per week:		
No alcohol	19.7	29.0
Up to 60 g of alcohol/week	41.8	40.4
61–240 g of alcohol/week	29.5	24.8
241–360 g of alcohol/week	4.1	3.2
360+g of alcohol/week	4.9	2.6
Total	100.0	100.0

[a] 4.4% with "no information" excluded from analysis.

Source: Statistische Quellenwerke der Schweiz, 1984 *(3)*

no unified programme in this field has ever been put forward, and measurements in this area have not been designed in the framework of such a national plan. Nevertheless, it is hoped that the efforts being made on several levels will have a significant impact on the fitness level of the population and also on the rates of morbidity and mortality from cardiovascular disease. As shown above, documentation of the need for further efforts and the monitoring of progress occur both in terms of a quantitative description of the progress of programme activities (e.g. number of fitness tracks installed, proportion of young people participating in compulsory sports lessons) and in terms of outcome measurements, in particular among the 19-year-old army conscripts. Progress has been slow, but at a time when more and more young people can afford their own motorcycles or cars, and when the distraction of television and video films offers a seductive alternative to physical exercise and sports, even the maintenance of past levels of endurance fitness or a small increase of 2.4% show that the endeavours to promote health and fitness meet with some success and are worth pursuing.

The same can be said of the advancement of sports among middle-aged adults. Although trend data showing an increase in physical fitness levels of the population are not available yet, the number of people participating in popular running events and using fitness tracks is increasing, and there is a growing awareness among the population that the level of physical fitness and, hence, of health potential at all ages can be considerably improved if enough time is devoted to leisure-time sports.

References

1. **Howald, H. et al.** Körperliche Aktivität und Leistungsfähigkeit in 4 Schweizer Städten. *Schweizerische medizinische Wochenschrift,* **111** (Suppl. 12): 47–55 (1981).
2. Turnprüfung bei der Aushebung 1977. *Statistische Quellenwerke der Schweiz,* vol. 662. Berne, Bundesamt für Statistik, 1980.
3. Turnprüfung bei der Aushebung 1982. *Statistische Quellenwerke der Schweiz,* vol. 765. Berne, Bundesamt für Statistik, 1984.
4. **Autorengruppe Nationales Forschungsprogramm 1A.** Gesundheitserzieherische Interventionen in Aarau: Übersicht und Vorgehen. *Sozial- und Präventivmedizin,* **25**: 280–286 (1980).
5. **Howald, H. et al.** Konzeption und Evaluation eines einfachen Fitnesstests. *Schweizerische Zeitschrift für Sportmedizin,* **23**: 57–92 (1975).
6. **Astrand, P.O. & Rodahl, K.** *Textbook of work physiology.* New York, McGraw-Hill, 1977.
7. **Lange Andersen, K. et al.** *Fundamentals of exercise testing.* Geneva, World Health Organization, 1971.
8. **Dressendorfer, H.** Oxygen requirements of postcoronary and competitive marathon runners during road running. *Journal of sports medicine,* **19**: 15–22 (1979).
9. **Marti, B. et al.** Maximale aerobe Kapazität und anaerobe Schwelle bei 16 km Volksläufern. *Schweizerische Zeitschrift für Sportmedizin,* **33**: 41–46 (1985).
10. **Abelin, T. et al.** Smoking and physical fitness. *In:* Fontana, F., ed. *Tobacco and youth.* University of Padua, Institute of Hygiene, 1982.

11.12 An investigation of the effects of daily physical activity on the health of primary school pupils in South Australia — *T. Dwyer, W.E. Coonan, D.R. Leitch, B.S. Hetzel & R.A. Baghurst*

This chapter, like the previous one, is concerned with the measurement of physical functioning. This subject was covered in Chapter 7.2 by Lange Andersen & Rutenfranz. Here, the authors demonstrate the health benefits gained by schoolchildren from a daily physical education programme.

It is apparent that children in industrial countries are at high risk of entering a state of positive energy balance in the long term *(1)*. This is likely to be due in part to a sedentary lifestyle, including considerable periods of time spent watching television *(2)*. This energy imbalance leads to obesity and in middle age is a significant risk factor for the occurrence of coronary heart disease and various forms of cancer *(3)*.

Recent studies of coronary heart disease risk factors in childhood have also demonstrated significant relationships between indices of obesity such as the Quetelet index (weight/height^2) and skinfold thickness with diastolic blood pressure and lipoprotein *(4)* at an early age.

The possibility of modifying these various health risk factors in children has arisen from studies of daily physical activity programmes in schools.

Previous studies conducted in Belgium, Canada and France on the effects of physical activity programmes in schools have reported a wide range of physical, psychological and academic benefits *(5)*. However, these studies were not well controlled and information on the selective effects of different types of physical activity was not sought. In particular, the possible effects of increased cardiopulmonary efficiency (endurance fitness) have not been distinguished from those resulting from the acquisition of motor skills.

In September 1978 a randomized trial involving more than 500 grade-5 pupils (mean age 10.2 years) was initiated in 7 Adelaide primary schools to investigate these issues.

Two intervention groups took part in different daily physical activity programmes, while a control group maintained a relatively inactive school routine. This phase of the study lasted for 14 weeks, measurements being made at commencement and completion.

The assessment included selected coronary heart disease risk factors (endurance, fitness, body fat, blood pressure, plasma cholesterol, triglycerides and high-density lipoprotein cholesterol) *(6–8)*, as well as measures of academic performance and psychological functioning.

Following the findings of the first phase of the study *(9)*, the schools involved decided to adopt daily physical activity as part of the school curriculum. Two years after the initial study, in 1980, further measurements were conducted among grade-5 pupils in 5 of the original 7 schools. These 1980 grade-5 pupils, unlike the 1978 grade-5 pupils, had therefore been participating in daily physical activity programmes for up to 2 years.

The results of the initial randomized trial (Phase I) and of the comparison between grade-5 pupils in 1978 and grade-5 pupils in 1980 (Phase II) are presented here.

Methods

Grade-5 (10-year-old) pupils from 7 Adelaide metropolitan primary schools participated in Phase I of the study. These schools were selected from an initial self-selected group that indicated a willingness to become involved. Further selection was made to ensure a broad distribution of ethnic and socioeconomic groups on the basis of information provided by the South Australian Education Department. In each of the 7 schools there were 3 classes, each of which was randomly allocated to one of 3 study groups (for fitness, skill and control, respectively). The non-participation rate of pupils was less than 5%.

The control group maintained the traditional programme, comprising 3 half-hour periods of physical education per week. The focus of teaching was to develop skill and competence levels in minor games, without particular emphasis on intense or prolonged endurance activities. The skill group had a programme content identical to that of the controls; however, the duration and frequency of exercise was increased to $1\frac{1}{4}$ hours daily, including 15 minutes in the early morning. The fitness group had a programme with the same duration, frequency and content as that of the skill group, but particular emphasis was placed on the intensity at which games activities were carried out, the aim being to raise the heart rate.

Intervention took place over 14 weeks, during which classes were kept under close observation by the investigators to ensure adherence to the programme. In the week preceding the intervention period, and in the week following completion, study measurements were made of a number of factors related to physical health, psychosocial functioning and academic performance.

The personnel performing the physical measurement and marking the psychosocial questionnaires and academic tests were unaware of the study group allocation of pupils. The same testers made pre- and post-intervention measurements. In the case of skinfold thickness and blood pressure, two trained observers performed each set of measurements respectively. Measurements on individual pupils were performed at the same time of day on both occasions.

The physical measurements performed were:

(*a*) height and weight; the Body Mass Index (Quetelet) (weight/height^2) was also calculated;

(*b*) four skinfold thicknesses — biceps, triceps, subscapular, and supra-iliac, using a Harpenden skin caliper;

(*c*) blood pressure, measured on the left arm with the child sitting, after a five-minute rest;

(*d*) endurance fitness — measured as physical work capacity (PWC) on a Monark bicycle ergometer at a heart rate of 170 (PWC 170);

(*e*) plasma total cholesterol, high-density lipoprotein cholesterol, and triglycerides were estimated in a subsample of 74 pupils — a fitness and a control class from two volunteer schools.

Full details of the methods are described elsewhere *(10)*.

The results of two tests of academic performance and rating inventory completed by teachers on pupils' classroom behaviour are also presented here. The academic tests were the ACER arithmetic test *(11)* and the GAP reading test *(12)*.

The teacher's ratings of classroom behaviour were recorded on the KAB Child Behaviour Scale *(13)*, consisting of a series of 18 items rated according to 5-point scales. The items cover social and work aspects of classroom behaviour. Ratings were summed to yield a total score for each child.

After a review of the findings of Phase I, the study school decided to continue with daily physical activity as a regular part of the curriculum.

In spring 1980 a random sample of 216 grade-5 pupils in 5 of the initial 7 schools were subjected to the same set of physical measurements that their predecessors had undergone 2 years previously, with the exception of blood lipids measurement. As the resources available were limited, assessment was restricted to 5 rather than 7 schools. Again the non-participation rate was low: less than 7%. The protocol used for the measurements in 1978 was rigorously followed for all study parameters. In the case of blood pressure, skinfold thickness, height and weight, the same observers as those used in Phase I performed the measurements.

The only academic performance measure repeated in Phase II was the ACER arithmetic test. Psychological measures were not included.

Results

Phase I

Changes during the intervention period in physical work capacity at a heart rate of 170 per kg body weight (PWC 170/kg), body fat and blood pressure in each of the study groups are summarized in Table 1. Changes for girls and boys were very similar and therefore they have been grouped throughout the analysis. There were no significant differences in the initial values for the various measurements.

All groups gained in endurance fitness as measured by PWC 170/kg, although the gain was greatest in the fitness groups. The latter also

Table 1. Changes in endurance fitness (PWC 170/kg), skinfold thickness and blood pressure in 10-year-old boys and girls following a daily physical education programme over 14 weeks in South Australian primary schools

		Mean ± 2SD		
		Control	Skills	Fitness
PWC 170/kg (Kpm/min/kg)	Initial value	10.88 ± 0.19	10.45 ± 0.19	10.57 ± 0.20
	Change	1.24 ± 0.15	1.66 ± 0.16	2.42 ± 0.14[a]
Four skinfold thicknesses (mm)	Initial value	37.25 ± 1.30	36.71 ± 1.33	37.36 ± 1.36
	Change	0.93 ± 0.46	0.39 ± 0.33	−1.26 ± 0.40[a]
Blood pressure (mmHg)				
Systolic	Initial value	102.98 ± 0.82	102.60 ± 0.79	101.95 ± 0.80
	Change	−1.08 ± 0.92	−1.23 ± 0.74	−1.19 ± 0.83
Diastolic	Initial value	62.32 ± 0.77	63.09 ± 0.68	63.37 ± 0.70
	Change	−1.54 ± 0.97	−4.72 ± 0.74	−3.80 ± 0.83

[a] Significant differences between changes in the three groups.

Note. Changes for boys and girls grouped, as no difference apparent.

experienced a significant decline in the sum of four skinfold thickness measurements. There was no significant change in systolic or diastolic blood pressure, and no significant differences between the groups were noted in the lipid measurements.

Table 2 gives details of the changes which took place in academic performance: the ACER arithmetic test, the GAP reading test, and the teachers' ratings of classroom behaviour. It shows that there were no significant differences between the treatment groups in respect of either of the academic performance measures. However, the measured classroom behaviour of the fitness and skill groups improved to a significantly greater extent than that of the controls. This observation may have been affected by the teachers' awareness of the fact that their pupils were involved in an intervention.

Phase II

The results of measurements of grade-5 pupils in 1980 are presented. The findings are given as comparisons between 1980 pupils and 1978 pupils from the same schools prior to the Phase I intervention. The demographic characteristics of the 1978 and 1980 pupils were similar *(10)*.

The 1980 pupils, both males and females, were superior as far as PWC 170/kg was concerned (Table 3). Examination of the differences in PWC 170, unadjusted for body weight, gave the same results.

There was a significant decrease in body fat in both sexes, as measured by the four skinfold thicknesses (Table 3). There was also a reduction in the proportion of overweight pupils in 1980 *(10)*.

The Body Mass Index (BMI) was also examined as an index of body fat. The results confirmed the findings from the sum of four skinfold thickness measurements, the 1980 pupils having lower BMIs (i.e. 17.35 in 1978 and 17.19 in 1980). This difference was not statistically significant, however.

Both systolic and diastolic blood pressures were lower in the two sexes in 1980, although the difference was statistically significant only for diastolic pressure in males.

Table 4 records the mean scores in the ACER arithmetic test. Although the 1980 value was higher than that for 1978, the difference was not statistically significant.

Discussion

These data provide strong evidence that children who engage in a daily exercise programme in the school setting derive health benefits from such exercise. They also suggest that the prospects of maintaining a successful programme in the long term at an average school are good, despite the practical difficulties that must be faced in the field.

Phase I of the study demonstrated that it was possible to reduce body fat and improve endurance fitness with a daily physical activity programme, particularly if the time was spent primarily on vigorous activities (Table 1). There was some indication that diastolic blood pressure had also

Table 2. Effects of daily physical activity: summary of changes in academic performance and classroom behaviour scores

		Mean ± 2SD		
		Control	Skills	Fitness
Arithmetic scores	Initial	105.20 ± 2.51	102.55 ± 2.45	101.42 ± 2.35
	Change	10.89 ± 1.29	10.54 ± 1.03	12.33 ± 1.09
Reading age (months)	Initial	122.18 ± 1.22	120.03 ± 1.12	121.64 ± 1.21
	Change	4.41 ± 0.72	3.89 ± 0.78	3.37 ± 0.79
Teachers' rating of classroom behaviour	Initial	37.34 ± 1.18	46.81 ± 1.45	41.79 ± 1.29
	Change	1.66 ± 0.74	9.32 ± 0.88	6.87 ± 1.07[a]

[a] Significant differences between changes in the three groups.

Table 3. Comparison of measures of health status
in 10-year-old South Australian schoolchildren in 1978 and 1980

	Sex	Mean ± 2SD	
		1978	1980
PWC 170/kg (Kpm/min/kg)	Males	11.68 ± 0.17	14.36 ± 0.23[a]
	Females	9.55 ± 0.17	11.94 ± 0.25[a]
Sum of four skinfold thicknesses (mm)	Males	31.90 ± 1.09	28.62 ± 1.08[a]
	Females	40.24 ± 1.20	36.23 ± 1.44[a]
Blood pressure (mmHg)			
Systolic	Males	102.61 ± 0.87	100.29 ± 1.10
	Females	101.92 ± 0.98	100.30 ± 1.28
Diastolic	Males	63.09 ± 0.77	55.68 ± 0.98[a]
	Females	60.66 ± 0.85	58.46 ± 1.13

[a] Significant difference between measures in 1978 and in 1980.

Table 4. Results of the ACER arithmetic test in 10-year-old South Australian schoolchildren in 1978 and 1980

	Year	Mean ± 2SD
Arithmetic score	1978	101.89 ± 1.64
	1980	105.62 ± 2.18

fallen. Significant changes in lipids and lipoproteins were not observed. Possible reasons for this have been discussed previously *(9)*.

What was uncertain after this phase of the study was whether the gains made in a closely monitored experimental setting over 14 weeks could be sustained in the long term outside this artificial framework. The results at the end of Phase II suggest that they can be (Table 3). An increase in endurance fitness and a decrease in body fat were observed in both boys and girls when comparisons were made between grade-5 pupils of 1978 and 1980. There was also a decline in blood pressure, particularly diastolic (although this only reached significance in males), confirming the trends in Phase I. Lipids were unfortunately not measured, so it is not possible to determine whether the lack of any changes in Phase I was due to the study period being insufficient.

Another possibility must be considered before inferring that the exercise programme was responsible for the physical changes observed. These changes may merely reflect secular trends in children in the community at large, occurring coincidentally with the study period. However, the magnitude of the changes suggests that this possibility may be discounted.

Unfortunately there were no control schools with which to make comparisons in Phase II. No schools participating in Phase I were asked specifically to delay adopting the daily physical activity curriculum, and all decided to introduce it. There were differences, nonetheless, in the degree to which schools adhered to the suggested programme. One school was generally regarded as being particularly rigorous in its adherence and when the results for this school were examined independently it was found that the change in body fat levels exceeded that in any of the other schools.

The extent to which the results of this study can be extrapolated to other children in other schools must be considered. In favour of the findings being externally applicable is the fact that the children came from a broad cross-section of social classes and ethnic groups, and that 21 teachers from 7 different schools were involved. Even so, studies in other locations are necessary to demonstrate the external validity of this study. The findings of several investigations conducted to date are relevant in this respect.

Examining effects over a longer period, Mayer *(14)* showed that a reduction in levels of obesity among 350 obese primary and secondary school pupils taking part in a 10-month diet and exercise programme was maintained while the intervention continued, but was lost in the years following its cessation.

The potential health gains to be derived from a daily physical activity programme in schools, particularly with regard to obesity, thus seem considerable. However, schools are unlikely to introduce an extra item into the curriculum, regardless of the health benefits, if the academic performance of their pupils is likely to suffer.

The findings reported here with respect to academic performance are encouraging, but not conclusive. The demonstration of improved academic performance in association with increased physical activity, as reported in previous studies, was not clearly replicated. In Phase I no significant changes occurred in arithmetic or reading scores (Table 2), and although pupils in 1980 had slightly higher arithmetic scores than in 1978 (Table 4), the difference was not statistically significant.

In general, it would appear that academic performance, while not being improved, is not adversely affected, despite a reduction of at least 45 minutes in formal daily teaching time. However, further work is required on this important aspect.

The present results indicate substantial health benefits for 10-year-old children resulting from the daily physical education programme described. This programme has gained the enthusiastic support of school teachers and parents, so that in the two-year period following Phase I (in late 1978), which involved 7 schools, no fewer than 281 schools, or 60% of all primary schools in the state of South Australia, adopted the programme.

Acknowledgements

This chapter is based on material drawn from a paper in the *International journal of epidemiology (11)* and is used by kind permission of the Oxford University Press.

References

1. **Williams, C.L. et al.** Chronic disease risk factors among children: the Know Your Body Study. *Journal of chronic diseases,* **32**: 505–513 (1979).
2. **Miller, M.R. & Binns, C.W.** Cultural differences in children's TV viewing habits and implications for nutritional status. *Proceedings of the Nutrition Society of Australia,* **4**: 120–125 (1979).
3. **Hetzel, B.S.** Dietary differences and disease. *Medical journal of Australia,* **1**: 113–115 (1981).
4. **Khoury, P. et al.** Clustering and interrelationships of coronary heart disease risk factors in school children ages 6–19. *American journal of epidemiology,* **112**: 524–538 (1980).
5. **McDonald, A.** Experiments at Vanves and Brussels. *Australian journal of physical education,* **21**: 25–30 (1961).
6. **Morris, J.W. et al.** Vigorous exercise in leisure-time and the incidence of coronary heart disease. *Lancet,* **1**: 333–339 (1973).

7. **Stamler, J. et al.** Primary prevention of the atherosclerotic disease. *Circulation,* **42**: 55–59 (1970).
8. **Castelli, W.P. et al.** HDL cholesterol and other lipids in coronary heart disease. The co-operative lipoprotein phenotyping study. *Circulation,* **55**: 767–772 (1977).
9. **Dwyer, T. et al.** An assessment of the effects of two physical activity programs on coronary heart disease risk factors in primary school children. *Community health studies,* **3**: 196–202 (1979).
10. **Dwyer, T. et al.** An investigation of the effects of daily physical activity on the health of primary school students in South Australia. *International journal of epidemiology,* **12**: 308–313 (1983).
11. *ACER arithmetic test form C.* Victoria, Australian Council for Education Research, 1976.
12. **Forms, B. & McLeod, R.J.** *GAP reading comprehension test,* 3rd ed. Australia, Heinemann Educational, 1978.
13. **McGee, R.** Evaluation of processes and products. *In:* Logsdon, B.E. et al., ed. *Physical education for children: a focus on the teaching process.* Philadelphia, Lea & Febiger, 1977, pp. 288–316.
14. **Mayer, J.** Obesity during childhood. *In:* Winick, M., ed. *Childhood obesity.* New York, John Wiley & Sons, 1975, pp. 73–80.

12. Assessing health and monitoring progress: instruments for use at individual level

12.1 Easy-to-use charts for monitoring the nutritional status of children, using weight-for-height assessment — *D. Nabarro*

The issues raised by Falkner in his coverage of measures of growth and maturity of children (Chapter 7.1) are illustrated by the next example, which deals with the use of simple measures in developing countries. Weight-for-height charts provide an indicator that may be used to assess children's nutritional status on the basis of a single measurement, of particular value where the age of the child is not accurately known. Of particular interest and general relevance in the contribution is the careful consideration of chart design in order to increase its usefulness and acceptability.

The regular weighing of children aged under 5 years and the widespread use of weight charts for monitoring growth are important features of child health services throughout the world. This is especially the case in poorer countries, where auxiliaries, with limited technical resources, provide primary health care.

The identification of children with impaired growth is harder if serial weight measurements are not available. In many societies, children only come into contact with health services when their parents are concerned about their health. Community nutrition surveys, too, are often expected to describe nutrition status with information gained from single assessments of children.

In these situations, the child's nutritional status is usually assessed by comparing a measurable growth parameter (e.g. weight) with an international or national reference value for age. The weight is expressed as a percentage of the international reference weight, and the nutrition status can thus be graded: the lower the percentage, the more malnourished the child.

Gomez et al. *(1)* suggested a classification based on ranges of percentage weight-for-age values to describe the severity of malnutrition. However, Waterlow *(2)* has emphasized that the relationship between a child's weight and the reference weight-for-age provides an incomplete description of the nutritional status when the child is assessed at a single point in time. Waterlow distinguishes three groups of children who are underweight for age: those who are thin (wasted), those who are short (stunted), and those who are both thin and short (wasted and stunted). The distinction is relevant, as slowed skeletal growth (which leads to stunting) is a result of long-standing malnutrition, while thinness (or wasting) is normally a result of recent weight loss. A combination of these two processes causes a child to be both short and thin.

Acutely malnourished children usually need medical and nutritional help. If provided with the right treatment, they will regain lost weight rapidly *(3)*. Stunted children also face dangers, though it is less easy to reduce these through clinical or dietary interventions. Their chronic malnutrition reflects the poor social, economic and environmental conditions in which they live.

Nutritional Assessment

The weight-for-height index is used to assess the thinness of children. The child's weight is compared with the weight of a well nourished child of the same height (the reference weight-for-height). If the child's weight is less than 80% of this reference, then he is referred to as "wasted" in this paper. A child's stature can be assessed by comparing his height with the international reference height for that age. A child whose height is less than 90% of this reference figure is said to be stunted *(4,5)*.

There are slight variations in the average weight of children of the same height at different ages and some workers feel that these need to be taken into account when nutritional status is assessed *(6,7)*. In practice, however, weight-for-height can usually be treated as an age-independent nutritional index. This is important, as many parents do not know the ages of their children accurately enough for weight-for-age or height-for-age percentages to be calculated correctly. Weight-for-height is often the only nutritional index that can easily be determined.

The assessment of the thinness of young children and the identification of those who are wasted is a valuable technique for use in any situation where malnourished children are encountered. This is especially the case where there are limited resources and a need to focus on the children at greatest risk. Difficulties associated with assessing weight-for-height have had the result that the index for an individual child is rarely identified and used as an action-oriented indicator of nutritional status, either in health clinics or in field programmes. Sometimes too, the difficulty of weighing children and measuring their height in their homes makes it hard for field workers to obtain even the basic measurements required for weight-for-height assessment.

This chapter describes the development, design and use of wall charts that simplify the assessment of the percentage weight-for-height and thus help in the identification of wasted children.

The Weight-for-Height Wall Chart

In 1977, a child health programme was established in Dhankuta, East Nepal, by the Nepal Children's Organization and the Save the Children Fund (United Kingdom). Many children in the area suffered from protein-energy malnutrition. A simple procedure was required to enable the programme's health workers to identify those children in urgent need of nutrition intervention.

Most mothers did not know their children's ages accurately. However, a high proportion of the children from the area were obviously stunted. Thus, weight-for-age assessments alone did not give field workers sufficient information with which to identify malnourished children accurately. Weight-for-height assessment was also introduced and wasted children were given first priority for intervention.

Health workers were trained to measure a child's height at the same time as weighing the child and to calculate weight-for-height using the Harvard reference figures. They referred wasted children for nutrition rehabilitation, though only workers with a relatively high level of formal education were able to do this.

A simpler procedure for identifying wasted children was needed. Weight-for-height graphs were drawn on a wall as a life-size wall chart. Workers could then identify wasted children by standing them against the chart and reading their percentage weight-for-height values off the wall directly. Sections on the chart were coloured and workers were able to identify a child's percentage weight-for-height range by using a colour code. They did not have to read height numbers, perform manoeuvres with graphs or consult any tables to obtain this information. Workers who were able to weigh children were also able, with minimal training, to use the chart to identify wasted children.

Method of use

A prototype wall chart is shown in Fig. 1. The child has been weighed at 7 kg and placed standing in front of the chart, which is painted on tin and fixed to the wall of a village health clinic. His feet are together, legs are straight and arms are by his sides.

On the chart there are separate columns each marked with different weights at 0.5 kg intervals. The child has been placed so that he is standing immediately in front of the column with 7 kg marked at its base.

At the upper end of each column on the chart there are three different coloured zones. The heights of the panels above the ground are so arranged

Fig. 1. Prototype weight-for-height wall chart in use in a village children's clinic to assess the thinness of a 7 kg boy

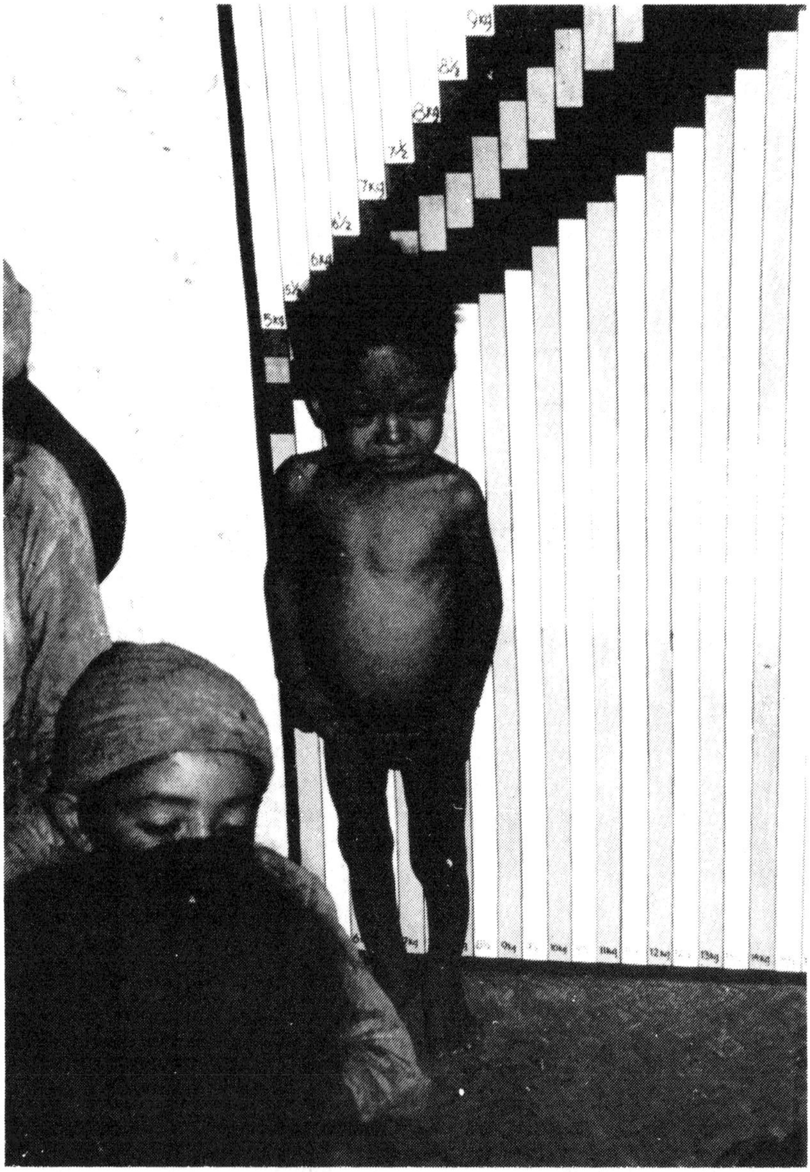

that the colour seen at the level of the top of the child's head in the column marked with the child's weight indicates the weight-for-height.

In Fig. 1, the head of the boy reaches the uppermost coloured zone of the 7 kg column, which indicates that his weight is between 70% and 80% of the reference weight-for-height and that he is wasted. The lowest colour zone indicates a weight that is between 90% and 110% of reference weight-for-height and the centre zone identifies children whose weight-for-height percentage is between 80% and 90%.

In order to ensure that a child's nutritional status is assessed as accurately as possible, the operator should check that the child stands upright and still. The operator's hand should be placed flat on top of the child's head parallel with the ground. The colour should be read off the chart at the point at which the operator's fingers touch the column marked with the child's weight.

Small children are often unwilling to stand still and remain in position while they are being measured. Two attendants are often needed to undertake the task satisfactorily. One person (e.g. the child's mother) has to hold the child in position and keep the limbs straight while the operator straightens the head and reads the weight-for-height colour off the chart.

The basis for the design

The wall chart can be constructed and used without the health worker having to understand the principles behind the design, or even the concept of weight for height as a nutritional index. However, anyone wishing to adapt the chart methods needs to understand the basis of the design. In the following example, two boys each weighing 10 kg are compared.

Fig. 2 shows two boys, A and B, each weighing 10 kg. Boy A, who is taller than boy B, is also the thinner of the two. Because he is thinner, he is more likely to be in need of immediate nutritional help than boy B, who is shorter, but of normal body build. Because they both weigh the same, their nutritional status cannot be distinguished by weighing alone. Boy A's height is 93 cm, boy B's is 80 cm.

In Fig. 2, the arrows marking the heights for which 10 kg will be 70%, 80%, 90%, 100% and 110% of standard weight-for-height, are indicated by lines behind the two boys. The positions of the tops of their heads can be compared relative to these lines. Then the ranges of percentages that include each child's own weight-for-height can quickly be determined. This is the basis of the wall chart design.

The ranges of height for which 10 kg would be 70–80%, 80–90% and 90–110% of the standard weights-for-height can be indicated by the use of different colours. One column is used for each weight value and the wall chart consists of a series of these columns.

Fig. 3 shows, diagramatically, the resulting wall chart and how such a chart could be used to assess the weight-for-height percentage values of boys A and B. Weight markings at the base of the columns make it easier for the measurer to identify the point where the child should stand. The widths of the columns can be varied: the wider they are, the easier the chart is to use.

Fig. 2. Comparison of boys A and B, each weighing 10 kg

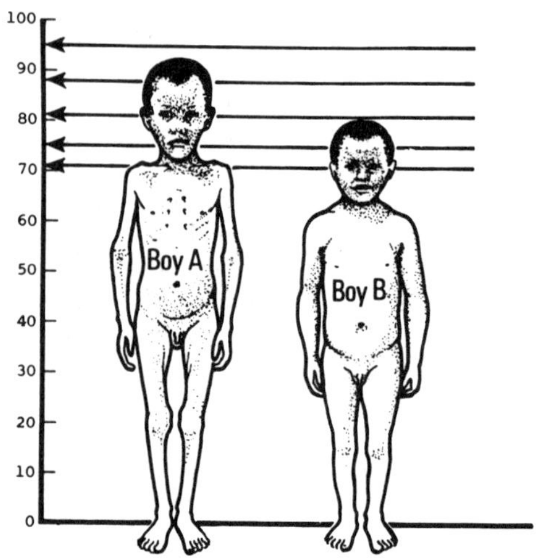

Note. The arrows mark the heights for which 10 kg will be 70%, 80%, 90%, 100% and 110% of standard weight-for-height.

The reference values for weight-for-height used in the chart were derived from the US National Academy of Science growth reference figures, which are recommended by WHO.

Construction

The chart can be drawn or painted on paper, plastic, tin or cloth and fixed to a clinic or house wall, or it can be painted directly onto the wall. The wall must be smooth, the floor in front of it level and the dimensions measured accurately, using a ruler or non-stretch tape measure. If the chart is on paper, plastic or cloth, the dimensions should be checked regularly.

Some workers may consider that a three-colour code is irrelevant and opt for two colours only. Others may prefer to use more than three colours so that the progress of a child undergoing nutrition rehabilitation can be followed. The choice of colours to indicate different zones at the top of the columns will depend on the significance of different colours in the location where the chart is used. The percentage weight-for-height values that indicate that a child needs help immediately may vary in different situations depending on the relative risks faced by thin or fat children and the resources available to help them.

Related applications

A number of additional applications of the technique have been developed, and some have still to be field tested. They include the following.

Fig. 3. Diagram of a full size weight-for-height wall chart in use for assessing boys A and B, whose standing positions are identified by floor markings on the floor in front of the chart

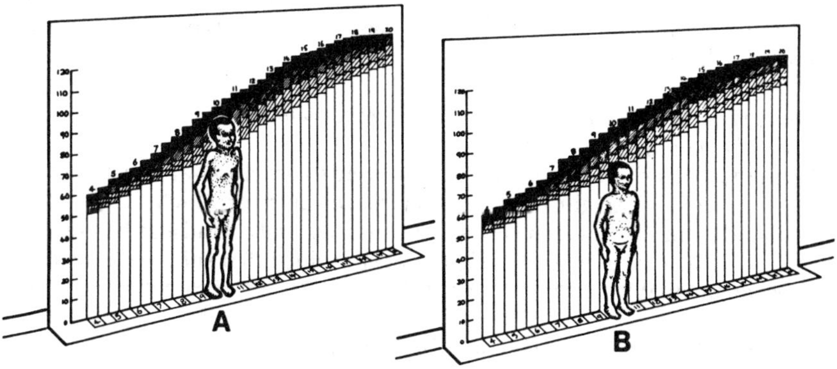

Fixing the weight-for-height chart to a stadiometer

Field workers using the weight-for-height chart have found that the reliability of assessments is increased by attaching the chart to a stadiometer with a fixed footboard and moving headboard. One such device, the "leanness board", has been field tested in India and found to give reliable assessments.

Assessment of weight as a percentage of standard weight-for-length

In practice, it is usually easiest, and in nutrition surveys it is desirable, to measure the length of children under 2 years old or less than 85 cm in length. This requires the construction of a length board. A weight-for-length chart can be drawn to help health workers assess children's weight-for-length. A weight-for-length chart suitable for fixing to the back of a length board has been designed. Health workers can use it for children who weigh between 3.5 kg and 8 kg. The chart has yet to be produced on a large scale.

Development of a weight-for-height wall chart suitable for use in temporary clinics

Detachable charts, which can be rolled up at the end of the day, have been printed on plastic. They are useful in temporary clinics, e.g. mobile village clinics set up in village leaders' homes. These detachable charts can be obtained through UNICEF.

A portable weight-for-height chart for field workers

For home visiting purposes, a readily portable version of the chart is needed. A chart for children weighing between 5 kg and 15 kg has been developed. It has very thin columns which are "stacked" on top of one another. These portable charts are supplied at low cost by Teaching Aids, London, United Kingdom.

Use of a weight-for-height wall chart for the early detection of obese children

A wall chart can also be used to help with the early detection of obese children. The columns can be divided into colour zones that indicate weights that are greater than the reference weight-for-height values, distinguishing children who are 90–110%, 110–120% and more than 120% of reference weight-for-height.

Development of wall charts using local reference values, or using cut-offs based on Z scores

The method described in this paper can be used to develop wall charts which are based on local weight-for-height reference values or which use cut-offs calculated from Z (Standard Deviation Unit) scores. It could also be used to develop charts based on local weight units provided that suitable reference figures are available.

Development of height-for-age wall charts to assess and identify stunted children

A different wall chart has been designed to ease the assessment of children's percentage height-for-age. Provided the children's ages are known, the charts can be used to identify children who are also stunted.

Use of the weight-for-height chart in field programmes

The Save the Children Fund has produced over 3000 copies of the original weight-for-height chart since it was first developed in 1978. These charts were all in use by 1982 and subsequently other agencies and governments have printed copies of the original chart or modifications based on local needs.

Various field trials have been conducted in which aspects of chart design and use have been tested *(8)*. They suggest that the chart is a valuable tool for nutritional assessment in a number of situations.

The charts are now used in child health clinics and health centres in Bangladesh, India and Nepal to help health workers assess children's nutritional status and identify children who urgently need nutritional therapy. Programme staff find the information obtained by using the chart very useful when making decisions about the kinds of treatment or advice to be offered. They particularly favour the chart when they do not have access to regular weight assessments.

The weight-for-height chart has proved to be an important tool for health workers in emergencies. For example, when the Karamoja area of Uganda was affected by severe drought in 1980, staff from international relief agencies used the chart to select those children who needed immediate intensive feeding and to differentiate them from children who would be offered supplementary feeds only. The chart proved to be particularly helpful in this respect because health workers could show community representatives the rationale behind their selections.

More recently (in 1982) workers at the National Institute of Nutrition, India, compared a variety of methods for assessing the nutritional status of children. They found that the most reliable and reproducible assessments were made when field workers used the weight-for-height chart. Charts have been incorporated in several child health and welfare programmes in South India. In Tamil Nadu, the State Government, with assistance from CARE, reproduced charts on plastic for use in the State nutrition programme.

Field workers' reactions to using the chart when surveying the nutritional status of populations are mixed. In 1982, an international agency used the charts (and the accompanying three-coloured recording cards) to document the nutritional status of children in different communities in Chad. They were able to identify those communities where there was a high prevalence of childhood malnutrition and directed relief efforts to them.

However, an experienced nutrition survey team working in North Africa has confirmed that field workers must be very careful when making nutritional assessments with the weight-for-height chart. The team reports that field workers frequently make errors when classifying children's nutritional status if they use the weight-for-height chart as it is. Classification errors can be reduced by modifying the way in which the chart is used. If a fixed footboard and moving headboard are attached to the chart, the number of errors made is substantially reduced. This modified weight-for-height chart can produce useful assessments in situations where field workers need to know whether children are wasted and are not easily able to calculate weight-for-height percentage values. (Surveyors would normally be advised to collect actual weight and height data from the children they examine.) Such a modified weight-for-height chart has been used in a number of different sites in India (the "leanness" board).

Conclusions

A single weight measurement provides relatively little information about a child's nutritional status, even if his age is known. The measurement of height as well enables workers to differentiate between wasted and stunted children. The weight-for-height chart is a device which helps field workers to assess the thinness of children whose weights are known. The nutritional index weight-for-height is used and wasted children are identified as those whose percentage weight-for-height is less than 80% of the reference figure. They will be the children who are likely to be in urgent need of help in any health or nutrition programme. Children also need to be given a physical examination to see whether there are other clinical signs of malnutrition or illness, as these, too, may indicate the need for urgent help.

In some situations, the relationship between thinness — or wasting — and risks to children's health has been established. In many societies, however, the risks associated with being thin are still not fully understood. The weight-for-height chart will enable workers to investigate the dangers associated with thinness. This information will assist programme planners who are trying to choose the most appropriate intervention points for thin children of different ages.

Assessment of the degree of thinness of a child provides additional information about the degree of urgency of nutrition intervention if thinness and wasting are associated with a high risk of the child becoming seriously ill or dying.

In children's clinics, weight or height measurements are usually imprecise. This may not matter when the wall chart is used, as it is only marked with 0.5 kg weight intervals. Imprecise height assessments were not considered to be a problem in the Dhankuta programme, where the wall chart was used to assist clinic workers in deciding on interventions. For nutrition purposes, however, design modifications can increase the reliability of assessment. These include height assessment with a moving headboard and the use of a more precise weighing machine; also, the provision of additional weight columns on the chart at intervals of less than 0.5 kg.

Results of the worldwide field testing of the weight-for-height chart *(8)* confirm that the chart technique is quickly learnt, measurements are performed in a straightforward manner and assessments can be made rapidly. The colour coding provides the health worker with a simple decision-making aid. The chart is of great practical value in emergency relief situations and for individual, action-oriented nutritional surveillance in a clinic or in a village, when regular weighing is not possible. It is useful as a teaching aid and as a means of involving mothers, children and health workers more closely in the improvement of their children's nutrition. More important, perhaps, is that the technique might enable more workers to study the risks associated with wasting in children in a number of different situations.

Those who have used the technique or who would like further information are invited to communicate with the author of this chapter, who will ensure that they are kept up to date with further developments.

References

1. **Gomez, F. et al.** Mortality in second and third degree malnutrition. *Journal of tropical paediatrics,* **2**: 77–83 (1956).
2. **Waterlow, J.C.** Classification and definition of protein calorie malnutrition. *British medical journal,* **3**: 566–569 (1972).
3. **Church, M.A.** Nutrition rehabilitation: an approach to the management and prevention of childhood malnutrition. *In:* Korte, R., ed. *Nutrition in developing countries. Proceedings of a seminar for German technical assistance personnel, Limuru, Kenya.* Eschborn, GTZ, 1978.
4. **Waterlow, J.C. et al.** The presentation and use of height and weight data for comparing the nutritional status of groups of children under the age of 10 years. *Bulletin of the World Health Organization,* **55**: 489–498 (1977).
5. **Waterlow, J.C.** Note on the classification of protein energy malnutrition in children. *Lancet,* **2**: 87–89 (1973).
6. **McLaren, D.S. & Read, W.W.C.** Weight/length classification of nutritional status. *Lancet,* **2**: 219–221 (1973).

7. **Cole, T.J.** A method for assessing age-standardised weight-for-height in children seen cross-sectionally. *Annals of human biology,* **6**: 249–268 (1979).

8. **Nabarro, D. et al.** *The weight-for-height chart project evaluation report 3, 1982/84.* London, Save the Children Fund, in association with the Department of Human Nutrition, London School of Hygiene and Tropical Medicine.

12.2 Guidelines for the design and use of weight-for-age growth charts — *G. Tremlett, H.J. Lovel & D. Morley*

This contribution by Tremlett et al., like the previous chapter, illustrates some of the points raised by Falkner in his coverage of measures of growth and maturity of children (Chapter 7.1). It focuses on the monitoring of the individual child's development over time by means of a weight-for-age chart, and emphasizes how these charts may be used to stimulate community involvement in the promotion of children's health and to provide summary measurements related to populations as well as to individuals. The chart presented here is of similar design to the WHO growth chart described by Falkner, and serves the same function. The chapter includes a discussion of features of chart design which should be considered in order to increase the usefulness and acceptability of such charts.

Is this child well nourished? Are the children in this community well nourished? Have they been immunized? What sicknesses have they had in the past? Growth charts are one means of answering these questions, so that the mother and the community health worker are able to identify the actions that need to be taken. The growth chart, as a home-based record, enables the mother to monitor her child's growth more accurately and more comprehensively. At the same time, the fact that the recording process is carried out by the community health worker stimulates contacts between the health worker and the mother on a regular basis, and not just when the child is ill. Growth charts also play an effective motivational and educational role in promoting child health as part of a primary health care approach.

The serial weighing and the recording of weight on weight-for-age charts is the most commonly used method of monitoring and supervising the growth of young children, as it is the most sensitive method of identifying those with nutrition and health problems.

Weight-for-age charts give a graphic representation of a child's weight according to age (Fig. 1). They can provide reliable data for evaluating specific interventions by individual families or health workers. In addition, where there is adequate coverage (80% or more of the children having well maintained weight charts), the charts can be used to monitor the level of growth on a community-wide basis and to evaluate the local and regional effectiveness of programmes *(1)*.

Fig. 1. Chart produced by Teaching Aids at Low Cost, United Kingdom.

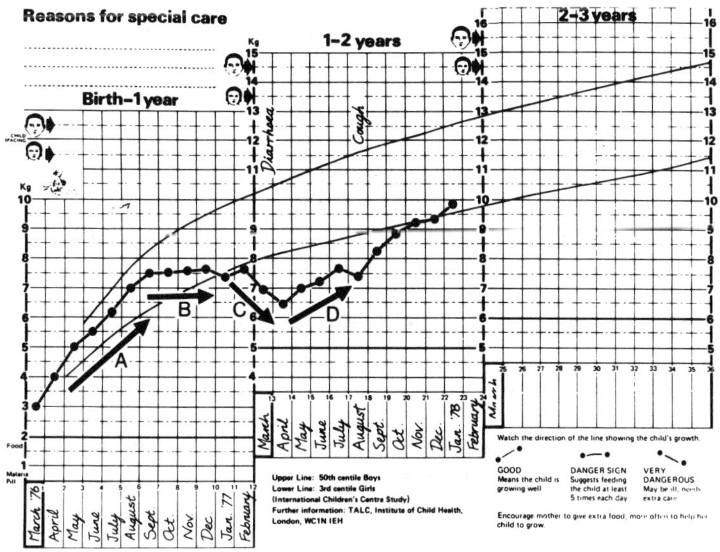

Note. This chart shows the use of heavily lined boxes for the child's birth month; the labelling and completion of the month boxes; the clarity of plotting the child's weight in the spaces, rather than on the vertical lines; the emphasis on the direction of the child's growth curve; and the usefulness of writing health problems, such as diarrhoea, on the chart so as to produce a graphic picture of the child's health and growth

Benefits of Using Growth Charts

At the individual and family level, charts provide a picture of a child's growth (with emphasis on the direction of the growth curve rather than on the child's weight in relation to any particular standard), and of the child's state of health in terms of nutritional and disease status.

The growth chart aims to be an educational tool for helping families to understand how diet and preventive health measures affect children's health, as well as a tool for motivating families to implement dietary and other changes if necessary. It also serves as a means of reassuring mothers that their children are doing well and are well cared for. The emphasis on the growth chart being kept by the mother underlines her vital function in the care of her child.

The growth chart should provide clear guidelines as to what is normal and what is abnormal growth, which children are at risk, which children need routine care and which need special care, and what preventive measures should be taken, and when (e.g. immunization).

Growth charts also provide a means of assessing the health status of a community in a form which can be fairly easily understood, so that everyone can be involved in deciding on appropriate interventions. As the charts are home-based, community groups can assess the health care they are receiving and cooperate with the health workers.

On a wider level, growth charts can provide reliable data for evaluating specific interventions at the community or regional level *(1)*. Their analysis will also enable health services to determine which children within a community are especially vulnerable and which can be helped, in such a way that limited resources can be directed towards those most in need.

Basic Components of Weight-for-Age Growth Charts

The basic components of growth charts may be summarized as:

(*a*) the *graph* on which a child's weight can be plotted against his age; on this graph there are usually a number of curves representing reference standards (see Fig. 1);

(*b*) *personal details:* the child's name, registration number and sex, the parents' names and address, and birth date;

(*c*) *potential risk factors or reasons for special care:* birth weight, problems calling for special care, and history of sibling health;

(*d*) *use of health services:* date first seen, immunization record and national schedule for immunizations;

(*e*) *other key factors which may affect growth:* breastfeeding, weaning diet, and child spacing;

(*f*) *other possible components:* treatment of diarrhoea and other common illnesses.

Using the Chart

Recording the child's age

On the child's first visit to a clinic, the health worker records the child's month of birth in each of the heavily lined boxes. Subsequent months are then written in by hand (Fig. 1).

Even if the exact date of birth is not known, a reasonable estimate can be made and used at each weighing. Thus the relative dates of different weighings are preserved and a useful observation of growth is obtained.

Interpreting the growth curve

This can be difficult, even for highly qualified staff. Growth reference lines have value in that they illustrate the shape of a child's growth curve. Almost any centile curve is equally useful, as the curves of centiles have essentially the same shape in all countries. Although many countries consider it desirable to use their own standards, there is little difference between the "elite" of different countries during their growth, and so the use of national standards does not bring many advantages.

In the past, the interpretation of the growth chart has concentrated upon a child's weight for its age at a particular point in time. Medical nutritionists now consider that a single weight-for-age measurement is a poor method of assessing a child's nutritional status. The present emphasis is thus upon the direction of the child's growth curve (Fig. 2 and 3) *(2)*. This is helpful for health workers, many of whom have difficulty in interpreting a child's growth. Often there has been a failure to recognize that a drop of 1 kg between the standard curves puts a child more at risk than a growth curve which runs parallel to, but just below, the third centile line.

Graphic presentation of a child's health

In addition to representing a child's growth by means of a growth curve, it is possible to give a graphic picture of the complex relationships between a child's diet, illnesses, social background and the birth interval, by writing on the chart, against the appropriate month, the relevant diseases or other factors, as in Fig. 1.

Marking appropriate boxes (see Fig. 4) to indicate specific problems is quick and simple and serves as a permanent reminder to the health worker of the questions to be asked to identify risk factors, particularly when a child is

Fig. 2. Three "growth curves" emphasizing the need to identify the cause of poor weight gain, the importance of showing the chart when talking to mothers and health workers, and the need for the health worker to explain the child's growth curve to the mother

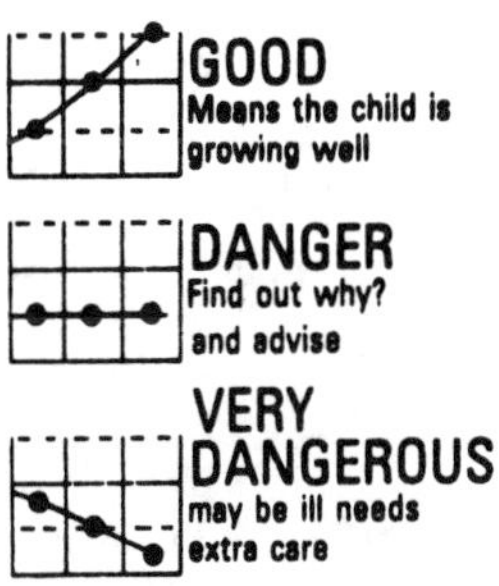
GOOD
Means the child is growing well
DANGER
Find out why? and advise
VERY DANGEROUS
may be ill needs extra care

Fig. 3. Three growth charts encouraging the mother to give extra food more often to help her child to grow

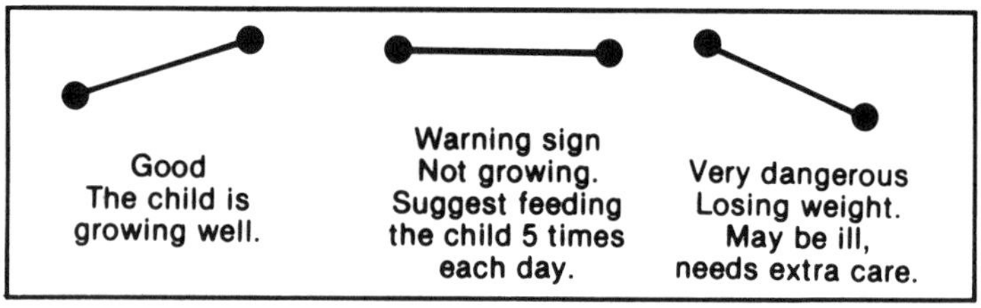
Good
The child is growing well.
Warning sign
Not growing.
Suggest feeding the child 5 times each day.
Very dangerous
Losing weight.
May be ill, needs extra care.

first seen at a clinic. However, the risk factors chosen must be appropriate for the area and the country.

In the first three months of life, particular emphasis needs to be placed on the 2.5 kg line, to draw attention to infants with a low birth weight and their progress in gaining weight during this period.

Many charts leave some space for recording the treatment provided, but this space is inadequate, especially as large writing is common to those whose level of literacy is low. Charts may be supplied with a separate treatment card. This is appropriate as it does not detract from the main message of the growth chart, which may otherwise become only a treatment record card.

Most charts allocate a space for immunizations on the reverse side of the growth chart or even (preferably) on the chart itself (Fig. 5). This provides a constant reminder and record not only for the health worker, but also for the mother, regardless of her level of literacy.

Fig. 4. List of risk factors

Reasons for special care	
Birth weight less than 2.5 kg	☐
Brothers or sisters undernourished	☐
Birth less than 2 years after last birth	☐
Twins	☐
3 or more children in family died	☐
Unsupported parent	☐

Fig. 5. Immunization illustrations on growth chart to remind mothers and health workers

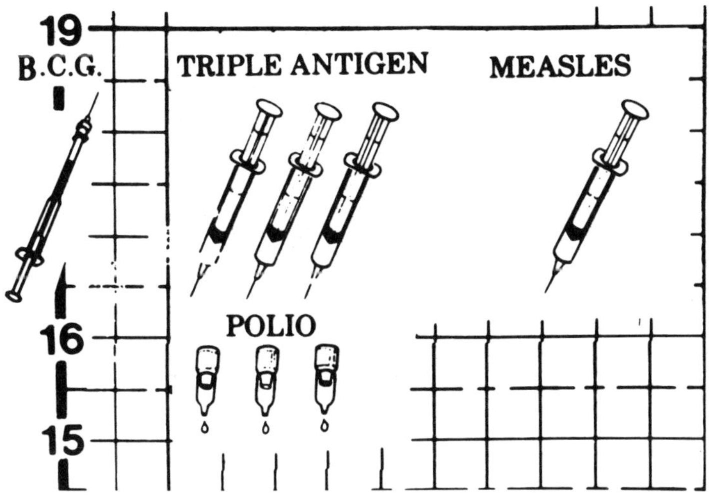

Many charts allocate space to record information on, for instance, breastfeeding, malaria prophylaxis, weaning practices, administration of deworming drugs, etc.

A simple record of birth spacing attitudes and practices can serve as a constant educational tool, and needs to be completed every month. However, some societies and persons find it unacceptable for their methods of contraception to be entered on the child's chart.

Use of the Growth Chart in Community Studies: the Malawi Example

Malawi is one of the poorest countries in Africa. It is, however, one of perhaps five countries (the others being Botswana, the Gambia, Lesotho and St Lucia) where clinic services and the use of charts are believed to have spread so widely that they are now available to over 75% of all children. This rapid improvement in Malawi was due in large measure to cooperation betwen voluntary agencies and government services.

As part of this development, a new record system was introduced, consisting of a simple register on a single sheet of paper (Fig. 6). The information was extracted from this for local use and also sent to a central statistical office for analysis. Great care was taken to ensure that the recording and reporting systems were as simple as possible. Before the systems were developed, they had been discussed with the people using them, so that accurate and useful data could be collected without undue expenditure of staff time.

Fig. 6. Part of an under-fives clinic attendance form

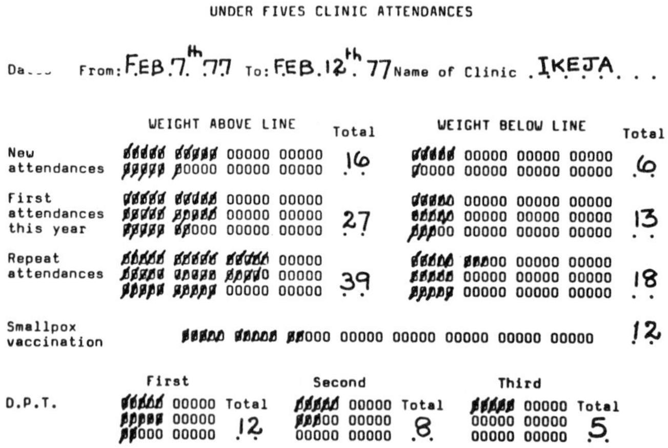

UNDER FIVES CLINIC ATTENDANCES

Da... From: FEB. 7th. 77 To: FEB. 12th. 77 Name of Clinic . IKEJA . . .

	WEIGHT ABOVE LINE Total	WEIGHT BELOW LINE Total
New attendances	16	6
First attendances this year	27	13
Repeat attendances	39	18
Smallpox vaccination		12

	First Total	Second Total	Third Total
D.P.T.	12	8	5

Note. A tally system is used and children whose weights fall below the lower line are recorded separately from those above it. Unlike most tally systems, this also records children seen on the first attendance in each calendar year. This is important, as the number of children receiving care from the clinic during the year can then be discovered.

The data on the sheet illustrated in Fig. 6 have many uses. The most valuable information is the proportion of all children attending the clinic who fall below the lower line. This is a most sensitive measure of nutritional state, as it varies even from month to month, according to the nutritional state of the children.

Establishing the proportion of children below the line will help to identify districts in most need of development, to measure the effects of crop failure and to evaluate the impact of any new development programme.

Instead of numbers being tallied according to "weight above line" or "weight below line", they may be tallied by "weight gain" or "weight loss". This method may have a slight advantage, in that it shows immediately the onset of famine in an area, but it has the disadvantage that the nutritional state of children attending different clinics cannot easily be compared.

Other Ways of Collecting Group Data

There are many simple ways of summarizing weight-for-age data as indicators of the nutritional status of a community or a group within it. For a single clinic, the following method is suggested.

1. The health worker responsible for making entries on individual weight charts is given additional training.

2. The health worker takes a separate weight chart, and writes on it "Clinic summary for [date]".

3. Then, as well as recording every weight on an individual weight chart, the health worker enters the identical weight on the clinic summary weight chart, and thus records all the weighings made in one day on the single summary chart (see Fig. 7). Separate charts should be used for males and females.

4. It is fairly simple to calculate the number of weights below the lower line as a proportion of the total weights recorded. If the standard chart is used, special plastic overlays are available from Teaching Aids at Low Cost (TALC), P.O. Box 49, St Albans, Herts AL1 4AX, United Kingdom.

Fig. 7. Chart showing weights of girls attending a clinic over a period of one week

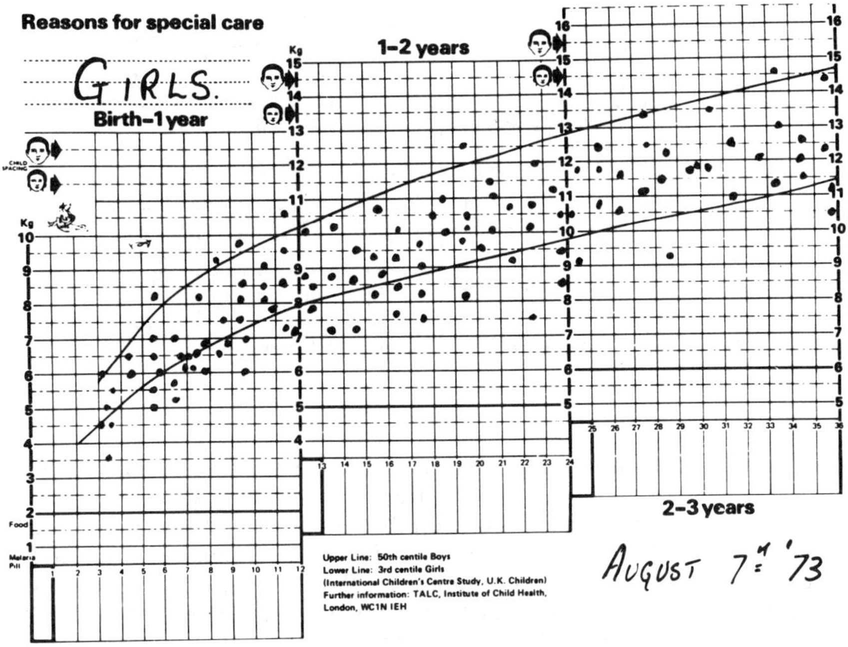

Note. A plastic overlay sheet (available from TALC, see text) can also be used to identify the number of girls below a certain standard.

Layout and Design

In order to make the chart as clear as possible, it is important to have all the information relating to the child's health and growth, including the child's name, immunization status, risk factors and disease problems on one side of the chart. The chart in Fig. 8 comes nearest to doing this, but it does not show immunizations. Also, some workers find that the use of a single line does not give enough guidance.

Fig. 8. Chart bringing together most of the essential information relating to a child's health, growth, risk factors and disease problems but excluding immunization status

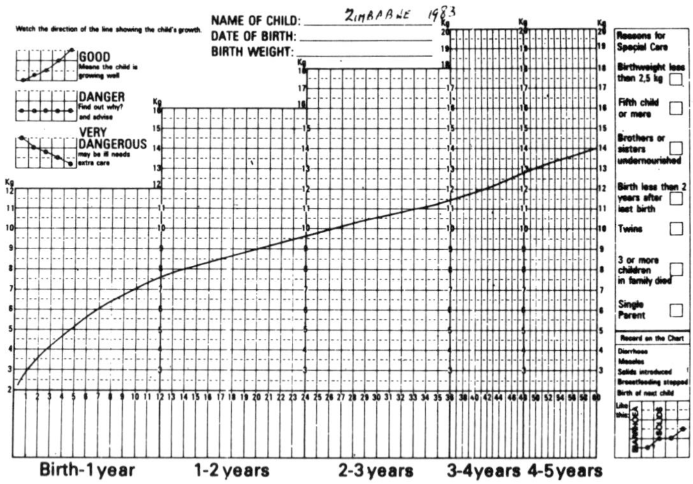

Health workers find it easier when each of the months is numbered. It may be clearer if all the years, i.e. 0–5, are presented on one side of the chart rather than years 4 and 5 appearing on the reverse side. However, placing years 4 and 5 on the reverse side does leave more space for details of the first 3 years to be written clearly and, as these are the key years, this is the layout most commonly adopted. It is much simpler to have the same chart for boys and girls than to have a different one for each sex.

Cards must be not only attractive but acceptable. A surprisingly large number of cards contain pictures, such as that reproduced in Fig. 9, which stigmatize mothers with malnourished children.

Charts that are attractive and well designed are more likely to be neatly completed and kept with pride by both the mother and the health worker. The most attractive charts are either yellow or white, with a glossy finish (which protects the chart from dirty fingerprints). Such yellow or white charts, with red or green printing, allow the worker's writing (usually in pencil or blue or black pen) to stand out clearly in contrast.

Fig. 9. Does it help to criticize mothers of malnourished children like this?

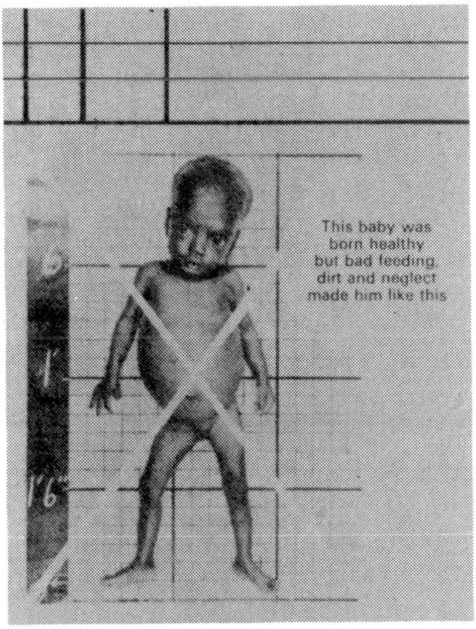

It is important to take into account the cultural significance of different colours when designing the charts. In western countries we have learned that red indicates danger while green signifies "go ahead, there are no problems", as in our traffic-light system. In many Asian countries, red would be more appropriate to signify health and green would be regarded as unfavourable.

Most charts are printed on cards of adequate thickness to withstand five years of handling, provided that they are protected in plastic bags. These plastic bags should be at least 2 cm wider and 5 cm longer than the folded card. Some cards are made of plasticized paper. This material cannot be torn, can be written on, is easily cleaned, and does not require a protective plastic bag. When mass-produced, such cards cost 40% more than those made of cardboard; however, there may be savings, particularly as plastic bags would not be required.

The size of charts is most important. A4 size (210 mm × 297 mm) would appear to be the most satisfactory in terms of economy and ease of use. Larger cards are often attractive. However, they are more easily damaged, as they are more likely to be folded for easier carrying — or they may not be carried at all. In addition, these large cards take up too much space on a table which may already be crowded with medicines, etc.

Challenges to the Effective Use of Growth Charts

Weight-for-age growth charts are not easy to understand and use; both doctors and persons with relatively little formal education have difficulties in using them. Those responsible for designing cards should consider the needs and level of understanding of less experienced workers rather than of doctors. The layout, especially of the graph, should be as clear and as simple as possible, but even the simplest designs are not always easy to grasp and require substantial training, especially in relation to the charting of the child's weight. Appropriate training materials need to be developed for this purpose *(3)*. Some, such as a flannelgraph series ("Teaching nutrition in the savannah of West Africa", six flannelgraphs by Gill Gordon), a set of slides ("Charting children's growth", by D. Morley, F. Savage and H.J. Lovel) and a book on the use of growth charts *(2)* are available from TALC at the address given on page 551.

Many clinic workers find it difficult to adjust to the use of a record card which is home-based and "belongs" to the mother rather than to the clinic.

In order to develop a clear picture of a child's growth and development, a long-term commitment is necessary on the part of the mother, so that she brings her child in regularly for weighing. A reciprocal commitment is required on the part of the health personnel, namely, to provide services which are credible, acceptable and readily available, and to share information with the family. The growth chart is one means by which the mother can be made to feel that her child is welcomed by the health worker and the health care system; for her it is a "passport" to health for her children.

Some of these problems are outside the scope of this paper, but the use of a clear, simple and well structured growth chart can help to overcome some of them. A chart that cannot be understood will not be used.

References

1. *How are the children growing? Collection and analysis of weight-for-age data growth charts about groups of children.* New York, UNICEF, 1982.
2. **Morley, D. & Woodland, M.** *See how they grow – monitoring child growth for appropriate health care in developing countries.* London, Macmillan, 1979, p. 27.
3. **Lovel, H.J. et al.** How mothers measure growth. Community dimensions for expanded growth monitoring in Ghana. *Assignment children,* **65/68**: 275–291 (1984).

12.3 Positive health status measurement and clinical application — *M.E. Harnly & G.Z. Williams*

As discussed by Goldberg & Dab in Chapter 7.5, there have been many attempts to construct complex indices of health status. The next example includes an attempt to derive a single *index measure through the use of a "health profile questionnaire". This is a self-administered questionnaire, information from which is used to derive seven different health scales relating to medical events, general wellbeing (perceived health), psychological wellbeing, physical activity, nutrition, alcohol use and smoking. An overall health status score is obtained by a combination of the seven scales. The authors give detailed examples of how the particular health category scales derived may be used in health counselling at an individual level. There may, however, be reservations about the technical complexity of the methods described in this chapter and how this may affect the extension of such measurements to communities and the usefulness of the approach in different surroundings.*

At the Institute of Health Research, San Francisco, chemical and haematological constituents of serum are measured and information on lifestyles and health history is collected annually in a non-infirm population of 2000. The primary objective in collecting this information is to study the health of the non-infirm individual and to determine whether, in the absence of disease, changes in good or "positive" health are reflected in serum constituents. To address this specific question, it was first necessary to define gradations in health by developing a quantitative and valid method for measuring positive health status. More generally, however, the measurement of positive health status enhances the process of health evaluation and health improvement. In the clinical setting, health measurements provide consistent and quantitative health evaluations and therefore a framework for intervention advice and procedures.

To measure health status, one must decide what data should be incorporated in the measurement. There is much speculation in medical literature over what constitutes positive health. While there are established definitions for death and specific diseases, which may be verified physiologically, the concept of optimum health cannot be tested in the same way. In the absence of a consistent, precise definition, it was necessary to accumulate a wide range of questionnaire data which might prove to be descriptive of healthy functioning. Professional expertise and a review of available health questionnaires indicated that the appropriate range of responses would be encompassed by collecting information in seven areas: medical events, general wellbeing (perceived health), psychological wellbeing, physical activity, nutrition, alcohol use and smoking.

To collect this information, a self-administered questionnaire, the health profile questionnaire, was devised. Each question in the health profile questionnaire attempts to produce the maximum amount of information while minimizing the time required to respond. For example, in the physical activity section the respondent is asked to identify which of 58 sports he/she performs and then, for each sport performed, to state how long and how often the sport is performed and if he/she competes. The questionnaire has a total of 117 questions which convert during data processing to 1334 separate variables. The methods described here were developed to consolidate these variables into measurements of health status. Major modification of the initial method was necessary to generate measurements that were valid for the individual and therefore clinically useful.

Health Status Measurement

To make a precise evaluation of an individual's positive health status on the basis of questionnaire data, scales must be established, i.e. an algorithm is established for converting an individual's many responses into one number, a score that positions the individual on a numerical health continuum or scale. The scale has an established range: low scores reflect low health status and high scores reflect high health status and, by implication, an optimum or high level of positive health. To preserve the integrity of the health profile questionnaire data and for the sake of conceptual simplicity, one scale was established for each of the seven health categories. Having separate health category scales allows health to be evaluated on the basis of each category alone. Ultimately, the seven health scale scores may be combined in one overall health status score, which could reflect the overall positive health status of an individual.

Establishing an algorithm for converting questionnaire responses into health category scale scores requires that each questionnaire item or variable, e.g. cigarette smoking, be assigned a numerical weight (item weight) representing the item's importance to health status in relation to all other items in the particular health category scale. If an item merits more than a yes/no response, e.g. the number of packs of cigarettes smoked per day, then numerical weights (response weights) must also be assigned to each response level within an item. Once item and response weights have been established, the algorithm for converting questionnaire responses into health category scale scores consists of matching a respondent's answers with the response weights, multiplying these response weights by their corresponding item weights, and then summing the products across all items in the particular scale category.

The assignment of item and response health weights is a difficult task, due to the absence of a reference point or a definition of optimum health. There are reports of weight designations for questionnaire responses relative to the risk of death or specific disease *(1)*. Such an approach incorporates responses that are unrelated to positive health status, e.g. wearing a seat belt while driving. Weighting relative to death or specific disease could not serve, in the authors' judgement, as a substitute for establishing weights relative to optimum health. A review of the literature revealed three types of method that can be adapted for health weighting: equal weighting, preference judgement and the indicator method. These three methods have been used, for the most part, in weighting illness symptoms relative to healthy functioning.

The first method, equal weighting, sidesteps the task of health weight assignment, assuming that each item contributes equally (e.g. the Cornell Medical Index *(2)*). The second method, preference judgement, relies on a panel of health professionals to rate each item in proportion to the degree that, in their opinion, it contributes to health *(3,4)*. According to this method, healthy functioning is defined by professional judgement. Because the weights generated depend on the expertise and experience of the judges, they vary greatly *(5)* and may or may not reflect a contribution to physiological health. The third approach, the indicator method, uses statistical methodology and an independent measure of health status to establish health weights. For example, Chambers et al. used discriminate function analysis to establish weights for physical symptoms in proportion to the symptom's ability to differentiate groups of healthy and unhealthy individuals as assessed by physicians *(6)*.

The health profile questionnaire item and response health weights were generated by a combination of preference judgement and the indicator method. This procedure is unique and innovative, because a physiological definition of healthy functioning is used not only to establish item weights (the indicator method), but also to validate and refine the response rates within each item which were initially based on the judgement of a four-member panel. Details of the methods used have been documented *(7)*.

Unfortunately, these methods generated scale scores which were neither statistically nor conceptually accurate when applied to individuals who had not been used for weight establishment. If the scale scores calculated for these new respondents could statistically differentiate the healthy/unhealthy dichotomy, then the scoring procedures could be considered statistically valid. The results of this analysis were not uniform. The overall health scale and three of the seven health category scales, notably lifestyle scales — physical activity, alcohol use and nutrition — could make this differentiation at a statistically significant level ($P < 0.01$). This result substantiated the item and response weighting procedures. However, four of the scales — smoking, general wellbeing, psychological wellbeing and medical events — could not make this differentiation, were not statistically valid and should theoretically be eliminated. Elimination of these scales was not a feasible option; health measurements or evaluations based on the three health habit scales alone would obviously be inaccurate. Furthermore, discriminate function analysis indicated that 45 out of 62 items should be eliminated from the scales. As a result, the generated scale scores had little variability and therefore did not measure the range of positive health that had been conceptualized. For example, there remained one item in the general wellbeing scale: "Do you generally feel healthy?". Because 88% of participants reported that they did feel healthy, they received the same high general wellbeing score. Because accurate scores could not be generated for each individual, scale scores calculated using the established weights could not be used clinically.

Despite the inaccuracy displayed by the scale scores, computer-generated reports that list the individual question responses in English have been invaluable clinically, although they are somewhat unwieldy. Preliminary data analysis has revealed that particular health habits, e.g. cigarette smoking, are correlated with specific chemical constituents. Given this direct confirmation of the health profile questionnaire's utility, it has been decided to modify the health weight establishment procedures and perform them again. Modifications are being made to include additional physiological factors such as percentage of body fat, heart rate and blood pressure response to graded bicycle ergometric stress, and pulmonary vital capacity and forced expiratory volume. These additional data should generate more valid scoring algorithms. Collection of the physiological data is complete and analyses are in progress.

Clinical Application

While collection of more comprehensive data is in progress, a mechanism for providing the participant with health evaluation is needed. After an individual has completed an annual test series, even though participating in a study, he/she is entitled to a professional interpretation of the results in an understandable format. Because health status scale scores and corresponding ranges provide the participant with this information in a consistent and efficient manner, the health scale methodology was reviewed for alternative health weighting procedures that would allow interim health status scores to be calculated. The response weights that reflected professional expertise (preference weights) were appropriate for clinical use. What had not been determined was whether these weights, when used together and in conjunction with item weights, had a valid relationship to a physiological definition of healthy functioning. The preference weights are, in fact, partially validated, in that the weights within each item are correlated with physiological health. Thus, health scores generated by the use of preference weights would, at the minimum, present a professional interpretation of an individual's health status in a quantitative and consistent manner.

To obtain scale scores utilizing preference judgement response weights, an individual's responses within a scale category are matched to the corresponding preference weights, and these weights are then summed into a scale score. Summing of the preference response weights assumes that the judges not only weighted each item relative to other responses in the same item but also relative to other responses in other items of the category. After summing of the preference weights, the scales are transformed (adding a constant and then multiplying by another constant) in such a way that all scales have a range of 1 to 100. A computer-generated output that displays the scale scores and ranges is given to the participant (see Fig. 1).

Presentation of this output to the participant has been useful during health counselling. Scale scores, supplemented by the computer-generated

Fig. 1. Computer-generated output displaying scale scores and ranges

```
UPDATE  HEALTH INDEX: SUMMARIZES EVENTS  SINCE YOUR FIRST TEST SERIES

NAME: WALTER X. NNNN      SSN: 599nnnnnn  DATE: 2/18/86    UPDATE #:4

                             HEALTH STATUS
                       HEALTH ZONE            RISK ZONE        DANGER
======================================================================
MEDICAL EVENTS: 100                    95                    82
  12/77: 90       |                     |        *           |
   2/79: 96       |                  *  |                     |
   1/80: 96       |                  *  |                     |
   2/81: 99       | *                   |                     |
   2/82: 46       |                     |                     |     *

GENERAL WELLNESS:100                   80                    70
  12/77: 85       |               *     |                     |
   2/79: 85       |               *     |                     |
   1/80: 90       |         *           |                     |
   2/81: 92       |       *             |                     |
   2/82: 75       |                     |          *          |

PSYCH WELLNESS  100                    83                    58
  12/77: 76.9     |                     |   *                 |
   2/79: 77.7     |                     |  *                  |
   1/80: 88.4     |               *     |                     |
   2/81: 86.8     |                 *   |                     |
   2/82: 88.4     |               *     |                     |
======================================================================


UPDATE HEALTH INDEX:  SUMMARIZES LIFESTYLE HABITS  SINCE FIRST SERIES

NAME:  WALTER X. NNNN      SSN: 599nnnnnn   DATE: 2/18/86   UPDATE #4

                            HEALTH HABITS

                     HEALTH ZONE           RISK ZONE        DANGER
======================================================================
NUTRITION:    100                    70                    56
  12/77: 66     |                     |    *               |
   2/79: 62     |                     |            *       |
   1/80: 64     |                     |        *           |
   2/81: 64     |                     |        *           |
   2/82: 60     |                     |                 *  |

TOBACCO:      100                    95                    87
  12/77: 100    *                     |                    |
   2/79: 100    *                     |                    |
   1/80: 100    *                     |                    |
   2/81: 100    *                     |                    |
   2/82: 100    *                     |                    |

ALCOHOL:      100                    72                    44
  12/77:  44    |                     |                    *
   2/79:  48    |                     |                 *  |
   1/80:  48    |                     |                 *  |
   2/81:  46    |                     |                  * |
   2/82:  98    | *                   |                    |

PHYSICAL ACTIVITY:
             100                     48                    24
  12/77:  47.8  |                     *                    |
   2/79:  48.4  |                     *                    |
   1/80:  82.2  |    *                |                    |
   2/81:  77.8  |       *             |                    |
   2/82:  18.4  |                     |                    |    **
======================================================================
```

listing of questionnaire responses, allow the health counsellor to identify readily areas that need improvement. The authors' experience in personal interviews with participants is that a large majority have been stimulated to modify habits by the act of responding to the questionnaire and by the presentation and interpretation of the scale scores. Further, the graphic display of annual results allows both improvement and undesirable trends to be easily visualized and recognized. Improvement in scores year by year reinforces the participant's determination to further improve his/her health habits.

Presentation of raw scores to the participant often generated a request for a verbal interpretation of the scale scores, analogous to a request for the interpretation of a glucose or cholesterol value. Initially, this query was answered with percentiles. However, the use of percentiles led to erroneous interpretations. For example, many participants jog and therefore those who jog 10–15 miles a week rank in the 50th percentile of the study population. Presentation of this percentile often leads the participant to the erroneous conclusion that he/she is half-way to ideal exercise habits. As an alternative, scores were grouped, on the basis of professional judgement, into healthy/risk/danger zones. (These zones are shown in Fig. 1.) Scale scores that fall into the danger zone are considered to indicate potentially harmful habits and lifestyles and the need for immediate intervention; those scores that fall into the risk zone indicate that the participant might benefit from a modification of habits and lifestyles; and scale scores that fall into the healthy zone indicate ideal health habits and status. It is explained to the participant that the zone limits are not absolute and are for general guidance.

The participant is also presented with a linear record of the annual serum test results. This chronological display may reveal trends which, if they persist, may indicate developing pathology. Such progressive changes call for intervention with a view to reversing or stabilizing the digression. When intervention leads to modifications in health habits, and these changes are subsequently documented in scale scores and reflected in laboratory test results, the participant is motivated and reinforced to continue the health habit modification. For example, a female participant, B.E., at entry into the health profile programme, possessed test results and scale scores that were within the established healthy zones. Domestic stress caused increased alcohol consumption. Her serum gamma-glutamyl transferase (GGT) rose gradually from 29 to 50. The graphic display of progressive intolerance by her liver (high GGT values) and an explanation of the probable consequences motivated her to reduce her alcohol intake substantially; this, in turn, started lowering the enzyme (see Table 1). Observation of this encouraging effect caused her to virtually abstain and the GGT is returning to her previous normal values.

Two further examples of participants' health scale scores and serum test results are given in Table 2. B.W., at entry, smoked, ate heavily, and was sedentary except for spurts of intense activity in his job (fire-fighting). Two years after entry he had stopped smoking, improved his diet, reduced his alcohol consumption, and had started running five days a week. The second

Table 1. A participant's yearly GGT[a] values and health scale scores

Year	GGT U/L	Health category scale score[b]				
		Alcohol use	Psychological wellbeing	General wellbeing	Nutrition	Exercise
1977	29	70	60	70	30	40
1978	50	50	40	30	20	40
1979	44	90	70	40	60	90
1980	27	86	72	82	62	72
1981	38	87	65	57	60	97

[a] GGT = gamma-glutamyl transferase.

[b] Scores are based on the scale 0–100; lower scores indicate low health status, i.e. high alcohol intake, high stress, low health perception and little exercise. Note that high alcohol intake precedes high GGT values.

Table 2. Examples of participants' yearly health scale scores and test results

Participant	Date	Health scale score[a]			Serum test results	
		Exercise	Alcohol	Nutrition	Serum cholesterol (mg/dl)	Triglycerides (mg/dl)
B.W.	March 1977	27	68	58	225	160
	October 1979	100	87	60	172	74
	November 1980	100	87	68	185	98
A.T.	April 1979	90	10	60	227	97
	April 1980	40	30	30	244	112
	May 1981	0	46	56	289	154
	May 1982	13	68	56	324	199

[a] Scores are based on the scale 0–100 for no exercise to vigorous exercise, poor to excellent nutrition, and high alcohol consumption to absention.

example illustrates the opposite trend: rising cholesterol and triglycerides due to a reduction in exercise and improper nutrition. A.T., a 43-year-old male, is being strongly advised to correct the hazardous levels in his blood fats by means of appropriate modifications in his diet and exercise habits.

Conclusion

Different methods of assigning health weights to questionnaire items and responses have been presented. One method has been adapted for health status evaluation as stipulated by professional expertise. Only by the consistent application of quantitative measures can time-related trends be identified and professional evaluation be kept uniform. Weights may be modified to reflect new knowledge and to allow for different professional opinions. Computer-generated reports allow response weights to be modified easily and consistently in past questionnaire responses.

Acknowledgements

Anne M. Seifert guided the development and structure of the questionnaire. Allan Bostrom, University of California, San Francisco, developed the statistical analyses. This research was partially supported by a grant from the Institute of General Medical Sciences, National Institutes of Health.

References

1. **Hall, J.H. & Zwemer, J.D.** *Prospective medicine.* Indianapolis, Methodist Hospital of Indiana, 1979.
2. **Brodman, K. et al.** The Cornell Medical Index. *Journal of the American Medical Association,* **140**: 530 (1949).
3. **Gilson, B.S. et al.** The sickness impact profile: development of an outcome measure of health care. *American journal of public health,* **65**(12): 1304 (1975).
4. **Patrick, D.L. et al.** Methods for measuring levels of well-being for a health status index. *Health services research,* **8**: 228–245 (1973).
5. **Blischke, W.R. et al.** Successive intervals analysis of preference measures in a health status index. *Health services research,* **10**: 181–198 (1975).
6. **Chambers, L.W. et al.** The development and application of indexes of health: general methods and a summary of results. *American journal of public health,* **67**: 423–428 (1977).
7. **Williams, G.Z. & Harnly, M.E.** Health status and health habits assessment. *Medical informatics,* **7**(3): 197–204 (1982).

13. Applications in research and development of methods

13.1 Retrospective determination of a child survival ratio suited to Third World situations — *D.H.J. Blom*

Demographic indicators used in developing countries tend to be difficult to collect and calculate, however simple the underlying concept (e.g. infant mortality). They also tend to rely on direct measurement of mortality. The indicator proposed here has the conceptual advantage of measuring survival, and the practical advantage of being relatively simple to calculate. It should be noted that the index described suffers from a drawback in the form of its dependency on the age of the mother, which limits its use for comparisons between women with different levels of gravidity. It should, however, still prove useful for comparisons between different locations and across time.

With the introduction of primary health care programmes in many areas of the Third World, there is an increasing need for indicators of the health situation in the populations concerned. In particular, indicators based on easily obtainable data are required, that can be used to assess needs prior to the introduction of programmes and, subsequently, to evaluate the impact of programmes. As many primary health care programmes focus on reducing infant and child mortality, there is a special need for indicators of child survival. The problem is that in many areas reliable data on vital statistics are not available, so that other sources of information have to be used. This chapter presents a method for the construction of a "child survival index" based on information obtained from mothers. It was originally developed for use in antenatal clinics, but was later extended to include data from village surveys as well. An earlier version of a child survival index based on the same data was published previously.[a]

The Child Survival Ratio

Antenatal clinic data usually include information about the number of past pregnancies of each woman, as well as the number of children still alive. The difference between the two figures represents the number of pregnancies that resulted in death. If only live births are asked for, deaths include neonatal deaths, infant deaths and deaths in childhood. If all pregnancies are considered, deaths include, in addition, abortions and stillbirths.

The survival ratio is determined by dividing, for each group of women who have the same number of previous pregnancies, the mean number of their children alive at the time of the interview by the number of previous pregnancies (or births). This ratio describes the survival experience of products of conception or of children born in the population of women attending the antenatal clinic during a period of time. If attendance rates at antenatal clinics are high, the ratio can be expected to reflect the population experience rather reliably.

When information based on clinic data is not representative, the same method of construction of survival ratio can also be applied on the basis of information gained in field interviews with samples of mothers.

Preliminary Results

The method has been applied to the maternity data of a district hospital in Zambia. The results are given in Table 1.

The table shows an increase in the mean number of children from the first to the second period, probably indicating better attendance at the antenatal clinic by older women in the second period. As other information suggests, about 50% of the women attended a clinic at least once in the first period, compared with about 75% in the second period. At about the same time, a survey was conducted among women in a group of villages some 25 km from the hospital and in a control group of women visiting the hospital antenatal and under-fives clinics. The material included gravidity status, allowing the number of previous pregnancies and numbers of children alive to be determined. These are shown in Table 2.

Both tables should be regarded only as an illustration of the calculation method and for several reasons (e.g. small sample sizes and lack of representativeness) they do not permit valid conclusions to be drawn about the health status of this particular population.

---

[a] **Blom, D.H.J.** Objective indicators of health in Western Zambia. *Social science and medicine,* **15B**: 395–398 (1981).

Table 1. Child survival ratio for women giving birth at the district hospital, June 1973 – December 1974 and January 1975 – May 1976

No. of previous pregnancies	June 1973 – December 1974				January 1975 – May 1976			
	No. of women	No. of children alive	Mean no. of children alive	Survival ratio (%)	No. of women	No. of children alive	Mean no of children alive	Survival ratio (%)
0	111	—	—		119	—	—	
1	87	68	0.8	78.2	71	64	0.9	90.1
2	56	88	1.6	78.6	64	111	1.7	86.7
3	58	139	2.4	79.9	59	139	2.4	78.5
4	49	146	3.0	74.5	53	171	3.2	80.7
5	38	149	3.9	78.4	49	215	4.4	87.8
6 or more	86	442	5.1	—	70	432	6.2	—
Total	485	1032			485	1132		

Table 2. Child survival ratio for women attending a hospital clinic, compared with village women

No. of previous pregnancies	Hospital clinic group				Village women			
	No. of women	No. of children alive	Mean no. of children alive	Survival ratio (%)	No. of women	No. of children alive	Mean no. of children alive	Survival ratio (%)
0	42	—	—		—	—	—	
1	43	33	0.8	76.7	3	3	1.0	100.0
2	41	60	1.5	73.2	7	9	1.3	64.3
3	27	52	1.9	64.2	20	48	2.4	80.0
4	22	72	3.3	81.8	10	29	2.9	72.5
5	22	86	3.9	78.2	19	71	3.7	74.7
6 or more	51	279	5.5	—	22	101	4.6	—
Total	248	582			81	261		

Discussion

The child survival ratio described here allows for insights into pregnancy outcome and infant and child survival based on data that can be easily obtained in antenatal clinics and cross-sectional interview surveys. Of course, its reliability depends on whether the women can remember their pregnancies, distinguish between their own and other women's children, and count the number of children alive. Any local taboos on giving information about one's children will also affect the reliability of results. It is obviously essential that the person asking the questions should fulfil such conditions as speaking the local language and belonging to the right tribal group.

Although the survival ratio reflects child survival rather directly, care has to be taken not to allow erroneous conclusions. Only information for women with the same parity should be compared, unless a parity-corrected survival ratio is computed. And even if parity is comparable, the age of the woman plays a role, because children of older women will most probably be older and have been at risk of dying for a longer time than children of younger women. Secondly, as the survival ratio is based on information supplied by the mothers, it will not take into account the survival experience of children whose mothers have died. As these children usually have a poorer prognosis than children whose mothers are alive, the survival ratio can be expected to overestimate the child survival experience of the entire population.

The survival ratio as presented in Tables 1 and 2 refers to all pregnancies, including those ending in abortion or stillbirth. As information about abortions may be rather unreliable, it may be preferable to include only those pregnancies that have resulted in a recognizable child (dead or alive) and to interpret the survival ratio accordingly.

Finally, any comparison of survival ratios based on information obtained from different populations of women calls for the usual caution to be exercised with regard to representativeness and comparability.

Conclusions

In view of the growing emphasis on primary health care programmes and the need to evaluate their impact regularly, there is a corresponding need for objective health indicators which take into account the specific situation in rural areas of the Third World. The survival ratio proposed above may give useful insights into the extent of such problems as death from gastrointestinal diseases in infants and young children, and the extent of improvements associated with the introduction of new preventive or therapeutic methods, without requiring longitudinal data collection procedures. In areas where antenatal clinic attendance is high, representative survival ratios may even be based on information routinely available from clinic records.

13.2 Assessment of quality of life and life satisfaction in a community health and social survey — *J. Krupinski*

"Quality of life" indicators have been developed for many countries. The example presented here combines an attempt at the measurement of quality of life with self-assessment of a population, using a standardized questionnaire. It does not address specific hypotheses and does not present comparative population data, and the methods are probably too labour-intensive to be widely applicable. However, both the standardized questionnaire and the measurement techniques applied to the answers can be adapted to other sociocultural settings.

One of the main objectives of epidemiological and sociomedical studies has been to investigate the relationship between health and social factors and the association between the latter and specific diseases or disorders. With the growing availability of computers, studies of social indicators were given fresh impetus to relate health data to the social profile of specific areas *(1–4)*.

"Hard" social data are of less use than in the past when examining morbidity rates in developed countries. It is not sufficient to relate ill health simply to poverty, unemployment, lower social class or overcrowding, although these factors still play a very important role in the developing countries of Asia, Africa and South America. In the world's industrialized countries a new concept, "quality of life", has been introduced and adopted in sociological publications. However, it is often unclear what is meant by the term "low quality of life", as many users of that concept have attempted to attach to it their own values. Some have stressed the negative aspects of boring and repetitive jobs, life in the "anonymous" environment of large cities or suburbia, the obsessive watching of television programmes, and so on. Others have identified quality of life with the wellbeing of people *(5,6)*, with personal happiness *(7)* and even with positive mental health *(8)*.

In the belief that people themselves should decide how they would like to live and whether they are satisfied with various aspects of their life, the study group wished to avoid the use of yet another measure of psychological wellbeing. Thus, a two-pronged approach was adopted in the health and social survey of the north-west region of Melbourne, Australia, a working-class area with a total population of 235 000, comprising both areas with predominantly Australian and British-born populations and areas with a high concentration of non-British immigrants *(9)*. On the one hand, it was desirable to use objective indicators of quality of life; these included social characteristics, such as work, income and housing. In addition, a time budget study was carried out to determine how much time people spent each week on specific activities. On the other hand, the study team wished to ascertain people's subjective perceptions of their lives in greater depth than was possible using the general "satisfied/dissatisfied" categorization. In the survey, Otto's idea of comparing the importance attached to specific aspects of life with their actual presence *(6)* was developed. As the main aim of the survey was to determine the health status of the population, it was possible to relate the quality-of-life indices to the morbidity of the population studied.

Method

A 2% sample of dwellings was drawn according to a stratified sampling frame prepared by the Australian Bureau of Statistics. Full interviews were obtained in 977 of the 1254 households selected, a total of 3105 persons being covered altogether. Of the 189 households which refused, short door-step interviews were obtained from 97, to determine whether they differed significantly from respondents.

Final-year medical students carried out a traditional medical interview, presented the results to their physician and psychiatrist supervisors, and made, in consultation with them, a physical or psychiatric diagnosis, if such was warranted, using the International Classification of Diseases. For psychiatric disorders, in addition to diagnosis, an index of psychological disturbance was calculated on the basis of the frequency and severity of specific symptoms. The morbidity data were compared with information on the use of health services by respondents. Information also included details of household composition, ethnic origin, education, occupation, employment, income and housing conditions. Thus, it was possible to relate the socio-demographic variables to the health findings.

All respondents over the age of 12 years were asked to provide information on the time they had spent on specific activities during the week preceding the survey interview. All the activities were coded in terms of their type and the time spent on them, both on weekdays and at weekends.

The questionnaire used to measure perception of life by the population covered areas such as life in general, work, school and housing; each area consisted of a series of items which respondents were asked to check in terms of the degree of importance they allotted to them. The same items were then presented in a different order and respondents were requested to check whether these statements were true of their actual life situation.

Three forms of the questionnaire were used. For children aged 12–14 years, only "school" was covered; for students aged 15 and over, "life in general", "school" and "housing" were included, whereas, for all the others, "work" was substituted for "school". Those not in the workforce (housewives, pensioners) did not fill in this part of the questionnaire. Thus, the number of responses for a specific area depended on the number of interviewees for whom this area was relevant. To ensure the participation of all the main ethnic groups in the district surveyed, Italian, Greek and Yugoslav translations of the questionnaire were also provided.

In order to determine the clustering of particular items in each area, the factoring method described by Nie et al. *(10)* was applied. Seven main factors were extracted from "life in general", four from "work" and "school", and two from "housing" (Fig. 1).

Factor scores were calculated for every subject in each area. The complete estimation method was not used, as it is based on a zero mean score for each factor and does not allow for a comparison of the values given to specific factors. As weighted and unweighted scores were almost identical, the latter were used in further analysis; the score for each factor was defined as a simple unweighted mean of the item scores for this factor, measuring the way in which each respondent perceived the importance of each area.

In order to determine the extent to which each specific factor was fulfilled in the lives of respondents, the importance score of each factor was first recoded as follows.

Factor stated by respondent to be not important, or slightly important:	0
Factor stated by respondent to be moderately important:	1
Factor stated by respondent to be very important:	2
Factor stated by respondent to be extremely important	4

The occurrence of each item belonging to a specific factor in the life of the respondent was recorded as + 1, its absence as – 1 and a fifty-fifty answer earned an occurrence score of 0. The products of the importance score by the occurrence score could therefore range from – 4 (non-occurrence of an item considered as extremely important) to + 4 (the occurrence in real life of such an aspect) through intermediate values of – 2, – 1, + 1, + 2. The unweighted mean of these products constituted the "fulfilment index" of each factor. If the fulfilment index was equal to or greater than + 2, it was assumed that the desires of the subject were fulfilled. A value between 0 and + 2 was equated with a neutral response. A negative value of the index indicated non-fulfilment of the respondent's aspirations in a particular area. Slight non-fulfilment was equated with an index not lower than – 1, moderate with an index value lower than – 1 but not lower than – 2, while a value of the index lower than – 2 implied extreme non-fulfilment of the expressed wishes.

Time Budget Study

As time budget studies have been carried out in several countries, within the framework of a multinational comparative time budget research project *(11)*, it was not felt necessary to provide in this chapter the results of this part of the study. Full details are contained in the published report on the survey *(9)*. The main finding was the difference between males and females regarding the number of hours spent on gainful and other work. Adult males spent, on average, some 40 hours on work outside the home and, in addition, an hour on gainful work on their own premises. Up to 12 hours a week were spent on work around the house, gardening and shopping by middle-aged men. In contrast, females spent only about 20 hours on gainful work, but they spent, on average, over 40 hours on home duties and, of these, 10 or more hours at weekends. If shopping, gardening and work around the house are added, it becomes clear that an average adult woman was involved in 45 hours' work, in addition to the 20 hours' work outside the home. The average data conceal the particularly heavy burden of women in full-time work, who spent 80 hours weekly on their work in and outside the home, as compared with 55 hours weekly spent on household chores by female respondents with home duties only.

It is noteworthy that the time spent on specific activities did not appear to influence the health status of respondents.

Importance of Specific Aspects of Life

Table 1 provides information on the importance of specific aspects of life, presented in each area in the order of the importance attached to them by the respondents.

With regard to life in general, "family", "material security" and "freedom from worries" top the list in terms of importance, while "recreation" and, especially, "beliefs and ideas" do not seem to be perceived as very important. No clear distinctions were perceived between specific factors in the work and school areas, but in housing, "house with a garden" was much more highly valued than "flat better than neighbours'".

For all areas of life in general, females tended to obtain higher scores than males, except for "recreation" which was more important for males, and "beliefs and ideas" which were equally undervalued by both sexes. In the work area, only "freedom from pressure" was more important for females than for males, while no sex differences were noted for the three other work factors. More males than females preferred a "house with a garden", while a "flat" was less strongly rejected by females than by males.

In terms of age, no differences were noted in the perception of the importance of the family, except for elderly males, who saw it as slightly less important than did other age and sex groups. All the age groups equally regarded "freedom from worries" as very important, the elderly males even more so than the others. "Material security" was considered very important by all age groups, including young people under the age of 18. "Personal relations" were more highly valued by the very young and by very old people, while the perceived importance of "recreation" decreased with age. Young people, especially young females, put greater stress on the importance of "dependence" in work, although the same age group also favoured work "independence"; this is, to some extent, contradictory.

The perceived importance of "working conditions" decreased with age, while no age differences were noted with regard to "freedom from pressure". "House with a garden" was most appreciated by middle-aged subjects, while youngsters rejected flats to a lesser degree than other age groups.

Age-standardized rates have been used to measure the influence of variables such as education, occupation and ethnic origin on the perceived importance of the specific area. Education seems to be most relevant to "recreation": the higher the level of education, the more important "recreation" is. The importance of "personal relations" increases with lower

Fig. 1. Results of factor analysis

Life in general[a]

Factor 1: Personal relationships

Having good friends
Contact with relatives you like
Being accepted and liked by people with whom you come into contact
Knowing that you can always get help if you have a problem

Factor 2: Recreation

Participation in sport
Active membership of an organization or club
The time and opportunity to do things you very much want to do
The opportunity to travel
Having a paid job

Factor 3: Material security

Enough money to live according to the standard you desire
The chance to save money for an emergency
The kind of accommodation which meets your needs

Factor 4: Freedom from worries

Freedom from worries about your family or others close to you
Freedom from health worries (concerning yourself)
Freedom from conflicts with relatives or other people
Self-confidence

Factor 5: Useful work

Having enough to do
Being of use to others

Factor 6: Family life

Having children of your own (now or later)
A troublefree and happy marriage (or similar relationship, e.g. boy-friend, girl-friend)

Factor 7: Beliefs and ideas

Commitment to certain political ideas
A non-religious belief which may give meaning to life
A strong religious belief

Work

Factor 1: Dependence

Precise instructions on what you are expected to do
The certainty that you can get advice and help with your work (whenever you need it)
Good mates or colleagues to work with
The feeling that the people you work for appreciate your work
The knowledge that you can remain in your job as long as you like

Factor 2: Independence

Work which makes you feel you are doing something worthwhile
Work which is interesting to you
The chance to work according to decisions of your own

Fig. 1 (contd)

Factor 3: Working conditions

Good pay
Attractive working conditions, e.g. heating, cooling, meal facilities
Opportunity for advancement or promotion

Factor 4: Freedom from pressure

Freedom from pressure (caused by too much work)
A job which has hours of work which suit your other responsibilities and commitments

School

Factor 1: Peer activities

A school with a large playground
A school in which you have the chance to make many friends
A mixed school (boys and girls)
A school where you can take an active part in sporting activities opf your choice

Factor 2: School rules

A strict school with rules that are clearly laid down
A school where you are told what you have to do

Factor 3: Educational setting

A school where teachers are friendly and interested in you
A school which will allow you to continue your education beyond high school to a university, college, etc.
A school where you can choose which classes you want to attend

Factor 4: Closeness

A school which is close to your home
A school which is small enough for everyone to know each other

Housing

Factor 1: House with garden

A house with a backyard or garden
A house with a place where you can work at your hobbies
A house which you own or can eventually own some day
A house which provides an indoor play area for the children

Factor 2: Flat better than others'

A self-contained flat or apartment
A house which is bigger and better than your neighbours'
A house which provides you with a room of your own where you can shut yourself off from the rest of the family

[a] Items included in each factor had a factor loading of more than 0.3 on the particular factor. These loadings have not been indicated here.

Table 1. Importance of selected aspects of life

	Mean score	Not important (%)	Slightly important (%)	Moderately important (%)	Very important (%)	Extremely important (%)
Life in general						
Family	3.3	1.9	3.4	14.8	36.6	43.4
No worries	3.2	0.3	3.6	23.4	58.8	14.0
Material security	3.1	0.7	3.9	25.7	51.1	18.6
Personal relations	2.9	0.8	6.6	33.6	50.0	9.0
Useful work	2.7	2.2	8.0	34.6	43.0	12.3
Recreation	2.4	4.4	19.9	49.8	24.4	1.4
Beliefs and ideas	1.4	28.8	40.5	25.9	4.3	0.4
Work						
Independence	3.0	0.9	4.9	26.7	51.7	15.8
Dependence	2.8	0.9	10.7	36.1	46.1	6.3
Working conditions	2.7	3.2	12.1	40.7	37.1	6.9
Freedom from pressure	2.6	4.0	13.3	35.4	36.6	10.8
School						
Educational setting	2.9	1.8	10.1	33.6	41.9	12.5
Peer activities	2.7	1.9	13.9	36.2	42.1	5.9
Closeness to home	1.9	11.5	31.7	37.8	15.1	3.9
Rules	1.7	22.2	30.4	32.2	12.3	2.9
Housing						
House with garden	2.9	0.6	9.4	33.7	48.1	8.2
Flat better than neighbours'	0.9	25.7	62.2	9.9	2.0	0.2

educational standards. Other aspects of life in general do not seem to be related to the level of education. However, there is a strong relation between the level of education and the two work factors "dependence" and "independence": the better educated are more interested in an independent job and less in a dependent one, while the opposite is true for those with less education.

Occupational hierarchy affects only one of the "life in general" factors, namely "useful work", the importance of which increases as one goes up the occupational hierarchy. "Material security" is less important for professional and unskilled workers than for those in the middle ranges of the occupational hierarchy: professional people are less interested in "personal relations" than the other occupational categories.

In contrast, occupational hierarchy significantly affects the perception of all work factors. The importance of "work independence" increases with occupational hierarchy, while the opposite is true with regard to "work dependence". Working conditions are most important for clerical and skilled workers, while professional and managerial workers are less interested in "freedom from pressure".

No clearcut patterns have emerged in terms of ethnic background. The differences between specific ethnic groups were larger than differences between immigrants and Australian-born respondents, and it is rather difficult to explain why Greeks were more interested than eastern Europeans in "personal relations" and why Italians were less interested than other groups in "material security" and "freedom from worries". The differences in the perception of the importance of specific work factors by particular ethnic groups were more closely related to their occupational status than to cultural differences.

Of the factors relating to school, the importance of school rules decreased with both occupational hierarchy and the educational level of respondents, whereas the value of the educational setting was seen as more important by senior students. No differences were found in terms of the perception of the two housing factors.

Fulfilment

Table 2 shows the distribution of respondents in terms of the degree of fulfilment in specific areas. As can be seen, the highest rate of fulfilment was reported for "family", followed by "useful work" and "personal relations". The highest non-fulfilment was apparent in the areas of "material security" and "freedom from worries". The factors considered least important, "beliefs and ideas" and "recreation", had, by definition, the lowest proportions of those scoring high, both on non-fulfilment and fulfilment.

With regard to work, "independence" achieved the highest score for fulfilment, while the opposite was true of "working conditions". For schoolchildren, "peer activities" scored the highest percentage for fulfilment, whereas " a school close to home and small enough for everyone to know each other" provided the highest percentage of dissatisfaction. As nine out of ten respondents preferred a house to a flat, the fulfilment of this desire

Table 2. Fulfilment of selected aspects of life

	Fulfilment	Neutral	Non-fulfilment		
			Slight	Moderate	Extreme
Life in general					
Family life	57.7	34.8	1.0	3.4	3.1
Peer relations	29.7	61.5	5.1	3.0	0.7
Useful work	28.5	67.5	1.2	1.3	1.5
Freedom from worries	21.5	60.6	6.1	8.3	3.5
Material security	13.9	60.4	10.1	9.8	5.8
Recreation	5.8	61.2	22.4	9.0	1.6
Beliefs and ideas	1.9	75.3	19.1	3.4	0.3
Work					
Independence	30.6	54.1	7.5	5.4	2.4
Freedom from pressure	20.8	59.4	5.3	7.1	7.4
Dependence	20.0	62.2	14.9	2.6	0.3
Working conditions	10.4	62.4	13.4	8.2	5.6
School					
Peer activities	23.7	63.9	8.4	2.7	1.3
Educational setting	18.8	56.6	15.4	4.6	4.6
Closeness to home	6.8	57.3	16.2	11.0	8.7
Rules	6.7	85.7	4.6	2.0	1.0
Housing					
House with garden	33.7	51.3	6.6	5.1	3.3
Flat better than others'	1.3	78.3	14.3	5.4	0.7

depended only on the type of house inhabited by them. The analysis of the level of fulfilment in terms of selected demographic and social variables did not provide any clearcut patterns which would indicate their influence on satisfaction or dissatisfaction in specific areas.

Relation to Health

The study team tried to determine the relation of ill health, as measured by physical and psychiatric diagnosis, to several social and familial factors. The main feature which emerged was the lack of association between social class (as measured by the position of the head of household in the occupational hierarchy) and the prevalence of physical and psychiatric conditions. This was especially evident among the elderly. Some ethnic groups (Italians) had fewer heart disorders and reported fewer psychological problems than did the Australian-born and the British immigrants. Australians consumed more alcohol than other ethnic groups, the lowest rates being found among southern Europeans and respondents, especially females, originating from the Middle East. On the other hand, lifestyles and the microenvironment had a considerable influence on the health of subjects. Smoking was clearly related to respiratory diseases. An association was also demonstrated between smoking and a history of abortion, abnormal menstrual loss and dysmenorrhoea. In children, the only significant factor was the association between behavioural and emotional problems and psychological disturbances in one or both parents.

The time spent on specific activities did not seem to influence the prevalence of either physical or psychological disorders. Except in the severely handicapped, it was not possible to establish any association between the time budget and ill health.

The only significant result was that people with hobbies had fewer psychological disturbances than those who had no hobbies. However, the small number of respondents with hobbies and the fact that they were quite different from respondents in general did not permit any conclusions to be drawn from the statistically significant association. The amount of time spent watching television did not relate to the rate of psychological disturbance.

On the other hand, marked associations were found between, on the one hand, the level of fulfilment in specific areas and, on the other hand, the prevalence of psychiatric disorders and the level of psychological disturbance as measured by a disturbance score. This association was noted for all factors except "beliefs and ideas" which, as has been shown, was not an important factor for the vast majority of respondents. In the area of "useful work", only those with extreme non-fulfilment had a significantly higher prevalence of psychiatric diagnoses and of moderate and severe disturbance scores. In the areas of "family life", "personal relations", "recreation" and "material security", this relation was much more marked: there were twice as many persons with psychiatric diagnoses in the non-fulfilled groups as in those with a positive fulfilment score. The psychological disturbance score discriminated even more clearly in this respect (see Table 3).

Table 3. Psychological disturbances in terms of fulfilment in specific areas (percentage of all subjects)

Level of fulfilment	No. of subjects	Psychological disturbance scale				Percentage with psychiatric diagnosis	
		None	Mild or moderate	Severe			
Useful work							
Extreme non-fulfilment	53	26.4	56.6	17.0	*	20.8	NS
All other	1813	39.5	54.9	5.6		14.8	
Family life							
Non-fulfilment	127	36.2	51.2	12.6		21.3	
Neutral	367	34.1	58.1	7.9	*	15.8	*
Fulfilment	1199	40.4	55.3	4.2		12.9	
Personal status							
Non-fulfilment	158	29.1	57.6	13.3		22.2	
Neutral	1448	39.7	55.0	5.3	*	13.8	***
Fulfilment	211	45.5	51.7	2.8		11.4	
Recreation							
Extreme non-fulfilment	27	14.8	66.7	18.5			
Non-fulfilment	155	32.3	60.0	7.7	*	19.2[a]	**
Neutral	1214	38.5	55.4	6.1		14.3	
Fulfilment	323	48.9	48.6	2.5		10.2	

Level of fulfilment	No. of subjects	Psychological disturbance scale				Percentage with psychiatric diagnosis	
		None	Mild or moderate	Severe			
Material security							
Non-fulfilment	441	30.2	59.8	10.0		19.3	
Neutral	1040	42.1	53.1	4.8	*	13.5	*
Fulfilment	238	40.3	55.4	4.2		10.5	
Freedom from worries							
Substantial non-fulfilment	212	21.7	58.5	19.8		30.7	
Slight non-fulfilment	116	28.4	62.0	9.5		22.5	
Neutral	300	30.7	62.4	7.0	*	16.0	*
Fulfilment	1006	44.3	52.8	2.9		12.9	
Extreme fulfilment	154	58.5	40.2	1.3		6.5	

[a] 19.2% calculated on 182 (= 27 + 155) subjects.

Note. Chi-square test used to determine significance of difference: * $P < 0.05$; ** $P < 0.025$; *** $P < 0.01$. Divisions by level of fulfilment presented only if showing statistically significant differences in psychiatric disturbance scale.

The largest differences in terms of fulfilment were noted for the "freedom from worries" factor, where the rates both of psychiatric diagnoses and of moderate and severe psychological disturbances were five times higher in the non-fulfilled group than in those with high fulfilment scores.

Discussion

The study has proved that it is feasible to assess in intensive population surveys how people live and what is their subjective approach to quality of life.

At the time when this survey was already in progress, other authors *(12, 13)* published works on social indicators and quality of life. Their main approach was to determine overall happiness and satisfaction with life, as well as satisfaction with specific areas, and to determine which attributes of a specific area contributed to overall satisfaction with it. Finally, the level of wellbeing or happiness was related to specific social or demographic characteristics. Zautra et al. *(14)* included their techniques in a study of dimensions of the quality of life in the community, while Kammann et al. *(15)* measured "happiness" and the "sense of wellbeing" in a New Zealand population sample.

The present survey was not limited to finding out whether people were happy or satisfied with specific aspects of life, but tried to determine the levels of fulfilment of their aspirations. While there was an association between level of fulfilment and degree of satisfaction within specific areas, determination of the level of fulfilment was much more discriminating than the simple satisfaction/dissatisfaction question; at the same time, it provided greater insight into the aspirations of the respondents in terms of the type of life they would like to live. It is felt, therefore, that the method employed in this survey provides a satisfactory measure of quality of life. Its further development could include an increase in the number of areas studied and the number of statements describing each area. The value of the method lies in the fact that the respondent does not know the socially accepted answers and does not feel under pressure to respond positively to the questions being asked.

Finally, the findings indicate that the prevalence of psychiatric disorders is less related to the objective way of life than to whether people live or do not live according to their wishes. These findings are in agreement with the results of Otto's original study *(6)*, which regarded the discrepancy between desires and the actual life situation as stressful factors leading to a higher prevalence of psychosomatic symptoms.

References

1. **Armstrong, A.F. & Wearing, A.J.** *Social indicators for Victoria, Stage One.* Melbourne, University of Melbourne, 1979 (Monograph in Public Policy Studies, No. 1).
2. **Armstrong, A.F. & Wearing, A.J.** *Social indicators for Victoria, Stage Two.* Melbourne, University of Melbourne, 1981 (Monograph in Public Policy Studies, No. 2).

3. **Bauer, R.A., ed.** *Social indicators.* Cambridge, MA, MIT Press, 1966.
4. **Organisation for Economic Co-operation and Development.** *Measuring social well-being: a progress report on the development of social indicators.* Paris, OECD, 1976.
5. **Bradburn, N.M.** *The structure of psychological wellbeing.* Chicago, Aldine, 1969.
6. **Otto, R.** *Patterns of stress, symptoms awareness and medical help seeking among men and women in selected occupations.* Thesis, La Trobe University, Melbourne, 1976.
7. **Bradburn, N.M. & Caplovitz, D.** *Reports on happiness.* Chicago, Aldine, 1965.
8. **Beiser, M. et al.** Assets and affects: a study of positive mental health. *Archives of general psychiatry,* **27**: 545–549 (1972).
9. **Krupinski, J. & Mackenzie, A.** *The health and social survey of the northwest region of Melbourne.* Mental Health Authority, 1979 (Special publication No. 7).
10. **Nie, H.N. et al.** *Statistical package for the social sciences,* 2nd ed. New York, McGraw-Hill, 1975, pp. 480–485.
11. **Szalai, A. et al.** *The use of time: daily activities of urban and suburban populations in twelve countries.* The Hague, Mouton, 1973.
12. **Andrews, F.M. & Whitey, S.B.** *Social indicators of well-being: American perceptions of life quality.* New York, Plenum Press, 1976.
13. **Campbell, A. et al.** *Quality of American life: perceptions, evaluations and satisfaction.* New York, Russell Sage Foundation, 1976.
14. **Zautra, A. et al.** The dimensions of life quality in a community. *American journal of community psychology,* **5**: 85–97 (1977).
15. **Kammann, R. et al.** Properties of an inventory to measure happiness (and psychological health). *New Zealand psychologist,* **8**: 1–12 (1979).

13.3 Measurements for evaluating health promotion programmes: a practical illustration — *I.W. McDowell*

This example deals with the measurement of health status through the construction and use of indices, as discussed by Goldberg & Dab in Chapter 7.5. It describes the proposed use of several different complex indicators aimed at measuring changes in health behaviours in different interrelated areas in connection with an experimental health promotion programme, "Healthstyles", takin place in Ottawa, Canada. The measures include the Bradburn scale, the modified health locus of control scale, scoring systems based on the content (fat, fibre, sugar and salt) of food consumed, and exercise level in terms of overall energy expenditure. The paper also discusses the question of reference standards and norms for the various indicators used. There is, however, no attempt to derive a single index measure.

Evaluating Health Promotion Programmes

If one accepts that health implies more than the absence of disease, it follows that health cannot be promoted solely by disease prevention. For many years, modification of risk factors has been the main approach to preventing chronic diseases in industrial countries; this approach is conceptually simple and also relatively easy to evaluate by recording changes in smoking, blood pressure or weight. Increasingly, however, the practical and logical limitations of this approach are being recognized. In practice, it is difficult to encourage people to stop smoking, to lose weight or to control their blood pressure, and improving one risk factor may at times lead to a deterioration in another. The results of recent risk factor modification trials seem to suggest that these tactics are often not sufficient to prevent disease and to promote health. As the risk factor modification approach is replaced by programmes which tackle the chain of causation one stage earlier by altering the precursors of the risk factors themselves, the task of the evaluator becomes more complex. Measurements of risk factors only reflect one aspect of the goals of health promotion programmes, and measurements may also be needed of more abstract qualities, such as stress levels, coping abilities, self-esteem and quality of life.

To illustrate the types of difficulty faced in evaluating health promotion, an experimental programme called "Healthstyles", conducted in Ottawa, Canada, will be described. This programme aims at encouraging its clients to assume personal responsibility for their health and to recognize that the physical, mental, spiritual and social aspects of personal health are interdependent. As a health promotion rather than a disease prevention trial, it does not address any particular disease and is based on several concepts that set it apart from risk factor intervention trials. The programme focuses not so much on lowering risk factors directly as on modifying (by increasing personal awareness) the causes which give rise to risk factors. Each person who smokes, drinks or overeats is presumed to do so for particular reasons, and no single approach is expected to suit all participants. The programme content is therefore flexible and emphasizes the autonomy and responsibility of each participant in making changes in his or her own lifestyle.

"Healthstyles" does not motivate participants by emphasizing risks, but by stressing the immediate, positive gains to be derived from changes in health-linked behaviour. The preliminary goals of the programme are, therefore, to increase personal awareness of the attitudes and beliefs which influence behaviour, to increase self-acceptance and to develop the skills necessary to change behaviour. A second set of goals, which follow from those above, specify changes in risk behaviour. They include: eliminating smoking, encouraging the appropriate use of alcohol, developing sound exercise and eating patterns, and managing stress healthfully. These goals are viewed as interdependent and closely related to the theme of self-responsibility. A third set of programme goals, which derive from these changes, include reductions in acute, minor morbidity, together with changes in the use of medical care, perhaps including an increase in the use of preventive services.

The evaluation of a programme of this type requires measurements at each stage in this sequence of outcomes; it should also analyse the process of change, showing which elements in the programme have been effective and for which type of person. The analysis of data will therefore search for interactions between attributes of the client and the success of the various parts of the programme. The evaluation uses a longitudinal design in which 600 experimental participants are each matched with two controls, giving a sample size of 1800. Measurements are taken at baseline, 3, 12 and 18 months. The majority of data are collected by questionnaire, while blood pressure, body weight and height are measured at baseline and at 18 months. To evaluate whether the model implied by the hierarchy of outcomes has, in fact, been attained, the data analysis will examine how far changes in psychological and motivational variables were followed by modifications in risk factors and how far this affected the use of medical services. The evaluation will combine data of various types, from simple physical measurements to questions on abstract concepts, such as coping with stress, and also computerized data at the provincial level on medical care use. As might be expected, a project of this type has encountered numerous practical problems, and the steps taken to overcome some of these are outlined below.

Measuring Qualitative Outcomes

Several of the immediate outcomes of this study cannot readily be expressed in quantifiable terms, e.g. healthy stress management, self-responsibility and self-awareness. The first response of the evaluator is often to decry such objectives as not measurable, although they form a central part of this type of programme. To concentrate the evaluation only on measuring changes in quantifiable risk factors is to avoid the issue: one cannot then judge whether improvement was a consequence of changes in coping and stress management or whether the opposite occurred and the change in behaviour actually raised stress levels.

Two types of approach have been used to measure stress and coping: a simple description of the response to a stressful event ("I work harder than usual", "I worry a lot") or a measurement of the results of this response in terms of positive or negative feelings. The present study employs both approaches, a check list of stress reactions and a summary of overall feelings, using the Bradburn scale *(1)*. The modified health locus of control scale has also been used to measure self-responsibility *(2)*. The Bradburn questions have been extensively used as a brief survey indicator of psychological wellbeing and describe the feelings that occur as a result of confronting the problems of daily living. Bradburn's ten questions are also used as a basis for a brief summary of the success of each person's coping strategies. There are several advantages to the questions: they are widely used, so that results may be compared with data from other studies, they cover both positive and negative feelings, and Bradburn provided a clear conceptual expression of the purpose of the scale. The conceptual formulation emphasizes the independence of negative and positive responses: they are not simply the converse of each other, and each may be associated with different variables in the web of disease causation *(3)*. This corresponded well with the study team's view that removing the causes of disease would not necessarily imply creating health.

While this measurement appears to hold some theoretical benefits, it is often the case that health indices do not succeed in measuring precisely what they were intended to, and Bradburn's questions have been quite widely criticized *(4)*. The evaluator is then confronted with a choice between altering certain of the questions in an attempt to improve them or to use a measurement tool he knows to be imperfect. There seems to be little advantage in altering individual questions piecemeal, since comparability with other studies would thus be lost. The study team therefore retained the scale intact, although recognizing the need for an improved method. The principal refinements they identified as desirable would include making further subdivisions to the positive and negative dimensions and would distinguish the general responses from those which are specific to a particular circumstance. The clinical interpretation of each question also needs to be clarified. Until more adequate measurement methods are developed, the evaluation will remain descriptive in nature, and it will be necessary to rely on rather crude methods of statistical analysis.

Diet and Physical Activity

The assessment of diet has always presented serious practical problems, and there still seem to be few acceptable ways to record food intake using a self-assessment questionnaire. Although complex computer programs exist for translating consumed foods into nutrient constituents, the basic problem of obtaining an accurate estimate of what was eaten remains. This problem is closely related to the cost of data collection: the cost of administering and analysing three- or seven-day dietary diaries is high, and the marginal returns on such an investment in terms of greater accuracy become debatable. Compliance with diary methods may also be low, especially for the control group. Because of these problems, it was decided to use a single-day dietary recall. This provides only a crude sample for any individual, but can show patterns of change over time in large groups of respondents. The design of a dietary recall form is critical. The respondent is first asked to record all the foods and drinks he consumed the previous day and then to check through a long list of commonly eaten foods to aid his recall. A scoring system is used, based on the estimated fat, fibre, sugar and salt content per serving of each food mentioned in the list, and these scores are cumulated across all the foods eaten. A similar approach is used for estimating exercise level, in which a check list of various types of physical activity records which type of exercise was performed in the previous week and for how long; these estimates are weighted according to metabolic equivalence scores for each activity and summed to give an estimate of overall energy expenditure *(5)*.

Reference Standards

The participants in the programme are volunteers, and unfortunately a random allocation to experimental and control groups could not be used. Although the relatively weak design, using matched controls, has been strengthened by matching for several variables, including sex, age, education, feelings of stress, smoking status and an aggregate score based on five other risk factors, there are serious problems inherent in statistical analyses of non-randomized studies. Furthermore, the comparison of experimental and control groups does not help in interpreting the magnitude of any contrast observed. One way to strengthen the interpretation of study outcomes is to relate them to population norms and percentile distributions for the measurements used. This raises no problem for physical measurements, such as body weight, for which reference standards are widely available. With regard to other outcome indicators, however, often less is known about population norms, and so in a preliminary stage of the study the study team sought to derive reference standards from nationally representative data. Re-analyses of data from the national Canada Health Survey *(5)* provided reference data on most health risk factors and on some psychological variables. For example, age/sex standards for the Bradburn questions discussed above were derived. These took the form both of simple response frequencies to each question (shown in Table 1 in the work by McDowell & Praught *(3)*) and also of percentile distributions for the overall score on the Bradburn scale. The percentile charts show very slight contrasts between the sexes, and a slight narrowing of the spread between the tenth and ninetieth percentiles with increasing age. Just as a child's growth may be evaluated by reference to Boston standards, the interpretation of the experimental results will be strengthened by expressing them in terms of changes from one population percentile to another.

Many well established questionnaires have been applied in national surveys. However, those who analyse the data frequently do not report percentile distributions of scores in the way commonly used in reporting anthropometric standards. Such information would be of great benefit in interpreting the results of small-scale studies. Emphasis should also be placed on using the same question wording as that employed in any available large comparative study; this also simplifies the cumulation of results from several such studies using meta-analysis techniques *(6)*.

Data Management

To solve the practical problems of managing the periodic data collection for a project which follows 1800 people over 18 months (subjects enter the study at different starting dates), the Statistical Analysis System of computer programs *(7)* was used to issue reminders and to update and check the data file.

The present project also illustrates the technical problem of linking information on intermediate outcomes with outcomes such as the use of health services. Obtaining accurate data on the use of medical services is usually difficult, but because doctors in Ontario are paid for each service they provide, a government computer system stores details of every consultation. Thus, tabulations can be prepared showing the rates of selected types of consultation in the experimental and control groups. Because of the need to retain the confidentiality of medical records, it is not possible to link changes in risk factors to medical care use by individuals, but group analyses will be prepared to compare experimental and control cases. It will also be possible to make a cost–benefit analysis of the programme in terms of the reduced cost of care for members of the experimental group.

Conclusion

The limited success of risk factor reduction programmes in controlling chronic disease in industrialized countries has encouraged the development of more intensive programmes, which present additional challenges of measurement to their evaluators. While measurement of traditional risk factors such as smoking or blood pressure can be achieved quite simply, others, such as exercise and diet, are more complex. As the focus of a programme shifts away from inherently quantifiable risk factors and also incorporates measurements of stress and coping, a different order of complexity arises. Where a programme tackles several risk factors, the burden of data collection for evaluation purposes increases, and it is often necessary to sacrifice accuracy of measurement in areas such as diet in order to contain the costs of the study. With stress measurements, which formed a crucial goal of the programme described, there appears at present to be no satisfactory middle-range measurement that lies somewhere between a crude numerical stress rating-scale and a very detailed interview assessment describing and evaluating the type of response to stress. As with many measurements in the field of health, the qualities assessed do not readily fall into simple dichotomous scales that indicate good or bad responses; it cannot be ascertained exactly how much stress is appropriate for each individual.

The prospects for improving this situation are uncertain. Research has led to some progress, but efforts are at present somewhat uncoordinated. There is, for example, no discipline of health measurement equivalent to psychometrics or econometrics; the journals in which relevant measurement methods are described span the social sciences, medicine and disciplines such as business and administration *(8)*. More work is needed to refine existing instruments, establish reference standards and publicize the measurements available. In this field, the dictum that science lags behind progress is true, in large measure because scientists have not yet established ways to measure and evaluate the innovations taking place in health promotion.

References

1. **Bradburn, N.M.** *The structure of psychological well-being.* Chicago, Aldine, 1969.
2. **Wallston, K.A. & Wallston, B.S.** Development of the multidimensional health locus of control (MHLC) scales. *Health education monographs,* **6**: 160–170 (1978).
3. **McDowell, I. & Praught, E.** On the measurement of happiness. An examination of the Bradburn Scale in the Canada Health Survey. *American journal of epidemiology,* **116**: 949–958 (1982).
4. **Cherlin, A. & Reeder, L.O.** The dimensions of psychological wellbeing: a critical review. *Sociological methods research,* **4**: 189–214 (1975).
5. **Health and Welfare Canada.** *The health of Canadians: report of the Canada Health Survey.* Ottawa, Minister of Supply and Services, 1981.
6. **Glass, G.V. et al.** *Meta-analysis in social research.* Beverly Hills, CA, Sage Publications, 1981.
7. **Roy, A.A., ed.** *SAS user's guide: basics.* Cary, NC, SAS Institute, 1982.
8. **McDowell, I. & Newell, C.** *Measuring health: a guide to rating scales and questionnaires.* New York, Oxford University Press, 1987.

13.4 A measure of perceived health: the Nottingham health profile — *J. McEwen, S.M. Hunt & S.P. McKenna*

This chapter describes the "Nottingham health profile", a self-administered questionnaire designed to measure perceived health and the extent to which health problems affect normal activities. Perceived health is examined in terms of six different areas: sleep, physical activity, energy, pain, emotional reactions and social isolation. The chapter illustrates some of the different uses that can be made of the profile by considering some of the results that have been obtained when using it as a population survey tool. The subject matter of this example relates to the earlier chapter by Goldberg & Dab (7.5) on complex indices of health status. Once again it is important to note that there is no attempt in the contribution that follows to derive a single *index measure.*

Various trends in western society over the past 50 years have combined to call into question traditional notions of health care and the provision of health services. While some of these trends stem from changes in the nature of medical problems, inputs from philosophy, social and behavioural sciences and politics have also been influential. Patterns of health and disease have changed dramatically in western countries, and the difficulty in relating health services to need is clearly demonstrated in both these and the developing countries. Every country has its share of chronically ill and handicapped children, adults and elderly people. In addition, there is considerable deviation from good health, mainly of a less severe or dramatic nature, that is never brought to the attention of health professionals. In addition, the almost universal lack of evaluation of health services, in terms of their impact and performance, has led to calls for means of assessing the extent to which the health needs of communities have been, or could be, met.

Evaluation of services, whether at national, community or clinical level, is attracting increasing interest, partly because the focus of attention is shifting to the quality of life rather than its quantitative aspects, and partly because of growing concern over the rising cost of service provision. It seems, therefore, that there is now in western countries and will soon be in other parts of the world a need to answer crucial questions about how predictions can be made concerning the demand for health services and the extent to which these services actually improve health status. It has been known for some years that voluntary utilization of health and other services is, by and large, based upon the perception by the client that he or she needs help or advice, rather than upon some more "objective" set of clinical criteria. Moreover, satisfaction with the care received is often based upon different factors from those used by the physician.

Thus, perceived need is of crucial importance when assessing the efficacy and delivery of services at a local level, and it is also of great value when planning for different patterns of health requirements and resource allocation.

There is abundant evidence that consumers are good judges of their own feelings of discomfort or distress. Measures of perceived health can provide an important complement to routinely collected statistics because they give direct information on experienced malaise or wellbeing which can, in turn, supply the basic data required for determining goals in health care and assessing how far such goals have been achieved *(1)*.

Information on how people themselves feel about their health, as opposed to professional definitions of morbidity, is scarce, and there is an absence of direct measures of differences in health status between various groups or communities. Since it is perceived and not necessarily actual problems that lead to demands for health care, a measure of perceived health which is reliable, valid and sensitive to change would seem to be an essential component of planning for health care, and would also provide a means of monitoring the effects of health care.

There have been many attempts to develop a standard measure of self-assessed health for use as a population survey tool, in the hope that it would be capable of measuring the health status of whole populations at particular points in time, or providing reliable repeated measures over time, and of assessing the efficacy of health care, particularly through its capacity to detect change.

The development of a measure of self-assessed health inevitably involves problems of definition, measurement, weighting, reliability, validity, sensitivity and applicability. Examples of instruments which have been extensively tested in North America are the Sickness Impact Profile, the Cornell Medical Index and the General Index of Well-Being *(2–4)*. Indices or scales for measuring health perceptions have also been produced by Ware *(5)* and Kaplan et al. *(6)*.

An indicator of hospital performance based upon self-assessment of disability and distress has been developed in London *(7)* and a self-assessed disability indicator based upon perception and social values has been used in the measurement of outcomes of treatment and allocation of resources *(8)*. Information on experienced symptoms has been presumed to be related to need and gathered by the use of standardized instruments *(9, 10)*. The General Household Survey, which is in routine use in the United Kingdom, also asks for general health ratings and information on days of acute sickness *(11)*.

There are a number of criticisms which can be made of existing self-report measures of health status, although not all the following comments apply to each instrument. First, they are often long and complicated, with ambiguous statements; second, scoring and weighting for seriousness often reflect the values of the physician, not the layman; third, the measures may be focused on too narrow an area, such as disability; and fourth, where the answers are summed to a single score or index, this could have been derived in many different ways and involve the addition of scores from areas not logically connected, such as physical morbidity and appetite. Finally, the emphasis is on measuring negative aspects of health; such measures may, nevertheless, be used to detect gains in health when used on populations over time.

A tool for the survey of populations, as Culyer *(12)* has pointed out, should not be too sophisticated, because of the difficulty of interpreting responses and standardizing scores. It must be sensitive enough to assess the health needs of the population and specific enough to evaluate health care provision for special groups. It must also be understood by a large majority of potential respondents, short and simple to answer, cheap to administer and score, and above all valid and reliable.

Bearing such considerations in mind, an attempt has been made to produce a completely new measure of perceived health which would be simple to use, yet fairly comprehensive.

Development

The research team started work in 1975, on a "quality of life" measure (a sociomedical indicator) which would describe the typical effects of ill health: physical, social and emotional. The reasons for developing the measure were:

— to provide some assessment of a person's need for care which was not based upon purely medical criteria;

— to enable the subsequent evaluation of care provided for persons in need;

— to develop an indicator which could be used for surveying a population's health status.

The team conducted 768 interviews with patients who had various acute and chronic ailments. A total of 2200 statements were extracted, in which the typical effects of ill health were described. The statements were grouped into categories according to the function described: sleeping, eating, movement, social life, emotional reactions, and so on. The wording of each statement was scrutinized to avoid redundancy, ambiguity and esoteric expressions and to ensure suitability according to reading age. This reduced the number of statements to 138.

Combinations of these remaining statements were used in a number of pilot studies on different populations, further reducing the number of statements and refining those that remained. A final pool of 82 items covering 12 function areas was obtained. These items had indicated their value in reflecting subjective states and providing a measure of perceived impairment *(10,13,14)*.

The development of the existing instrument into a "population survey tool" required statements to be re-examined, retested and analysed, using the following criteria:

— there should be no statements containing negatives;

— statements should be easy to understand, unambiguous and easy to answer;

— statements should be answerable by "yes" or "no";

— language should conform to standards of a minimum reading age.

Items which met these standards were tested on patient and nonpatient groups, and those which proved satisfactory were retained *(15)*. The final version was called the Nottingham Health Profile and consists of two parts.

The Nottingham Health Profile

Part I of the profile comprises 38 statements which met the stringent criteria defined above and which best reflected health problems. They fall into six areas: sleep, physical mobility, energy, pain, emotional reactions, and social isolation.

The statements in each section have been weighted, using the Thurstone method of paired comparisons *(16)*. The weights reflect the perceived severity of the items: the higher the score, the poorer the perceived health status. Thus, on each section a score of 100 indicates that the respondent has checked every statement and has the worst possible subjective health allowed by the questionnaire. The ceiling of 100 is the sum of the derived and adjusted weights and was chosen arbitrarily to allow comparisons between sections.

Part II of the profile consists of seven statements relating to those areas of daily life most often affected by health: paid employment, looking after the home, social life, home life, sex life, hobbies and interests, and holidays.

For both parts, the respondent simply indicates "yes" or "no" according to whether the statement applies to him or her "in general". In Part I, the maximum score on any section is 100. Such a score would indicate that the respondent has every problem listed in that section. Statements in Part II are scored thus: 1 for an affirmative response and 0 for a negative. Attempts to weight those items were unsuccessful, since there was no consistent agreement by respondents about the relative severity of a problem in one area (e.g. sex life) as opposed to another (e.g. paid employment).

Administration

The profile was designed to be self-administered. It is also possible to read out the statements to individuals who have sight or reading problems. The profile can either be administered to an individual or be completed by individuals at a group session. Studies in which the profile has been sent by post have yielded response rates of between 68% and 93%. Its success as a postal questionnaire is highly dependent upon the population that is being sampled, appropriate preparatory discussions, and the content and source of the covering letter.

The profile can be used with populations aged 16 years and over and requires a minimum reading age of 10 years.

The scoring and analysis of the results are described in a manual which can be obtained from the authors. This contains a format suitable for analysis, using the book *Statistical package for the social sciences (17)*. Preliminary age, sex and social class norms are included in the manual, although it is intended that further studies will be used to provide an enlarged sample for the calculation of norms.

Testing

The profile has been tested for face, content and criterion validity among groups of elderly people of differing clinical condition *(18)*, patients consulting their general practitioners *(19)*, firemen *(20)*, mine rescue workers *(21)*, pregnant women *(22)*, patients undergoing minor surgery *(23)* and fracture victims *(24)*. Two further studies *(25,26)* established the reliability (or consistency over time) of profile scores. Table 1 shows some comparative scores in Part I.

These studies indicated that the profile was a highly valid and reliable indicator of subjective health in the physical, social and emotional domains and a useful guide to the extent to which health problems were restricting customary daily activities, and also that it can be used with a wide range of people and age groups. It was sensitive to change and capable of detecting gains or losses in perceived health.

A population survey

The validity and reliability of the profile having been established, it was necessary to gauge its usefulness and acceptability as a survey tool. As previously mentioned, studies using it as a postal questionnaire had yielded high response rates, but these were from motivated, chronically ill patients. Accordingly, and in the light of a report on continuing social inequalities in health status in the United Kingdom *(27)*, a study was set up whereby the profile would be used to examine social class differentials in perceived health by taking a random sample of patients from the records of a group practice in Nottingham. Questionnaires, together with a covering letter and a prepaid reply envelope, were posted to 3200 persons. A follow-up questionnaire was sent to non-responders 10 days after the original and a final response rate of 68% was obtained.

An analysis by social class showed that differentials in perceived health reflect overall patterns of morbidity as calculated from routinely collected vital statistics. Respondents in social classes IV and V (the lower socioeconomic groups) had significantly higher scores on emotional reactions, sleep and social isolation than did respondents of the same age in classes I, II and III. Similarly, in Part II lower socioeconomic groups were more likely to have more areas of their lives affected by health problems. Tables 2 and 3 illustrate these findings.

Examination of the score patterns in Part I of the profile shows that, in general, sex differences are not consistent, but are more pronounced in some age groups than in others; this tends to support the view that it is actual differences in perceived health status which account for different scoring rather than a difference in the tendency to report health problems and distress, particularly in the socio-emotional spheres. In general, perceived health declines with age. Although pain, physical mobility, energy and sleep

Table 1. Mean scores on sections of Part I of the profile for selected groups

	Mine rescue workers	"Fit" elderly	Pregnant women		Patients with minor non-acute conditions	Fracture victims	Patients with peripheral vascular disease	Elderly who are chronically ill	Patients with osteoarthrosis
			18 weeks	37 weeks					
Energy	0.99	4.06	31.4	39.6	24.2	25.79	30.3	37.98	63.2
Pain	1.37	1.05	2.1	11.2	15.9	6.58	22.6	29.16	70.8
Emotional reactions	1.25	3.28	15.7	15.7	14.7	13.65	13.9	15.13	21.3
Sleep	4.21	0.68	11.3	28.3	18.7	27.96	24.7	32.09	48.7
Social isolation	0.38	1.34	6.4	6.2	5.1	7.99	9.2	12.80	12.5
Physical mobility	0.54	1.91	7.3	26.0	7.3	27.62	22.0	29.16	54.8

Table 2. Mean scores on Part I of the profile, by social class (males and females, all ages)

	Social class					
	I (n = 76)	II (n = 279)	IIIN (n = 249)	IIIM (n = 467)	IV (n = 165)	V (n = 61)
Energy	10.25	10.63	15.69	15.84	18.58	13.49
Pain	3.00	4.70	6.84	7.60	6.51	8.24
Emotional reactions	9.74	8.42	9.00	9.89	14.41	13.07
Sleep	7.60	9.86	14.83	15.95	20.89	22.29
Social isolation	4.98	3.78	4.50	4.27	7.51	5.45
Physical mobility	3.05	3.12	5.58	6.42	5.20	7.66

Table 3. Part II of the profile: percentage of affirmative responses on areas of daily life being affected by health problems, by social class (males and females, all ages)

	Social class					
	I (n = 76)	II (n = 279)	IIIN (n = 249)	IIIM (n = 467)	IV (n = 165)	V (n = 61)
Problems with:	(%)	(%)	(%)	(%)	(%)	(%)
Paid employment	5.2	6.1	8.0	8.1	9.7	21.3
Jobs around the home	6.5	9.6	15.3	13.5	15.1	9.8
Social life	5.2	6.4	12.8	11.3	12.1	16.3
Personal relationships	7.9	5.0	7.2	8.8	11.5	6.5
Sex life	10.5	12.2	13.6	13.7	12.1	8.1
Hobbies and interests	10.5	7.2	14.4	13.3	15.1	16.3
Holidays	6.2	3.9	11.2	11.1	14.5	6.5

scores all show an increase, scores on social isolation and emotional reactions are relatively low, suggesting adaptation to physical problems experienced with age. The findings were interpreted as suggesting a greater vulnerability to social and economic stresses among younger people in lower socioeconomic groups, with some adaptation and resignation occurring after middle age *(28)*.

Results from Part II suggested that, as people get older, health problems begin to affect more areas of their daily lives and women are inclined to report more effects than men at all ages. The pattern of findings from this study confirmed the ability of the profile to extract meaningful and valid data. Although the response rate to the mailed questionnaire (68%) was disappointingly low, a comparison of respondents with census data for the area showed that they were representative of the population in relation to age, sex, marital status and type of housing. The best explanation for non-response is that people who did not return the questionnaire saw it as inapplicable to them because they did not have any of the problems on the questionnaire. This is an issue which will be mentioned again.

A later use of the profile in a population survey was carried out, using it as part of an interview schedule in a study of comparative health care in two London boroughs. In this case a response rate of 71% was achieved, non-response being due mainly to failure to make contact with selected households. An incidental finding of this study was that the Nottingham Health Profile was less susceptible to interviewer bias than the General Household Survey *(29)*.

Currently, the profile is being used as one of several outcome measures of a heart transplant programme; in clinical trials of cancer therapies and to predict needs for counselling in cancer patients; as a measure of rehabilitation success in stroke patients; in a survey of health at work; in studies of the unemployed; in responders and non-responders to an invitation for breast cancer screening; and in studies of housing conditions.

Advantages of the profile

1. It is suitable for use in a wide range of situations, from individual clinical interviews to large-scale population surveys.

2. It has a high degree of validity and reliability.

3. It is easy and cheap to administer.

4. It takes only a short time to complete and is highly acceptable to respondents.

5. It is easy to score and compute, particularly if the *Statistical package for the social sciences (17)* is used.

6. Scores can be compared graphically.

7. It can be used to measure perceived health status and adds a further dimension to the assessment of specific medical conditions of ill health.

8. Since the profile does not ask directly if people have *health* problems, it is more likely to pick up people who are ill or at risk but who do not perceive their problems as being related to health.

9. Since the items in the profile refer to problems, not symptoms, there is less opportunity for respondents to "medicalize" psychological or social stress.

Limitations of the profile

1. The items in Part I represent rather severe problems. This was found necessary to avoid large proportions of the population affirming the statements, with consequent loss in sensitivity. This does mean that some individuals who are suffering discomfort may not be identified by the profile.

2. "Normal" populations or those with minor ailments may affirm few statements in some sections. This makes it difficult to compare the scores or to demonstrate change.

3. An improvement in the health of "zero scorers" cannot be shown by the profile, although in fact they may be feeling better than on the previous occasion when they answered the questions.

4. The profile does not attempt to cover all possibilities. Despite this, the statements are selected to sample the whole range of health problems.

5. The scores in Part II are a combination of two functions: whether or not the respondent has a health problem and, if so, whether it is affecting any part of the specified area. This should not be taken to mean that an area may not be affected even when the individual has no health problem. Also, individuals who are having problems, say at work, may attribute them to ill health, whether or not this is the case.

6. Part I involves six scores and Part II a further seven. Analysis can, therefore, become cumbersome if large numbers of other variables need to be taken into account. The profile does not provide one global measure for a population, since combining scores in a single index was judged inappropriate.

7. The profile measures health by its absence, by focusing on negative aspects of health. This may deter people who do not have any of the stated problems from responding, especially to mailed questionnaires.

It is the opinion of the authors that the best use of the profile at present is with selected populations who are known, or believed, to have acute or chronic health problems, so that the vast majority of people sampled will respond beyond a minimum level of scoring. When this is the case, perceived gains in health or deteriorations can be assessed with some accuracy, as can the unmet needs of the population. For example, by taking a population known to be at risk, or of a certain level of morbidity, and standardizing for age, sex and class differences, one may use information on perceived health to investigate differentials related to the use of services or to the allocation of resources to special groups.

Future developments

Attempts are at present under way to remedy the major limitations of the profile, i.e. the tendency of potential zero scorers not to respond and the ambiguities associated with Part II. Versions of the profile are being tested which have more positive statements interspersed among the original ones, for example, "I sleep soundly most nights" and "I have plenty of energy". These statements will not be scored, since this would entail repeating a whole series of validity and reliability tests, but they will enable almost every respondent to give some affirmative responses, will provide a greater incentive to return the questionnaire and will make the profile less negative in tone.

In addition, the reseach team is experimenting by placing the former Part II at the front of the questionnaire and simply asking if any of the areas are affected; this is followed by a check list of possible influences on the areas, only one of which is health (e.g. financial worries, marital problems).

It should be noted that the instrument was developed, tested and applied in the United Kingdom. An attempt to produce an Arabic version was unsuccessful, due primarily to translation problems and to the lack of salience of items in the culture concerned, particularly statements in the socio-emotional domain *(30)*. On the other hand, a version suitable for use in North America has been developed, and currently the questionnaire is being adapted for use in France, Italy, Spain and Sweden.

The language in which the items comprising the profile are expressed fulfils many of the requirements for producing English expressions that can be successfully translated *(31)*, for example the use of simple sentences in the active voice and the avoidance of the subjunctive. Nevertheless, in an instrument which is based upon the perceptions of ordinary people the use of some colloquialisms and culture-specific concepts is inevitable. Some retesting, piloting and reformulation will probably be necessary before it can be used confidently in countries with other cultures.

Conclusion

Bearing in mind the foregoing comments and assuming the definition of appropriate samples and populations, the Nottingham Health Profile is appropriate for use in the following ways:

— as an outcome measure for group comparisons;

— as a survey tool with specified groups;

— as an adjunct to the clinical interview.

In the field of health services research, it is envisaged that the profile will be able to contribute to:

— the identification of individuals and groups who may be in need of care, for example those who fail to utilize, or who underutilize, services;

— the development of social policy, by helping to determine the allocation of resources;

— the pre-test and post-test design of evaluations of medical/social intervention;

— mass aspects of the evaluation of health and social services;

— the identification of consumer concerns;

— a theoretical understanding of the relationship between different subjective responses to comparable pathologies.

The profile is not intended to be a substitute for morbidity and mortality statistics or other refined indices, but an adjunct to them. Routine data can be enriched by the input of data specially collected from target populations or even from the population as a whole. In order to aid decision-making for health care, it will be necessary to have a range of indicators which can be used to delineate more clearly needs and problems in the community. Measures of perceived and objective needs as the means of evaluating services should be built into all health information.

References

1. WHO Technical Report Series, No. 472, 1971 (*Statistical indicators for the planning and evaluation of public health programmes*).
2. **Bergner, M. et al.** The sickness impact profile: conceptual formulation and methodology for the development of a health status measure. *International journal of health services,* **6**(3): 393–415 (1978).
3. **Broadman, K. et al.** The Cornell medical index and health questionnaire 11 as a diagnostic tool. *Journal of the American Medical Association,* **145**: 152–157 (1951).
4. **Wan, T.I.H. & Livieratos, B.** Interpreting a general index of subjective well-being. *Milbank Memorial Fund quarterly,* **56**: 531–536 (1978).
5. **Ware, J.E.** Scales for measuring general health perceptions. *Health services research,* **11**: 396–415 (1976).
6. **Kaplan, R.M. et al.** Health status: types of validity and the index of well-being. *Health services research,* **11**: 478–507 (1976).
7. **Rosser, R.M. & Kind, P.** A scale of valuations of states of illness, a social consensus. *International journal of epidemiology,* **7**: 347–357 (1978).
8. **Williams, R.G.A. et al.** Disability: a model and measurement technique. *British journal of preventive and social medicine,* **30**: 71–78 (1976).
9. **Hannay, D.R.** Symptoms prevalence in the community. *Journal of the Royal College of General Practitioners,* **28**: 492–499 (1978).

10. **Martini, C.J.M. & McDowell, I.** Health status: patient and physician judgement. *Health services research,* **11**(4): 508–575 (1978).
11. **Office of Population Censuses and Surveys, Social Survey Division.** *The General Household Survey.* London, H.M. Stationery Office, 1973 (introductory report).
12. **Culyer, A.J.** Need values and health status measurement. *In:* Culyer, A.J. & Wright, K.G., ed. *Economic aspects of health services.* London, Martin Robertson, 1978, pp. 9–31.
13. **McDowell, I. & Martini, C.J.M.** Problems and new directions in the evaluation of primary care. *International journal of epidemiology,* **5**: 247–250 (1976).
14. **McDowell, I. et al.** A method for self-assessment of disability before and after hip replacement operations. *British medical journal,* **2**: 875–879 (1978).
15. **Hunt, S.M. et al.** *Measuring health status.* London, Croom Helm, 1986.
16. **McKenna, S.P. et al.** Weighting the seriousness of perceived health problems using Thurstone's method of paired comparisons. *International journal of epidemiology,* **10**: 93–97 (1981).
17. **Nie, H.N. et al.** *Statistical package for the social sciences,* 2nd ed. New York, McGraw-Hill, 1975.
18. **Hunt, S.M. et al.** A quantitative approach to perceived health status: a validation study. *Journal of epidemiology and community health,* **34**: 281–286 (1981).
19. **Hunt, S.M. et al.** Nottingham Health Profile: subjective health status and medical consultations. *Social science and medicine,* **15A**: 221–229 (1981).
20. **McKenna, S.P. et al.** Looking at health from the consumers' point of view. *Occupational health,* **32**: 350–355 (1980).
21. **McKenna, S.P. et al.** Absence from work and perceived health among mine rescue workers. *Journal of the Society of Occupational Medicine,* **31**: 151–157 (1981).
22. **Backett, E.M. et al.** *Health and quality of life.* Report of the Social Science Research Council, London, 1981.
23. **Hunt, S.M. et al.** Subjective health assessments and the perceived outcome of minor surgery. *Journal of psychosomatic research,* **28**: 105–114 (1984).
24. **McKenna, S.P. et al.** Changes in the perceived health of patients recovering from fractures. *Public health (London),* **98**: 97–102 (1984).
25. **Hunt, S.M. et al.** Reliability of a population survey tool: a study of patients with osteoarthrosis. *Journal of epidemiology and community health,* **35**: 297–300 (1981).
26. **Hunt, S.M. et al.** Subjective health status of patients with peripheral vascular disease. *Practitioner,* **226**: 133–136 (1982).
27. **Department of Health and Social Security.** *Inequalities in health.* London, H.M. Stationery Office, 1980 (report of a research working group).
28. **Hunt, S.M. et al.** Social inequalities and perceived health. *Effective health care,* **2**: 151–159 (1985).

29. **Curtis, S.** *Intra-urban variations in health and health care: the comparative need for health care: survey of Tower Hamlets and Redbridge. Volume 1. Adult morbidity and service use.* London, Health Research Group, Department of Geography and Earth Science, Queen Mary College, 1984.
30. **Hunt, S.M.** Cross-cultural issues in the use of socio-medical indicators. *Health policy,* **6**: 149–158 (1986).
31. **Werner, O.T. & Campbell, D.** Translating, working through interpreters and the problem of decentering. *In:* Narrol, R. & Cohen, R., ed. *A handbook of method in cultural anthropology.* New York, American Museum of Natural History, 1970.

13.5 A primary care programme of health promotion in Cali, Colombia — *O.I. Rojas,* A. Alzate & R. Guerrero*

This description of an integrated programme carried out in Cali, Colombia, with the aim of improving existing levels of coverage for primary health care and welfare assistance, illustrates some of the simple measures that are applicable in the field of personal protection discussed in Chapter 8.1 by Brzeziński & des Fontaines. It does not, however, include a full evaluation of the programmes implemented, and this makes it difficult to draw definitive conclusions about the applicability elsewhere of the approaches discussed.

The failure of existing health services to meet people's basic health needs has led to the development of primary health care programmes of different types and characteristics in most underdeveloped countries. The introduction of biological and sociocultural factors as essential features of risk classification has allowed health planners and epidemiologists to identify the individuals and population groups who are more likely to develop a disease or pathological condition. Human, technical and physical resources will then be allocated according to the levels of risk.

Despite the fact that risk criteria have allowed a much clearer definition of priority groups, there exists a wide gap between the policies and general principles relating to health and the actual accessibility and availability of services to those priority groups. This situation was recognized by a team of health planners in Cali, Colombia, in 1979, when they decided to set up a programme aimed at improving the existing levels of health and welfare services coverage by means of an integrated programme that would put forward a model for the provision of primary health care and welfare assistance to an estimated population of 250 000.

This chapter describes a model in which assignment of resources is made on the basis of biological and social risk criteria. It also discusses the management process and evaluation in terms of coverage and performance of the components of the model. Issues concerning equity and intersectoral collaboration are included in the evaluation of the model.

General Description of the Setting

Four government institutions (two from the health sector, one from the planning sector and one university) agreed to coordinate actions, strategies and resources in an integrated programme to improve the provision of health care and welfare assistance to the urban poor in the city of Cali, Colombia.

Cali is situated in the south-west of Colombia, has a population of about 1.3 million, and has undergone rapid growth caused, among other factors, by massive migration of the rural population. The disorderly movement towards the city has led to the development of poor neighbourhoods or shanty towns, in which, it is believed, one third of the population of Cali lived by 1979.

The general mortality rate for Cali was 5.7 per 1000 population in 1979. One half of all deaths in the city were caused by motor vehicle accidents, hypertensive heart disease, diarrhoea and enteritis, and pneumonia. The infant mortality rate in the same year was 37 per 1000 live births, and the rate for the whole country was around 80 per 1000 *(1)*. Seventy-five per cent of urban households had a piped water supply, while only 65% of the population enjoyed the benefits of a sewage system *(2)*.

The Municipal Secretariat of Health is theoretically responsible for the health care of 70% of the population. The remaining 30% are covered by the social security scheme and related organizations (18%) and the private sector (12%).

For the provision of health care the city has been divided into four areas, each with a population of about 250 000. The hospital health centre is the referral point for between 5 and 8 health centres and health posts, and the hospital health centre's director is the main health authority in each area. Since 1976 a regionalized scheme for the provision of health care has been operating in the city. Yet it was estimated that approximately one third of the city population, those in the poorest strata, did not receive any health care at all.

Welfare assistance in the city is the responsibility of the Colombian Family Welfare Institute. In 1979 the Institute ran 50 nurseries in Cali, which were attended by only 4700 children under 5 years of age, an extremely low coverage of about 3% of preschool-age children.

The Colombian Family Welfare Institute collects 2% of the total payroll revenue from private and government sectors, and a need to devise new strategies to improve its level of coverage was felt at that time.

Since 1960, government bodies and the Universidad del Valle had been carrying out innovative and useful joint programmes in the health field. These programmes led to the development of new strategies for the provision of health care by means of domiciliary services, reassignment of functions and use of personnel with limited training *(3)*.

Planning the Programme

In 1979 the Municipal Secretariat of Health proposed that the Colombian Family Welfare Institute set up a programme to improve existing levels of coverage in the health and welfare services. Central issues at that time were the low levels of service coverage provided by each of the institutions, equity as a crucial factor determining the availability and accessibility of services and general concern about the constant increase in the costs of the services provided.

The programme objectives were as follows:

(*a*) to provide comprehensive care for families, especially children, comprising the most vulnerable group (250 000) in the population of Cali;

(*b*) to extend the coverage of services provided by the participating institutions by rationalizing the provision of services and encouraging the use of new methods in the delivery of care;

(*c*) to promote community involvement by making the household the basis for the provision of services and encouraging the development of community groups to study and analyse the situation and find solutions capable of meeting the needs of children and families.

The strategies decided upon to meet these objectives were:

(*a*) organization of efforts and community participation as the basis for generating social change and ensuring the continuity of the programme;

(*b*) the use of the at-risk approach to define and orient the activities according to different levels of priority;

(*c*) the use of a regionwide system in which the household is the lowest level of the pyramid for either health care or welfare assistance, with increasing levels of complexity from health posts to health centres, regional hospital and university hospital;

(*d*) emphasis on adaptating activities to the limited resources available, the use of auxiliary manpower and appropriate technologies, and maximum reliance on local materials;

(*e*) the development of a permanent information and evaluation system for monitoring programme performance.

The Model

Classification of risk

Families living in the area covered by the programme were classified according to three different levels of risk: high, medium and low. The classification took into account a series of variables traditionally associated with health, i.e. number of vaccine doses applied, spells of diarrhoea, water supply and sanitation of household, date of the last menstrual period, and nutritional status of children. At the same time, social variables such as occupation of the head of the household, existence of child labour, single motherhood, and exposure of children to physical violence or moral danger were included.

One of the outstanding features of the classification was that it allowed a first-hand evaluation of the "family risk" by means of a weighted average of the sum of the health and welfare variables; in this way it was easy to ascertain whether families were subject to a high, medium or low level of risk *(4)*.

Households in the high- and medium-risk categories were to be provided with a more thoroughgoing follow-up and visited at least three times a year; low-risk families were to be visited twice a year.

Human resources

The following criteria were suggested to community organizations to help them select and recruit health and welfare promoters:

- women aged between 25 and 35 years;
- leadership characteristics;
- at least two years of secondary school attendance;
- residence in the area where the programme is to be developed;
- experience in community work;
- experience in health or welfare work;
- skills in communication.

Seventy candidates, all resident in the programme area and most of them proposed by community organizations, took part in the selection procedure that included, among other features, a spelling test, a formal interview, a psychological test of behaviour and a field test.

Thirty-eight candidates (54.2%) fulfilled all the selection requirements and 17 (24%) were rejected, either because of failure in the test or because they did not meet the minimum requirements; 15 candidates (21%) dropped out at an early stage in the selection process.

A training course was designed to cover two main subjects: health care and welfare services. A period of 4 weeks was assigned to health care and 3 weeks to welfare content respectively. After a seven-week course, 23 of the 38 original candidates had satisfactorily passed the different tests to become health and welfare promoters.

Indicators and criteria

A series of measurable indicators and criteria were chosen to evaluate the programme's performance and impact. Information concerning indicators was to be gathered through routine recordings of the programme's information system. This would allow continuous monitoring of activities, of the implementation of objectives and of problems arising, for which adjustments were necessary.

The list of indicators was as follows:

- levels of coverage with regard to health care and welfare activities;
- response to referral;
- community involvement as shown by the contribution made in respect of labour, materials, security and maintenance of premises, etc.;
- number and characteristics of community groups dealt with by the promoters;
- coverage of activities directed to specific groups of women;
- number and characteristics of activities aimed at the high-risk population, e.g. home visits, welfare activities.

A set of criteria was selected to determine whether the indicators were reflecting the achievement of objectives. With regard to coverage of high-risk families, for example, a minimum of 3 home visits per year per family was scheduled. A mean duration of 50 minutes per visit and an average of 2 community groups per week per promoter were programmed.

According to the schedule, the promoter would allocate her working time (8 hours per day) as follows:

— 50% to home visits, for activities such as detection, classification, health education, referral, nutritional surveillance, etc.;

— 40% to work with community groups;

— 10% to planning the working day and filling in records.

A coverage of 60% or more for health care activities, such as antenatal and postnatal care, nutritional surveillance, family planning and response to referral, was considered a good cut-off point for evaluating the level of attainment of objectives in the first year. As far as welfare activities were concerned, a 40% level of coverage and response to referral was selected.

With regard to community involvement, characteristics such as internal organization, representativeness and democracy in the selection of the members were considered appropriate criteria for classifying community organizations existing in the programme area, and for predicting the degree of commitment to the project. The willingness of community organizations to contribute with labour and materials and cooperate in the recruitment and selection of promoters were also indicators of community commitment to the programme.

Operation of the model

The household was taken as the operational base of the programme. The health and welfare promoters selected were the front-line workers with responsibilities for the promotion of health, detection, referral and preventive activities, as well as work with community groups.

The promoters were to refer all pregnant women, family planning acceptors and malnourished children to the health auxiliaries working at the health posts. They might also refer cases needing welfare assistance to the local units that the Colombian Family Welfare Institute set up at the primary level. Furthermore, each promoter had to hold meetings with two community groups each week. These groups met once a week to discuss health-related problems or to hold an educational session on antenatal care or the improvement of nutrition. In both activities, i.e. home visiting and community group organization, the target population was defined as all women of reproductive age and children aged less than 5 years.

Health and welfare promoters were assisted by traditional health auxiliaries (4 years' high school plus 2 years' technical training). These auxiliaries worked in the health posts and were responsible for antenatal and postnatal care and family planning advice.

Most of the activities of the promoters were carried out at the domiciliary level, whereas the activities of health auxiliaries combined home visits with work in health posts.

A technical support team of 6 professionals with intermediate level training, 3 social workers from the Colombian Family Welfare Institute and 3 registered nurses from the Municipal Secretariat of Health was appointed to provide support for the programme's field activities. The members of the team had responsibility for the selection and training of field personnel. They also supervised and coordinated field work.

A public health physician from the Municipal Secretariat of Health was responsible for managing the programme and implementing the policies and guidelines decided upon by a steering committee. He also had to ensure that activities were carried out in accordance with the proposed objectives. The steering committee itself was made up of the directors of each of the participating institutions, and a coordinating committee gave institutional and political support to the programme.

The following ratios of health and welfare personnel to numbers of inhabitants were established:

— 1 registered nurse and social worker per 60 000 inhabitants;

— 1 health and welfare promoter per 3500 inhabitants;

— 1 health auxiliary per 7500 inhabitants;

— 1 statistician (technician) per 33 000 inhabitants.

Regionalization and referral system

Regionalization was seen as a means of integrating preventive and curative activities, and it was also considered important to encourage the appropriate use of services which, together with the early detection of morbidity, ensured better attention through the different levels of care. The various manpower categories were felt to be more effectively deployed in a regionalized system.

The integration of health and welfare services at the local level eventually led to the change of designation of "health posts" to "local units" under the programme. Seven local units were organized, covering an area with 100 000 inhabitants as the initial step in expanding the coverage of services to 250 000 people. The regionalized scheme is summarized in Fig. 1.

Community involvement

A series of strategies and activities was devised to achieve community participation. The initial approach was made through existing community organizations known as *juntas comunales.* When this was not possible, political organizations or other groups working in the community were contacted.

The main activities included individual talks with community leaders, meetings with community organizations and community gatherings to which all the people living in a neighbourhood were invited. A list of organizations and community groups was drawn up for each neighbourhood, together with a list of grocery stores that might be used as food

Fig. 1. Regionalized health and welfare system

TERTIARY CARE

SECONDARY CARE

PRIMARY CARE

Health centre

Health	*Welfare*
Outpatient clinics	Legal advice
Minor surgery	Psycho-logical advice
Health education	Day care (nurseries)

Health post

Colombian Family Welfare Institute units

Health	*Welfare*
First aid	Community groups' activities
Vaginal smear	
Family planning	
Supple-mentary feeding programme	

Household

Health and welfare

Detection and identification

Classification of risk

Diagnosis and treatment (self-care)

Follow-up, control and referral

Health education

Health and welfare promotion

Top of page here.

University Hospital

Colombian Family Welfare Institute Regional Office

Health	*Welfare*
Highly specialized services	Adoption procedures
	Legal protection of the child
	Psychological orientation

General Hospital

Colombian Family Welfare Institute Zonal Unit

Health	*Welfare*
Outpatient and inpatient care	Civil registration
Specialized services	Food allowance issues
X-rays	Family conflicts
Emergency services	Legal actions

distribution points within the supplementary food component of the programme. Community organizations were briefed on the scope of the programme and asked to collaborate in recruiting candidates for posts in health and welfare promotion.

Evaluation of the Model and Results

The results of the first stage of the programme, designed to cover a population of 100 000, are as follows.

Scheduled v. actual performance of health promoters

Table 1 compares the scheduled and the actual results of the programme's first stage.

Table 1. Scheduled v. actual performance of health promoters in first stage of programme

	Scheduled	Actual
Duration of programme stage	4 months	10 months
Time assigned to home visits	50%	55%
Time assigned to community groups	40%	30%
Time assigned to filling in records	10%	15%
Field work personnel	30	26
Ratio of promoter to population	1 : 3500	1 : 4038
Community groups dealt with per promoter per week	2	1
Time assigned to continuing training	4 hours per month	8 hours per month

This stage lasted 10 months, 2.5 times longer than the period forecast. The time assigned to activities with community groups showed a 20% shortfall resulting from an increase in the time spent on home visits and filling in records. The ratio of promoter to population also showed an increase of 538 in the number of persons covered by each promoter. The time devoted to continuing training was twice as much as had been scheduled.

Classification of risk

With regard to health variables, 85% of the population was classified as being at low risk, 14% at medium risk and 1% at high risk. As far as welfare variables were concerned, 12% of the population was classified as being at high risk. The total risk (sum of health risks and welfare risks) showed 10% of the population to be at high risk, 10% at medium risk and 80% at low risk.

Community participation

Table 2 gives a summary of the points of agreement reached with community organizations. Four of the seven communities in which local units were set up had community bodies, e.g. *juntas comunales* and health committees, that were considered to be fairly well or strongly developed according to characteristics such as democracy in the selection of their members, internal organization and representativeness. These same organizations agreed to collaborate by providing buildings, labour, materials, security and maintenance of premises. Most groups agreed to cooperate in the establishment of a distribution network for the supplementary feeding programme and the recruitment of candidates for selection as health and welfare promoters.

A total of 23 community groups continued to meet until the end of the year. Most of the groups in the local units were formed by expectant mothers and mothers of malnourished children; a few consisted of neighbours who met to seek solutions to community problems such as garbage collection and the establishment of vegetable gardens.

Nutritional surveillance by the promoters

Of a total of 13 359 children detected (representing 92% of the 14 455 who were eligible), a nutritional assessment was made in 12 871 cases (89%). Among those classified, 10 047 (75.2%) were considered normal and 2824 (21%) were found to be malnourished.

At the time of the survey, 321 children (2.4%) were found to be slightly malnourished and 762 (5.7%) to be severely malnourished. No significant differences were found in the prevalence rates of malnutrition in the seven local units of the programme.

Activities for eligible women

A total of 13 822 women of reproductive age were identified and classified by the promoters. This number represents 55.6% of the total population of women between 15 and 44 years of age (24 877) living in the area covered by the programme.

The proportions of women who were found pregnant or thought to be pregnant were 6.2% and 6.0% respectively; 22.1% of women were found not to be exposed to the risk of pregnancy (widows, single, or having undergone tubal ligation). Thirty-seven per cent of the eligible women were family planning acceptors and 29% did not use family planning methods at all. The rates of acceptance of family planning did not show marked differences from unit to unit, nor was a difference in pregnancy rates found between the units.

Classification of users of welfare services

A total of 14 685 persons needing welfare assistance of some kind were identified. Among the kinds of problem encountered, 9488 (64.6%) fell into the category of cases needing legal advice, orientation on the use of welfare services, etc.; 10% of the total came under the heading of "abandonment". Family conflict and behavioural problems accounted for 5.8% and 5.9% of the cases respectively.

Table 2. Points of agreement reached with community organizations

Local unit	Community organization	Community contribution					Food programme	Recruiting of promoters
		Building	Labour	Materials	Security	Maintenance		
No. 1	Poor	—	—	—	—	—	+	—
No. 2	Strong	+	+	+	+	+	+	+
No. 3	Poor	—	—	—	—	—	—	—
No. 4	Strong	+	—	—	+	+	+	+
No. 5	Strong	+	+	—	+	+	+	+
No. 6	Fair	+	—	—	+	+	+	+
No. 7	Poor	—	—	—	—	—	+	+

Key: + = agreed to contribute; — = did not agree to contribute

Functioning of the referral system

A total of 3524 cases needing care at different levels of the health system were referred by the promoters; almost 72% (2526) received care. There were differences in the degree to which the local units satisfied the referral demand. The response rates varied between a minimum of 48% and a maximum of 84%. As far as welfare assistance was concerned, only 618 cases (22.3%) received care out of a total of 2768 cases referred during the year.

Coverage attained by health auxiliaries

Table 3 shows the levels of coverage attained in the different types of service provided by health auxiliaries. Of a total of 25 134 people detected as being in need of these services, 17 753 (70.6%) were kept under surveillance during the one-year period. The coverage attained varies, according to the service, from 76.5% for prenatal care to 56.3% for family planning.

Table 3. Coverage attained by health auxiliaries within the health care component

Service		Population in need	Population covered	Coverage (%)
Antenatal care		851	651	76.5
Postnatal care		748	508	68
Nutrition surveillance	<1 year	3 101	2 400	77.4
	1-4 years	11 354	9 083	80
Family planning		9 078	5 111	56.3
Total		25 132	17 753	70.6

Range of services provided

The programme provided a wide range of services through the seven local units (see Table 4). Antenatal and postnatal care was available at four units, family planning, immunization and treatment of common illnesses at three, and nutrition surveillance, health education and first aid at all seven.

Welfare service orientation was adequately provided in three of the local units and partially in the other ones. The work of promoters with community groups showed promising results in five unit areas.

Discussion

The programme described above represented a successful effort in institutional collaboration between health and welfare agencies. Undoubtedly, a

Table 4. Range of services provided by primary units

Services	Local unit						
	1	2	3	4	5	6	7
Antenatal care	+	p	+	—	—	+	—
Postnatal care	+	p	+	—	—	+	—
Family planning	+	—	+	—	—	+	—
Immunizations	+	—	+	—	—	+	—
Treatment of common illnesses	+	—	+	—	—	+	—
Nutrition surveillance	+	+	+	+	+	+	+
Health education	+	+	+	+	+	+	+
First aid	+	+	+	+	+	+	+
Welfare service orientation	+	p	+	p	p	+	p
Work with community groups	p	+	+	+	+	+	p

Key: + = fully provided; — = not provided; p = partially provided

strong political will is necessary for this coordination to be achieved. In the present case, the backing of the Mayor of Cali and other public figures at the national level was of great value.

It is not an easy task to evaluate levels of implementation and the achievement of objectives. In the case of this programme, evaluation was built in as an integral part of the project's information system and one of the problems that had to be solved early on in the field work was that statistical records were too complex and their preparation consumed much more time than had been initially foreseen.

The importance of using social indicators to define a high-risk or priority target population was confirmed. An increase of 1–10% in the high-risk group was observed when the social indicators were applied in addition to the others.

Community participation was, in general, very good when judged by the various indicators referred to in Table 2.

The follow-up to the programme has shown that the same *juntas comunales* which participated in the selection of promoters have been providing most of the support with regard to the security and maintenance of the local units. The more active groups still working 18 months after the start of the programme were those whose appointed promoters had not dropped out. Of the 23 community groups run by promoters appointed by the *juntas comunales,* 10 were engaged in a range of public amenity activities at the end of 1981. The authors strongly believe that participation in the selection of the promoters was crucial to the success of the programme. Promoters were always considered members of their respective communities.

From an analysis of the procedures involved in setting up the programme, it is clear that a number of difficulties arise when different government bodies agree to coordinate efforts and resources to solve a particular problem. Among the identified constraints that made the launching of the programme difficult were inter-institutional jealousy, political interference, different levels of commitment among the participating institutions, and bureaucracy. All these constraints affected in one way or another the functioning of the various committees responsible for planning and developing the programme.

One of the main difficulties at the stage of community survey and contacts was the dominance of some community organizations by political parties. The programme's staff had a very hard time trying to make them aware of the importance of the programme and the impossibility of the programme being conducted according to party-political criteria.

The introduction of a continuing training programme which was needed to fill gaps in the training course, especially in the area of welfare assistance and work with community groups, effectively reduced the time available for performing field work.

Another important fact established when the programme was in its third month was that the statistical forms were too complex and their completion required much more time than had initially been foreseen.

The data on health service coverage are encouraging, especially when one bears in mind that, prior to the launching of the programme, the municipal health services were covering a maximum of 30% of the population in need. The different levels of attainment of objectives for health care and welfare services, though expected, may well reflect the difficulties experienced by the two main supporters of the programme, the Municipal Secretariat of Health and the Colombian Family Welfare Institute. For instance, a regionalized schedule for the provision of health services was easily developed, whereas it took more than 8 months to set up an equivalent scheme for the provision of welfare services.

References

1. **Municipal Secretariat of Health, Cali.** [*Annual report on activities.*] Cali, Epidemiology and Statistics Unit, 1981 (mimeographed document) (in Spanish).
2. **Municipal Planning Department.** [*Five-year investment programme for the health sector, Cali, 1981-1985.*] Cali, 1980 (mimeographed document) (in Spanish).
3. **Aguirre, A.** [*Care of mothers and children under five, with emphasis on primary care.*] Cali, Universidad del Valle, Division of Health, Ministry of Public Health, Secretariat of Public Health, 1978 (in Spanish).
4. **Rojas, O.** *Evaluation of the primary health and welfare programme in Cali, Colombia.* Thesis. London School of Hygiene and Tropical Medicine, 1981.

13.6 Indicators for assessing the impact of safe water supplies on health and health promotion: the Jhansi Impact Study — *R.N. Srivastava & B.L. Verma*

Evaluation of the impact of water supply and sanitation programmes has tended to focus on the measurement of reductions in mortality and morbidity from water-related diseases, and on reductions in the amount of work required to obtain sufficient water for personal and household purposes. This chapter describes a study that utilizes these traditional forms of measurement but which also investigates the use of possible indicators related to positive improvements in health and quality of life. Sufficient results are not yet available to validate these indicators and it remains to be seen whether they will prove to be generally useful. This study, therefore, should be regarded very much as a research exercise, since the emphasis should eventually be on the selection of a few relatively simple but powerful indicators relevant to the particular local context.

Strategies for health for all by the year 2000 emphasize the importance of the provision of safe water supplies in the programme for the promotion of health. Efforts to achieve this are leading to substantial investments in water supplies, particularly in the rural areas of developing countries.

The general scope of the measurement of health impacts of safe water supplies is laid down in the report of a World Bank Expert Panel on measurement of health benefits of investment in water supplies *(1)* and the World Bank's research publication on village water supply *(2)*. One of the strongest arguments put forward for investments in water supply is the improvement of people's health. Assessment of the impact of safe water supplies on health status is expected in itself to improve the effectiveness of such supplies, thereby providing information on health promotion.

The current study is a longitudinal follow-up of the health status of two populations provided with a continuous and abundant supply of safe (piped) water and of another, comparable, group (control) which is using traditional water sources. Details of the study design, methods and operational plan have been set out in its Protocol (Srivastava, R.N., unpublished document).

The pre-intervention health status of the study population and control villages has been established in baseline survey reports (Srivastava, R.N. et al., unpublished observations, 1982, 1983). The health status of the populations of these villages has been continuously monitored since the intervention to supply piped water in the study villages began in 1983. The aim here is to review the indices of health and health promotion used in the study, including those related to other aspects of water supply. Results, however, are as yet fully available only on pre-intervention health status.

Methods

The development and use of indicators to measure the impact of safe (piped) water supply on health and health promotion call for the systematic collection, compilation and processing of data. The methods adopted in this study are summarized below.

Population and area

The study is being carried out among the population of three villages which are representative of the area and, as far as possible, similar in their population size, socioeconomic conditions, habits, traditional sources of water supply, etc. These villages are Shahjahanpur, Tahlaur and Datawali/Barnaya, situated at a distance of about 70 km from the city of Jhansi (Uttar Pradesh) within the area of the primary health unit of Moth.

Interventions

These foresaw that in 1983, Shahjahanpur (population 2081) be provided with a piped water supply and related health education, and Tahlaur (population 2086) receive a piped water supply, health education and technical expertise for the construction of domestic soakage pits; however, the supply of piped water was in fact delayed until late 1985. In the control village of Datawali/Barnaya (population 1752) no intervention was foreseen until the close of the study.

Data collection

The study began in October 1980. Since then, various data on the study and control villages have been collected each year; details are given below.

Census

Initially, mapping of each village house and numbering of households, wells/handpumps and other drinking-water sources was carried out. This was followed by a door-to-door census of households to obtain basic data on family members, water sources and means of excreta disposal. Data on births, deaths and migrations are also continuously recorded in these villages.

Assessment of health status

Health status is assessed by means of surveys of water-related diseases, (enteric fever, acute diarrhoeal diseases (diarrhoea, dysentery and gastroenteritis), infectious hepatitis, conjunctivitis, trachoma and scabies) and by monitoring nutritional status (considering only the height and weight of children aged less than 10 years).

Prevalence surveys are conducted after the census each year to study point prevalence of water-related diseases. Height, weight and the prevalence of intestinal parasites in stools of children under 10 years of age are also studied in this survey. *Incidence surveys* of the water-related diseases, excluding trachoma, are carried out through weekly household visits. Field investigators residing in the respective villages collect data under the guidance of a full-time epidemiologist. The clinical assessment of cases is based on the cardinal signs/symptoms as observed by the field investigators. Doubtful cases are confirmed by the epidemiologist. Stool samples, as far as possible, are also collected from cases of enteric fever and acute diarrhoeal diseases for culture examinations.

Assessment of behavioural patterns
The behavioural patterns related to water collection, transportation, storage, usage and personal hygiene are studied regularly on the basis of participant observations, questionnaires and inventory methods with the help of a resident anthropologist, assisted by a field investigator, in the study and control villages.

In addition, observations on the quantities of water drawn and used for different purposes have also been made each season (since January 1981) in each of the villages to supplement anthropological observations. Such data are collected discretely each season for 12 hours (6 a.m. – 6 p.m.) in each household.

Monitoring of water quality
For each drinking-water source, the physical and chemical qualities are monitored every six months and the bacteriological quality once a month. The sanitary status of all traditional drinking-water sources is also assessed once a year.

Cost–benefit analysis
Data are also collected on the cost of the piped water supply scheme (capital cost, maintenance cost, current capital cost/operating cost of the existing system) and its benefits (reduction in the cost of medical care and treatment and in indirect social costs, etc.) in order to attempt a cost–benefit analysis of the piped water supply programme.

Data maintenance and analysis
Data are maintained systematically in family folders for each village and year at the headquarters office of the project. Every year, data are stored on magnetic tapes and processed for analysis on the computer.

Results and Discussion

Choice of indicators of health and health promotion
The choice of indicators of health and health promotion for measuring the health impact of water supply and sanitation programmes is affected by the nature of the investigations (retrospective, cross-sectional, prospective), the sources of data (clinic/hospital, surveys), the resources available, the level of expertise, the adequacy of sample size, the variables under study and the

degree of precision desired in the estimates. The validity and sensitivity of the indices also need to be considered.

Indices of health and health promotion used in the Jhansi Impact Study

Health promotion indices

Some nutritional indices, namely mean height and weight for age, height as a percentage of standard height for age, weight as a percentage of standard weight for age, and weight as a percentage of standard weight for height, are being recorded in an attempt to measure improvement in nutritional status. The last of these, being independent of age, is likely to prove the most useful.

Indices for measuring behaviour and practices conducive to health

The results of observations and interviews on domestic and personal hygiene practices are recorded on different point scales. These are scored in increasing order of magnitude according to the desirability of the practices. The classification of total score produces different hygienic groups. The following indices are used.

Domestic hygiene index. Assessment of domestic hygiene is performed through subjective observations and interviews concerning items such as water storage and use methods, condition and cleanliness of the house, signs of defaecation present inside the house and use of soap by family members. Answers are recorded on a 2-point scale in terms of "yes" and "no", and are scored as either 1 or 0. Details are given in Fig. 1.

Personal hygiene index. This includes answers recorded on 3-point scales (poor, satisfactory and good) on cleanliness with regard to 10 major personal variables. Answers are scored in increasing order from 1 to 3. The individual's hygienic status is categorized on the basis of the total score. Details of the assessment variables are shown in Fig. 2.

Quality-of-bathing index. Bathing habits are studied in terms of 5 major variables: time spent, quantity of water used, use of soap, scrubbing and cleansing body during bathing, and drying body using a clean towel or cloth, on the basis of actual observations. This is possible in the study situation as, in most instances, both males and females bathe in the open. Details of the scores assigned for each of the variables and the derivation of the index of bathing quality are shown in Fig. 3.

Other indices. Other indices based on practices or behaviour include the washing of hands with soap after defaecation and before meals, the cleaning of hands, mouth and teeth after meals, and the frequency of bathing, particularly in the summer or during the rainy seasons.

Indices relating to water availability, quality and use

Ratio of families/population to drinking-water sources. This gives an idea of the average number of families/persons taking water from one

Fig. 1. Criteria for assessing domestic hygiene

Note: This proforma is filled in according to actual observations as far as possible. If necessary, answers to the questions may be gathered by interviewing the head of the household.

Village:	Date:
Household head:	Time:
	Family Code No.:

		Yes/no
1. Are there separate clean vessels for storing drinking-water in the family?	Score	1 0
2. Are drinking-water vessels of the family kept covered?	Score	1 0
3. Is water taken out from water vessels by dipping hands without cleaning them?	Score	0 1
4. Is cooked food properly covered and protected from house-flies?	Score	1 0
5. Is soap used for washing hands by family members after defaecation?	Score	1 0
6. Are signs of defaecation present inside house?	Score	0 1
7. Is the drainage system of the family dwelling satisfactory?	Score	1 0
8. Is the inside of the house satisfactorily cleaned?	Score	1 0

Family hygienic status is classified according to the total score over the eight questions, as follows.

Score	*Hygienic status*
0–3	Poor
4–6	Satisfactory
7–8	Good

Fig. 2. Criteria for assessment of individual hygiene

Note: An individual's hygienic status is assigned according to the total score over the ten items as follows.

Score	*Hygienic status*
0–15	Poor
16–25	Satisfactory
≧26	Good

Variables considered	Good (score: 3)	Satisfactory (score: 2)	Poor (score: 1)
1. Teeth	Regular daily cleaning with brush in the morning Cleaning every day after meals Shining teeth	Irregular brushing in the morning No cleaning after meals Partially yellow teeth	Teeth trimmed and yellow Presence of foul smell in mouth Never brushed
2. Tongue	Regular cleaning in the morning and after meals Reddish and clean tongue	Irregular cleaning Whitish and partially cleaned	Never cleaned Presence of foul smell Presence of white layer on tongue
3. Gums	Regular cleaning No swelling and pain Clean and reddish gums	Irregular cleaning in morning and after meals Occasional pain and swelling	Never cleaned in morning or after meals Frequent swelling and pain
4. Eyes	Properly cleaned Good eyesight No swelling, redness or discharge	Cleaned Satisfactory eyesight Presence of partial redness/discharge	Dirty eyes Weak eyesight Presence of discharge, redness or swelling

Fig. 2 (contd)

Variables considered	Good (score: 3)	Satisfactory (score: 2)	Poor (score: 1)
5. Hands	Regular cleaning with soap particularly after defaecation Clean hands	Irregular cleaning Cleaning of hands by soil after defaecation Soap seldom used	Very dirty hands No use of soap Cleaning of hands after defaecation by water only
6. Nails	Cutting of nails once a week or more often Very clean nails	Cutting of nails once a fortnight Satisfactorily cleaned nails	No regular cutting of nails Large, dirty nails Nails cut once a month or less often
7. Hair	Daily cleaning and combing Regular washing with soap at least once a week Proper oiling	Washing of hair with soap once a fortnight Irregular oiling and combing of hair Hair cleaned mainly by soil	No use of soap Hair cleaned once a month or less often Seldom oiled and combed
8. Clothes	Regular weekly cleaning with soap Clean and ironed clothes	Irregular cleaning of clothes with soap Clothes satisfactorily cleaned No ironing	No use of soap in washing Occasional washing Dirty clothes

9. Face	Daily washing Use of soap for cleaning face at least once a day Daily/alternate day shaving	Washing of face without soap Shaving once a week Face satisfactorily cleaned	Dirty face, shaves once a fortnight Irregular shaving
10. Arms (skin)	Daily washing Use of soap Clean arms	Irregular cleaning Occasional use of soap Arms satisfactorily cleaned	Rarely cleaned No use of soap Dirty arms

Fig. 3. Criteria of scoring for the index of quality of bathing[a]

Actual time spent bathing	Adequate/Inadequate 1 0
Quantity of water used in bathing	Adequate/Inadequate 1 0
Use of soap during bathing	Yes/No 2 0
Scrubbing/cleansing of body during bathing	Adequate/Inadequate 1 0
Use of clean towel after bathing	Yes/No 1 0

Note: Bathing quality is classified on the basis of the total score for the five items as follows.

Score	*Bathing quality*
0–2	Poor
3–4	Satisfactory
≧5	Good

[a] To be filled in at home.

drinking-water source and the availability of the latter in a locality. This is defined as $1 : a/b$, where a = families/persons and b = drinking-water sources available. (Some comparative pre-intervention results for study and control villages are shown in Table 1.)

A decreasing ratio between families/populations and drinking-water sources would indicate ready availability of water. This may influence people's behaviour in relation to water use, which in turn may have an impact on health.

Index for measuring sanitary status of drinking-water sources. Data on eight factors related to the construction and site conditions of the source, presumed to play an important role in determining its sanitary status, were collected and observations for each factor were assigned scores ranging from 0 to 3, according to the increasing sanitary status, and sources classified on the basis of total score. Details are given in Fig. 4. Examples of differences in the sanitary status of the sources studied are shown in Table 2. This index is indicative of the pollution potential of water from the source.

Table 1. Ratios between available drinking-water sources and total families/population in study and control villages, 1981

Village	Ratio between:	
	drinking-water sources and families	drinking-water sources and population
Shahjahanpur	1 : 27	1 : 139
Tahlaur	1 : 18	1 : 95
Datawali/Barnaya	1 : 14	1 : 76

Water quality index. Whereas physical and chemical qualities of water reflect the likelihood of pollution, bacteriological quality indicates the extent of pollution. In the assessment of water quality, total scores based on the sanitary status of the source and the physical, chemical and bacteriological qualities of water were first worked out for each source. Details of how scores for physical, chemical and bacteriological quality were assigned are given in Fig. 5. The final score was then calculated by the following formula:

Final score = (sum of scores on sanitary status of site/construction, physical and chemical quality indexes) × (bacteriological score)

Suitable grouping of final scores for each source gives an index of water quality (examples of pre-intervention measurements for two of the villages are shown in Table 3). Separate indices, however, based on construction/site conditions and chemical and physical qualities, as well as an index based on the bacteriological quality of water, can also be used.

Mean quantities of water drawn per family/person. This index gives an idea of the average quantity of water drawn from the sources in a day (24 hours) for various purposes per family/person. Its purpose is to measure the availability and adequacy of water for various uses. It is defined as c/d, where c = the total amount of water collected from various sources by a group of families in a day, and d = the number of families/persons within the above group present on the same day.

The quantities of water drawn in a day (24 hours) in the study and control villages in winter 1981 are set out in Table 4.

Mean quantities of water used per family/person. This gives an idea of the average amount of water used for all purposes per family/person in one day. It measures the amount of water actually used for all purposes, and is defined as e/f, where e = the total amount of water used for all purposes in a day by a group of families/persons, and f = the number of families/persons present on that day.

Fig. 4. Assessment of sanitary status of drinking-water sources

Note: This proforma is filled in according to actual observations as far as possible.

Village: Date:

Name of drinking-water source: Drinking-water source code:

1. Construction		pukka	semi-pukka	kutcha	
	Score	3	2	1	
2. Platform around the source		raised, cemented	bricks without cement	dilapidated condition	absent
	Score	3	2	1	0
3. Nature of inner lining		not applicable[a] or cemented bricks	bricks only	bricks in ruined condition	absent
	Score	3	2	1	0
4. Presence of drain around the source for used water		pukka	semi-pukka	kutcha	absent
	Score	3	2	1	0
5. Whether source is covered		yes/no			
	Score	2 1			
6. Pollution due to human activities		absent	suspected	present	
	Score	3	1	0	
7. Pollution due to ground sources		absent	suspected	present	
	Score	3	1	0	

8. Smell from water		pleasant	unpleasant	objectionable
	Score	2	1	0
9. Taste of water		pleasant	unpleasant	objectionable
	Score	2	1	0
10. Other visible sources of pollution		absent	suspected	present
	Score	2	1	0
Total score:				

[a] For handpump.

The sanitary status of the water source is then classified according to the total score on the ten items, as follows.

Score	*Sanitary status*
0–4	Very poor
5–9	Poor
10–14	Satisfactory
15–19	Good
20–26	Excellent

Table 2. Sanitary status of drinking-water sources in study and control villages, 1981

Sanitary status (total score)	Drinking-water source			
	Well[a]		Handpump[b]	
	No.	%	No.	%
Very poor (≦4)	0	—	0	—
Poor (5–9)	18	45.0	1	5.0
Satisfactory (10–14)	21	52.5	17	85.0
Good (15–19)	1	2.5	2	10.0
Excellent (≧20)	0	—	0	—

[a] Open, dug.

[b] Bored, shallow.

Similarly, indices based on mean quantities of water used for specific purposes, such as drinking, bathing, washing parts of the body (e.g. hands and face), washing clothes and work in the kitchen are also calculated.

As these indices measure the quantities of water used for all purposes, an increase in the quantities used would indicate behavioural changes resulting from the easy availability of water, and this may have an impact on health status.

Mortality and morbidity indices

Several mortality indices are in use. These include the crude death rate, age/sex-specific death rates, the infant mortality rate, the child mortality rate (ages 1–4 years) and cause-specific death rates.

Morbidity indices recorded include annual incidence rates (for both persons and episodes) and point prevalence rates for enteric fever, acute diarrhoeal diseases, infectious hepatitis, trachoma, conjunctivitis and scabies.

A reduction in the incidence and prevalence rates of water-related diseases in the study villages compared with the control village after the water

Fig. 5. Assessment of water quality based on physical, chemical and bacteriological examinations

Village:	Date:
Water source type:	Water source code:

A. Scoring criteria based on physical/chemical examination results

Variable considered	Assigned score		
	Acceptable 2	Tolerable 1	Rejectable 0
1. Turbidity (units on J.T.U. scale)	≦2.5	>2.5–10.0	>10.0
2. Colour (units on platinum cobalt scale)	≦5.0	>5.0–25.0	>25.0
3. Taste	pleasant	unpleasant	objectionable
4. Odour	pleasant	unpleasant	objectionable
5. pH	7.0–8.5	6.5–6.9 or 8.6–9.2	<6.5 and >9.2
6. Total dissolved solids (mg/l)	≦500	>500–1500	>1500
7. Total hardness as $CaCO_3$ (mg/l)	≦200	>200–600	>600
8. Fluoride as F (mg/l)	≦1.0	>1.0–1.5	>1.5
9. Nitrite as NO_2 (mg/l)	0	—	>0
10. Nitrate as NO_3 (mg/l)	≦45	—	>45
11. Chloride as Cl (mg/l)	≦200	>200–1000	>1000
Total score:			

B. Scoring criteria based on bacteriological examination results

Variable considered	Assigned score	
	Acceptable 1	Objectionable 0
1. Coliform count (MPN/100 ml)	<3	≧3
2. *E. coli* (MPN/100 ml)	0	>0
Total score:		

Table 3. Quality of handpumped water[a] in Tahlaur and Datawali/Barnaya

Status of source (final score)	Village: Tahlaur No.	Tahlaur %	Datawali/Barnaya No.	Datawali/Barnaya %
Unsafe (≦ 19)	4	30.8	3	42.8
Suspect (20–39)	2	15.4	1	14.4
Safe (≧ 40)	7	53.8	3	42.8

[a] Based on combined scores for sanitary status, physical, chemical and bacteriological qualities according to examinations undertaken in August 1981.

Table 4. Quantities of water drawn in one day in the study and control villages, winter 1981

Village ($n^a = 10$)	Average amount of water drawn (in litres): Well, Per family	Well, Per capita	Handpump, Per family	Handpump, Per capita
Shahjahanpur	245	31	369	46
Tahlaur	198	29	223	35
Datawali/Barnaya	328	47	290	34

[a] No. of families studied.

supply intervention started in 1985 would indicate the impact that the safe water supply programme is having. The study should come to an end in late 1988.

Conclusion

The impacts of change on health and social functioning are difficult to define and measure, even when the evaluation study design is well conceived. Consequently, many aspects of health which need to be studied by means of direct measures are at times evaluated using indirect measures or process measures. For example, it is rather difficult to measure the amount of energy expended on water collection and transport; however, one can easily measure the time spent and the distance travelled by those fetching water. Furthermore, as population-based data on morbidity and mortality can easily and with reasonable accuracy be collected in the rural areas of the developing countries, the indices considered for evaluating the impact of water supply programmes on health often depend more heavily on health status indices than on health promotion indices. This has also been the case in the present study.

In evaluation studies on a water supply programme such as the present one, the use of only a few indices that provide accurate qualitative information on various aspects of the total health of people is highly desirable. One such method is the use of mathematical modelling. Models based on stochastic and deterministic approaches have been suggested by Verma et al. *(3,4)* and Cvjetanovic et al. *(5)* for measuring the health impacts of disease eradication and health improvement measures, respectively. These models can well be used for the present purposes. The application of stochastic models like the one developed by Chiang & Cohen *(6)* for measuring the level of health in impact studies would be highly useful, provided relevant data are available. This model provides one single value to indicate the level of health of a community, after considering both "negative" and "positive" aspects of the total health spectrum.

References

1. **International Bank for Reconstruction and Development.** *Measurement of health benefits of investment in water supplies:* report of an Expert Panel. Washington, 1976 (P.U. Report No. PUN 20).
2. **Saunders, R.J. & Waxford, J.J.** *Village water supply — economics and policy in the developing world.* Baltimore, Johns Hopkins University Press, 1976.
3. **Verma, B.L. et al.** Mathematical models and their applications in medicine and health. *Health and population — perspectives and issues,* **4**(1): 42–58 (1981).
4. **Verma, B.L. et al.** Longevity benefits of malaria eradication in India — a stochastic model and its application. *Annals of the National Academy of Medical Sciences (India),* **17**(2): 90–101 (1981).

5. **Cvjetanovic, B. et al.** Epidemiological model of typhoid fever and its use in the planning and evaluation of anti-typhoid immunization and sanitation programmes. *Bulletin of the World Health Organization,* **45**(1): 53–75 (1971).
6. **Chiang, C.L. & Cohen, R.D.** How to measure health — a stochastic model for an index of health. *International journal of epidemiology,* **2**(1): 7–12 (1973).

13.7 Health care data collection and information system in Kasongo, Zaïre — *W. van Lerberghe, P. Mercenier & H. van Balen*

Appropriate provision and management of services is of vital importance, particularly when resources are severely limited. The example presented here shows how a system of routine data collection used in just such a situation, in Zaïre, can form the basis for decisions on the provision and management of services. The chapter illustrates, in a very practical way, many of the general points relevant to the discussion of strategies for the collection of information (Chapter 9).

The ultimate aim of health services research is utilitary: to develop services that provide an optimal level of health care and in particular of primary health care to the population. However, under operational circumstances the health services manager tends to look at health services research (and at the data collection it implies) as at a luxury, and thus may quite justifiably feel that this research can be done only if the marginal effort for data collection required is sufficiently small to be justified by the gain of knowledge, taking into account all the pressing immediate tasks of keeping the machine rolling and responding to demand. Likewise, the primary health care nurse in a health centre is more concerned with patient and health centre management than with the collection of data for, say, policy evaluation.

A health services research programme will thus have to "piggyback" its data collection on that required for the functioning of the service itself, disturbing it as little as possible, and obtaining the relevant information with as marginal an effort as possible. The bulk of available information will consist of routine data. In other words, the normal functioning of the health service has to be recognized as a constraint to data collection, a constraint which is mandatory if relevance is to be ensured.

These are the constraints to which data collection in the Kasongo Project was subjected: its primary function was to be operational, and only at a second level were the data to be used for research purposes in testing the underlying organizational principles and hypotheses.

The Context

The Kasongo area is an administrative area of about 200 000 inhabitants in eastern Zaïre. Of this total, some 30 000 live in the town of Kasongo itself, the rest in some ten or so villages of between 2000 and 5000 inhabitants or in smaller communities. The major source of income is agriculture.

The Kasongo Public Health Project *(1)* has overall responsibility for health care in the area, and aims at obtaining a satisfactory coverage of the target population with integrated and continuous care *(2)*. Planning is based on a compromise between the health service's assessment of needs and the expressed demands of the population. The medical service is based on a two-tier structure consisting of a decentralized network of health centres responsible for providing individual primary health care, both curative and preventive, and for maintaining contact with the community, and a reference level in the form of the town hospital. The total budget allocated to the project amounts to about US $3 per head of population per year. Each health centre covers about 10 000 inhabitants. It is run by a team of one auxiliary nurse, one medicosocial aide and one orderly, and one clerk who is responsible for the major part of the paperwork. Each health centre is supervised by one of the five doctors of the project who also run the hospital. Jointly with the senior nursing staff, they constitute a steering committee which manages the health system.

Usefulness of Collected Data

The data that are routinely collected in Kasongo are used at three levels. The core of data gathering is the information system for patient management. This body of available data is topped up to provide an instrument for health unit management. Finally, these data are used and completed for health system management and research purposes. These levels of utilization of data in Kasongo are shown in Table 1.

Patient management

The nucleus of information gathering in the health centre is the information kept on individual clients. It consists of individual summary cards (which are kept in a file of household records) and operational record cards.

The operational record cards are where the information that is essential for decision-making is kept during episodes considered to be significant: high-risk periods (children under five, pregnant women, women at risk of dangerous pregnancies and under contraceptive control) and certain chronic conditions (tuberculosis, leprosy, trypanosomiasis, malnutrition, etc.). Their chief aim is to improve rational patient management and continuity of care.

The summary card contains the individual information available on each patient: it summarizes the episodes, past or current, considered significant for the patient's health in the longer term. This may include such items as vaccination status, the presence of sickle-cell trait, a history of caesarean section, etc. These summary cards are intended to improve the integration and comprehensiveness of care; even if a mother brings her child with a specific demand for curative care, the summary card permits an immediate check on whether the child is eligible for some preventive or promotive programme. This avoids compartmentalization between, for example, the vaccination and nutrition programmes: every contact with any

Table 1. Levels of utilization of data in Kasongo

Level of utilization	Basic input	Instrument of synthesis	Effort marginal to that required for patient management	Benefit
Patient management	Standardized instructions Census	Summary card in household record Operational record		Improved quality of (preventive and curative) care
Health unit management	Household records Operational records Routine output data	Monthly activity report	Record routine output data (clerk) Make and discuss the monthly activity report (1–2 hours per month for team and supervisor) Supervision (supervisor) (1 day per 10 000 inhabitants per month)	Improved health unit management
System management and research	Monthly activity report Supervision notes Data on resource utilization	Synthesis by steering committee	System monitoring and evaluation as a part of the normal duties of cadre personnel	Smoothed articulation of different levels Adjustment of procedures and approaches
		Specific studies	Analysis of operational records and/or surveys, both requiring an extra time input from cadre personnel	Check of the validity of specific techniques and approaches (relevance, impact, potential for reproducibility)

individual is taken as an opportunity to link up the whole range of relevant care, be it curative, preventive or promotive.

These summary cards are stored in the household record, which is filed according to a geographical classification. This permits a more collective dimension to the individual contact; for example, the recruitment of children for the under-fives programme when a mother comes to the antenatal clinic, or the identification of specific family or social problems. One of the ways of establishing a file of household records would be to register patients as they present at the health centre. In Kasongo the file is established during a census conducted by the health centre. It is further updated as families move into the area and come to register themselves. However, it is not the establishment of an exhaustive file of household records that prompted these censuses. The main reason was to establish contact with the population in order for them to learn about the potential and limitations of the health centre, to give sufficient information to permit participatory discussion about the health centre system, and for the nurse to get to know the population and its problems. The census therefore satisfies the constraint to information gathering which was specified at the start, that of direct operational usefulness. The usefulness of establishing this direct contact with the population was felt to justify the fairly high cost of the operation: it requires the investment of 2–3 months of the nurses' time.

The system of household records and operational record cards at the health centre is complemented by a series of measures to ensure information flow in cases where a patient has to be transferred to referral level: the referral letter informs the referral level about patient background and reasons for referral, and the referral level uses it to send the relevant information about the patient back to the health centre. The health centre remains the place where all information from both levels on preventive and curative care is generated; the instrument is the household record.

This patient management system is relatively simple but its handling requires some time. The danger therefore existed that, with limited human resources, either the paperwork would not be done correctly or this logistic work would encroach too much upon the operational work. In both cases quality of care would suffer. The use of a clerk, whose salary is supported by the community, made it possible to have sufficient logistic support and time for the nurse to deliver quality care.

Health unit management

Part of the workload and achievement data required for adequate health unit management is readily available from the operational record cards for under-fives, or other patient management tools. For certain activities extra data on service outputs have to be collected: the number of consultations, of home visits, of decisions taken with the health committee, etc. This data gathering has been kept to a minimum, is carried out chiefly by the clerk, and has to do with such items as are clearly important for day-to-day planning of the work (ordering of supplies, establishing a work schedule, etc.) for the discussions with the community (financial balance, extension of coverage, etc.) and for identification of problems, for example, with continuity of care (completion of vaccination schedules, of leprosy treatment, etc.).

It should be noted that the fact that the file of household records is based on a census of the population makes it possible to relate the data to population figures; for example, vaccination or antenatal care workload data can be transformed into information on coverage. The census data, which are regularly updated by recording vital events and by validity checks every few years, are sufficiently reliable for decision-making, even if they might not be accurate enough for detailed epidemiological or demographic analysis. The geographical classification of the household records allows for a spatial dimension to the population-related figures.

The mere recording of such data at health centre level does not automatically mean that they will actually be used for the health unit management. In fact, in many situations in developing countries these routine data are often not used at all — one of the causes of their frequent obvious unreliability. In order to permit the health unit to effectively use this data, an extra instrument had to be introduced — the activity report. For a small effort, the activity report permits collected data to be presented in a form that is more easy to interpret than the raw data in the different registers.

It should be stressed that the primary function of this report is operational and not one of transfer of information to higher hierarchical levels. The report is not limited to the presentation of the raw data on workload. It explicitly calls for calculations of coverage of curative care, vaccination, and antenatal and under-fives clinics, or for calculations of vaccination regularity. The raw data are digested into a form that is directly relevant to decision-making at health centre level, and this is done at the health centre itself. There are numerous small indications that at least some of the health centre nurses use these reports as a tool to analyse their situation, leading, for example, to proposals for mobile antenatal and under-fives clinics for remote villages where they consider the coverage to be unsatisfactory.

The activity report is usually made in collaboration with the health centre supervisor, and takes about 1–2 hours per month. The small extra effort it requires is well offset by its usefulness: it permits better planning of the health unit's work, offers immediate feedback to health centre personnel about the development of their activities, and provides the supervisor with a data base that may be of use in supervision.

Health system management and measurement of health

For health system management purposes data from different health centres have to be centralized and compared, and they have to be combined with information from the referral level (hospital and central logistic services). The steering committee then uses the available information in different ways.

Monitoring of workload data for resource allocation

The central question here is that of the allocation of (scarce) resources. The relevant information comes from two sides: on the one hand from the health centre activity reports, which are centralized every three months; on the other hand from the central structures (pharmacy, logistic services, etc.). The information for these purposes is handled by auxiliary administrative personnel, and then transmitted to the steering committee. This subsequently provides both central structures and peripheral users with feedback concerning resource utilization, and thus enables its correction where necessary.

One example concerns drug utilization. Every 3–6 months the pharmacy prepares a list of the quantities of certain selected drugs which have been provided to the health centres, corrected for the number of new patients seen in each centre. Besides giving information on patterns of drug consumption, the presentation of this information provides an automatic mechanism through which overconsumption of drugs can be identified and restrained.

Monitoring of achievement at health centre level

The relevant information is found in the health centre activity reports; the principal indicators monitored concern coverage, utilization of preventive and curative services, and contact with the community. The mere figures from the activity report, however, give an incomplete image of what is going on in the health centres, and have to be supplemented with information from the supervisions. It is only an instrument such as the steering committee that can measure such elusive phenomena as progress in the establishment of a dialogue with the community. The health centre activity reports give the number of health committee meetings held. With an additional effort one could look at the meetings' minutes to quantify specific interventions or actions undertaken at these committee meetings. The most sensitive indicator, however, is the absence, in the health centres with a functioning health committee, of the continuous (financial, personnel and other) problems and incidents that characterize the others. The main impact of such a committee indeed seems to reside in the solving of problems at a stage where they are not yet important enough to disrupt normal functioning.

It is at such levels that the steering committee as it exists in Kasongo is most useful. It regroups people who work at both referral and health centre level, and this eases the synthesis of information and the identification of problems and bottlenecks, which can then be further analysed.

Specific evaluation of certain strategies or activities

Up to this point all data gathering and utilization had an essentially operational function: making the system work at the interface with community and individual clients, at health unit level and at health system level. With little additional effort it is possible to go further and make specific evaluations of certain strategies or activities.

One example is the evaluation of the standardized referral procedures that have been introduced at health centre level. Over a certain period the doctor's opinion was asked on the children referred by three health centres — had the nurse correctly followed the referral strategy and had the referral been justified by the child's condition? The results are shown in Table 2. By means of this evaluation, it was possible to assess where the system worked well and where it did not, and if the latter was the case, whether this was due to faulty construction or faulty application of the referral strategies.

Table 2. Referral to hospital of children seen at urban health centres, 1975

	Health centre			Total
	1	2	3	
Number of consultations	1826	859	2419	5104
Number sent to hospital	222	133	173	528
(As a percentage of consultations)	(12%)	(15%)	(7%)	(10%)
Number presenting at hospital	201	127	159	487
(As a percentage of those sent)	(91%)	(95%)	(92%)	(92%)
Number properly sent, with benefit to patient	143	75	112	330
(As a percentage of those presenting)	(71%)	(59%)	(70%)	(68%)
Number wrongly sent, strategy incorrectly applied	21	20	9	50
(As a percentage of those presenting)	(10%)	(16%)	(6%)	(10%)
Number wrongly sent, strategy not justified	26	18	22	66
(As a percentage of those presenting)	(13%)	(14%)	(14%)	(14%)
Number with information lacking	11	14	16	41
(As a percentage of those presenting)	(5%)	(11%)	(10%)	(8%)

Other examples are the analysis of the available data on tuberculosis control activities, which confirmed that their integration in the primary health care package in Kasongo is not only feasible but improves effectiveness and efficiency *(2)*, and the analysis of the risk indicators for antenatal screening in Kasongo *(3)*.

Such evaluations are possible on the basis of routine data or with limited additional data collection. They have an epidemiological dimension as they can be related to defined population groups (although for detailed epidemiological analysis the denominator has to be refined). Nevertheless, there are two restrictions.

The first is that they require significant effort, if not for data collection, at least for data analysis. This additional effort for the analysis of routine data is often difficult to obtain from overworked field workers who have other priorities.

The other limitation is that the information remains limited to either health service functioning or the health service/population interface. If one wants information on the impact of health care activities in terms of direct measurement of the population's health status, the routine data have to be complemented by surveys *(4)*. The general feeling is, however, that these require a relatively large effort, whilst being of less immediate operational relevance.

In fact, this limitation to the service/population interface may well be an advantage, as it focuses analysis on those aspects of health care delivery that may be vulnerable to action from the health system manager. The health system as it is conceived in Kasongo is based on a compromise between planning from top to bottom (the technocrat's input in the choice of activities) and from bottom to top (the health care demand as input in the choice of activities). This also means that the research focuses on those aspects of health care for which a dialogue with the population is being started, and therefore might be vulnerable to action from the community. Measurement of health and health promotion is thus put in an action–research rather than in an academic context.

References

1. **Equipe du Projet Kasongo.** Le Projet Kasongo, une expérience d'organisation d'un système de soins de santé primaires. *Annales de la Société belge de médecine tropicale,* **60**(Suppl.): 1–54 (1981).
2. **Kasongo Project Team.** The impact of primary and secondary health care levels on tuberculosis control activities in Kasongo (Zaïre). *Bulletin of the International Union against Tuberculosis,* **57**: 150–155 (1982).
3. **Kasongo Project Team.** Antenatal screening for foetopelvic dystocias. *Journal of tropical medicine and hygiene,* **87**: 173–183 (1984).
4. **Kasongo Project Team.** Influence of measles vaccination on survival pattern of 7–35-month-old children in Kasongo, Zaïre. *Lancet,* **1**: 764–767 (1981).

14. Application of indicators for monitoring progress towards health for all by the year 2000

K. Uemura

This chapter describes the indicators that have been accepted by the Member States of WHO as tools for assessing progress towards the goal of health for all by the year 2000. Although the indicators deal with multiple aspects of health, very few actually concentrate on the areas of health promotion and protection that form the focus of this book. The common framework and format mentioned in the chapter presents one possible approach to the evaluation of indicators.

In 1979, the Thirty-second World Health Assembly launched the global strategy for health for all by the year 2000, and invited the Member States of WHO to act individually in formulating national policies, strategies and plans of action for attaining this goal, and collectively in formulating regional and global strategies.

The global strategy *(1)* was adopted by the Thirty-fourth World Health Assembly in May 1981. The Health Assembly invited the Member States to formulate or strengthen, and implement, their strategies for health for all accordingly, and to monitor their progress and evaluate their implementation, using appropriate indicators to this end.

In May 1982, the Thirty-fifth World Health Assembly approved the plan of action for implementing the global strategy *(2)*. This plan of action calls on the regional committees and the World Health Assembly to monitor progress in implementing the regional and global strategies every two years, and to evaluate the effectiveness of the regional strategies every six years and update them as necessary.

According to the plan, the Member States submitted a first monitoring report in 1983 on implementation of their strategies and a first evaluation report in 1985. Regional monitoring and evaluation reports, prepared on the basis of national reports, were submitted to the regional committees in the same years. Global monitoring and evaluation reports, prepared by consolidating the six regional reports, were reviewed by the World Health Assembly in 1984 and 1986, respectively.

In view of the relatively short time that had elapsed since the strategies for health for all were launched, countries concentrated in these reports on the monitoring and evaluation of the *relevance* of their health policies to the attainment of the goal of health for all, and on the *progress* made in the initial phases of implementation. In this process, the main emphasis has been placed on finding out to what degree strategies have already been formulated and are actually being carried out, and on indicating wherever possible reasons or factors that are facilitating or impeding progress. In addition, an effort has been made to collect information, to the extent possible, on the twelve global *indicators* agreed upon by the Health Assembly.

A common framework and format was prepared to facilitate the monitoring and evaluation of national, regional and global strategies *(3,4)*. The documents, whose basic aim was to enhance monitoring and evaluation by the countries of progress made in implementing their national strategies, were also intended to enable them to present the results of monitoring and evaluation in a uniform fashion so that these results could be used to prepare regional and global syntheses.

The Twelve Global Indicators

The twelve indicators were agreed on as a minimum for assessing the strategy for health for all at the global level. These indicators were selected through a process of active consultation at the country, regional and global levels, by successively sifting the lists of indicators relevant at each level so as to arrive at a minimum global list applicable to a large number of Member States.

Since world average values for indicators have little meaning, global indicators are expressed in terms of the number of countries as follows.

1. The number of countries in which *health for all has received endorsement as policy at the highest official level,* e.g. in the form of a declaration of commitment by the head of state; allocation of adequate resources equitably distributed; a high degree of community involvement; and the establishment of a suitable organizational framework and managerial process for national health development.

2. The number of countries in which *mechanisms for involving people in the implementation of strategies have been formed or strengthened, and are actually functioning,* i.e. active and effective mechanisms exist for people to express demands and needs; representatives of political parties and organized groups such as trade unions, women's organizations, farmers' or other occupational groups are participating actively; and decision-making on health matters is adequately decentralized to the various administrative levels.

3. The number of countries in which *at least 5% of the gross national product is spent on health.*

4. The number of countries in which *a reasonable percentage of the national health expenditure is devoted to local health care,* i.e. first-level contact, including community health care, health centre care, dispensary care and the like, excluding hospitals. The percentage considered "reasonable" will be arrived at through country studies.

5. The number of countries in which *resources are equitably distributed,* in that the per capita expenditure as well as the staff and facilities devoted to primary health care are similar for various population groups or geographical areas, such as urban and rural areas.

6. The number of countries in which *the number of developing countries with well defined strategies for health for all, accompanied by explicit resource allocations, whose needs for external resources are receiving sustained support from more affluent countries.*

7. The number of countries in which *primary health care is available to the whole population, with at least the following:*

— safe water in the home or within 15 minutes' walking distance, and adequate sanitary facilities in the home or immediate vicinity;

— immunization against diphtheria, tetanus, whooping cough, measles, poliomyelitis and tuberculosis;

— local health care, including availability of at least 20 essential drugs, within one hour's walk or travel;

— trained personnel for attending pregnancy and childbirth, and caring for children up to at least 1 year of age.

8. The number of countries in which *the nutritional status of children is adequate, in that:*

— at least 90% of newborn infants have a birth weight of at least 2500 g;

— at least 90% of children have a weight for age that corresponds to the reference values given in Annex 1 to the book *Development of indicators for monitoring progress towards health for all by the year 2000 (5).*

9. The number of countries in which *the infant mortality rate for all identifiable subgroups is below 50 per 1000 live births.*

10. The number of countries in which *life expectancy at birth is over 60 years.*

11. The number of countries in which *the adult literacy rate for both men and women exceeds 70%.*

12. The number of countries in which *the gross national product per head exceeds US $500.*

Each of these indicators expressed in terms of the number of countries is constructed on the basis of the corresponding data for individual countries. For example, indicator 1 is based on the information as to whether each country has endorsed health for all as its policy (yes/no) and indicator 9 on the actual infant mortality rate recorded in each country.

The desired level of each indicator mentioned above represents the global level of reference that *all* countries will strive to attain collectively. The attainment of that level, however, may not suffice as the target for individual countries. Some countries will wish to aim at more demanding targets in their national strategies, such as a level of infant mortality far below 50 per 1000 live births.

However limited the selection of the global indicators has been for global use, a few innovative features are seen that had not been taken into account in many of the attempts made in the past when choosing indicators for international use. First, the use of indicators directly linked with policy and programme objectives and numerically expressed reference values is a relatively new approach. Second, the global indicators try to relate to the broad concepts of health and several of them concern intersectoral aspects. Third, they include also indicators of health promotion and disease prevention, such as indicators 7 and 8, besides those focusing on the negative aspects of health.

Regional Indicators

Some of the six WHO regions have adopted additional indicators for use in monitoring and evaluating the respective regional strategies.

In the Eastern Mediterranean Region, 14 indicators have been adopted besides the global indicators. Some of these are proxy indicators such as government or public expenditures (proxy to indicator 3); disaggregated indicators such as indicators 5, 6 and 7 separately for urban and rural areas; and supplementary indicators such as annual incidence rate of the target diseases for immunization and maternal mortality rate (supplement to indicator 7). Two new indicators added are natural population increase and unemployment rates.

In the Western Pacific Region, seven indicators have been adopted in addition to the global indicators. They comprise indicators of community involvement, per capita calorie and protein availability, maternal mortality, incidence of the target diseases for immunization, and population growth rate.

Intensive efforts have been made in the European Region in establishing a series of regional targets for the strategy for health for all. In 1984 the WHO Regional Committee for Europe adopted 38 such targets covering a wide range of concerns such as prerequisites and basic needs for health, healthy life and reduction of disease, disability and premature death, lifestyles, environment, appropriate health care, health research, and managerial support for health development. Corresponding to these targets, search was made for suitable indicators to measure progress, resulting in the adoption of a provisional list of some 65 "essential" indicators (which include the twelve global indicators) and a number of optional indicators. The list contains many indicators measuring various aspects of health promotion and protection *(6)*.

Outcome of Monitoring in 1983 and Evaluation in 1985

In the global monitoring undertaken in 1983, 122 of the then 160 Member States of WHO presented national progress reports. In 1985, 148 of the 166 Member States submitted national reports. Their distribution according to WHO region is shown in Table 1.

Many of the reports, however, failed to include concrete information on the twelve global indicators. The status of reporting in 1985 on each indicator by countries by WHO region is summarized in Table 2. It is seen that reporting was most frequently on the "traditional" indicators such as infant mortality (indicator 9) and life expectancy (indicator 10) but much less frequently on some other indicators. No doubt many countries were unable to generate data on some of the indicators, but it was also clear from the information available to the WHO secretariat through various other channels that some countries did not make use of all the relevant data existing in the countries. In particular, intersectoral exchange of information, which is needed in relation to some of the indicators, appears to be very inadequate. Some steps have been taken by many countries to make special efforts to assemble the required information from sectors other than health in the first evaluation of the strategy for health for all in 1985.

From the national reports produced in 1983 and 1985 the following general conclusions may be drawn.

- The strategies and plans of action have received national, regional and global attention, and the Member States have been active in their formulation and implementation. There was a significant increase in the number of Member States that prepared reports in 1985, but the reports were often not as complete or accurate as they should have been. The reports often suffered from a lack of detailed and precise information on many of the important aspects which were crucial to the national strategies. At the regional and global levels, synthesis and consolidation of the available information lent itself to only a very general overall assessment of the progress being achieved.

- The common framework and format played a generally positive role in facilitating reporting. However, in view of the difficulties experienced by some of the countries in its application, as well as in providing information on the twelve global indicators, the document has since been revised so as to provide improved tools for monitoring and evaluation, including further explanatory notes on these indicators.

Table 1. Number of reports received from Member States in 1983 and 1985, by WHO region

Region	Monitoring in 1983			Evaluation in 1985		
	No. expected	No. received	Coverage (%)	No. expected	No. received	Coverage (%)
African	43	37	86	44	42	95
American	31	19	61	34	20	59
Eastern Mediterranean	23	22	96	22	22	100
European	35	21	60	35	35	100
South-East Asian	11	11	100	11	11	100
Western Pacific	17	12	71	20	18	90
All regions	160	122	76	166	148	89

Table 2. Number of countries reporting on global indicators in 1985, by WHO region

Global indicator	WHO region						Total
	African	American	Eastern Mediterranean	European	South-East Asian	Western Pacific	
1	41	20	21	35	11	16	144
2	33	23	22	35	11	16	140
3	24	27	20	35	10	13	129
4	21	8	15	15	9	14	82
5[a]							
6[a]							
7[b]	37	34	22	33	11	8	145
8[b]	30	28	18	34	8	16	134
9	43	34	22	32	11	17	159
10	43	34	22	33	11	18	161
11	36	33	21	32	9	16	147
12	24	27	20	35	10	13	129

[a] Results not analysed because of heterogeneous reporting by countries.

[b] Some countries did not report on all components (subindicators).

- While a high level of political sensitization appears to have taken place and health policies appear to have been oriented to achieve greater coverage of the population through primary health care, it was not clear whether health was receiving a high priority in national sociopolitical and economic development policies.

- A number of countries still have to formulate detailed plans of action with specific objectives, targets and a projection of resources for the achievement of these objectives. Most found it difficult to estimate the resources now going to their health sector, i.e. indicator 3, which is required in a review of existing resources, an analysis of overall needs, and plans for mobilization of resources from national and external sources.

- Countries appear to be making efforts to review and reorient their health systems to extend primary health care services. Available information is, however, inadequate to assess how effective these efforts have been in achieving improved coverage of the population. Several crucial issues still remain largely unresolved. Among these are: the establishment of effective linkages among the different levels of the health care system so that they are really supportive to primary health care; effective coordination of activities dealing with the essential elements of primary health care; planning and training of health manpower consonant with the needs of the health system; and strengthening of national capabilities for carrying out a suitable managerial process for health development, including the collection, analysis and utilization of information in support of the process.

- National experience in stimulating a greater degree of community involvement and participation of other sectors in health appears to point to the need for real decentralization and delegation of authority to the intermediate and local levels of health administration and the communities. Some countries have made no or very little effort to involve the communities or have found it difficult to involve other sectors effectively.

- The reports indicate a trend towards increased cooperation in health development among countries. Available information on indicator 6, however, does not permit an assessment of trends in transfer of financial resources from the richer to the poorer countries, and especially the least developed ones.

- In spite of its limitations, the monitoring process yielded useful information on the efforts of governments to implement their national strategies for health for all by the year 2000. What is even more important at this stage is that a process for monitoring progress at national, regional and global levels has been set in motion. Improvement of the process will help in analysing factors that are facilitating or impeding the development of national strategies, and suggest areas for supportive or developmental action to enhance and facilitate national health development.

References

1. *Global strategy for health for all by the year 2000.* Geneva, World Health Organization, 1981 ("Health for All" Series, No. 3).
2. *Plan of action for implementing the global strategy for health for all.* Geneva, World Health Organization, 1982 ("Health for All" Series, No. 7).
3. *Common framework and format for monitoring progress in implementing the strategies for HFA/2000.* Geneva, World Health Organization, 1982 (unpublished document DGO/82.1).
4. *Evaluating the strategies for health for all by the year 2000 — common framework and format.* Geneva, World Health Organization, 1984 (unpublished document DGO/84.1).
5. *Development of indicators for monitoring progress towards health for all by the year 2000.* Geneva, World Health Organization, 1982 ("Health for All" Series, No.4).
6. *Targets for health for all.* Copenhagen, WHO Regional Office for Europe, 1985.

15. Health promotion: concepts and principles[a]

In January 1984 a new programme in health promotion was established in the WHO Regional Office for Europe. It is the first programme of its kind in WHO, and its development has had strong support from Member States. Planning began in 1981, since when a number of meetings, bringing together people from professional and academic disciplines and consumer groups, have helped to clarify the special approach of such a programme *(1–4)*.

This chapter is designed to clarify some of the most important issues related to the development of policy and programmes in health promotion. It is not intended as a final statement, but as a focus for discussion on which to base the development of health promotion activities in Europe. It is clear that the development of priorities and practices for health promotion depends on the prevailing economic and cultural conditions. In each country, region and district, health promotion should involve the full participation of all people in the development of their health.

At a general level, health promotion has come to represent a unifying concept for those who recognize the need for *change* in the ways *and* conditions of living, in order to promote health. Health promotion represents a mediating strategy between people and their environments, synthesizing personal choice and social responsibility in health to create a healthier future.

The basic resources for health are income, shelter and food. Improvement in health requires a secure foundation in these basics, but it also requires information and life skills; a supportive environment that provides opportunities for making healthy choices among goods, services and facilities; and conditions in the economic, physical, social and cultural environments (the "total" environment) that enhance health.

Principles

Health promotion is the process of enabling people to increase control over, and to improve, their health. This perspective is derived from a conception of "health" as the extent to which an individual or group is able to realize

[a] This chapter is based on the summary report of the Working Group on Concepts and Principles of Health Promotion, held at the WHO Regional Office for Europe, Copenhagen on 9–13 July 1984.

aspirations and satisfy needs, and to change or cope with the environment. Health is, therefore, seen as a resource for everyday life, not the objective of living; it is a positive concept emphasizing social and personal resources as well as physical capacities.

1. *Health promotion involves the population as a whole in the context of everyday life, rather than focusing on people at risk for specific diseases.* It enables people to take control over, and responsibility for, their health as an important component of everyday life — both as spontaneous and as organized action for health. This requires full and continuing access to information about health and how it might be sought for by *all* the population, using all available methods of dissemination.

2. *Health promotion is directed towards action on the determinants or causes of health.* Health promotion, therefore, requires the close cooperation of sectors beyond the health services, reflecting the diversity of conditions that influence health. Government, at both local and national levels, has a unique responsibility to act appropriately and in a timely way to ensure that the "total" environment, which is beyond the control of individuals and groups, is conducive to health.

3. *Health promotion combines diverse, but complementary, methods or approaches,* including communication, education, legislation, fiscal measures, organizational change, community development and spontaneous local activities against health hazards.

4. *Health promotion aims particularly at effective and concrete public participation.* This requires the further development of problem-defining and decision-making life skills, both individually and collectively.

5. While health promotion is basically an activity in the health and social fields, and not a medical service, *health professionals — particularly in primary health care — have an important role in nurturing and enabling health promotion.* Health professionals should work towards developing their special contributions in education and health advocacy.

Subject Areas

Health promotion best enhances health through integrated action at different levels on factors influencing health — economic, environmental, social and personal. Given these basic principles, an almost unlimited list of issues for health promotion could be generated: food policy, housing, smoking, coping skills, social networks. The general subjects for health promotion may be grouped in the following areas.

1. The focus of health promotion is *access to health:* to reduce inequalities in health and to increase opportunities to improve health. This involves changing public and corporate policies to make them conducive to

health, and involves reorienting health services to the maintenance and development of health in the population, regardless of current health status.

2. The improvement of health depends on the development of *an environment conducive to health,* especially in conditions at work and in the home. Since this environment is dynamic, health promotion involves monitoring and assessment of the technological, cultural and economic state and trends.

3. Health promotion involves the *strengthening of social networks and social support.* This is based on the recognition of the importance of social forces and social relationships as determinants of values and behaviour relevant to health, and as significant resources for coping with stress and maintaining health.

4. The predominant way of life in society is central to health promotion, since it fosters personal behaviour patterns that are either beneficial or detrimental to health. The promotion of lifestyles conducive to health involves consideration of personal coping strategies and dispositions as well as beliefs and values relevant to health, all shaped by lifelong experiences and living conditions. *Promoting positive health behaviour and appropriate coping strategies* is a key aim in health promotion.

5. Information and education provide the informed base for making choices. They are necessary and core components of health promotion which aims at *increasing knowledge and disseminating information* related to health. This should include: the public's perceptions and experiences of health and how it might be sought; knowledge from epidemiology, social and other sciences on the patterns of health and disease and factors affecting them; and descriptions of the "total" environment in which health and health choices are shaped. The mass media and new information technologies are particularly important.

Dilemmas

Health-related public policy will always be confronted with basic political and moral dilemmas, as it aims to balance public and personal responsibility for health. Those involved in health promotion need to be aware of possible conflicts of interest both at the social and the individual level.

1. *There is a possibility with health promotion that health will be viewed as the ultimate goal incorporating all life.* This ideology, sometimes called healthism, could lead to others prescribing what individuals should do for themselves and how they should behave, which is contrary to the principles of health promotion.

2. Health promotion *programmes may be inappropriately directed at individuals at the expense of tackling economic and social problems.* Experience

has shown that individuals are often considered by policy makers to be exclusively responsible for their own health. It is often implied that people have the power to completely shape their own lives and those of their families so as to be free from the avoidable burden of disease. Thus, when they are ill, they are blamed for this and discriminated against.

3. *Resources, including information, may not be accessible to people in ways which are sensitive to their expectations, beliefs, preferences or skills.* This may increase social inequalities. Information alone is inadequate; raising awareness without increasing control or prospects for change may only succeed in generating anxieties and feelings of powerlessness.

4. *There is a danger that health promotion will be appropriated by one professional group and made a field of specialization to the exclusion of other professionals and lay people.* To increase control over its own health the public requires a greater sharing of resources by professionals and government.

Priorities for the Development of Policies in Health Promotion

Health promotion stands for the collective effort to attain health. Governments, through public policy, have a special responsibility to ensure basic conditions for a healthy life and for making the healthier choices the easier choices. At the same time, supporters of health promotion within governments need to be aware of the role of spontaneous action for health, i.e. the role of social movements, self-help and self-care, and the need for continuous cooperation with the public on all health promotion issues.

1. *The concept and meaning of "health promotion" should be clarified at every level of planning,* emphasizing a social, economic and ecological, rather than a purely physical and mental perspective on health. Policy development in health promotion can then be related to and integrated with policy in other sectors, such as work, housing, social services and primary health care.

2. *Political commitment to health promotion* can be expressed through the establishment of focal points for health promotion at all levels — local, regional and national. These would be organizational mechanisms for intersectoral, coordinated planning in health promotion. They should provide leadership and accountability so that, when action is agreed, progress will be secured. Adequate funding and skilled personnel are essential to allow the development of systematic long-term programmes in health promotion.

3. In the development of health promotion policies, there must be *continuous consultation, dialogue and exchange of ideas* between individuals and groups, both lay and professional. Policy mechanisms must be established to ensure opportunities for the expression and development of public interest in health.

4. *When selecting priority areas for policy development a review should be made of:*

— indicators of health and their distribution in the population

— current knowledge, skills and health practices of the population

— current policies in government and other sectors.

Further, the possible options should be assessed on the grounds of:

— expected impact on health

— economic constraints and benefits

social and cultural acceptability

— political feasibility.

5. *Research support is essential for policy development and evaluation* to provide an understanding of influences on health and their development, as well as an assessment of the impact of different initiatives in health promotion. There is a need to develop methods for research and analysis, in particular to devise more appropriate approaches to evaluation. The results of research should be disseminated widely and comparisons made within and between nations.

The Ottawa Charter

The first International Conference on Health Promotion in Industrialized Countries was held in Ottawa, Canada on 17–21 November 1986. The Conference, jointly organized by Health and Welfare Canada, the Canadian Public Health Association and the World Health Organization, put theory into practice. Over 200 participants from 38 countries developed a plan of action based on the concepts and principles of health promotion. The Ottawa Charter for Health Promotion was the result of these efforts.

Establishing the fundamental condition and resources for health as peace, shelter, education, food, income, a stable ecosystem, sustainable resources, social justice and equity, the Charter sets out three basic elements of action for health promotion:

— advocacy for health

— enabling people to achieve their full health potential

— mediating between different interests in the pursuit of health.

Furthermore, the Charter identifies and defines the main areas for action in the future development of health promotion:

— building a healthy public policy

— creating supportive environments

— strengthening community action

— developing personal skills

— reorienting health services.

More than a milestone in health promotion, the Ottawa Charter represents a turning point from health care to health. Health is created and lived by people within the settings of their everyday life. The Charter affirms that health is created by caring for oneself and others, by being able to take decisions and have control over the circumstances of one's life, and by ensuring that the society one lives in creates conditions for the attainment of health by all its members. Caring, holism and ecology are essential issues in developing strategies for health promotion.

Conclusions

The concept of health promotion is positive, dynamic and empowering making it rhetorically useful and politically attractive. By considering the recommended principles, subject areas, dilemmas and policy priorities it is hoped that future activities in the health promotion field can be planned, implemented and evaluated more successfully. Further developmental work is clearly required and this chapter, together with others in this book, indicates some of the major priorities and starting points for such work.

References

1. **Kickbusch, I.** Involvement in health: a social concept of health education. *International journal of health education*, **24**(Suppl.4): 1–15 (1981).
2. *Lifestyles and living conditions and their impact on health:* report of a meeting. European Monographs in Health and Health Education Research No. 5, 1983.
3. **Hatch, S. & Kickbusch, I., ed.** *Self-help and health in Europe: new approaches in health care.* Copenhagen, WHO Regional Office for Europe, 1983.
4. *Health promotion.* European Monographs in Health and Health Education Research No. 6, 1984.